NAPERVILLE, ILLINOIS

This publication is designed to provide accurate and authoritative information in regard to the subject matter covered. It is sold with the understanding that the publisher is not engaged in rendering legal, accounting, or other professional service. If legal advice or other expert assistance is required, the services of a competent professional person should be sought.—*From a Declaration of Principles Jointly Adopted by a Committee of the American Bar Association and a Committee of Publishers and Associations*

All brand names and product names used in this book are trademarks, registered trademarks, or trade names of their respective holders. Sourcebooks, Inc., is not associated with any product or vendor in this book.

Published by Sourcebooks, Inc.
P.O. Box 4410, Naperville, Illinois 60567-4410
(630) 961-3900
Fax: (630) 961-2168
www.sourcebooks.com

Printed and bound in the United States of America.
TR 10 9 8 7 6 5 4 3 2

Dedication

Special thanks to my daughter, Jennifer, and my grandchildren. They are absolutely fabulous and bring me more fun and happiness than seems humanly possible.

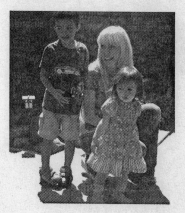

Acknowledgments

Special thanks for help on this book goes to:

Camilla Pierce, my dear sister who jumped in and gave me many hours of assistance.

Jennifer San Luis, my precious daughter who is always by my side in everything I do—and my biggest cheerleader.

Greg Munoz, my very special man who went above and beyond to make sure I got this book finished on time.

David Nordin, my lifelong friend who kept me on track and offered much-needed support.

Chris Fleming, my Houston galpal who kept reminding me that I'd completed tough projects before—and that I would finish this one, too.

Ed and Elizabeth Knappman of New England Publishing Associates, who have supported me over the years with good advice, good book projects, and a great deal of help

Dominique Raccah, Bethany Brown, Tara VanTimmeren, Rachel Jay, and the sales force of Sourcebooks for making this book successful—one more time!

And best wishes to you parents out there who are searching for the perfect name for those babies you'll love and cherish. Have a terrific time raising your kids—it's the most important thing you'll ever do!

Be Gentle When Baby-Naming
(Birth Names Are Nonreturnable)

When it comes to baby-naming, are people:

A. Just wackier these days?
B. More imaginative?
C. Less hamstrung by tradition and convention?

Because I'm a baby-name-book author, people ask me this question all the time. Those who are in the process of thinking up a name experience shock and awe when they hear the amazing names coming down the pike these days. They have never been weirder or wilder. Consider Denim, Sunny-Bebop, Moxie Crimefighter, Strawberry, and Diva-Muffin. Need I say more?

This doesn't mean that "substantial" names have lost their footing entirely. The top names on Social Security Administration lists for recent years still have scads of Michaels, Jakes, Joshuas, Emmas, Christines, and Elizabeths. It's clear that many U.S. parents continue to take the safe route when they're naming their babies.

But we do have a greater number of risk-taking parents, and that's because the name game simply has fewer boundaries today. Parents-to-be are creating names, pulling names from other cultures, and even choosing interesting words to use as names. So, when we're told that a girl's name is Lennox or a boy's name is Lyfe, it doesn't surprise us. Or when movie stars name their kids Pilot Inspektor, Trixiebelle, or Plenty, few of us are blown away by the news.

Will Fluffy Like Her Name at 5, 15, and 50?

Psychiatrists and psychologists tell us that people who grow up with odd names aren't always happy about their parents' creative nature. The results of having an off-the-wall name typically go like this:

> People (teachers, peers) seldom say your name.

> No one can spell your name.

> When you're introduced to someone, the other person is likely to say "*What?*" They don't recognize the name as legit, and they need clarification.

Fun-Fun-Fun Till Your Daddy Takes Your Name Book Away

We also know that sublime craziness always spawns occasional bursts of brilliance. These trends are good examples.

Parents' and grandparents' surnames as first

names: Park, Karcher, Santeene, Kemper, Cooper, Kyler, Mackenzie, Romaine, and Simms.

Foreign names for girls (Lennox, Britta, Shabina) and for boys (Magni, Jens-Eric, Romano)

Seasonal names (Harvest, Summerly, Autumn)

A parent's special interest (late crocodile hunter Steve Irwin's daughter Bindi Sue was named for two of his favorite pets)

Place names (Ireland, Dubai, Montana, Wichita, Dallas, Austin, Savannah)

When Does It Go Too Far?

Shampooya. I truly think the parents should have bypassed that idea. Same goes for Snarla. And *Dijonnaise*? This mom definitely took her pregnancy cravings (mayonnaise and Dijon mustard) too far.

As Will and "Mike Boogie" of the alliance Chill Town (TV's *Big Brother*) joked to galpals Erika and Janelle, "Hey, let's name our baby Chillia for Chill Town." Inventing names has become an American hobby—signed, sealed, delivered.

In essence, today's Nameanistas make up a baby-naming club, with celebrity members like Brad and

Angelina (Maddox, Zahara, Shiloh Nouvel), Tom and Katie (Suri), and Gwen Stefani and Gavin Rossdale (Kingston) at the helm. It's a trend that continues to take on a life of its own, with creative parents expressing themselves dramatically and emphatically—clearly living large.

What's In, What's Out
While we'd all agree that baby-naming has become pretty raucous, some practices get a big thumbs-down while others have takers nationwide.

What's In:

> **Fancy/odd spellings for ordinary names.** Once frowned upon, this has been done so much it has become acceptable. Look at Dilana, Dyanne, Lantz, and Tary.

> **Grandparent-type names.** Harry, Homer, Gladys, Mabel, Hazel, and Charlie are back and going strong. And how about Bub-Jo?

> **Tough boy names.** Stone, Rock, and Crash may not remind us of future CEOs, but they're big nonetheless. Travolta's son Jett may have set the pace for this trend.

> **Fun names.** Banjo and Scout—both from star parents—are pretty darn cute but don't expect

to hear these names in the boardroom or the White House.

Foreign names. Cool ones abound, like Theani (Greek), Nalini (Hawaiian), and Atessa (Scandinavian).

Substantial names. The top 100 still reign supreme—if in doubt, pick one out!

Biblical names spelled backward. This trend suits people who like Biblical names but don't want to go with Luke, David, Leah, or Sarah.

What's Out:

Multisyllable names. These are too hard to say and too cumbersome for little kids. Do you think Shyrilalanease is going to feel comfortable with her name?

Hard-to-pronounce names. Kids have too much trouble with these in school.

Anything-as-a-name. Trust me, you can't just take any old word and call it a name.

One thing's for sure: baby-naming has changed dramatically, from being a necessity to a full-time, fun-filled hobby. Today, anyone can become a member fun-filled hobby. Today, anyone can become a member of the club populated by Brangelina and TomKat. The common denominator is that each couple has a tiny tot who's the center of their universe—and they want to give that baby the best name imaginable. Personally, I give that idea a hearty thumbs-up!

Note to Reader:

Find within the text the most popular names of 2005 for boys and girls designated by: ●

Find within the text the top twin names of 2005 for boys and girls designated by: ●

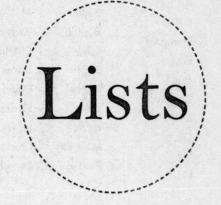

Lists

Dickensian Names

Girls	Boys
Ada	Arthur
Belle	David
Caroline	Ebenezer
Clara	Edwin
Dora	Fagin
Emma	Gaspard
Estella	Nicholas
Fanny	Oliver
Kate	Pip
Lizzie	Uriah

Future Notorious Criminals

Girls	Boys
Baden	Al
Bonnie	Badger
Ethel	Charlie
Heidi	Clyde
Jezebel	David
Leslie	Hannibal
Lizzie	Jeffrey
Mary Kay	Leopold
Patti	Orenthal James
Sadie	Ted

Names from John Hughes Movies

Girls	Boys
Allison	Andrew
Amanda	Blane
Andie	Brian
Brenda	Bryce
Caroline	Cameron
Claire	Chet
Kristy	Ferris
Lisa	Jake
Samantha	Richard
Sloane	Ted

World Leaders

Girls	Boys
Angela	Fidel
Beatrix	George
Condoleezza	Hu
Elizabeth	Hugo
Gloria	Jacques
Golda	Oscar
Mary	Tony
Michelle	Vincente
Portia	Vladimir
Ruth	Winston

Soap Opera Names

Girls	Boys
Alexis	Alex
Blair	Austin
Brooke	Dean
Cricket	Dillon
Elise	Drake
Kendall	Grant
Maeve	Jake
Morgan	Luke
Reva	Mac
Tabitha	Reginald

As Seen on TV

Girls	Boys
Carrie	Alex
Charlotte	Chandler
Cristina	Derek
Izzie	George
Meredith	Jack
Miranda	Joey
Monica	Preston
Rachel	Raymond
Phoebe	Ross
Samantha	Will

Horror Movie Names

Girls	Boys
Annie	Chucky
Audrey	Damien
Baby Jane	Freddie
Blair	George
Carol Anne	Hannibal
Carrie	Jack
Charlotte	Jason
Emily Rose	Michael
Regan	Norman
Rosemary	Robbie

Names That Will Get Your Kid into Harvard

Girls	Boys
Abigail	Charles
Caroline	Edward
Dalton	Franklin
Doris	Gregory
Elizabeth	Henry David
Josephine	John
Katherine	Leonard
Leda	Ralph Waldo
Margaret	Theodore
Ruth	Wallace

Names That Look Good in a Heart-Shaped Tattoo

Girls	Boys
Bambi	Bobby
Charlene	Butch
Darla	Chance
Denyse	Malik
Genene	Mashawn
Mom	Prince
Mona	Slim
Rosalita	Snake
Stella	Tony
Theresa	Viggo

First Ladies and Presidents

Girls	Boys
Abigail	Abraham
Claudia	Andrew
Dolly	Benjamin
Eleanor	Dwight
Hillary	James
Jacqueline	John
Lucretia	Theodore
Martha	Thomas
Mary Todd	Winston
Sarah	Zachary

Names That Might Give Your Child a Complex

Girls	Boys
Calliope	Apollo
Clio	Ares
Daphoneel	Aristotle
D'Echon	Elton
Erato	Jebus
LaDaune	Hermes
Thalia	Plato
Sappho	Socrates
Urania	Zeus
Zydeco	Zury

Names That Used to Be Just Nicknames for Other Names but Can Now Be Names by Themselves

Girls	Boys
Angie	Bill
Ann	Dan
Jen	Jake
Jessie	Jon
Jill	Matt
Julie	Mike
Kate	Pat
Lori	Sam
Maggie	Steve
Pam	Will

Celebrity Baby Names

Girls	Boys
Apple	Blanket
Coco	Brooklyn
Hailie Jade	Jett
Hazel	Maddox
Ireland	Noah
Lily-Rose	Phinnaeus
Melody	Prince Michael
Shiloh	Rafferty
Suri	Ryder
Zahara	Sean Preston

Very Southern

Girls	Boys
Dolly	Atticus
Dusty	Billy Ray
Fannie	Carter
Flannery	Garland
Harper	Jackson
Loretta	Jefferson Davis
Nadine	Otis
Priscilla	Rhett
Scarlett	Robert Lee
Sherlene	Vernon

Go Either Way Names

Bailey	Parker
Cameron	Pat
Casey	Phoenix
Devin	Riley
Drew	Robin
Hayden	Ryan
Jamie	Sam
Jessie	Shannon
Jordan	Sidney
Morgan	Tyler

Names That Your Children Will Shorten or Change

Girls	Boys
Charmaine	Augustus
Constance	Cornelius
Evangeline	Claybel
Gwendolyn	Donovan
Lucretia	Emmanuel
Magdalena	Roderick
Nanette	Roosevelt
Penelope	Solomon
Rosalinda	Wilfredo
Roxanna	Woodrow

Couch Potatoes of the Future

Girls	Boys
Aspen	Bo
Barbie	Diego
Birdie	Donny
DeeDee	Gino
Dodie	Kato
Happy	Malik
Lark	Rip
Precious	Sonny
Sunny	Tino
Trixie	Tyson

People You Would Call If Your Car Broke Down

Girls	Boys
Amy	Aaron
Bethany	Brent
Carrie	Chris
Elle	Devin
Heather	Forrest
Lynn	Hunter
Olena	Jack
Sofie	Keller
Trusteen	Leo
Ximena	Werner

Most Likely to Succeed

Girls	Boys
Addison	Butler
Blythe	Firoozeh
Camille	Gavin
Emma	Kaufman
Erin	Keane
Jessalyn	Mitchell
Leanne	Norton
Nahla	Patton
Rebecca	Teague
Taylor	Thorne

Future Cleopatras and Don Quans

Girls	Boys
Bridget	Bret
Chandi	Chance
Coco	Duncan
Kimana	Fernando
Laya	Jaret
Mia	Jase
Nicolae	Luke
Rita	Santino
Sierra	Tolbert
Tanisha	Viggo

Swimming Pools, Movie Stars

Girls	Boys
Charlize	Antonio
Demi	Ashton
Drew	Damon
Fiona	Denzel
Halle	Fabrice
Portia	Hudson
Reese	Kiefer
Selma	Liam
Thora	Marc
Uma	Russell

Names That Are So Last Week

Girls	Boys
Betty	Al
Delores	Dennis
Edith	Frank
Frances	Gary
Loretta	Harvey
Maureen	Jerry
Myrna	Juwon
Priscilla	Ken
Stacy	Marvin
Tiffany	Rick

Future Trendsetters

Girls	Boys
Austene	Barkan
Chiara	Calum
Corianna	Clarke
Evette	Dario
Kathlaya	Jelani
Nicks	Kamal
Rivers	Kenji
Selia	Massimo
Tanis	Rainier
Viviana	Zade

Star Wars Nerds of the Future

Girls	Boys
Arye	Boleslav
Brana	Brainard
Devane	Challen
Gert	Cornel
Keira	Dickey
Margot	Gray
Nell	Jensen
Skylar	Keever
Sonora	Marshall
Talisa	Warren

You Just Don't Like This Kid, Huh?

Girls	Boys
Antigone	Ambrose
Bathsheba	Dakarai
Elspeth	Gershom
Flannery	Godfrey
Millicent	Humphrey
Minerva	Ignatius
Muriel	Marmaduke
Thomasina	Mortimer
Ursula	Thelonius
Zuwena	Wolfgang

Will Work in a Funeral Home

Girls	Boys
Angelita	Cecil
Atu	Dyer
Cloudy	Fritz
Decena	Mervyn
Elna	Night
Justine	Patch
Honor	Stone
Psyche	Taber
Vivica	Talmadge
Yeva	Walter

Future Authors

Girls	Boys
Austen	Cervantes
Bronte	Chaucer
Browning	Cummings
Grisham	Dickens
Harper	Dryden
Kipling	Foster
Millay	Grimm
Patricia	Milton
Sadie	Swift
Whittier	Wordsworth

Boy or Girl, They'll Be Shy

Barney	Engelbert
Bruce	Eustace
Chester	Ewan
Dabney	Fagan
Dudley	Fairfax
Durwood	Gomer
Edgar	Lenna
Edward	Percy
Elwood	Priscilla
Emory	Warren

People and Places

Girls	Boys
Bali	Aberdeen
Capri	Bexley
Flanders	Billings
Georgia	Cyprus
Ireland	Dodge
Jordan	Elam
Lansing	Gobi
Odessa	Rainier
Persia	Sydney
Savannah	Yukon

The Next Tammy Faye Bakers and Billy Grahams

Girls	Boys
Alma	Abbott
Athena	Cedric
Bernadette	Coley
Capricia	Cornelius
Dinah	Crist
Irma	Darius
Rikina	Dayne
Sondra	Felix
Tabitha	Malcolm
Valorie	Wyatt

Law Enforcement of the Future

Girls	Boys
Carni	Bruno
Darla	Frank
Holly	Gary
Janet	Guard
Lori	Justice
Marg	Law
Micah	Mace
Obedience	Rocko
Paige	Stu
Tiawanna	Wayne

Pop Stars of Tomorrow

Girls	Boys
Becca	Amadeo
Blondelle	Calden
Dyana	Carlos
Jasmine	Diego
Liliana	Gabe
Lourdes	Heath
Renee	Jude
Roxanne	Ransom
Shae	Starr
Shyla	Tarek

Slimy Senators

Girls	Boys
Annaca	Bradlee
Cloris	Colt
Faulk	Deshan
Ganine	Harv
Karnit	Nixon
Luba	Magee
Mavis	Olveny
Ramba	Orest
Salmone	Theodorist
Utica	Wilbret

Something's Just Not Right with These Names

Girls	Boys
Breezy	Butler
Delite	Delete
Fashion	Elmo
Liberty	Excell
Michelin	Fabio
Oceana	Gomer
Panther	Nimrod
Promise	Rebel
Sweetpea	Young
Vixen	Ziggy

Evil Knievel's

Girls	Boys
Alyx	Avery
Austin	Colombo
Elkie	Dagan
Kiera	Fitz
Kita	Geronimo
Lena	LeBron
Mare	Hughey
Raven	Mustafa
Ree	Rossano
Seneca	Sergio

They'll Party Like It's 1999 (Not That They Saw That Year)

Girls	Boys
Cat	Bucky
Donica	Derrick
Gaby	Deshon
Idam	Erold
Maisha	Favian
Paisley	Lynus
Paris	Niko
Rose	Sparky
Sand	Tabor
Tandy	Vorris

May Induce ADD

Girls	Boys
Bianca	Ace
Brandi	Dino
Gia	Eddie
Kawana	Jerome
Rochelle	Lance
Suzy	Mikey
Mandy	Rocky
Tara	Troy
Vida	Vito
Yvette	Yarb

Shameless Flirts

Bebe	Miranda
Bliss	Pixie
Bunny	Poppy
Chica	Precious
Dusky	Queenie
Fluffy	Rabbit
Jandy	Schmoopie
Jinx	Skip
Lily	Sunny
Merrilee	Trixie

Future Talk Show Hosts

Girls	Boys
Calliope	Carr
Dominique	Chazz
Grisham	Doran
Kaley	Gavin
Livia	Judson
Meloni	Landon
Pfeiffer	Montgomery
Tana	Ronan
Tessa	Seaton
Wyoming	Trev

Tomorrow's Tree-Huggers

Girls	Boys
Aida	Basye
Beatrice	Dorian
Connie	Jovan
Daphne	Kemper
Giovanna	Loring
Jorie	Marquis
Jeannie	Nolan
Jolyn	Rhys
Kelsi	Rumford
Sarita	Silas

Resurrected from the Past

Girls	Boys
Annette	Atticus
Ava	Charlie
Belle	Dexter
Hazel	Gill
Inez	Mitchell
Isabel	Monty
Kyra	Oscar
Lydia	Stanley
Polly	Wilbur
Trudy	Wyatt

Curies and Einsteins

Girls	Boys
Amira	Brody
Cyd	Grail
Delfina	Hadwin
Greer	Isaac
Isolde	Jute
Madelon	Kelvis
Nombeko	Lucan
Olwen	Marvell
Pandora	Pirney
Rhonwen	Thanos

Fly Girls and Fly Boys

Girls	Boys
Anora	Brody
Cabot	Canyon
Delaney	Dominic
Gia	Farley
Kelby	Jacek
Mamie	Keary
Posada	Nagel
Rorley	Renny
Shantel	Spencer
Waverly	Taz

Future Motivational Speakers

Girls	Boys
Brie	Booker
Cherie	Clayton
Donica	Garreth
Hallie	Heston
Kaven	Jennings
Lilia	Kester
Mackenzie	Macdowell
Mara	Pippin
Piper	Simms
Romola	Zane

Tomorrow's Beautiful People

Girls	Boys
Anise	Anka
Donella	Canyon
Estelle	Dagan
Grazia	Faxan
Jonica	Fabron
Mardi	Gabor
Monet	Tyee
Paulina	Umar
Rue	Vachel
Sloan	Xenos

Doctors and Lawyers

Girls	Boys
Athena	Bryant
Bryce	Dimitri
Catrice	Fowler
Elaine	Judd
Freda	Lister
Greta	Mason
Jane	Niles
Miriam	Philip
Suzanne	Reagan
Victoria	Sabin

Family Names

Girls	Boys
Briley	Afton
Childers	Brandt
Gilmore	Corbitt
Golden	Deagan
Kearney	Greer
Lane	Halliwell
Margery	Laskey
Payton	Orton
Reeve	Prescott
Somers	Rollins

Young Republicans

Girls	Boys
Barbara	Ari
Condoleezza	Arnold
Gale	Calvin
Jenna	Charlton
Katherine	Gerald
Laura	Mazal
Lynne	Newt
Nancy	Orrin
Peggy	Rudy
Tammy	Spiro

Young Democrats

Girls	Boys
Chelsea	Barack
Eleanor	Carter
Geraldine	Delano
Gloria	Jefferson
Hillary	Lyndon
Jacqueline	Moore
Madeleine	Rubin
Rosalynn	Theodore
Shaney	Walter
Tipper	Wesley

Tomorrow's County Western Stars

Girls	Boys
Annie	Austin
Cassidy	Beau
Cheyenne	Cody
Dakota	Dallas
Dixie	Emmett
Harlee	Jesse
Montana	Rusty
Olivia	Shane
Ruby	Stetson
Sierra	Wyatt

Future Supreme Court Justices

Girls	Boys
Campbell	Atticus
Carlisle	Carlson
Dana	Jack
Joanna	Lawrence
Kendra	Noble
Madison	Preston
Mason	Reese
Parker	Ryder
Sloan	Samuel
Terese	Sandford

Nobel Prize Winners

Girls	Boys
Alva	Archer
Christiane	Cordell
Gabriela	Desmond
Jane	Emil
Marie	Linus
Nadine	Niels
Pearl	Peyton
Sigrid	Roald
Teresa	Seamus
Toni	Sinclair

Architects of the Future

Girls	Boys
Alana	Art
Deandra	Jay
Ernestine	Liam
Grace	Royce
Hannah	Sage
Justine	Sebastian
Katy	Shaw
Penelope	Smith
Stella	Sterling
Treece	Victor

A Name for All Seasons (and Weather)

Autumn	Sky
Cloudy	Snow
Equinox	Soleil
Fog	Spring
Grey	Storm
Holly	Summer
Misty	Sunshine
Noel	Typhoon
Rain	Windy
Season	Winter

Simply Unforgettable

Allegra	Momo
Aura	Montague
Bai	Prince
Hyacinth	Rivers
King	Santeene
Lake	Schmoopie
Leelee	Spirit
Lindberg	Symphony
Madonna	Trocky
Poppy-Honey	Wyclef

The Cool Kids

Girls	Boys
Ava	Britt
Emma	Cam
Gina	Cody
Lexi	Dylan
Lindsay	Heath
Madison	Hunter
Morgan	Ian
Piper	Julian
Reese	Max
Taylor	Tyler

Tomorrow's O'Keeffe's and Picasso's

Girls	Boys
Alexis	Ballard
Caramia	Eduardo
Emelle	Francesco
Kavita	Hector
Mona	Justinian
Neva	Laurent
Prema	Maximilian
Regine	Oscar
Skyler	Paulo
Tallulah	Sebastian

What Did You Say Your Name Was?

Adjanys	Lovella
Bego	Nimrod
Blue	Oak
Bucko	Pity
Bukola	Rudow
Dix	Swell
Edju	Tiago
Idarah	Tilla
Kermit	Zap
Kiwa	Zone

An Exotic Flare

Girls	Boys
Cherokee	Desiderio
Kimone	Diego
Lakesha	Enrique
Laurent	Francesco
Philomena	Gabriel
Rania	Gaston
Rhiannon	Hansel
Saffron	Jacques
Sequoia	Javier
Simone	Johann

Future Mob Bosses

Angelo	Louis
Aniello	Lucky
Antonio	Michael
Craddock	Nicky
Dominick	Paulie
Frank	Ralph
Gotti	Salvatore
James	Sonny
John	Stephen
Joseph	Vincent

Safe (and Just a Touch Boring)

Girls	Boys
Betty	Bob
Carol	Ed
Jane	Guy
Jill	Henry
Mary	Joe
Nancy	John
Patty	Paul
Sally	Ralph
Sarah	Rick
Sue	Tom

Poetry in Motion

Girls	Boys
Anne	Collins
Barrett	Dylan
Edna	Ezra
Emily	Goethe
Gertrude	Langston
Gwendolyn	Ogden
Maya	Percy
Millay	Ralph Waldo
Parker	Sandburg
Sylvia	Tennyson

Might Get Made Fun of on the Playground

Girls	Boys
Cocoa	Adolf
Feather	Ashley
Gay	Boris
Hortense	Bucky
Lez	Farley
Ruta	Farr
Sesame	Flabia
Sweetpea	Haywood
Taffy	Jericho
Teddi	Titus

All the Colors of the Rainbow

Girls	Boys
Azura	Amarillo
Burgundy	Blue
Ciara	Brinley
Iona	Forest
Melina	Grey
Peridot	Hunter
Saffron	Red
Scarlet	Russet
Sienna	Sable
Xanthe	Whitey

Babies as Advertisements

Girls	Boys
Arden	Clavin
Campbell	Carter
Charmin	Duncan
Claiborne	Gianni
Cristal	Giorgio
Harley	Hugo
Jemima	Isaac
Lexus	Kenneth
Mercedes	Merrill
Stella	Morton

Mini Music-Makers

Allegra	Harper
Aria	Kalliope
Baird	Kyrie
Bongo	Lyra
Cadence	Melody
Canon	Octavia
Chantal	Odele
Citare	Pitch
Gloria	Song
Harmony	Viola

Lifelong Bachelors and Bachelorettes

Girls	Boys
Bertha	Amos
Clementine	Cyrus
Ernestine	Ebenezer
Gladys	Engelbert
Heloise	Felix
Hortense	Gaylord
Mavis	Lester
Maude	Mortimer
Millicent	Otis
Phyllis	Sigmund

Will Become the Boo Radley of the Neighborhood

Antigone	Galatea
Balfour	Gawain
Bark	Goliath
Bizzo	Lady
Bird	Lazarus
Chantilly	Obedience
Cloudy	Orson
Echo	Rambo
Ecstasy	Stoli
Shaff	

Cut Ups of Tomorrow

Girls	*Boys*
Bara	Chappelle
Channing	Conan
Chevy	Dawber
Ellen	Farrell
Fey	Hartman
Gilda	Komic
Goldie	Pryor
Gracie	Rodney
Ruri	Wilder
Tissy	Woody

Future Queens and Kings

Girls	*Boys*
Anastasia	Alexander
Antoinette	Constantine
Catherine	Felipe
Cleopatra	Hussein
Eleanor	Juan Carlos
Elizabeth	Louis
Grace	Napoleon
Haya	Rainer
Sonja	Royal
Victoria	Wenceslas

Pretty as a Picture (or Sculpture)

Beatrice
Cindy
Danae
Hyacinth
Irene
Jackie
Jacob
Jeremiah
Joseph Roulin
Lazarus
Madonna
Magdalen
Marie
Marcus Aurelius
Mona Lisa
Olympia
Salome
Theresa
Tiger
Venus

Top Twins' Names
of 2005

1. Jacob, Joshua
2. Matthew, Michael
3. Daniel, David
4. Faith, Hope
5. Ethan, Evan
6. Taylor, Tyler
7. Isaac, Isaiah
8. Joseph, Joshua
9. Nathan, Nicholas
10. Madison, Mason
11. Hailey, Hannah
12. Madison, Morgan
13. Alexander, Andrew
14. Elijah, Isaiah
15. Jordan, Justin
16. Mackenzie, Madison
17. Alexander, Nicholas
18. Caleb, Joshua
19. Emma, Ethan
20. Jonathan, Joshua
21. Emily, Ethan
22. Alexander, Benjamin
23. Andrew, Matthew
24. Benjamin, Samuel
25. James, John
26. Matthew, Nicholas
27. Brandon, Brian
28. Ella, Emma
29. Alexander, Zachary
30. Dylan, Tyler
31. Hannah, Sarah
32. Madison, Matthew
33. Christian, Christopher
34. Faith, Grace
35. Jacob, Jordan
36. Jacob, Matthew
37. Jaden, Jordan
38. Alexander, Anthony
39. Brandon, Bryan
40. Emily, Sarah
41. Ethan, Nathan
42. Jacob, Joseph
43. Jordan, Joshua
44. Landon, Logan
45. Olivia, Sophia
46. Ashley, Emily
47. Elizabeth, Emily
48. Elizabeth, Katherine
49. Jeremy, Joshua
50. John, Joseph
51. Nathan, Noah
52. Nicholas, Noah
53. Nicholas, Zachary
54. Alexander, Christopher

55. Christopher, Michael
56. Jacob, Zachary
57. Jason, Justin
58. Abigail, Allison
59. Amy, Emily
60. Andrew, Nicholas
61. Benjamin, William
62. Christopher, Nicholas
63. Ella, Ethan
64. Gabriella, Isabella
65. Isabella, Sophia
66. Jeremiah, Joshua
67. Megan, Morgan
68. Samuel, Sophia
69. Aidan, Ava
70. Alexander, Alexis
71. Andrew, Anthony
72. Andrew, Ethan
73. Andrew, William
74. Ava, Olivia
75. Caleb, Jacob
76. Jacob, Nicholas
77. Jacob, Ryan
78. Jake, Luke
79. Jayden, Jordan
80. John, William
81. Mark, Matthew
82. Natalie, Nathan

83. Nathaniel, Nicholas
84. Ryan, Tyler
85. Abigail, Emily
86. Anna, Emma
87. Anthony, Michael
88. Anthony, Nicholas
89. Austin, Justin
90. Benjamin, Jacob
91. Brian, Brianna
92. Christopher, Matthew
93. Daniel, Samuel
94. Gabriel, Michael
95. Haley, Hannah
96. Jada, Jaden
97. Jayden, Jaylen
98. Jonathan, Joseph
99. Kyle, Ryan
100. Logan, Lucas
101. Logan, Luke
102. Matthew, Ryan
103. Parker, Payton
104. Parker, Peyton
105. Reagan, Riley
106. Tanner, Tyler

Most Popular Names of 2005

Boys

1. Jacob
2. Michael
3. Joshua
4. Matthew
5. Ethan
6. Andrew
7. Daniel
8. Anthony
9. Christopher
10. Joseph
11. William
12. Alexander
13. Ryan
14. David
15. Nicholas
16. Tyler
17. James
18. John
19. Jonathan
20. Nathan
21. Samuel
22. Christian
23. Noah
24. Dylan
25. Benjamin
26. Logan
27. Brandon
28. Gabriel
29. Zachary
30. Jose
31. Elijah
32. Angel
33. Kevin
34. Jack
35. Caleb
36. Justin
37. Austin
38. Evan
39. Robert
40. Thomas
41. Luke
42. Mason
43. Aidan
44. Jackson
45. Isaiah
46. Jordan
47. Gavin
48. Connor
49. Aiden
50. Isaac
51. Jason
52. Cameron
53. Hunter

54. Jayden
55. Juan
56. Charles
57. Aaron
58. Lucas
59. Luis
60. Owen
61. Landon
62. Diego
63. Brian
64. Adam
65. Adrian
66. Kyle
67. Eric
68. Ian
69. Nathaniel
70. Carlos
71. Alex
72. Bryan
73. Jesus
74. Julian
75. Sean
76. Carter
77. Hayden
78. Jeremiah
79. Cole
80. Brayden
81. Wyatt

82. Chase
83. Steven
84. Timothy
85. Dominic
86. Sebastian
87. Xavier
88. Jaden
89. Jesse
90. Devin
91. Seth
92. Antonio
93. Richard
94. Miguel
95. Colin
96. Cody
97. Alejandro
98. Caden
99. Blake
100. Carson

Most Popular Names of 2005

Girls

1. Emily
2. Emma
3. Madison
4. Abigail
5. Olivia
6. Isabella
7. Hannah
8. Samantha
9. Ava
10. Ashley
11. Sophia
12. Elizabeth
13. Alexis
14. Grace
15. Sarah
16. Alyssa
17. Mia
18. Natalie
19. Chloe
20. Brianna
21. Lauren
22. Ella
23. Anna
24. Taylor
25. Kayla
26. Hailey
27. Jessica
28. Victoria
29. Jasmine
30. Sydney
31. Julia
32. Destiny
33. Morgan
34. Kaitlyn
35. Savannah
36. Katherine
37. Alexandra
38. Rachel
39. Lily
40. Megan
41. Kaylee
42. Jennifer
43. Angelina
44. Makayla
45. Allison
46. Brooke
47. Maria
48. Trinity
49. Lillian
50. Mackenzie
51. Faith
52. Sofia
53. Riley

54. Haley
55. Gabrielle
56. Nicole
57. Kylie
58. Katelyn
59. Zoe
60. Page
61. Gabriella
62. Jenna
63. Kimberly
64. Stephanie
65. Alexa
66. Avery
67. Andrea
68. Leah
69. Madeline
70. Nevaeh
71. Evelyn
72. Maya
73. Mary
74. Michelle
75. Jada
76. Sara
77. Audrey
78. Brooklyn
79. Vanessa
80. Amanda
81. Ariana

82. Rebecca
83. Caroline
84. Amelia
85. Mariah
86. Jordan
87. Jocelyn
88. Arianna
89. Isabel
90. Marissa
91. Autumn
92. Melanie
93. Aaliyah
94. Gracie
95. Claire
96. Isabelle
97. Molly
98. Mya
99. Diana
100. Katie

Most Popular Names of the 1950s

Girls	Boys
1. Mary	1. Michael
2. Linda	2. James
3. Patricia	3. Robert
4. Susan	4. John
5. Deborah	5. David
6. Barbara	6. William
7. Debra	7. Richard
8. Karen	8. Thomas
9. Nancy	9. Mark
10. Donna	10. Charles
11. Cynthia	11. Steven
12. Sandra	12. Gary
13. Pamela	13. Joseph
14. Sharon	14. Donald
15. Kathleen	15. Ronald
16. Carol	16. Kenneth
17. Diane	17. Paul
18. Brenda	18. Larry
19. Cheryl	19. Daniel
20. Elizabeth	20. Stephen
21. Janet	21. Dennis
22. Kathy	22. Timothy
23. Margaret	23. Edward
24. Janice	24. Jeffrey
25. Carolyn	25. George

Most Popular Names of the 1960s

Girls	Boys
1. Lisa	1. Michael
2. Mary	2. David
3. Karen	3. John
4. Susan	4. James
5. Kimberly	5. Robert
6. Patricia	6. Mark
7. Linda	7. William
8. Donna	8. Richard
9. Michelle	9. Thomas
10. Cynthia	10. Jeffrey
11. Sandra	11. Steven
12. Deborah	12. Joseph
13. Pamela	13. Timothy
14. Tammy	14. Kevin
15. Laura	15. Scott
16. Lori	16. Brian
17. Elizabeth	17. Charles
18. Julie	18. Daniel
19. Jennifer	19. Paul
20. Brenda	20. Christopher
21. Angela	21. Kenneth
22. Barbara	22. Anthony
23. Debra	23. Gregory
24. Sharon	24. Ronald
25. Teresa	25. Donald

Most Popular Names of the 1970s

Girls	*Boys*
1. Jennifer	1. Michael
2. Amy	2. Christopher
3. Melissa	3. Jason
4. Michelle	4. David
5. Kimberly	5. James
6. Lisa	6. John
7. Angela	7. Robert
8. Heather	8. Brian
9. Stephanie	9. William
10. Jessica	10. Matthew
11. Elizabeth	11. Daniel
12. Nicole	12. Joseph
13. Rebecca	13. Kevin
14. Kelly	14. Eric
15. Mary	15. Jeffrey
16. Christina	16. Richard
17. Amanda	17. Scott
18. Sarah	18. Mark
19. Laura	19. Steven
20. Julie	20. Timothy
21. Shannon	21. Thomas
22. Christine	22. Anthony
23. Tammy	23. Charles
24. Karen	24. Jeremy
25. Tracy	25. Joshua

Most Popular Names of the 1980s

Girls	*Boys*
1. Jessica	1. Michael
2. Jennifer	2. Christopher
3. Amanda	3. Matthew
4. Ashley	4. Joshua
5. Sarah	5. David
6. Stephanie	6. Daniel
7. Melissa	7. James
8. Nicole	8. Robert
9. Elizabeth	9. John
10. Heather	10. Joseph
11. Tiffany	11. Jason
12. Michelle	12. Justin
13. Amber	13. Andrew
14. Megan	14. Ryan
15. Rachel	15. William
16. Amy	16. Brian
17. Lauren	17. Jonathan
18. Kimberly	18. Brandon
19. Christina	19. Nicholas
20. Brittany	20. Anthony
21. Crystal	21. Eric
22. Rebecca	22. Adam
23. Laura	23. Kevin
24. Emily	24. Steven
25. Danielle	25. Thomas

Most Popular Names of the 1990s

Girls	Boys
1. Ashley	1. Michael
2. Jessica	2. Christopher
3. Emily	3. Matthew
4. Sarah	4. Joshua
5. Samantha	5. Jacob
6. Brittany	6. Andrew
7. Amanda	7. Daniel
8. Elizabeth	8. Nicholas
9. Taylor	9. Tyler
10. Megan	10. Joseph
11. Stephanie	11. David
12. Kayla	12. Brandon
13. Lauren	13. James
14. Jennifer	14. John
15. Rachel	15. Ryan
16. Hannah	16. Zachary
17. Nicole	17. Justin
18. Amber	18. Anthony
19. Alexis	19. William
20. Courtney	20. Robert
21. Victoria	21. Jonathan
22. Danielle	22. Kyle
23. Alyssa	23. Austin
24. Rebecca	24. Alexander
25. Jasmine	25. Kevin

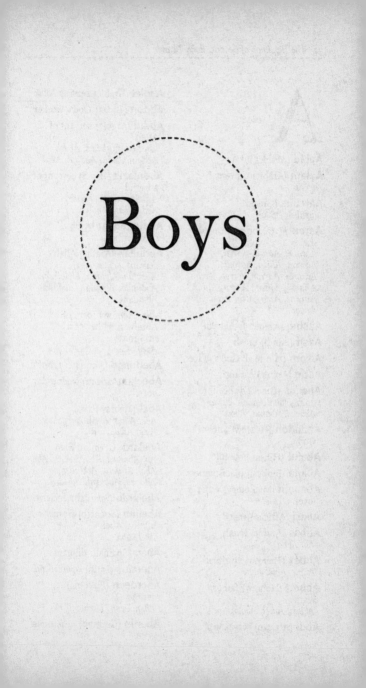

Boys

A

Aabid (Arabic) loyal

Aalam (Arabic) universal spirit

Aarcuus (Greek) rambunctious

Aaron ✿ (Hebrew) revered; sharer
Aahron, Aaran, Aaren, Aareon, Aarin, Aarone, Aaronn, Aarron, Aaryn, Aeron, Aharon, Ahran, Ahren, Ahron, Aranne, Aren, Arin, Aron, Arron

Aashiq (Arabic) fights evil

Aasif (Hindi) brash

Aasim (Hindi) in God's grace

Aatiq (Arabic) caring

Abacus (Greek) device for doing calculations; clever
Abacas, Abakus, Abba

Abaddon (Hebrew) knows God

Abahu (Hindi) hopeful

Abana (Biblical) place name

Abanobi (Mythology) water lover

Abasi (African) strict

Abbas (Arabic) harsh
Ab, Abba

Abbey (Hebrew) spiritual
Abbie, Abie, Abby

Abbott (Hebrew) father; leader
Abbitt, Abott, Abotte

Abdi (African) serves well

Abdiel (Arabic) serving Allah

Abdon (Greek) God's worker

Abdul (Arabic) servant of Allah
Ab, Abdal, Abdeel, Abdel, Abdoul, Abdu, Abdual, Abul

Abdulaziz (Hindi) servant of a friend
Abdelazim, Abdelaziz, Abdulazaz, Abdulazeez

Abdul-Jabbar (Arabic) comforting

Abdullah (Arabic) Allah's servant
Abdalah, Abdalla, Abdallah, Abdualla, Abdulah, Abdulla, Abdulahi

Abe (Hebrew) form of Abraham: father of a multitude
Abey, Abie

Abednego (Aramaic) faithful

Abeeku (African) wednesday-born

Abel (Hebrew) vital
Abe, Abele, Abell, Abey, Abie, Able, Adal, Avel

Abelard (German) firm
Ab, Abalard, Abbey, Abby, Abe, Abel, Abelerd, Abelhard, Abilard, Adalard, Adelard

Abelardo (Spanish) decisive

Abelino (Spanish) from biblical Abel
Abel, Able

Aben (Spanish) diligent

Abercius (Latin) open mind

Aberdeen (Place name) serene
Aber, Dean, Deen

Aberlin (German) ambitious

Abhay (Indian) unafraid

Abhijit (Indian) winner

Abi (Turkish) family's oldest brother

Abiah (Hebrew) child of Jehovah
Abia, Abiel, Abija, Abijah, Abisha, Abishai, Aviya, Aviyah

Abiasaph (Biblical) loyal to God

Abidan (Biblical) God judges him

Abidla (Arabic) worshipping

Abiezer (Hebrew) father's light

Abihu (Biblical) believer

Abijah (Hebrew) God's gift
Abish

Abilene (Place name) town in Texas; good old boy
Abalene, Abileen

Abimael (Biblical) loves God

Abimbola (African) destined for riches

Abimelech (Hebrew) believer

Abinadab (African) tuesday-born

Abioye (African) he loves God

Abir (Hebrew) strong
Abeer

Abisia (Hebrew) God's gift; gifted child
Abixah, Absa

Abisoye (African) believer

Able (French) strong

Abner (Hebrew) cheerful leader
Ab, Abnir, Abnor, Avner, Ebner

Aboo (African) father; wise

Abosi (African) remembered

Abraar (Hebrew) fathers many

Abraham (Hebrew) father of a multitude
Abarran, Abe, Aberham, Abey, Abhiram, Abie, Abrahim, Abrahm, Abram, Bram, Ibrahim

Abram (Hebrew) form of Abraham: father of a multitude
Abe, Abrams, Avram, Bram

Abrasha (Hebrew) father

Abraxas (Spanish) bright
Aba

Abs (Hebrew) form of Absalom: my father is peace
Abe

Absalom (Hebrew) my father is peace
Abe, Abs, Absalon, Avshalom

Absolon (French) form of Absalom: my father is peace

Abundiantus (Latin) plentiful
Abbondanzio, Abbondazio, Abbondio

Abundio (Spanish) living in abundance
Abun, Abund

Acacius (Latin) blameless

Ace (Latin) one; unity
Acer, Acey, Acie

Acencion (Spanish) ascends

Ace-Shane (American) gracious God is first

Achaea (Biblical) good ancestry

Achard (French) dark mind

Achilles (Greek) heroic
*Achill, Achille, Achillea,
Achillios, Ackill, Akil, Akili,
Akilles*

Acho (Greek) loud

Acisclo (Spanish) frantic

Acisclus (Greek) from the
river god Achelous

Ack (Scandinavian) peaceful

Acker (American) oak tree
Aker

Ackerley (English) born of
the meadow; nature-loving
*Accerley, Ackerlea, Ackerleigh,
Ackersley, Acklea, Ackleigh,
Ackley, Acklie*

Actium (Biblical) place name

Acton (English) sturdy; oaks
Acten, Actin, Actohn, Actone

Adad (Mythology) stormy

Adael (Hebrew) decorated by
God

Adair (Scottish) negotiator
Adaire, Adare, Ade

Adal (German) noble man
Adall, Adel

Adalai (Hebrew) my witness

Adalard (German) brave

Adalberto (Spanish) bright;
dignified
Adal, Berto

Adam ✪ (Hebrew) first man;
original
*Ad, Adahm, Adama, Adamo,
Adas, Addam, Addams, Addie,
Addy, Adem, Adham*

Adamson (Hebrew) adam's
son
*Adams, Adamsen, Adamsson,
Addamson*

Adan (Irish) bold spirit
*Aden, Adin, Adyn, Aidan,
Aiden*

Adar (Hebrew) fire; spirited
Addar

Adarsh (Spanish) first man
(Adam)

Adbeel (Biblical) crowned

Add (Greek) steadfast

Addae (African) the sun

Addis (English) form of
Addison: Adam's son
Addace, Addice, Addy, Adis

Addison (English) adam's
son
Ad, Addis, Adison, Adisson

Addo (Spanish) amazing

Addy (German) awesome;
outgoing
Addey, Addi, Addie, Adi

Ade (German) form ofm of
Adel: royal

Adebayo (African) joyfully
born

Adeeb (African) twelfth son

Adel (German) royal
Adal, Addey, Addie, Addy

Adelaido (Latin) adorned

Adelante (Spanish) brave

Adelard (German) brave
*Adalar, Adalard, Addy, Adel,
Adelar, Adelarde*

Adelmo (German) protects
others

Adelpho (Greek) breathes
Adelfo

Aden (Irish) fiery

Adeniyi (Biblical) believer

Adeone (Welsh) royal
Addy, Adeon

Adeoye (Latin) God-given

Adewale (Welsh) in flight; soars

Adhinav (Indian) newest

A'Dhron (American) warm

Adi (Arabic) fair

Adigun (American) distinctive

Adilson (Jewish) son of justice

Adin (Hebrew) good-looking
Adan

Adina (Biblical) slight

Adio (African) devout

Adir (Hindi) lightning

Adit (Sanskrit) bright

Aditya (Sanskrit) sun

Adlai (Hebrew) ornamented
Ad, Addy, Adlay, Adley, Adlie

Adlay (Hebrew) God's haven
Adlei, Adley

Adler (German) eagle-eyed
Ad, Addler, Adlar

Admer (English) noble

Adna (Hebrew) physical

Adnee (English) loner
Adni, Adny

Ado (American) respected
Ad, Addy

Adofo (German) sly

Adolf (German) sly wolf
Ad, Adolfe, Adolph

Adolphus (German) noble wolf
Adulphus, Adolfus

Adom (African) blessed

Adomas (African) blessed

Adonai (Biblical) my Lord

Adonaldo (Spanish) baby of hope

Adonijah (Hebrew) believer

Adonis (Greek) gorgeous Aphrodite's love in mythology
Addonis, Adon Adones, Adonnis, Adonys, Andonice

Adoren (Hebrew) my Lord

Adorjan (Welsh) birdlike

Adrastos (Mythology) tenacious

Adrian ✿ (Latin) wealthy; dark-skinned
Adarian, Ade, Addie, Adorjan, Adrain, Adreeyan, Adreian, Adreyan, Adriaan, Adriane, Adriann, Adrien, Adrion, Adron, Adryan, Adryon, Aydrien, Aydrienne

Adriano (Italian) wealthy
Adriannho, Adrianno

Adrie (Hungarian) leader of men

Adriel (Hebrew) God's follower
Adrial, Adryel

Adrien (French) form of Adrian: wealthy; dark-skinned
Ade, Adriene, Adrienn

Adya (Russian) man from Adria

Adyn (Irish) manly
Adann, Ade, Aden, Aidan, Ayden

Adzel (Native American) fruitful

Aedan (Welsh) fire; fiery temperament

Aedron (Welsh) fiery

Aegle (Mythology) light

Aemilios (German) nobility

Aeneas (Greek) worthy of praise
Aineas, Aineias, Eneas, Eneis

Aeolus (Greek) ruler of the winds

Aerin (Welsh) berry

Aeron (Mythology) masculine god

Aesoh (Biblical name spelled backward) revered

Aeson (Mythology) steady

Afan (Russian) form of Afanasy: forever

Afanasy (Russian) forever
Afanasi

Afdhaal (Arabic) quiet

Affie (Arabic) pure

Afililio (Hispanic) commentator

Afra (Arabic) pale red hair

Afton (English) dignified
Affton, Aftawn, Aften

Afzal (Arabic) best

Agaf (Greek) martyr

Agamemnon (Greek) slow but sure
Agamem

Agapito (Spanish) loving

Agapius (Greek) love

Agaue (Greek) worker

Aggie (English) works the soil

Aggis (Asian) good

Aglay (Russian) splendid

Agnar (Irish) purity

Agricola (Irish) farms

Agripino (Hispanic) grieves

Agron (Spanish) farmer

Agrona (Celtic) combative

Aguayo (Spanish) smart

Agueda (Spanish) gives

Agueleo (Greek) wise one

Agurs (Spanish) good; often a girl's name

Agus (Spanish) form of Agustin: dignified

Agustin (Latin) dignified
Aguste, Auggie, Augustin

Agustive (Spanish) thoughtful

Ahab (Hebrew) father's brother; sea captain in *Moby Dick*

Ahaziah (Hebrew) beloved

Ahearn (Irish) horse tender
Ahearne, Aherin, Ahern, Aherne, Hearn

Aherin (Hebrew) held on high
Aharon, Ahern, Aherne

Ahimelech (Biblical) religious support

Ahmad (Arabic) praised man
Achmad, Achmed, Ahamad, Ahamada, Ahamed, Ahmaad, Ahmaud, Amad, Amahd, Amed

Ahmed (Arabic) praised man

Ahmoz (African) praised

Ahsan (Hindi) gracious

Ahsan (Arabic) grateful

Ahti (Mythology) water god

Ahura (Mythology) wise

Aiah (Biblical) shepherd

Aidan ○ ◉ (Irish) fiery spirit
Adan, Aden, Adin, Aiden, Aydan, Ayden, Aydin

Aided (Irish) spirited

Aigars (Russian) content

Aignan (Greek) pure

Aijalon (Biblical) place name

Aiken (English) hardy; oak-hewn
Aicken, Aikin, Ayken, Aykin

Ailbhe (Irish) saint

Ailill (Irish) small; elfin

Ailred (English) spiritual

Aimery (German) leader
Aime, Aimerey, Aimeric, Amerey, Aymeric, Aymery

Aimo (Scandinavian) plenty

Aino (Scandinavian) the best one

Ainsley (Scottish) in a meadow
Ainsleigh, Ainslie, Ansley, Ainslee, Ainsli, Aynslee, Aynsley, Aynslie

Ainsworth (English) joyful

Aiolos (Greek) fleet

Aisha (Arabic) living; typically a female name

Aiwar (Arabic) form of Anwar: shining

Aiyetoro (African) destined for a peaceful life

Ajani (African) victorious

Ajax (Greek) daring
Ajacks

Ajay (American) spontaneous
A.J., Aj, Ajah, Ajai

Ajmal (African) depressed

Akan (Biblical) blessed

Akando (Asian) smart boy

Akar (Hindi) lightning
Akara

Akash (Indian) of the sky

Akbar (Hindi) muslim king; giving

Akbar (Indian) king

Ake (Scandinavian) inherits

Akeem (Arab) form of Hakim: brilliant
Ackeem, Ackim, Akieme, Akim, Hakeem, Hakim

Akevy (Hebrew) form of Akiva: cunning

Aki (Scandinavian) blameless

Akil (Arabic) intelligent
Ahkeel, Akeel, Akeyla, Akhil, Akiel, Akili

Akilles (Greek) form of Achilles: heroic

Akim (Russian) loved by God
Achim, Ackeem, Ackim, Ahkieme, Akeam, Akee, Akeem, Akiem, Akima, Arkeem

Akinori (Japanese) spring flower

Akins (African) brave

Akira (Japanese) intellectual

Akiva (Hebrew) cunning
Akiba, Kiva

Akram (Arabic) kind

Akren (American) in jeopardy

Aksel (Scandinavian) calm

Akwasi (African) hopes

Akwete (African) second-born twin

Al (Irish) form of Alexander: great leader; helpful; form of Alan: handsome boy

Aladdin (Arabic) believer
*Al, Ala, Alaa, Alaaddin,
Aladdein, Aladean, Aladen*

Alain (French) form of Alan
and Allen: handsome boy
*Alaen, Alainn, Alayn, Allain,
Alun*

Alair (Gaelic) happy
Alaire

Alan (Irish) handsome boy
*Ailin, Al, Aland, Alen, Allan,
Allen, Alley, Allie, Allin, Allyn,
Alon, Alun*

Alander (American)
argumentative; cogitative

Alando (Spanish) form of
Alan: handsome boy
*Al, Alaindo, Alan, Aland,
Alano, Allen, Allie, Alun,
Alundo, Alyn*

Alanson (Celtic) son of Alan;
handsome
Alansen, Alenson, Allanson

Alarcon (French) dominant

Alarcon (German) rules

Alaric (German) ruler
*Alarick, Alarik, Aleric, Allaric,
Allarick, Alric, Alrick*

Alasdair (Scottish) form of
Alastair: strong leader
*Al, Alaisdair, Alasdaire,
Alasdare, Alisdair, Allysdair*

Alastair (Scottish) strong
leader
*Alaistair, Alasteir, Alastere,
Alastaire, Alastor, Aleistere,
Alester, Alistair, Allaistar,
Allastair, Allastir, Alystair*

Alaster (American) form of
Alastair: strong leader
Alaste, Alester, Allaster

Albair (Welsh) rules

Alban (Latin) white man;
from Alba's white hill
*Abion, Albain, Albany, Albean,
Albee, Albein, Alben, Albi,
Albie, Albin, Alby, Auban*

Albanse (American) form of
Albany: town in New York;
restless
*Alban, Albance, Albanee,
Albany, Albie, Alby*

Albany (American) town in
New York; restless
Albanee, Albanie

Albe (Latin) from Alba's
white hill

Alberic (German) ruler;
tough
Albric

Albert (German)
distinguished
*Al, Alberto, Alberts, Albie,
Albrecht, Alby, Ally, Aubert*

Alberto (Italian)
distinguished
Al, Albert, Bertie, Berto

Albie (German) form of
Albert: distinguished
Albee, Albi, Alby

Albie (German) form of
Albert: distinguished

Albion (Greek)
old-fashioned
Albionne, Albyon

Albis (Spanish) unaware

Alby (Irish) white

Alcario (Spanish) delight

Alcide (Spanish) spirited

Alcippe (Greek) strong horse

Alcordia (American) in
accord with others
Alcord, Alkie, Alky

Alcott (English) cottage-
dweller
*Alcot, Alkokt, Alkott, Allcot,
Allcott, Allkot, Allkott*

Aldee (American) friend

Aldegundo (Spanish) old
soul

Alden (English) wise
Al, Aldan, Aldin, Aldon, Elden

Alder (English) revered; kind

Aldest (Last name used as
first name) great

Aldo (Italian) older one; jovial
Aldoh

Aldor (Spanish) elder

Aldorse (American) form of
Aldo: older one; jovial
Al, Aldo, Aldorce, Aldors

Aldous (German) wealthy
Aldis, Aldus, Aldas

Aldred (English) advisor;
judgmental
Al, Aldrid, Aldy, Alldred, Eldred

Aldren (English) old friend
*Al, Aldran, Aldie, Aldrun,
Aldy, Aldryn*

Aldrich (English) wise advisor
*Aldie, Aldric, Aldrick, Aldridge,
Aldrige, Aldrish, Aldritch,
Alldric, Alldrich, Alldrick,
Alldridge, Eldridge*

Aldrin (English) old ruler

Aldwin (English) old friend

Aldyn (Irish) veteran

Alec (Greek) high-minded
Al, Aleck, Alek, Alic

Alecs (Scandinavian) defends
man

Aleden (English) old friend

Alejandro ✪ (Spanish)
defender; bold and brave
*Alejandra, Alejo, Alex,
Alexjandro*

Alek (Russian) form of
Aleksei: defender; brilliant
Aleks

Aleka (Slavic) form of Alex:
great leader; helpful

Aleksander (Greek and
Polish) defender
Alek, Sander

Aleksei (Russian) defender;
brilliant
Alek, Alik, Alexi

Aleksey (Russian) smart

Aleman (Spanish) protects

Alemet (African) world leader

Aleppo (Place name)
easygoing
Alepo

Aleric (Scandinavian) rules all
Alarik, Alerick, Alleric, Allerick

Aleron (French) the knight's
armor; protected

Alessandro (Italian) helpful;
defender
Allessandro, Alessand

Alessio (Italian) defensive

Alex ✪ (Greek) form of
Alexander: great leader;
helpful
Alax, Alecs, Alix, Allax, Allex

Alexander ✪ ✆ (Greek)
great leader; helpful
*Al, Alec, Alecsander,
Aleksandar, Aleksander,
Aleksandur, Alex, Alexandar,
Alexandor, Alexandr, Alexis,
Alexxander, Alexxxander,
Alexzander, Alisander,
Alixander, Alixandre*

Alexandros (Greek) form of Alexander: great leader; helpful
Alesandros, Alexandras

Alexdann (Hawaiian) helpful

Alexis (Greek) form of Alexander: great leader; helpful
Alexace, Alexei, Alexes, Alexey, Alexi, Alexie, Alexius, Alexiz, Alexy, Lex

Alf (Italian) form of Alfonso: bright; prepared

Alfa (Spanish) first

Alfalfa (Botanical) sprite

Alfeo (Italian) different

Alfeus (Hebrew) follower
Alpheus

Alfie (English) form of Alfred: counselor
Alf, Alfi, Alfy

Alfon (Spanish) bright

Alfonso (Spanish) bright; prepared
Alf, Alfie, Alfons, Alfonsin, Alfonso, Alfonsus, Alfonz, Alfonza, Alfonzo, Alfonzus, Alphonsus, Fons, Fonzie, Fonzy

Alford (English) wise

Alfred (English) counselor
Al, Alf, Alfeo, Alfie, Alfrede, Alfryd

Alfredo (Italian) alf
Alfie, Alfreedo, Alfrido

Algas (English) has spears

Alger (German) hardworking
Algar, Allgar

Algernon (English) man with facial hair
Al, Algenon, Alger, Algie, Algin, Algon, Algy

Algernon (English) mustached

Algia (German) prepared; kind
Alge, Algie

Algirdas (Scandinavian) chariot rider; believer

Algo (American) lovable

Ali (Arabic) greatest
Alee, Aly

Ali-Baba (Literature) from *A Thousand and One Nights*; cunning

Alicio (Spanish) noble; dignified

Alick (English) defends

Alim (Arabic) musical

Alipi (Spanish) calm

Alipio (Spanish) place name

Alireza (Hebrew) joyful

Alirio (Spanish) alert

Alisander (Greek) form of Alexander: great leader; helpful
Alisander, Alissander, Allisandre, Alsandair, Alsandare, Alsander

Alisen (Irish) honest

Allan (Irish) form of Alan: handsome boy
Allane, Allayne

Allard (English) brave man
Alard, Ellard

Alleem (American) bold

Allegheny (Place name) mountains of the Appalachian system; grand
Al, Alleg, Alleganie, Alleghenie

Allen (Irish) handsome boy
Al, Alen, Alley, Alleyn, Alleyne, Allie, Allin, Allon, Allyn, Alon

Allett (BIblical) hides

Allie (Arabic) divine

Allington (English) calm

Allward (Polish) brave

Almagor (Hebrew) courageous

Almar (German) strong
Al, Almarr, Almer

Almedia (Spanish) place name

Almee (German) ruler

Almere (American) director
Almer

Almez (Spanish) dependable

Almo (American) form of Elmo: gregarious

Almodad (Biblical) sturdy

Almon (Biblical) place name

Almund (Botanical) from almond; wise

Alois (Czech) famous warrior
Aloysius, Aloisio

Alonzo (Spanish) enthusiastic
Alano, Alanzo, Alon, Alonso, Alonza, Alonze, Elonzo, Lon, Lonnie

Alouis (French) sun king

Aloys (French) king

Aloysius (German) famed
Alaois, Alois, Aloisius, Aloisio

Alpar (Hindi) champions downtrodden

Alpheus (Hebrew) form of Alfeus: follower
Alphaeus

Alphin (German) leads first

Alphonse (German) distinguished
Alf, Alfonse, Alphons, Alphonsa, Alphonso, Alphonzus, Fonsi, Fonsie, Fonz, Fonzie

Alpin (Scottish) man from alpine area

Alps (Place name) climber
Alp

Alquince (American) old; fifth
Al, Alquense, Alquin, Alquins, Alquinse, Alqwence

Alrick (German) leader
Alrec, Alric

Alston (English) serious; nobleman
Allston, Alsten, Alstin

Alsworth (English) from a manor; rich

Alta (Latin) high; elevated
Al

Altair (Scottish) defender

Altan (Turkish) dawn

Altarius (African American) form of Altair: defender
Altare, Altair, Altareus, Alterius, Alltair, Al

Altemease (Turkish) dawn light

Alter (Hebrew) old; will live to be old

Altilio (Spanish) bright

Altman (German) wise
Altmann, Atman

Alton (English) excellent; kind
Allton, Altawn, Alten, Altyn

Altonio (Spanish) form of Antonio: superb

Altus (Latin) form of Alta: high; elevated
Al, Alta

Alula (Latin) winged

Alun (Welsh) adored

Alva (Hebrew) intelligent; beloved friend
Alvah

Alvado (Spanish) fair

Alvah (Biblical) high God

Alvan (Biblical) friend

Alvar (Spanish) careful
Alvaro, Alver

Alvarado (Spanish) peacemaker
Alvaradoh, Alvaro, Alvie, Alvy

Alvaro (Spanish) just
Alvaroh, Alvarro, Alvey, Alvie, Alvy

Alvern (English) old friend
Al, Alverne, Alvurn

Alvim (Slavic) pale friend

Alvin (Latin) light-haired; loved
Alv, Alvan, Alven, Alvie, Alvy, Alvyn

Alvin-Don (American) combo of Alvin and Don

Alvis (American) form of Elvis: all-wise
Al, Alviss, Alvy

Alvord (Greek) cautious

Alwin (German) form of Alvin: light-haired; loved
Allwyn, Alwyn, Alwynn, Aylwin

Alzado (Arabic) forlorn

Amaan (African) loyal
Aman, Amman

Amable (French) amiable

Amac (Mythology) wise

Amadayus (Invented) form of Amadeus: God-loving
Amadayes

Amadeo (Italian) blessed by God; artistic

Amadeus (Latin) God-loving
Amad, Amadayus, Amadeaus, Amadei, Amadio, Amadis, Amado, Amador, Amadou, Amedeo, Amodaos

Amado (Spanish) loved
Amadee, Amadeo, Amadi, Amadis, Amadus, Amando

Amadour (French) loved
Amador, Amadore

Amadus (Latin) adores God
Amandus

Amal (Hebrew) hardworking; optimistic
Amahl, Amhall

Amalek (Biblical) place name; works hard

Amancio (Spanish) faithful

Amandeep (Hindi) light of peace
Amandip, Amanjit, Amanjot, Amanpreet

Amando (Spanish) God-loving

Amandor (Spanish) affectionate

Amanus (Biblical) place name

Amar (Arabic) making a home
Amari, Amario, Amaris, Ammar, Ammer

Amaramto (Latin) beauty does not fade

Amarbir (Spanish) forevermore

Amardeep (Indian) loved

Amarillo (Place name) town in Texas; in Spanish
Amarille, Amarilo

Amarion (Hebrew) believes in God

Amasa (Hebrew) carries a heavy load

Amathus (Biblical) place name

Amato (Italian) loving
Amahto, Amatoh

Amaury (Spanish) slanted; power

Amazu (Hebrew) burdened

Ambert (Arabic) golden boy

Amblin (English) of nobility

Ambrel (Spanish) amber

Ambrogia (Italian) everlasting

Ambrose (German) everlasting
Amba, Ambie, Ambroce, Ambrus, Amby

Ambrosio (Spanish) everlasting

Ambrus (Slavic) immortal

Ameer (Arabic) rules

Amer (Spanish) leader

America (Place name) patriotic

Americo (Spanish) patriotic
Ame, America, Americus, Ameriko

Amerigo (Italian) ruler; name of Italian explorer
Amer, Americo, Ameriko

Amery (Arabic) regal birth
Amory

Ames (French) friendly
Aims

Amias (Latin) devoted to God
Amyas

Amichai (Hebrew) my nation lives

Amiel (Hebrew) my people's God
Ameal, Amheel, Ammiel

Amin (Arabic) honorable; dependable
Aman, Ameen

Amine (Arabic) honest

Amir (Arabic) royal; ruler
Ameer, Amire

Amiren (American) leader

Amit (Hindi) forever;
Amitan, Amreet, Amrit

Amiti (Japanese) endless friend

Ammen (Mythology) hides

Ammiel (Biblical) adventurer

Ammon (Irish) hidden
Amnon

Amodeo (Invented) loving

Amol (Hebrew) perseveres

Amon (Egyptian) secretive

Amor (Latin) love
Amerie, Amoree, Amori, Amorie

Amor (Spanish) loving

Amory (German) home ruler
Amery, Amor

Amos (Hebrew) strong
Amus

Ampah (African) certainty

Amparo (Spanish) winding

Ampy (American) fast
Amp, Ampee, Ampey, Amps

Amram (Biblical) uplifted

Amran (Biblical) spirited

Amund (Scandinavian) fearless

Amyas (Latin) lovable
Aimeus, Ameus, Amias, Amyes

An (Chinese) peaceful; safe
Ana

Anah (Biblical) the answer

Anaitis (Mythology) pure

Anamim (Biblical) windy

Anan (Irish) outdoorsy
An, Annan

Ananan (Biblical) hopes

Anand (Hindi) delightful
Ananda, Anant, Ananth

Ananiah (Biblical) place name

Ananias (Biblical) pious

Anant (Indian) forever

Ananta (Sanskrit) forever

Anarolio (Spanish) called forth

Anas (Czech) born again

Anast (Russian) born again

Anastasius (Greek) reborn
Anas, Anastagio, Anastas, Anastase, Anastasi, Anastasio, Anastastios, Anastice, Anasticius, Anastisis, Athanasius

Anatole (French) exotic
Anatol, Anatoli, Anatolijus, Anatolio, Anatoly, Anitolle

Anatu (Hebrew) water

Ancel (French) creative
Ance, Ancell, Anse, Ansel, Ansell

Andalf (Norse) leads with staff

Andel (Scandinavian) honored

Ander (English) form of Andrew: manly and brave

Anders (Swedish) masculine
Ander, Andersen, Anderson, Andirs, Andries, Andy

Ando (Slavic) form of Andrew: manly and brave

Andrade (Scandinavian) manly

Andrae (Slavic) form of Andrew: manly and brave

Andras (French) form of Andrew: manly and brave
Andrae, Andres, Andrus, Ondrae, Ondras

André (French) masculine
Andra, Andrae, Andre, Anrecito, Andree, Aundré, Andrei

Andreas (Greek) masculine
Andrieas, Andries Adryus, Andy

Andrej (Slavic) masculine; manly

Andren (English) masculine

Andrere (Greek) manly

Andres (Spanish) macho
Andras, Andrés, Andrez, Andy

Andre-Shaun (French) combo of Andre and Shaun; kind boy
Kind boy

Andretti (Italian) speedy
Andrette, Andy

Andrew ✿ ✝ (Greek) manly and brave
Aindrew, Anders, Andery, Andi, Andie, Andreas, Andres, Andrews, Andru, Andrue, Andy, Audrew

Andrick (Scandinavian) masculine

Andromache (Greek) manly

Andronek (Greek) wins

Andronico (Italian) victor

Andronicus (Greek) clever

Andros (Polish) masculine
Andris, Andrus

Andru (Greek) form of Andrew: manly and brave
Andrue

Andrzej (Polish) manly

Andy (Greek) form of Andrew: manly and brave
Andee, Andie

Anekin (Slavic) manly

Aner (Biblical) well-born

Aneurin (Welsh) golden child
Aneirin

Anfanio (Spanish) secretive

Anferny (American) variation of Anthony
Andee, Anfernee, Anferney, Anferni, Anfernie, Anfurny

Angel ✿ (Greek) angelic messenger
Ange, Angele, Angell, Angie, Angy

Angelberto (Spanish) shining angel
Angel, Angelbert, Bert, Berto

Angelo (Italian) angelic
Ange, Angelito, Angeloh, Angelos, Anglo, Anjelo

Angharad (Welsh) loving

Angits (Celtic) divine

Angle (Word as name) spin doctor
Ange, Angul

Anglin (Greek) angelic
Anglen, Anglinn, Anglun

Angra (Mythology) dark spirit

Angra (Mythology) dark spirit

Angus (Scottish) standout; important
Ange, Angos, Aonghas

Anh (Vietnamese) smart

Anibal (Spanish) brave noble

Aniceto (Spanish) invincible

Anick (Hebrew) gracious

Anlello (Italian) risk-taker

Anil (Hindi) air
Aneel, Anel, Aniel, Aniello

Aniol (Polish) angel
Ahnjol, Ahnyolle

Anju (Indian) younger

Anka (Polish) gracious; stems from Anna

Ankoma (African) last-born child

Ankur (Indian) blooms

Annan (African) second; from Annar

Annatto (Botanical) tree; tough
Annatta

Anndo (Scandinavian) protects

Annibale (Phoenician) form of Hannibal: leader

Anniel (Biblical) angel

Annis (English) God's gift

Anok (Slavic) reliable

Anolus (Greek) masculine
Ano, Anol

Anrue (American) masculine
Anrae, Anroo

Ans (Scandinavian) dramatic

Anscom (English) awesome
man
Anscomb

Ansel (French) creative
Ancell, Ansa, Anse, Ansell

Anselm (German) protective
Anse, Ansehlm, Ansellm

Anselmo (Spanish) protected
by God
*Ancel, Ancelmo, Anse, Ansel,
Anselm, Anzelmo, Selmo*

Ansgar (German) spear of
God

Anshel (Hindi) blessed
Anshel, Anshl

Anskar (German) brusque

Ansley (English) loner
*Anslea, Anslee, Ansleigh,
Anslie, Ansly, Ansy*

Anson (German) divine male
Anse, Ansonn, Ansun

Anssi (Scandinavian)
protected

Antal (Latin) princely

Ante (Slavic) flourishes

Ante (Spanish) special

Antero (Greek) moves with
grace

Anthonisamy (Indian) form
of Anthony: priceless

Anthony ✪ ✞ (Latin)
priceless
*Anathony, Anothony, Anth,
Anthawn, Anthey, Anthoney,
Anthoni, Anthonie, Anthonio,
Anthyonny, Anton, Antony, Tony*

Antioch (Biblical) place name

Antioco (Spanish) best

Antipas (Greek) father

Antjuan (American) form of
Anthony: priceless

Antoan (Latin) form of
Anthony: priceless

Antoine (French) worthy of
praise
*Antone, Antons, Antos,
Antwan, Antwon, Antwone*

Antolin (Slavic) unusual

Anton (Latin) outstanding
Antan, Antawn

Antonce (African American)
form of Anthony: priceless
Antawnce

Antonio ✪ (Spanish) superb
*Antinio, Antonello, Antoino,
Antone, Antonino, Antonioh,
Antonnio, Antonyio, Antonyo,
Antonyia, Tony*

Antony (Latin) good
*Antawny, Antini, Antonah,
Antone, Antoney, Antoni,
Antonie, Anty, Tone, Tony*

Antran (Spanish) energetic

Antrinell (African American)
valued
Antrie, Antrinel, Antry

Antroy (African American)
form of Anthony: priceless
Antroe, Antroye

Antuane (Slavic) first

Antwan (American) form of
Antoine: worthy of praise
Antawan, Antawn, Anthawn,
Antowine, Antowne, Antown,
Antwain, Antwaine, Antwaion,
Antwane, Antwann,
Antwanne, Antwaun, Antwen,
Antwian, Antwine, Antwion,
Antwoan, Antwoin, Antwoine,
Antwon, Antwonn, Antwonne,
Antwuan, Antyon, Antywon

Antwone (American) form of
Antoine: worthy of praise
Antwonn

Anubis (Egyptian) royal

Anulf (Scandinavian) royal

Anwar (Arabic) shining
Anour, Anouar, Anwhour

Anwyl (Welsh) beloved
Anwyll, Anwell

Anyon (Latin) form of
Anthony: priceless

Anzelm (Polish) protective
Ahnzselm

Apatin (Slavic) aggressive

Apearen (Native American)
armed

Apen (Irish) likes horses

Aplin (American) strong

Apolinar (Spanish) manly
and wise
Apollo

Apolinard (Spanish) strong

Apolla (Greek) strong

Apollo (Greek) masculine; a
god in mythology
Apolloh, Apolo, Apoloniah,
Applonian, Appollo

Apolonio (Greek) form of
Apollo: masculine; a god in
mythology

Apostle (Greek) follower;
disciple
Apos

Apostolos (Greek) disciple
Apos

Apple (American) favorite;
wholesome
Apel

Aquan (Native American)
tranquil

Aquila (Spanish) eagle-eyed
Acquilla, Aquil, Aquilas,
Aquile, Aquilla, Aquillino

Aquileo (Spanish) warrior
Akweleo, Aquilo

Ara (Slavic) integrity

Arachne (Greek) spider

Aracin (Latin) ready; heaven's
gate

Araldo (German) army leader

Aralis (Hawaiian) godlike

Aralt (Irish) army leader

Aram (Syrian) noble;
honorable
Ara, Aramia, Arra

Aramis (French) clever
Airamis, Arames, Aramith,
Aramys, Aramyse, Arhames

Arann (Slavic) calm

Arbel (Biblical) prayerful

Arber (American) from arbor;
adorned

Arbet (Last name as first
name) high
Arb, Arby

Arbogast (German) covered

Arcana (Latin) esoteric
wisdom

Arcen (English) virile

Arceneaux (French) friendly; heavenly
Arce, Arcen, Arceno

Arch (English) form of Archie and Archibald: bold leader
Arche

Archard (English) bold

Archer (English) athletic; bowman
Arch, Archie

Archibald (German) bold leader
Arch, Archibold, Archie

Archie (English) form of Archibald: bold leader
Arch, Archi, Archy

Arcis (Spanish) from war god
Arecio

Ard (Thai) woodsy

Ardan (Latin) passion; eagle

Ardee (American) ardent
Ard, Ardie, Ardy

Ardell (Latin) go-getter
Ardel

Arden (Latin) ball of fire
Ard, Arda, Ardie, Ardin, Ardon, Arrden

Ardley (English) with dedication

Ardmohr (Latin) more ardent than others
Ard, Ardmoor, Ardmore

Ardolph (German) ardent

Ardor (French) loving

Ardouin (French) ardent

Arecin (French) smooth

Areeb (Arabic) passionate

Areeg (Welsh) gold

Arellano (Scandinavian) unique

Arelus (Latin) form of Aurelius: golden son

Aren (Dutch) form of Aaron: revered; sharer

Arenas (Spanish) eager

Arenda (Spanish) eager

Ares (Mythology) combats

Arethuse (Greek) excels

Arfel (Welsh) struggles

Argan (American) leader
Argee, Argen, Argey, Argi, Argie, Argun

Argento (Spanish) silver
Arge, Argey, Argi, Argy

Argeroula (Greek) shines

Argus (Greek) careful; bright
Agos, Arjus

Argyl (Irish) from Ireland; aware

Argyle (English) diamond pattern; planning
Argile

Ari (Greek) best
Ahree, Aria, Arias, Arie, Arih, Arij, Arri

Arian (Welsh) form of Arion: enchated man

Aribert (German) holy

Aribold (German) holy

Aric (English) leader
Aaric, Arec, Areck, Arick, Arik, Arric, Arrick, Arrik

Arie (English) God's lion

Ariel (Hebrew) God's spirited lion
Airel, Arel, Arell, Ari, Arie, Ariele, Arielle, Ariya, Ariyel, Arrial, Arriel

Aries (Greek) god of war;
mythology
Arees, Arie, Ariez

Arik (German) leads

Arik (Welsh) form of Erik:
powerful leader

Arild (Hebrew) God's lion

Arimas (Literature) form of
Aramis: clever

Arines (Spanish) strong

Ario (Spanish) warring
Ari, Arrio

Arioch (Biblical) dignity

Arion (Greek) enchanted man
*Ari, Arian, Ariane, Arien,
Arrian, Arie, Ariohn*

Arisbe (Spanish) believer

Arisodemos (Greek) best
person

Arist (Greek) God-fearing

Aristeo (Spanish) best
Aris, Aristio, Aristo, Ary

Aristeus (Greek)
quintessential

Aristides (Greek) son of the
outstanding
Ari, Aris, Aristidis

Aristides (Spanish) son of
the best

Aristophanes (Greek)
playwright

Aristotle (Greek) best man
*Ari, Aris, Aristie, Aristito,
Aristo, Aristokles, Aristotelis,
Aristottle*

Ariwin (Spanish) best friend

Arj (Welsh) white

Arjan (Hindi) one Pandavas
Arjun

Arkady (Russian) revered

Arkan (Scandinavian) king's
baby

Arkell (Scandinavian) of the
king

Arki (Greek) ruler

Arkos (Biblical) people's
master

Arkyn (Scandinavian) royal
offspring
*Aricin, Ark, Arkeen, Arken,
Arkin*

Arle (Irish) sworn
Arlee, Arley, Arly

Arledge (English) lives by a
lake
Arleedj, Arles, Arlidge, Arlledge

Arleigh (Irish) sworn
Arly

Arlen (Irish) dedicated
*Arl, Arlan, Arland, Arle,
Arlend, Arlin, Arlyn, Arlynn*

Arley (English) meadow-
loving; outdoorsy
Arleigh, Arlie, Arly

Arlindo (Italian) dedicated

Arlis (Hebrew) dedicated; in
charge
Arlas, Arles, Arless, Arly

Arliss (English) wise eyes

Arlo (German) strong
Arloh

Arlonn (Irish) sworn;
cheerful
Arlan, Arlann, Arlen, Arlon

Arlyn (Irish) form of Arlen:
dedicated

Arlys (Hebrew) pledged
Arlis

Arm (English) arm
Arma, Arman, Arme

Arman (German) army man; defender
Armaan

Armand (German) strong soldier
Armad, Armanda, Armando, Armands, Armanno, Armaude, Arme, Armenta, Armond, Ormand

Armando (Spanish) entertainer
Armand, Arme, Armondo

Armani (Italian) army; disciplined talent
Amani, Arman, Armanie, Armon, Armoni

Armel (French) royal; sturdy

Armen (Spanish) from Armenia
Arme, Arment, Armenta

Armetris (Greek) prepared; armed

Armineh (Armenian) from Armenia

Armino (Teutonic) warrior

Armitage (Last name as first name) safe haven
Armi, Armita, Army

Armon (Hebrew) strong as a fortress
Arman, Arme, Armen, Armin, Armino, Armoni, Armons

Armstrong (English) strong-armed
Arme, Army

Arnaud (French) strong
Arnaldo, Arnauld

Arnborn (Scandinavian) eagle-bear; animal instincts
Arn, Arne, Arnborne, Arnbourne

Arndt (German) strong
Arne, Arnee, Arney, Arni, Arnie

Arne (German) form of Arnold: ruler; strong
Arn, Arna, Arnel, Arnell

Arnell (American) strong

Arnette (Dutch) little eagle
Arnat, Arnet, Arnot, Arnott

Arnic (Scandinavian) eagle-eyed

Arnie (German) form of Arnold: ruler; strong
Arne, Arney, Arni, Arnny, Arny

Arno (German) farsighted
Arn, Arne, Arnoh, Arnou, Arnoux

Arnold (German) ruler; strong
Arnald, Arne, Arndt, Arnie, Arnoll, Arny

Arnome (Invented) powerful
Arnom

Arnon (German) eagle

Arnot (French) form of Arnold: ruler; strong
Arnott, Arnart, Arnett

Arnov (Slavic) resolved

Arnst (Scandinavian) eagle-eyed
Arn

Arnulfo (Spanish) strong
Arne, Arnie, Arny

Arocles (Greek) masterful

Aroldo (German) eagle; strong

Aron (Hebrew) generous
Aaron, Arron, Erinn

Aronon (Welsh) blond

Arpad (Hungarian) prince; sunny

Arper (Slavic) fruitful

Arquimides (Spanish) philosopher

Arran (Scandinavian) form of Aaron: revered; sharer

Arrigo (Italian) ruler

Arsenio (Greek) macho; virile
Arne, Arsen, Arsenius, Arseny, Arsinio, Arsonio

Arshad (Iranian) revered

Arshaq (Arabic) supports

Arsinoe (Biblical) place name

Arslan (Spanish) form of Arsenio: macho; virile

Arson (Greek) masculine

Art (English) bearlike; wealthy
Arte, Artie

Artax (Biblical) rules

Artemus (Greek) gifted
Art, Artemas, Artemio, Artemis, Artie, Artimas, Artimis, Artimus

Arthel (Slavic) royalty

Arthi (Scandinavian) masculine

Arthisus (Origin unknown) stuffy
Arth, Arthi, Arthy

Arthur (Celtic) bear; stone
Art, Arth, Arther, Arthor, Artie, Artor, Artur, Arty, Aurther, Aurthur

Artie (English) form of Arthur: bear; stone
Art, Artee, Arty

Artin (Slavic) form of Arthur: bear; stone

Artra (Scandinavian) bear boy

Arturo (Italian) talented
Art, Arthuro, Artur, Arture, Arturro

Arun (Hindi) the color of the sky before dawn
Aruns

Arund (Hindi) free spirit

Arundel (English) lives with eagles; soars

Arv (Scandinavian) worthwhile

Arvai (Hebrew) roams
Arve

Arvel (German) friendly

Arvid (Hebrew) full of wanderlust
Arv, Arvad, Arve, Arvie, Arvind, Arvinder, Arvydas

Arvin (German) friendly
Arv, Arven, Arvie, Arvind, Arvinder, Arvon, Arvy

Arvo (Spanish) friend

Arwen (German) friend
Arwee, Arwene, Arwhen, Arwy

Arwey (Welsh) priceless

Arwin (American) assertive friend

Ary (Hebrew) lion; fierce
Ari, Arye

Arya (Indian) analytical

Aryan (English) white

Asa (Hebrew) healer
Ase, Aza

As·d (Arabic) happy
Asaad, Asad, Asid, Assad, Azad

Asafa (Biblical) collector

Asbury (Last name used as first name) dignified

Ascencion (Spanish) ascends

Ascot (English) cottage-dweller

Asgar (Scandinavian) God's home

Ash (Botanical) tree; bold
Ashbey, Ashby, Ashe

Asha (Hebrew) fire

Asharious (Mythology) ashur

Ashbel (Hebrew) fiery god

Ashby (Scandinavian) brash
Ashbee, Ashbey, Ashie, Ashy

Asher (Hebrew) joyful
Ash, Ashar, Ashor, Ashur

Ashfaaq (Arabic) honorable

Ashford (English) spunky
Ash, Ashferd, Ashtin

Ashkenaz (Biblical) sincere

Ashley (English) smooth
*Ash, Asheley, Ashelie, Ashely,
Ashie, Ashlan, Ashlee, Ashleigh,
Ashlen, Ashlie, Ashlin, Ashling,
Ashlinn, Ashlone, Ashly,
Ashlyn, Ashlynn, Aslan*

Ashlin (English) form of Ashley: smooth

Ashmon (English) of the ash trees

Ashok (Indian) content

Ashraf (Arabic) honors others

Ashrin (English) of the ash trees

Ashton (English) handsome
Ashteen, Ashtin

Ashtoreth (Biblical) staunch

Ashur (Hebrew) happy

Ashvin (English) ash tree

Asifa (Hebrew) gathers

Askew (Last name used as first name) distinguished

Askia (American) worthy

Aslan (Literature) from CS Lewis's Narnia series; lionlike

Asmer (Last name used as first name) ash tree

Asmus (German) well-known

Asner (Hebrew) giving

Asriel (Hebrew) praised

Asshurim (Biblical) of the ash-tree land

Assir (Biblical) hawk-like

Aston (English) eastern
Asten, Astin

Aswin (English) from the land of ash trees

Atam (American) form of Adam: first man; original
Atame, Atom, Atym

Atanacio (Spanish) everlasting
Atan, Atanasio

Atanase (Spanish) forever

Atch (American) lively

Ateeq (Arabic) affectionate

Athan (Biblical) form of Dathan: fountain of hope

Athanasius (Greek) immortal
Atanasio, Atanas

Athar (English) lives on a farm

Atherton (English) coming from a farm

Athos (Greek) high

Atilano (Greek) strong

Atilio (Spanish) aggressor

Atinuwa (African) aware

Atkins (Last name as first name) linked; known
Atkin

Atlas (Greek) courier of greatness
Atlass

Atley (English) from the meadow
Atlea, Atlee, Atleigh, Atli, Attley

Aton (Egyptian) sun child

Ator (Scandinavian) born of thunder

Atropos (Greek) unbinding

Atsu (African) second-born twin

Atticus (Greek) ethical
Aticus, Attikus

Attila (Gothic) powerful
Atalik, Atila, Atilio, Atiya, Atlya, Att

Attillio (Italian) hero

Atul (German) good

Atwater (English) living by the water

Atwell (English) the well; full of gusto

Atwood (English) the woods; outdoorsy

Atworth (English) farmer

Atyab (Arabic) cultivated

Auberon (German) like a bear; highborn
Aube, Auberron, Aubrey

Aubert (German) leader
Auber, Aubey

Aubin (French) ruler; elfin
Auben

Aubrey (French/German) ruler
Aubary, Aube, Aubery, Aubree, Aubry, Aubury, Bree

Auburn (Latin) brown with red cast; tenacious
Aubern, Aubie, Auburne

Auday (American) strong

Audelon (French) wealthy

Auden (English) old friend
Aude, Audie

Audencio (Spanish) companion
Auden

Audie (German) strong man
Aude, Audee, Audi, Audiel, Audley

Audley (English) rich
Audlea, Audlee, Audleigh, Audly

Audon (Scandinavian) alone

Audran (American) purposeful

Audras (Scandinavian) having wealth
Audres

Audric (French) wise ruler

Audun (Scandinavian) form of Audon: alone

Audwin (English) rich

Augie (Latin) form of Augustus: highly esteemed
Aug, Auggie, Augy

August (Latin) determined
Auge, Augie

Augustine (Latin) serious and revered
Agostino, Agoston, Agustin, Aug, Augie, August, Augustene, Augustin

Augustive (Spanish) serious

Augusto (Spanish) respected; serious
Agusto, Augey, Auggie, Austeo

Augustus (Latin) highly esteemed
Aug, Auge, Augie, August

Aulderay (American) old soul

Aulie (English) form of Audley: rich
Awlie

Aurek (Latin) golden

Aurelius (Latin) golden son
Arelian, Areliano, Aurel, Aurey, Aurie, Auriel, Aury

Aureo (Spanish) gold; pleases

Ausburn (English) reddish-brown

Aust (American) form of Austin: serious and revered

Austin ❂ ❂ (Latin) form of Augustine: serious and revered
Astin, Aust, Austen, Austine, Auston, Austyn

Austreberto (Spanish) austere

Auther (American) form of Arthur: bear; stone
Authar, Authur

Autry (Latin) golden

Avanindra (Hindi) king of the earth
Avan

Avdis (Slavic) providential

Avelino (Spanish) nature-lover

Avenall (English) from the woods; calm
Avenel, Avenell

Avent (French) up-and-coming
Aventin, Aventino

Averill (French) april-born child
Ave, Averel, Averell, Averiel, Averil, Averyl, Averyll, Avrel, Avrell, Avrill, Avryl

Avery (English) soft-spoken
Avary, Ave, Aveary, Averey, Averie, Avry

Avi (Hebrew) springlike
Avian, Avidan, Avidor, Aviel, Avion

Aviaz (Hebrew) believer

Aviden (Hebrew) God judges him

Avinoam (Biblical) pleasant brother

Avion (French) flyer
Aveonn, Avyon, Avyun

Avison (Hebrew) believes

Avitol (Hebrew) vital

Aviv (Hebrew) spring

Aviv (French) vibrant

Avner (Hebrew) father of light
Avneet, Avniel

Avniel (Hebrew) God is my rock

Avon (Hebrew) spring birth

Avon (English) place name

Avram (Hebrew) almighty father
Arram, Avraham, Avrom, Avrum

Avren (Hebrew) uplifts God

Avrum (Yiddish) form of Abraham: father of a multitude

Avrylle (French) hunter
  Avryll

Axel (German) peaceful;
  contemporary
  Aksel, Ax, Axe, Axil, Axill, Axl

Axie (Scandinavian) peaceful
  child

Axton (German) town of
  peace; peacemaker

Ayal (English) highborn

Ayden (Turkish) knowing

Aydin (Irish) masculine

Aydinus (Slavic) knowing

Ayers (Last name as first)
  industrious

Aylen (Native American) joy

Aylmer (English) of noble
  birth

Aylward (English) guards
  best

Aylwin (Welsh) elf friend

Ayman (Arabic) fortunate

Ayo (African) happy

Ayson (Origin unknown)
  lucky
  Aison

Aytekin (American) friend

Azad (Arabic) lucky

Azael (Spanish) God-loved

Azar (Biblical) form of
  Azariah: aided by Jehovah

Azariah (Biblical) aided by
  Jehovah

Azeem (Arabic) cherished
  Aseem, Asim

Azeez (Arabic) strong

Azhar (Arabic) flourishes

Azi (African) a child

Azia (Biblical) powerful

Azim (Arabic) grandiose

Aziz (Arabic) powerful

Aziz (African) adorable

Azizi (African) beloved

Azmon (Biblical) place name

Azrae (Mythology) azrael

Azriel (Hebrew) the Lord's
  angel

Azuriah (Hebrew) aided by
  God
  Azaria, Azariah, Azuria

Azzie (Slavic) strong

Babak (Iranian) the father

Babar (Turkish) lion
  Baber

Babe (American) athlete

Babu (Hindi) fierce

Bacchus (Greek) reveler;
  jaded
  Baakus, Bakkus, Bakus

Bach (Last name as first
  name) talented
  Bok

Bachar (Hebrew) eldest

Bachir (Hebrew) oldest son;
  reliable
  Bachur

Bacon (English) literary;
  outspoken
  Baco, Bake, Bakon

Badar (Hindi) full moon

Bade (Welsh) wild boar

Baden (German) bathes; cleansed

Badge (American) moon-watcher

Badger (Last name as first name) difficult
Badge, Badgeant, Bage, Bagent

Badget (English) moon-loving

Badr (African) full moon; lucky

Badru (African) full moon; lucky

Baghai (Arabic) form of Bahij: delighted

Bagher (American) magnificent

Bagley (English) boy from the field

Bagor (English) fun

Baha (Arabic) splendid

Bahij (Arabic) delighted

Bahir (Arabic) magnificent

Bai (Chinese) white

Bailey (French) attentive
Baile, Baily, Baley, Baylie

Bainbridge (Irish) bridge; negotiator
Bain, Banebridge, Beebee

Baines (Last name as first name) pale
Baine, Baynes

Bainlon (American) form of Bailey: attentive
Bailey, Baily

Baird (Irish) singer/poet; creative
Bard, Bayrde

Bairon (Spanish) creative

Baka (Biblical) place name

Bakari (African) promising

Baker (English) cook
Baiker, Baykar

Bal (Hindi) strong

Bala (Hindi) young

Balan (Last name used as first name) childlike

Balan (Indian) youthful

Balbino (Italian) mumbler

Baldemar (Spanish) form of Balthasar: God save the king
Baldy

Balder (Scandinavian) good prince
Baldur, Baudier

Baldev (Hindi) strong God

Baldie (German) nickname for Baldwin: brave friend

Baldric (German) leader
Baldrick, Baledric, Bauldric

Baldridge (English) persuasive

Baldwin (German) steadfast friend
Baldwinn, Baldwynn, Bally

Balendin (Place name) balen

Baley (American) form of Bailey: attentive
Baleye

Balfour (Scottish) landowner
Balf, Balfore

Balfre (Spanish) brave

Balin (Hungarian) from Balint: strong and healthy

Balint (Latin) strong and healthy

Ballance (American) courageous
Balance, Ballans

Ballard (German) brave
Ballerd

Balraj (Hindi) strong king

Balthasar (Greek) God save the king
Bath, Bathazar

Balu (Hindi) young

Balun (English) bold friend

Balwin (Last name as first name) friendly; brave
Ball, Winn

Bamboo (Malay) botanical

BaNaire (Slavic) of God's peace

Banan (Irish) white

Bancroft (English) bean field; gardener
Banc, Bankie, Bankroft

Bandy (Origin unknown) gregarious
Bandee, Bandi

Banjo (Word as name)

Banks (Last name as first name) focused
Bank

Banning (Irish) fair-haired
Bannie, Banny, Bannyng

Bao (Chinese) prized boy

Baptist (Latin) one who has been baptized

Barak (Hebrew) lightning; success
Barrak, Barack

Baram (Hebrew) son of the people

Barclay (Scottish) audacious man; birch tree meadow
Bar, Barclaye, Bark, Barklay, Barky

Bard (Irish) singer
Bar, Barr

Barden (English) peaceful; valley-dweller
Bardon

Bardolf (German) wily hero

Bardrick (English) sings ballads
Bardric

Barek (English) flash

Barend (Scandinavian) bearlike

Baret-Carlyle (American) combo of Baret and Carlyle

Bargo (Last name as first name) outspoken
Barg

Bari (Irish) fair-haired

Baris (Slavic) calm

Barison (English) son of peaceful man

Baritta (Last name used as first name) able

Bark (English) form of Barker: handles bark; lumberjack
Birk

Barker (English) handles bark; lumberjack
Bark, Barkker

Barlaam (History) hermit

Barlam (Hebrew) giving

Barlow (English) hardy
Barloe, Barlowe

Barman (Last name as first name) bright; blessed
Barr

Barn (American) word as name; works in barns
Barnee, Barney, Barny

Barnabas (Hebrew) seer; comforter
Barn, Barnaby, Barnebus, Barney, Barnie, Barny

Barnaby (Hebrew) companionable
Barn, Barnabee, Barnabie, Barnie, Barny

Barnali (Last name used as first name) son of the gatekeeper

Barneo (Place name) barn boy

Barner (English) mercurial
Barn, Barnerr, Barney, Barny

Barnes (English) powerful; bear

Barnett (English) leader of men
Barn, Barnet, Barney

Barney (English) form of Barnett: leader of men
Barn, Barni, Barnie, Barny

Barnum (German) safe; barn
Barnham, Barnhem, Barnie

Baron (English) noble leader
Bare, Baren, Barren, Baryne

Barra (Irish) fair-haired

Barragan (Irish) fenced in

Barrance (Last name used as first name)

Barrett (German) strong and bearlike
Bar, Baret, Barett, Barette, Barry

Barrington (English) dignified
Bare, Baring, Berrington

Barry (Irish) candid
Barre, Barrie, Bary

Barryrex (American) combo of Barry and Rex

Bart (Hebrew) persistent
Bartee, Bartie, Barty

Bartelt (English) form of Bartholomew: friendly; earthy

Barth (Hebrew) protective
Bart, Barthe, Barts

Bartholomew (Hebrew) friendly; earthy
Bart, Barthlolmewe, Bartie

Bartlett (Last name as first name) motivated

Bartley (Last name as first name) rural man
Bart, Bartle, Bartlee, Bartli, Bartly

Bartley (Last name used as first name) rural man

Barto (Spanish) form of Bartholomew: friendly; earthy
Bartelo, Bartol, Bartoli, Bartolo, Bartolomeo

Barton (English) persistent man; Bart's town
Bart, Barty

Bartosz (Slavic) form of Bartholomew: friendly; earthy

Bartoz (Slavic) form of Bartholomew: friendly; earthy

Bartram (English) intelligent
Bart, Barty

Baruch (Hebrew) most blessed
Barry

Baruti (African) teaches

Basant (Arabic) smiling

Basford (American) charming; low-profile
Bas, Basferd, Basfor

Bash (American) party-loving
Bashi, Bashey, Bashy

Basil (Greek) regal
Basel, Basey, Basile, Bazil

Basim (Arabic) smiles
Bassam

Basir (Turkish) smart

Bass (Last name as first name) fish; charmer
Bassee, Bassey, Bassi, Bassy

Bassam (Arabic) smiles

Bassett (English) small man
Baset, Basett, Basey, Basse

Bastete (Egyptian) fiery cat

Bastian (Greek) respected
Bastien, Bastyun

Basye (American) home-based; centered
Base, Basey

Batch (French) from bachelor; unmarried man
Bat, Bats, Batsh

Bates (English) romantic
Bate

Baudelio (Spanish) bold

Baudoin (Latin) winning

Baudouin (French) bold friend

Bauer (French) small

Baul (Gypsy) slow-moving

Baurice (African American) form of Maurice: dark

Bavan (Welsh) evan's son

Bavol (Gypsy) windblown

Baxley (English) from the meadow; outdoorsy
Bax, Baxlee, Baxli

Baxter (English) tenacious
Bax, Baxey, Baxie, Baxther

Bay (English) hair of russet; vocal
Baye, Bayie

Bayard (English) russet-haired
Bay, Baye, Bayerd

Bay-Atlas (American) combo of Bay and Atlas; 7th from heaven

Baylon (English) from the bay; outdoorsman

Bayro (Spanish) from the barn

Bazel (French) form of Basil: regal

Bazooka (American) fun-loving; unusual
Bazookah

Bazzy (American) loud
Bazzee, Bazzi, Bazzie

Beacan (Irish) small boy
Beag, Bec, Becan

Beach (English) fun-loving
Bee, Beech

Beacher (English) pale-skinned; beech tree
Beach, Beachie, Beachy, Beecher

Beagan (Irish) small
Beagen, Beagin

Beale (French) attractive
Beal, Beally

Beall (English) handsome

Beaman (English) tends bees
Beamann, Beamen, Beeman

Beamer (English) musician
Beam, Beamy, Beemer

Bean (Scottish) lively
Beann

Beanon (Irish) good boy
Beinean, Beineon, Binean

Bear (Scottish) lively

Beara (American) athletic

Bearach (Irish) spearing
Bearchan, Bercnan, Bergin

Beasley (English) nurturing;
pea field
Beas, Beasie, Beesly

Beate (German) serious
*Bay, Baye, Bayahtah, Beahta,
Beahtae*

Beattie (Irish) happy

Beau (French) handsome
man
Beaubeau, Bo, Boo, Bow

Beauford (French) attractive
Beau, Beauf, Beaufort

Beaumont (French) attractive
and strong
Bo, Bomont, Bowmont, Beau

Beauregard (French) a face
much admired
*Beau, Beauregarde,
Beaurigard, Bobo*

Beaver (French) tenacious
Beav, Beever, Bevoh, Beave

Bebe (Spanish) baby
Be-Be

Becher (Hebrew) firstborn
Bee

Beck (English) stream; laid-
back
Bec, Becc, Becke, Becker, Bek

Becker (English) calm
Bekker

Becket (English) by the brook

Beckett (English) methodical
Beck, Beket, Bekette

Bede (English) prayerful
Bea, Bead, Beda, Bedah

Bedford (Last name as first
name) laid-back

Bedrich (Czech) rules
peacefully

Bedro (Spanish) form of
Pedro: dependable; rock
Bed

Bedros (Spanish) prays

Beebe (English) tending bees;
tenacious
B.B., Bee-be, Beebee

Beechum (English) of the
trees (beech)

Beeson (Last name as first
name) son of beekeeper; wary
Bees

Beggs (Last name as first
name) admired
Begg, Begs

Behlin (Spanish) from
Bethlehem

Behrad (Indian) form of
Bharat: fire

Beig (English) mouth

Beige (American) calm
Bayge

Beinish (Latin) form of
Benedict: blessed man

Beircheart (Welsh) spears

Bela (Hawaiian) beauty

Belden (English)
plain-spoken
*Beld, Beldene, Beldon, Bell,
Bellden, Belldon*

Beldon (English) pretty valley child

Belen (Greek) following the arrow's straight path

Belizario (Spanish) archer

Bell (French) handsome man

Bellamy (French) beautiful friend
Belamie, Bell, Bellamie, Bellmee, Belmy

Bellindo (German) ferocious; attractive
Balindo, Belindo, Belyndo

Bello (African) advocates Islam

Belman (English) handsome

Belmount (French) gracious
Belmon, Belmond, Belmonde, Belmont, Belmonta

Belosi (Slavic) humble

Belton (English) from a lovely town of bells
Beltan, Belten

Belvin (American) form of Melvin: friendly
Belven

Belvon (Welsh) smart

Bem (African) peaceful

Ben (Hebrew) form of Benjamin: son of the right hand; son of the south
Benjy, Bennie, Benno, Benny

Benaiah (Hebrew) God-built; wars
Benaya, Benayahu

Benammi (Biblical) comes into his own

Bence (American) form of Benson: son of Ben; brave heart
Bens, Bense, Binse

Bend (American) word as name; lithe

Bendell (Last name used as first name) loving
Ben

Bender (American) tweaker; diplomatic
Ben, Bend

Bendo (American) soothing
Ben, Bend

Benedict (Latin) blessed
Ben, Benedik, Benne, Bennie, Benny

Benes (Czech) blessed

Benesh (Yiddish) blessed

Bengt (Scandinavian) blessed

Beni (Slavic) blessing

Beniah (Hebrew) articulate
Benia, Benyah

Benicio (Spanish) adventurous
Benecio, Benito

Benigno (Latin) kind child

Benito (Italian) blessed
Benedo, Beni, Beno

Benjamin ✪ ✿ (Hebrew) son of the right hand; son of the south
Behnjamin, Ben, Benjamen, Benjamine, Benjie, Benjy, Benni, Bennie, Benny, Benyamin

Benjiro (Japanese) promotes peace

Bennell (Last name used as first name) blessed

Benner (English) blessed

Bennett (French) blessed
Ben, Benet, Benett, Bennet, Bennette, Benny

Benno (Italian) form of Ben:
son of the right hand; son of
the south
Beno

Benny (Hebrew) form of
Benjamin: son of the right
hand; son of the south
Benge, Benjy, Benni, Bennie

Benoit (French) growing and
flourishing
Ben, Benoyt

Benoni (Hebrew) sorrow

Bensey (American)
easygoing; fine
Bence, Bens, Bensee

Benson (Hebrew) son of Ben;
brave heart
Bensahn, Bensen

Bent (English) form of
Benton: formidable
Bynt

Bentley (English) clever
Bent, Bentlee, Leye

Benton (English) formidable
Bentan, Bentawn, Bentone

Benvenuto (Italian)
welcomed child
Ben

Benz (German) from
carmaker Mercedes-Benz;
upscale
Bens

Benzi (Hebrew) blessed

Beowulf (Literature) warrior

Ber (Hebrew) bear

Berar (French) speaks well

Berdy (German) bright

Beresford (English) place of
spears
Berresford

Berfit (Origin unknown)
farming; outdoorsman
Berf

Berg (German) tall; mountain
Bergh, Berj, Burg, Burgh

Bergen (Irish) little spear
man
Bergin, Birgin

Berger (French) watchful;
shepherd
Bergher, Bergie

Bergin (Swedish) loquacious;
lives on the hill
*Bergan, Berge, Bergen, Berger,
Bergin, Birgin*

Berj (Scandinavian) form of
Birger: helpful

Berk (Turkish) rough-hewn

Berkeley (English) idolized;
place name
*town in California, Berk,
Berkeley, Berki, Berkie, Berklee,
Berkley, Berklie, Berkly, Berky*

Berko (Hebrew) bear
Ber

Berks (American) adored
*Berk, Berke, Berkelee, Berkey,
Berkli, Berksie, Berkslee, Berky,
Birklee, Birksey, Burks, Burksey*

Berlon (German) loyal

Berman (German) steady
Bermahn, Bermen, Bermin

Bermudez (Spanish) place
name; battles

Bernabe (German) bold
*Bernabee, Bernabey, Bernaby,
Bernby, Bernebe, Berns,
Bernus, Burnby*

Bernal (German) bearlike
Bern

Bernar (Last name used as first name) hardy

Bernard (German) brave and dependable
Bern, Bernarde, Bernee, Bernerd, Bernie, Berny, Burnard

Bernardo (Spanish) brave; bear
Berna, Bernardo, Barnardoh, Berny

Bernave (American) form of Bernard: brave and dependable
Bernav, Bernee, Berneve, Berni

Bernd (German) bearlike
Bern, Berne, Bernee, Berney, Berny

Berndt (German) hardy

Berne (German) courageous
Bern, Berni, Bernie, Bernne, Berny

Berner (English) bearlike

Bernhard (German) brave

Bernie (German) brave boy
Bern, Berni, Berny, Birnie, Burney

Bernstein (Last name used as first name) brave

Berrios (Spanish) the berries

Berry (English) botanical; flourishing

Bert (English) shining example
Berti, Bertie, Berty, Birt, Burt

Berthold (German) bold ruler
Bert, Berthol, Berthuld, Berty, Bertolt

Berthrand (German) form of Bertram: outstanding
Bert, Berthran, Bertie, Bertrand, Berty

Bertil (Scandinavian) bright
Bertel

Bertin (English) form of Burton: protective; town that is well fortified
Berton, Burtun

Bertoldo (Spanish) ruler
Bert

Berton (American) form of Burton: protective; town that is well fortified
Bert, Bertan, Berty

Bertram (German) outstanding
Bert, Bertie, Bertrem, Bertrom, Berty

Bertrand (German) bright
Bert, Bertie, Bertran, Bertrund, Birtryn

Bertren (German) smart

Berts (English) bright

Bertus (Last name used as first name) child of Bert

Berty (English) form of Bert: shining example
Bert, Bertie, Burty

Bervick (American) upwardly mobile; brave
Bervey

Berwyn (English) loyal friend
Berrie, Berwin, Berwynd, Berwynne

Besley (Last name as first name) calm
Bes, Bez

Best (American) word as name; quintessential man
Beste

Betel (Biblical) man of God

Bethel (Hebrew) loves the house of God
Bethell

Bethuel (Biblical) religious

Bettis (American) vocal
Bettes, Bettus, Betus

Beuford (Last name as first name) form of Buford: diligent
Beuf, Bu, Bueford

Beval (Welsh) vivacious

Bevan (Welsh) beguiling
Bev, Bevahn, Beven, Bevin

Bevell (Last name used as first name) craftsman

Bever (English) form of Bevis: strong-willed

Beverly (English) from a stream of beavers; natural

Bevil (English) form of Bevis: strong-willed

Bevis (French) strong-willed
Bev, Bevas, Beves, Bevvis, Bevys, Bevyss

Bexal (American) studious
Bex, Bexlee, Bexly, Bexy

Bexley (Place name) distinguished

Bezalel (Biblical) loyal

Bhakati (Hindi) devoted man

Bhanu (Hindi) sun-loving

Bharat (Hindi) fire

Bhaskar (Hindi) shining

Bhupen (Indian) forest

Biaggio (Italian) stutters; unsure
Biage, Biagio

Bialas (Polish) white-haired
Bialy

Bicken (Last name used as first name) boy with ax

Bickford (English) wields an ax; chops

Bickley (Last name used as first name) boy with ax

Biffy (American) popular
Bibbee, Biff

Bigram (Origin unknown) handsome
Bigraham, Bygram

Bijou (French) jewel

Bijoy (Indian) winning

Biju (French) joy

Bilal (Arabic) selected one

Bill (German) form of William: staunch protector
Billi, Billie, Billy

Billings (Place name) sophisticated

Billy (German) form of William: staunch protector
Bilie, Bill, Billee, Billi, Billie, Bily

Binden (Last name used as first name) binds closely

Bindo (Italian) blessed

Bing (German) outgoing
Beng

Bingo (American) spunky
Bengo, Bingoh

Binh (Vietnamese) a part of the whole

Binkie (English) energetic
Bink, Binki, Binky

Binnie (American) devoted son

Bion (Greek) life

Birch (English) white and shining; birch tree
Berch, Bir, Burch

Bird (American) soaring
Byrd

Biren (American) form of
Byron: reclusive; small
cottage
Biran

Birger (Scandinavian) helpful

Birger (Scandinavian)
watchful

Birinder (Indian) devout

Birkett (English) living in
birches; calming
Birk, Birket, Birkie, Birkitt,
Burkett, Burkette, Burkitt

Birkey (English) from the
birch tree isle
Birkee, Birkie, Birky

Birley (English) outdoorsy;
meadow
Berl, Birl, Birlee, Birly

Birney (English) single-
minded; island
Birne, Birni, Birny, Burney

Birtle (English) from the hill
of birds; natural

Bish (Hindi) universal

Bishamon (Mythology)
japanese god of war and luck

Bishop (Greek) supervisor;
serving the bishop
Bish, Bishie, Bishoppe

Bix (American) hip
Bicks, Bixe

Bizzo (American) lively

Bjorn (Swedish) athletic
Bjarn, Bjarne, Bjonie, Bjorne,
Bjorny

Black (Scottish) dark
Blacke, Blackee, Blackie

Blackburn (Scottish) lives by
a brook; dark

Blade (Spanish) prepared;
knife
Bladie, Blayd

Blades (American) sporty

Blagden (English) likes the
dark valley

Blaine (Irish) svelte
Blain, Blane, Blayne

Blainen (American) pious

Blair (Irish) open
Blaire, Blare, Blayree

Blaise (French) audacious
Blasé, Blayse, Blaze

Blake ○ (English) dark and
handsome
Blaike, Blakey, Blakie

Blakeley (English) outdoorsy;
meadow
Blake, Blakelee, Blakely, Blakie

Blame (American) sad
Blaim, Blaime

Blanchard (Last name as first
name) white
Blan

Blanco (Spanish) light
Blancoh, Blonco, Blonko

Blandon (American) form of
Brandon: hill; high-spirited

Blanford (English) from the
gray ford
Blandford

Blank (American) word as
name; blank slate; open
Blanc

Blanket (Invented) security
Blank, Blankee, Blankett,
Blankey, Blankie, Blanky

Blanton (English) mild-
mannered
Blanten, Blantun

Blasio (Spanish) stutterer
Blaseo, Blasios, Blaze

Blaynn (Last name used as first name) form of Blaine: svelte

Blaze (English and American) daring
Blaase, Blaise, Blazey, Blazie

Blazej (Czech) stutters; insecure

Blazer (American) fiery

Bleddyn (Welsh) heroic

Blendan (Last name used as first name) edge

Bliss (English) happy
Blice, Blyss

Blithe (English) merry
Bly, Blye, Blythe

Blitzer (German) adventurous
Blitz, Blitze

Block (English) on the block; engaged

Blocker (Last name as first name) block
Bloc, Block, Blok

Bloo (American) zany

Blue (Color name) hip
Bleu, Blu

Blunt (Last name used as first name) candid

Blye (American) joyful
Blie

Bo (Scandinavian) lively
Beau

Boat (American) word as name; sea-loving
Bo

Boaz (Hebrew) strong; swift
Bo, Boase, Boaze, Boz

Bob (English) form of Robert: brilliant; renowned
Bobbi, Bobbie, Bobby

Bobby (English) form of Robert: brilliant; renowned
Bob, Bobbie, Bobi

Bobo (African) tuesday-born

Bocko (English) fair-haired

Bodaway (Native American) fire maker

Boden (French) communicator
Bodin, Bodun, Bowden

Bodhi (Chinese) founder of Ch'an Buddhism in China
Bodhee

Bodhi (American) form of Bodie: laid-back

Bodie (American) laid-back

Bodil (Scandinavian) living

Bodua (African) last one

Bodun (Scandinavian) shelter

Bodynam (Scandinavian) flourishes

Boele (Scandinavian) helpful

Bogan (Slavic) godlike

Bogart (German) bold
Bo, Bobo, Bogardte, Boge, Bogert, Bogey, Bogie

Bogdan (Polish) God's gift

Bogdari (Polish) gift from God
Bogdi

Boggle (American) confusing
Bogg

Boghos (Slavic) strong

Bogumil (Polish) loves God

Bohumil (Polish) favored by God

Bohus (Slavic) favored

Bojan (Czech) fighter

Bojesse (American) comical
Boje, Bojee, Bojeesie, Bojess

Bola (American) careful; bold
Bolah, Boli

Bolden (American) bold man
Boldun

Boleslaw (Polish) in glory
Boleslav

Bolin (Last name as first
name) bold
Bolen

Bolivar (Spanish) aggressive
Bolley, Bollivar, Bolly

Bolley (American) strong
Bolly

Bolton (English) town of the
bold

Bomani (African) fighter
Boman

Bon (French) good
Bonne

Bonam (English) decent

Bonar (French) gentle
Bonarr, Bonnar, Bonner

Bonaventura (Spanish) good
fortune
*Bona, Bonavento,
Buenaventura, Buenaventure,
Ventura*

Bonaventura (Italian) good
luck

Bonaventure (Latin) humble
*Bonaventura, Bonnaventura,
Buenaventure*

Bond (English) farmer;
renegade
Bondee, Bondie, Bondy

Bondee (English) close

Bongani (African) thankful

Bongo (American) type of
drum; musical
Bong, Bongy

Boni (Latin) fortunate
Bonne

Bonif (American) giving

Bonifacio (Spanish)
benefactor
Bona, Boni, Boniface

Bonner (American) good

Bono (Spanish) good
Bonno

Bonocorso (Italian) good
path

Bonsi (Italian) good

Bonyer (American) hopeful

Boo (Literature) recluse in *To
Kill a Mockingbird*

Booker (English) lover of
books
Book, Booki, Bookie, Booky

Boone (French) blessed; good
Boon, Boonie, Boony

Boonen (English) asset

Bootaan (Unknown) deserted

Booth (German) protective
Boot, Boothe, Boothie, Bootsie

Booth (Last name used as
first name) lives there

Boots (American) cowboy
Bootsey, Bootsie, Bootz

Booveeay (Invented) form of
Bouvier: elegant; sturdy; ox
Boo

Bordan (English) secretive; of
the boar
*Borde, Bordee, Borden, Bordi,
Bordie, Bordy*

Border (American) word as name; fair-minded; aggressive
Bord

Borg (Scandinavian) fortified; castle
Borge, Borgh

Borges (Last name as first name) labyrinthine

Borgey (Scandinavian) castle

Borim (Biblical) place name

Boris (Russian) combative
Boras, Bore, Bores

Borka (Slavic) battles

Bornami (Asian) conflicted

Borr (Russian) contentious

Bos (English) woodsman
Boz

Boscoe (English) woodsman

Boseda (African) sunday-born

Bosley (English) thriving; grove
Bos, Boslee, Boslie, Bosly

Bosor (Biblical) place name

Bosque (Russian) fighter

Bosser (Scandinavian) lively

Bost (Place name) from Boston
Bostt

Boston (Place name) distinctive
Boss, Bost

Bosvely (English) child from the grove

Boswell (English) well near woods; dignified
Bos, Bosswell, Boz, Bozwell

Botan (Japanese) long-living

Botolf (English) wolf; standoffish
Botof

Bouck (Last name used as first name) worldview

Bour (English) loves the stream

Bourbon (Place name) jazzy
Borbon, Bourbonn, Bourbonne

Bourey (Vietnamese) countryman

Bourne (French) planner; boundary
Bourn, Bourney, Bournie, Byrn, Byrne, Byrnie

Bouvier (French) elegant; sturdy; ox
Bouveah, Bouveay, Bouviay

Bovo (Last name as first name) macho
Bovoh

Bowen (Welsh) shy
Bowie, Bowin

Bowie (Irish) brash; western
Booie, Bowen

Bowing (Last name as first name) blond and young
Beau, Bo, Bow, Bowen

Bowlin (Irish) blond

Bowman (Last name as first name) young; archer
Bow

Bowry (Irish) form of Bowie: brash; western
Bowy

Boy (American) boy child of the family

Boyce (French) defender
Boice, Boy, Boyce

Boyd (Scottish) fair-haired
Boide, Boydie

Boydine (French) from the woods
Boyse

Boydine (American) God's gift

Boydon (Last name used as first name) fair-haired

Boyer (French) woodsman

Boyette (Last name used as first name) joyful

Boyko (Slavic) fearful

Boylingston (Last name used as first name) sedate

Boyne (Irish) cow; grows

Boysey (Last name used as first name) treasured

Bozarth (Last name used as first name) gifted

Bozidar (Polish) God's precious
Bovza, Bovzek

Brack (English) from the plant bracken; fine
Bracke

Bracken (English) plant name; debonair
Brack, Brackan, Brackin, Brackun

Brackson (English) son of Brack

Bracy (Last name used as first name) holding

Brad (English) form of Bradley: prosperous; expansive
Braddie, Braddy

Brada (American) steadfast

Bradan (English) open-minded
Braden, Bradin, Brady, Bradyn, Braedyn, Braid

Bradford (English) mediator
Brad, Brady

Bradley (English) prosperous; expansive
Brad, Bradie, Bradlee, Bradlie, Bradly

Bradshaw (English) broad-minded
Brad, Brad-Shaw, Bradshie

Brady (Irish) high-spirited
Brade, Bradee, Bradey

Brahma (Hindi) worshipful

Braid (English) form of Bradan: open-minded

Brain (Word as name) brilliant
Brane

Brainard (English) princely
Brainerd

Brait (American) in demand

Braith (Welsh) spotted

Brak (American) support

Bram (Hebrew) form of Abraham: father of a multitude
Brahm, Bramm

Bramb (Dutch) form of Abraham: father of a multitude

Bramly (English) brambles

Bran (Irish) raven; blessed
Brann

Brance (Welsh) dark

Branch (Latin) growing
Bran, Branche

Branco (Last name as first name) authentic
Brank, Branko

Brand (English) fiery
Brandd, Brande, Brandy, Brann

Brandeis (Czech) has a
charitable nature

Brandell (Last name used as
first name) beacon of light

Brando (American) talented
Brand

Brandon ♂ ♀ (English) hill;
high-spirited
*Bradonn, Bran, Brandan,
Brandin, Branny*

Brandt (English) dignified
Bran, Brandtt, Brant

Brandy (English) firebrand;
bold; brandy drink
*Brand, Brandee, Brandey,
Brandi, Brandie*

Brannon (Irish) bright-
minded
Bran, Brann, Brannen, Branon

Bransby (Last name used as
first name) beacon of light

Branson (English) persistent
Bran, Brans, Bransan, Bransen

Brant (English) hothead
Brandt

Brantley (English) proud
child

Brants (English) proud child

Brashier (French) brash
Brashear, Brasheer

Brasil (Irish) disagrees
Brazil, Breasal, Bresal

Bratcher (Last name as first
name) aggressive
Bratch

Bratumil (Polish) brother's
love

Braulio (Italian) from a
meadow

Braunsen (Last name used as
first name) son of brown-
haired man

Bravillo (Spanish) brave
Braville

Bravo (Italian) top-notch
Bravoh, Bravvo

Brawley (English) meadow
man

Brax (Spanish) scrappy

Braxton (English) worldly
*Brack, Brackston, Brax,
Braxsten, Braxt*

Bray (English) vocal
Brae

Brayan (Origin unknown) to
yell out
Brayen

Brayd (English) loyal

Brayden ♂ (English) effective
*Braedan, Braedon, Braydon,
Braydun*

Braylon (English) steadfast

Brayton (English) town of
Bray

Braz (American) mysterious

Brazan (American) mystery

Brazil (Portuguese) reddish
brown tree

Brecht (Last name as first)
playwright

Breck (Irish) fair and freckled
Breckie, Breckle, Brek

Brecken (Irish) freckled

Brede (Scandinavian) glacier;
cold heart

Breeahno (Invented) form of
Briano: strong man of honor

Breeon (American) strong

Breer (English) fine

Breeson (American) strong
Breece, Breese, Bresen

Breeze (American) happy
Breese, Breez, Breezy

Bref (American) brave

Brekett (Irish) freckled

Brencis (Russian) sad

Brendan (Irish) armed
Brend, Brenden, Brendie,
Brendin, Brendon

Brennan (English) pensive
Bren, Brenn, Brennen,
Brennon, Brenny

Brennan (Irish) raven

Brenson (Last name as first
name) disturbed; masculine
Brens, Brenz

Brent (English) prepared; on
the mountain
Bren, Brint

Brenton (English) forward-
thinking
Brent, Brenten, Brintin

Brenton (English) hill town
boy

Breslin (English) land of Bres

Brett (Scottish) man from
Britain; innovative
Bret, Breton, Brette, Bretton,
Britt

Brettson (American) manly
man; Briton
Brett

Brewer (English) brews

Brewster (English) creative;
brewer
Brew, Brewer

Breyen (Irish) strong;
aggressive
Brey, Breyan

Brian ○ ○ (Irish) strong
man of honor
Bri, Briann, Brien, Brienn,
Bry, Bryan

Briand (English) jolly

Briander (American)
inquisitive; rider of waves

Briano (Celtic) form of Brian:
strong man of honor

Briant (American) form of
Bryant: honest; strong

Briareus (Mythology) giant
with one hundred arms;
strong

Brice (Welsh) go-getter
Bryce

Brick (English) alert; bridge
Bricke, Brik

Brickle (American) surprising
Brick, Brickel, Brickell, Bricken,
Brickton, Brickun, Brik

Brider (English) of the bride

Bridgely (English) coming
from the bridge
Bridgeley

Bridger (English) makes
bridges
Bridge

Bridges (English) bridge boy

Bridon (English) bright-eyed

Brielton (English) briel town

Brig (English) punished

Brigdo (American) leader
Brigg, Briggy

Brigham (English) mediator
Brigg, Briggie, Briggs, Brighum

Brigham (English) place
name

Brighton (English) from the
shining town

Brike (American) creative

Briley (English) calm
Bri, Brilee, Brilie, Brily

Brill (English) climbs

Brimmer (English) hill

Brinden (English) tawny

Brinell (English) tawny

Brink (English) on the precipice

Brinkley (English) meadow on edge

Brinley (English) of the joyful meadow; sweet
Brindley, Brinly, Brynley, Brynly

Briscoe (Last name as first name) forceful
Brisco, Brisko, Briskoe

Brishen (English) craftsman

Bristol (English) place name

Britt (English) humorous; from Britain
Brit, Britts

Brittin (American) boy from Britain

Britton (English) loyal; from Britain

Brock (English) forceful
Broc, Brocke, Brockie, Brocky, Brok

Brockly (English) aggressive
Brocklee, Brockli, Broklee, Broklie, Brokly

Brockton (English) badger; stuffy
Brock

Brod (English) form of Broderick: broad-minded; brother
Broddie, Broddy

Brodall (Irish) rules

Brode (Irish) broad wall

Broder (Scandinavian) true brother
Brolle, Bror

Broderick (English) broad-minded; brother
Brod, Broddee, Broddie, Broddy, Broderic, Broderik, Brodric, Brodrick

Brodie (Irish) builder
Brode, Brodee, Brody

Brodny (Irish) falling aside; brash

Brodrick (Last name used as first name) ruler's son

Brogan (Irish) sturdy shoe; dependable
Brogann

Bromley (English) meadow of shrubs; unpredictable
Brom, Bromlee, Bromlie, Bromly

Bron (Irish) sadness

Bronc (Spanish) wild; horse
Bronco, Bronk, Bronko

Bronco (Spanish) wild; spirited
Broncoh, Bronko, Bronnco

Brondo (Last name as first name) macho
Bron, Brond

Brone (Irish) sorrow

Bronick (English) brown

Bronnie (American) brown

Bronson (English) brown's son
Bron, Brondson, Bronni, Bronnie, Bronny, Bronsan, Bronsen

Bronto (American) from
brontosaurus; thunderous
*Bront, Brontee, Brontey, Bronti,
Bronty*

Bronze (Metal) alloy of tin
and copper; brown
Bronz

Brook (English) easygoing
Brooke, Brookee, Brookie

Brooker (English) stream boy

Brooks (English) easygoing
Brookes, Brooky

Brosio (Spanish) son of the
stream

Brost (Spanish) able

Broughton (English) from a
protected place

Brow (American) snob
Browy

Brown (English) tan
Browne, Brownie, Browny

Brownie (American) brown-
haired
Brown

Brownlee (English) brown-
haired

Brownson (Last name used
as first name) son of Brown

Broylon (English) noble

Broze (American) soulful

Brubaker (English)
brown-haired

Bruce (French) complicated;
from a thicket of brushwood
Bru, Brucie, Brucy, Brue

Bruck (English) brown-haired

Bruder (Last name used as
first name)

Bruiser (American) tough
guy
Bruezer, Bruser, Bruzer

Brumley (French) smart;
scattered
Brum

Brundage (Last name used
as first name)

Brundo (Spanish) brown-
haired

Brune (German) brown-
haired

Bruni (German) brown-haired

Bruno (German) brown-
skinned
Brune, Brunne, Brunoh

Brunon (Polish) brown-
haired

Brush (American) confident

Bruton (Latin) brutal

Brutus (Latin) aggressive; a
bully

Bry (American) form of
Bryan: ethical; strong

Bryan ✪ ✆ (Irish) ethical;
strong
Brye, Bryen

Bryand (English) form of
Bryan: ethical; strong

Bryant (Irish) honest; strong
Bryan, Bryent

Bryce (Welsh) spunky
Brice, Bry, Brye

Brycen (English) fast

Brychan (Welsh) speckled

Brycy (Welsh) lively

Brydon (American)
magnanimous
*Bridon, Brydan, Bryden,
Brydun*

Brydson (American) well-liked

Brylee (American)

Bryn (Welsh) hill-dweller

Brynmor (Welsh) big hill

Bryon (American) form of Byron: reclusive; small cottage

Brys (Welsh) spotted

Brysen (English) son of Brice

Bryson (Welsh) bryce's son; smart
Briceson, Bry, Bryse

Bryton (Welsh) hill town

Bu (Irish) winner; form of Buagh

Bual (English) son of speed

Bubba (German) a regular guy
Bub, Buba, Bubb, Bubbah

Bub-Joo (Asian)

Buck (English) studly; buck deer
Buckey, Buckie, Bucko, Bucky

Buckingham (Last name used as first name) male deer

Buckley (English) outdoorsy; a meadow for deer
Buckey, Buckie, Bucklee, Bucklie, Bucks, Bucky

Bucko (American) macho
Bukko

Bucky (American) warmhearted
Buck, Buckey, Buckie

Bud (English) courier
Budd, Buddie, Buddy, Budi, Budster

Buddy (American) courier
Bud, Buddi, Buddie, Budi

Budington (English) awakened

Budrys (Spanish)

Buell (German) upward; hill
Bue

Buf (English) castle

Buffalo (American) tough-minded
Buff, Buffer, Buffy

Buffington (Last name used as first name) town of Buffing

Buford (English) diligent
Bueford, Bufe, Buforde

Bulgara (Slavic) hardworking
Bulgar, Bulgarah, Bulgaruh

Bulldog (American) rough-and-tough
Bull, Dawg, Dog

Bullock (Last name as first name) practical

Bulmarck (Spanish)

Bulmaro (Spanish) fair

Bumpus (Last name as first name) humorous
Bump, Bumpey, Bumpy

Bunard (English) good
Bunerd, Bunn

Bune (American) free

Bunyan (English) good and burly
Bunyan, Bunyen

Buran (American) complex
Burann, Burun

Burch (English) strong

Burchard (English) tree trunks; sturdy
Burckhardt, Burgard, Burgaud, Burkhart

Burdell (English) in the dell

Burdette (English) shielded

Burditt (Last name as first name) shy
Burdett, Burdette, Burdey

Burford (Last name as first name) from the water

Burge (English) form of Burgess: businessman
Burges, Burgis, Burr

Burgess (English) businessman
Berge, Burge, Burges, Burgiss

Burhan (Last name as first name) complex

Burke (German) fortified
Berk, Berke, Burk, Burkie

Burl (German) homespun

Burley (English) nature-lover; wooded meadow
Burl, Burlea, Burlee, Burli, Burly, Burr

Burnaby (English) brook man

Burne (English) lives by the brook
Bourn, Bourne, Burn, Byrn, Byrne, Byrnes

Burnell (English) of the brook
Burnel

Burnell (French) brown-haired

Burnett (English) by the small brook
Burnet, Burnitt

Burney (English) loner; island
Burn, Burne, Burnie, Burny

Burnie (American) form of Bernie: brave boy

Burnis (English) by the brook
Burn, Burnes, Burney, Burr

Burnis (English) brown-haired

Burr (English) prickly; brusque
Burry

Burrell (American) safe

Burrick (English) townsman
Bur, Burr, Burry

Burrin (English) safe haven

Burris (English) sophisticated; living in the town
Berris, Buris, Burr, Burres

Burston (English) safe haven

Burt (English) shining man
Bert, Bertee, Burtie, Burty

Burtard (English) from the stronghold town

Burton (English) protective; town that is well fortified
Burt, Burty, Brutie

Busby (Scottish) artist; village
Busbee, Busbi, Buzbie, Buzz, Buzzie

Busher (Last name as first name) bold
Bush

Buster (American) fun
Bustah

Bustos (Spanish) jovial

Butcher (English) worker
Butch, Butchy

Butler (English) directing the house; handsome
Butler, Butlir, Butlyr, Buttler

Buxton (Last name as first name) kind

Buz (Biblical) hateful

Buzz (Scottish) popular
Buzy, Buzzi, Buzzie, Buzzy

Byelo (Slavic) white

Byford (English) leaving the cottage; forever young

Byorn (American) form of Bjorn: athletic

Byram (English) stealthy; yard that houses cattle
Bye, Byrem, Byrie, Byrim

Byrd (English) birdlike
Bird

Byrne (English) loner
Birn, Birne, Byrn, Byrni, Byrnie, Byrny

Byrnett (Last name as first name) stable
Burn, Burnett, Burney, Burns, Byrne, Byrney

Byron (English) reclusive; small cottage
Biron, Biryn, Bye, Byren, Byrom, Byrone, Byryn

Cab (American) word as name
Cabby, Kab

Cabbon (Biblical) place name

Cabell (Last name as first name) spontaneous

Cable (French) rope-making boy; crafty
Cabel

Cabot (French) loves the water
Cabbott

Cabral (African) Tuesday's child

Cabree (Irish) rides

Cabrera (Spanish) able
Cabrere

Cacal (Last name used as first name) noisy

Cack (American) laughing
Cackey, Cackie, Cacky, Cassy, Caz, Kass, Kassy, Khaki

Cactus (Botanical) prickly
Cack, Kactus

Cadas (Biblical) place name

Cadby (Norse) spirited heritage

Caddock (Last name as first name) high spirits

Cade (English) stylish; bold; round
Cadye, Kade

Cadel (Welsh) fierce

Caden ✪ (English) spirited
Cadan, Cade, Cadun, Caiden, Kaden, Kayden

Cadman (Irish) fighter
Cadmann

Cadmar (Greek) fiery
Cadmarr

Cadmus (Greek) one who excels; prince
Cad, Cadmuss, Kadmus

Cadon (American) friendly

Cadou (Welsh) fights

Cady (American) forthright
Cadee, Cadey, Cadie

Cael (Irish) slim

Caesar (Latin) focused leader
Caeser, Caez, Caezer, Cesaro, Cezar, Seezer

Caetan (Irish) slim

Cage (American) dramatic
Cadge

Caglar (American) able

Cagle (Spanish) winner

Cailen (American) gentle
Kail, Kailen, Kale

Cain (Hebrew) aggressive
Caine, Cainen, Cane, Kain, Kane

Cairn (Welsh) stone; sturdy
Cairne

Caj (Scandinavian) from Gaius (Caesar's first name); masculine

Caja (American) close proximity

Cal (Latin) form of Calvin: bald
Callie, Kal

Calah (Scandinavian) outdoors

Calam (Scottish) peaceful

Calbert (American) cowboy
Cal, Calbart, Calberte, Calburt, Callie, Colbert

Calcher (American) peaceful

Calden (English) singer

Calder (English) stream; flowing
Cald, Kalder

Calderon (Spanish) stream; flowing
Cald, Kald, Kalder, Kalderon

Caldwell (English) refreshing; cold well

Cale (Hebrew) slim; good heart
Kale

Caleb ✪ ✞ (Hebrew) faithful; brave
Cal, Calab, Cale, Caley, Calie, Calub, Kaleb

Calek (American) fighter; loyal
Calec, Kalec, Kalek

Calen (Irish) slim
Cailun

Calendt (American) slim

Caler (English) promising

Caley (Irish) slender

Calf (American) cowboy
Kalf

Calfray (American) singer

Calhoun (Irish) limited; from the narrow woods
Cal, Calhoon, Calhoune, Callie

Calixto (Spanish) handsome
Calex, Calexto, Cali, Calisto, Calix, Callie, Cally, Kalixto

Call (Native American) flourish

Callahan (Irish) spiritual
Cal, Calahan, Calihan, Callie

Callard (Last name used as first name) thrives

Callie (American) form of Calvin: bald
Cal, Calley, Calli, Cally

Callistua (Greek) most beautiful man

Callo (American) attractive
Cal, Cally, Kallo

Cally (Scottish) peacemaker

Calman (Last name as first name) caring
Cal

Calno (Biblical) place name

Calum (Irish) cal
Callum, Calym, Calyme

Calv (American) form of
Calvert: respected; herding

Calvary (American) word as
name; herding all
Cal, Kal, Kalvary

Calvert (English) respected;
herding
*Cal, Calber, Calbert, Calver,
Kal, Kalvert*

Calvin (Latin) bald
Cal, Calvie, Kal

Cam (Scottish) form of
Cameron: mischievous;
crooked nose
*Camm, Cammey, Cammie,
Cammy, Kam*

Camara (African) instructs

Cambell (American) form of
Campbell: bountiful; crooked
mouth
*Cam, Cambel, Cammy,
Kambell*

Camberg (Last name as first
name) valley man
Cam

Cambio (Italian) short

Cambridge (Place name) city
in England; twisting; mover
Cambrydge

Camden (Scottish) conflicted
Cam, Camdan, Camdon

Camerero (Last name as first
name) charismatic

Cameron ✪ (Scottish)
mischievous; crooked nose
*Cam, Camaron, Camerohn,
Cami, Cammy, Camren,
Camron*

Camiel (Spanish) helps

Camilo (Latin) helpful; Italian
free, Cam, Camillo

Cammer (Spanish) hall
worker

Campbell (Scottish)
bountiful; crooked mouth
*Cambell, Cammie, Camp,
Campie, Campy*

Campillo (Spanish) form of
Camilo: helpful; Italian

Campion (English) champion

Camrin (American) form of
Cameron: mischievous;
crooked nose

Camron (Scottish) form of
Cameron: mischievous;
crooked nose
Camren

Can (Turkish) vibrant

Canaan (Biblical) spiritual
leanings
Cane, Kanaan, Kanan

Canada (Place name) from
Canada

Canal (Word as name)
waterway
Kanal

Candelario (Spanish) bright
and glowing
Cadelario

Cander (American) candid
*Can, Candor, Candy, Kan,
Kander, Kandy*

Candido (Spanish) pure;
candid
Can, Candi, Candide, Candy

Candle (American) bright;
hip
Candell

Cangelo (Spanish) vibrant

Canice (Spanish) seamless

Cannon (French) courageous
*Canney, Canni, Cannie,
Canny, Canon, Canyn,
Kannon, Kanon*

Cano (Scottish) attractive

Canow (American) like a
canon

Canten (American Indian)
hunter

Canute (Scandinavian) great
Knut, Knute

Canyon (Nature) hip

Capan (American) bird;
jaunty

Capi (American) high energy

Capon (American) bird;
captain

Capone (Last name used as
first name) risk-taker

Capote (Italian) bright

Cappy (French) breezy; lucky
Cappey, Cappi

Capua (Biblical) place name

Caractacus (Latin) bold

Carad (American) wily
Karad

Caradine (Spanish) birdlike

Caravaggio (Italian) painter

Caravale (Last name used as
first name) dear valley girl

Carballo (Spanish) explosive

Card (English) form of
Cardan: crafty; carder
Kard

Cardan (English) crafty;
carder
Card, Carden, Cardon

Cardente (Spanish) clarity

Cardente (Spanish)
craftsman

Carder (Last name used as
first name) confident

Cardew (Welsh) dark

Cardin (Irish) dark home

Cardoc (Welsh) loved

Cardozo (Spanish) supportive

Cardwell (English) craftsman
Kardwell

Carel (Dutch) free

Carew (Latin) runner
Currew

Carey (Welsh) masculine; by
the castle
Care, Cari, Cary, Karey

Cari (English) masculine
Care, Carie, Cary

Carino (Last name as first
name) strong

Carl (Swedish) kingly
Karl

Carland (Last name as first
name) land of free men

Carlin (Irish) winning
*Carlan, Carle, Carlen, Carlie,
Carly*

Carlisle (English) strengthens
Carl, Carly, Carlyle

Carlo (Italian) sensual; manly
Carl, Carloh

Carlon (Irish) form of Carl:
kingly
Karlon, Carlonn

Carlos ❂ (Spanish) manly; sensual
Carl, Carlo

Carlson (English) son of a manly man
Carls, Carlsan, Carlsen

Carlton (English) leader; town of Carl
Carleton, Carltan, Carlten, Carltown, Carltynne

Carmel (Hebrew) growing; garden
Carmell, Karmel

Carmello (Italian) flourishing
Carm, Carmel, Carmelo, Karmello

Carmi (Biblical) beloved son

Carmi (Italian) garden

Carmichael (Scottish) bold; Michael's follower
Car, Kar, Karmichael

Carmine (Italian) carmane
Carmin, Carmyne, Karmen, Karmine

Carmo (Italian) songs

Carmody (French) manly; adult
Carmodee

Carn (English) winner

Carneg (Slavic) horner

Carnell (Irish) victor
Car, Carny, Kar, Karnell, Karney

Carney (Irish) winner
Carn, Carnay Carnee, Carnie, Carny

Caro (Hungarian) horn boy

Carol (Irish) champion
Carroll, Carrol, Carroll

Carpus (Greek) bountiful

Carr (Scandinavian) outdoorsy
Car, Kar

Carrew (Latin) runner

Carrick (Irish) lives on rocky place

Carrier (Last name used as first name) growth

Carroll (German) masculine; winner
Carall, Care, Carell, Caroll, Carrol, Carrolle, Carry, Caryl

Carson ❂ (English) confident
Carr, Cars, Carsan, Carsen

Carsten (German) a Christian

Carswell (English) diligent

Cart (American) word as name; practical
Cartee, Cartey, Kart

Carter ❂ (English) insightful
Cart, Cartah, Cartie

Cartrell (English) practical
Car, Cartrelle, Cartrey, Cartrie, Cartrill, Kar, Kartrel, Kartrell

Cartwright (English) creative
Cart, Cartright, Kart, Kartwright

Carungay (Spanish) crass

Caruso (Italian) musically inclined
Karuso

Carvell (English) innovative
Carvel, Carvelle, Carver, Karvel

Carver (English) carver
Carve, Carvey, Karver, Karvey

Cary (English) pretty brook; charming
Carey

Casady (English) curly-haired

Casdeen (American)
assertive; ingenious
Kassdeen

Case (Irish) highly esteemed
Casey

Caseen (Dutch) together

Casel (English) boisterous

Casen (Last name used as
first name) bound

Casey (Irish) courageous
*Case, Casey, Casi, Casie, Kacie,
Kacy, Kase, Kaysie*

Cash (Latin) conceited
Casha, Cashe, Cazh

Cashmere (American)
smooth; soft-spoken
*Cash, Cashmeer, Cashmyre,
Kashmere*

Cashone (American)
cash-loving
Casho

Casiano (Latin) empty

Casimir (Polish) peace-loving
Casmer, Casmir

Casimiro (Spanish) famous;
aggressor
Casmiro, Kasimiro

Caslu (Biblical) turmoil

Casper (German) secretive
*Caspar, Casper, Caspey, Caspi,
Caspie, Cass*

Caspian (Place name) sea
near Iran; daring

Caspin (Biblical) place name

Cass (Irish) form of Cassidy:
humorous
Cash, Caz, Kass

Cassell (English) saintly

Cassian (Last name used as
first name) thinker

Cassidy (Irish) humorous
*Casidy, Cass, Cassadie,
Cassidee, Cassidie, Kasidy,
Kass, Kassidy*

Cassie (Irish) form of
Cassidy: humorous
Casi, Cass, Cassy

Cassius (Latin) protective
Cass, Casseus, Casshus

Cast (Greek) form of Castor:
eager protector
Casta, Caste, Kast

Castellan (Spanish)
adventurer

Caster (English) saint

Castern (Last name used as
first name) reliable

Castle (Last name used as
first name) sturdy

Casto (Mythology) form of
Castor: eager protector
Cass, Kasto

Casto (Spanish) star

Casto (Greek) truthful

Castor (Greek) eager
protector
Cass, Caster, Castie

Castulo (Spanish) aggressor
Castu, Kastulo

Cata (American) form of
Catarino: unflawed; perfect

Catarino (Spanish) unflawed;
perfect
Catrino

Cathal (Irish) leader

Cather (Last name used as
first name) virile

Cathmor (Irish) brave
warrior

Cato (Latin) zany and bright
Catoe, Kato

Catou (French) wise

Cauda (Biblical) place name

Caudell (Last name used as first name) pure

Caughtry (Welsh) fighter

Cavan (Irish) attractive man
Cavahn, Caven, Cavin

Cavance (Irish) handsome
Caeven, Cavanse, Kaeven, Kavance

Cavell (Last name as first name) opinionated
Cavil, Cavill

Cavin (Irish) safe; stylish

Cavinal (Irish) not of substance; hollow

Cawley (Last name as first name) brash

Cayce (American) form of Casey: courageous
Cace, Case, Kayce

Caycen (American) of the case

Cayern (Last name used as first name) makes cases

Cayetano (Spanish) feisty

Cayetano (Spanish) destiny

Cayeto (Spanish) survivor

Caynce (Invented) form of Cayce: courageous
Caincy, Cainse, Kaynse

Cayo (American) smart

Cazare (Last name as first name) daring
Cazares

Ceabron (Last name used as first name) giving

Cease (American) rowdy

Cebriane (Spanish) form of Cyprus: island south of Turkey; outgoing

Cebron (Spanish) generous

Cecil (Latin) unseeing; hard-headed; blind
Cece, Cecel, Cecile, Cecilio, Cicile

Cedar (Botanical) tree name; sturdy
Ced, Sed, Sedar

Cedric (English) leader
Ced, Ceda, Cedrick

Ceferino (Spanish) careful

Celedonio (Spanish) heavenly

Celius (Spanish) celestial

Celso (Italian) heavenly
Celesteno, Celestino, Celesto, Celestyno, Celsus, Selso

Celsorio (Last name used as first name) soars

Celum (Spanish) holly berries

Celumiel (Spanish) of the heavens
Celu

Celvan (Slavic) winning

Cemal (Arabic) handsome

Cender (Spanish) articulate
Peace

Cened (Slavic) wins

Cengiz (Inventive) weapon

Cenobio (Spanish) shy

Centola (Spanish) tenth child
Cento

Century (Invented) remarkable
Cen, Cent

Cerb (Greek) dark mind

Cerber (Mythology) three-headed

Cerbulo (Spanish) serene

Cerce (Greek) form of Circe; thinker

Ceres (Greek) loving

Cerf (French) buck

Cerlito (Spanish)

Ceron (Greek) thunders

Cerone (French) serene; creative
Serone

Cervacio (Spanish) serves

Cervando (Spanish) fawning

Cervant (Spanish) original

Cervantes (Literature) for the Spanish author; original
Cervantez

Cesaire (French) form of Caesar

Cesar (Spanish) leader
Cesare, Cezar, Zarr

Cesar-Vega (Spanish) combo of Cesar and Vega
Famed star

Cetrell (Spanish) centered

Chaban (American) form of Chabe: from Shabe in Bible

Chabe (Biblical) from Shabe in the Bible

Chacko (Spanish) form of Chico: boy

Chad (English) firebrand
Chadd, Chaddy

Chadburn (English) spirited

Chaden (English) battles

Chadley (English) cautions

Chads (English) aggressive

Chadson (English) son of Chad; comforts

Chadwick (English) warrior
Chad, Chadwyck

Chaffee (Last name as first name) bold adventurer

Chaggy (American) cocky
Chagg, Shagg, Shaggy

Chaicus (Biblical) strong

Chaika (Hebrew) life
Chaikeh, Chaikel, Chaiki, Chai

Chaim (Hebrew) life
Chai, Chayim, Haim, Hy, Hyman, Hymie, Khaim, Manny

Chaise (French) chases
Chayse

Chaker (Arabic) best

Chalen (American) strong

Chalfie (American)

Chalfin (Last name used as first name)

Challen (American) form of Allen: handsome boy

Chalmer (Scottish) the Lord's son
Chall, Chally, Chalmers

Chalmers (French) chambers; surrounded
Chalm

Chalmers (Scottish) Lord's child

Chamara (Asian) diligent

Chamb (American) messenger

Chambers (English) regal boy

Chamblin (American)
easygoing
Cham

Chan (Chinese) bright;
Vietnamese
truthful

Chanan (Hebrew) filled with
God's compassion

Chance (English) good
fortune; happy
*Chancey, Chanci, Chancy,
Chanse, Chanz, Chauncey*

Chancela (American)
dedicated

Chancellor (English) book
keeper
Chance, Chancey

Chand (Indian) sun

Chanda (Indian) brightness

Chandell (African American)
innovator
*Chandelle, Chandey, Chandie,
Shandel, Shandell*

Chanderkala (Hindi)
luminous

Chandler (English)
ingenious; French
*maker of candles, Chand,
Chandey, Chandlor*

Chandru (Indian) moon

Chaney (French) strong
*Chane, Chanie, Chayne,
Chaynee*

Chang (Chinese) free;
flowing

Chanina (Hebrew)
compassionate by virtue of
God

Channing (English) brilliant
Chann, Channy

Chanoch (Hebrew)
dedicated; loyal

Chantan (Indian) sparkle

Chante (French) singer
*Chant, Chanta, Chantay,
Chantie*

Chapa (Last name as first
name) merchant; spirited
Chap, Chappy

Chaparro (Spanish) from
chaparral southern landscape;
cowboy
Chap, Chaps

Chapel (Last name used as
first name) singer

Chapell (Hindi) spiritual

Chapen (French) clergyman
Chapin, Chapland, Chaplin

Chaplin (Last name used as
first name) pious

Chapman (English)
businessman
Chap, Chappy

Chappelle (French) of the
chapel

Char (French) truthful;
spiritual

Charilaos (Greek) giving

Charlem (English) of Charles

Charlemagne (French)
historic; King of the Franks
"Charles the great"

Charles ✪ (German) manly;
well-loved
*Charl, Charley, Charli, Charlie,
Charly, Chas, Chaz, Chazz,
Chuck*

Charleston (English)
charles's town; confident
Charlesten

Charlie (German) manly
Charl, Charley, Charli, Charly

Charlie-John (American)
combo of Charlie and John

Charlton (English) leader
*Charles, Charley, Charlie,
Charlt*

Charome (American)
masculine
*Char, Charoam, Charom,
Charrone, Charry*

Charon (Greek) mythological
ferryman of the underworld

Charro (Spanish) wild-
spirited cowboy
Charo, Charroh

Charudata (Hindi) beautiful

Charvaka (Hindi) form of
Charudata: beautiful

Chas (American) form of
Charles: manly; well-loved

Chase ○ (French) hunter
Chace, Chass

Chaskel (Hebrew) strong

Chason (French) hunts
Chansen

Chat (American) happy
Chatt

Chatham (Last name as first
name) serious

Chatsworth (English)
warrior's place

Chatwin (Last name as first
name) thoughtful

Chaucer (Literature) for
Geoffrey Chaucer;
distinguished
Chauce, Chauser

Chaudray (French) hopeful

Chauncey (English) fair-
minded
*Chance, Chancey, Chanse,
Chaunce*

Chausse (English) form of
Chauncey: fair-minded

Chavers (English) stern

Chavivi (Hebrew) beloved

Chavlier (French) elegant

Chayne (Scottish) swagger
Chane, Channe, Chay

Chaz (German) form of
Charles: manly; well-loved
Chas, Chazz, Chazzie, Chazzy

Ché (Spanish) form of José:
asset; favored
Chay, Shae, Shay

Ched (French) form of Shad:
joyful

Chee (American) high-energy
Che

Chekhov (Russian)
playwright; genius

Chen (Chinese) great

Cheney (French)
outdoorsman
Chenay, Cheney

Cheramy (American) form of
Jeremy: talkative
Cheramee, Charamie, Chermy

Cheran (Biblical) dearest

Chermon (French) my dear

Cherno (Slavic) black

Chesed (Biblical) difficult

Chesley (American) patient
Ches, Cheslee, Chez, Chezlee

Chesman (Last name used as
first name) hard

Chester (English) comfy-cozy
Ches, Chessie, Chessy

Chesterfield (English) field of Rochester; comforting

Chet (English) creative
Chett

Chetan (Indian) vibrant

Chetny (Native American) determined

Chetwin (English) winding road

Chevalier (French) gallant
Chev, Chevy

Chevalle (French) dignified
Chev, Chevi, Chevy

Cheven (Invented) playful
Chevy

Chever (Place name)

Chevery (French) form of Chevy: clever
Chev, Shevery

Chevy (French) clever
Chev, Chevi, Chevie, Chevv

Chew (Chinese) mountain

Chiamaka (African) God is good

Chibale (Hebrew) loving

Chick (English) form of Charles: manly; well-loved
Chic, Chickie, Chicky

Chico (Spanish) boy
Chicoh, Chiko

Chief (Word as name) leader

Chieko (Spanish) boy

Chiel (Hebrew) God lives

Chijoke (African) talented

Chikosi (African) the ruins

Chili (American) appetite for hot food

Chillen (American) form of Chilton: serene; farm

Chilton (English) serene; farm
Chill, Chillton, Chilly, Chilt

Chimanga (African) grain

Chimento (Italian) of the chimes

Chin (Korean) precious boy

Chip (English) chip off the old block; like father
Chipp, Chipper

Chiram (Hebrew) held in high esteem

Chiriga (Indian) lights the way

Chisholm (Place name) from Chisholm Trail: pioneer spirit
Chis, Chishom, Chiz

Chita (Spanish) fiery

Chito (American) fast-food eater; hungry
Cheetoh, Chitoh

Chiura (Italian) light; textured

Chiztam (Hebrew) imbued with God's strength

Chobi (Spanish) buddy

Chogie (Spanish) friendly

Choicey (American) word name; picky
Choicie, Choisie

Chombel (American) birdlike

Chonito (Spanish) friend
Chonit, Chono

Chopo (American) cowhand
Chop, Choppy

Choto (Spanish) kid
Shoto

Chotto (Last name as first name) child

Chovev (Hebrew) companion

Chow (Chinese) everywhere

Chris (Greek) form of Christopher: the bearer of Christ
Cris, Chrissy, Chrys

Christer (Norwegian) religious
Krister

Christian ♀ ♂ (Latin) follower of Christ
Chris, Christen, Christiane, Christyan, Cristian, Kris, Krist, Kristian

Christo (Spanish) christian

Christodoulous (Greek) filled with sweet love for Christ

Christop (Greek) christian

Christophe (French) beloved of Christ
Cristoph, Kristophe

Christopher ♀ ♂ (Greek) the bearer of Christ
Chris, Christofer, Crista, Cristopher, Cristos, Kit, Kristopher

Christopherson (English) son of Christopher; religious
Christophersen, Cristophersen, Cristopherson

Christos (Greek) form of Christopher: the bearer of Christ
Chris, Kristos

Chubby (American) oversized
Chubbee, Chubbey, Chubbi, Chubbie

Chuck (German) rash
Chuckee, Chuckey, Chuckie, Chucky

Chuckles (American) clown

Chucky (German) impulsive
Chuckey, Chucki, Chuckie

Chuey (Spanish) form of Charles: manly; well-loved

Chuhei (Japanese) shy

Chuna (Hebrew) warm

Chuneh (Hebrew) with the Lord's grace

Chunky (American) word name; large
Chunk, Chunkey, Chunki

Chur (American) form of Churchian: spirited

Churchian (American) spirited

Churchill (English) bright
Church

Chutar (Spanish) aiming for goals
Chuter

Chux (American) clear

Chuxin (American) clear

Chuyen (Native American) clear

Cian (Irish) old soul

Ciano (Irish) old

Cibab (German) giving

Cicero (Latin) strong speaker
Cice

Ciceron (Latin) chickpea

Cicil (English) shy
Cecil, Cice

Cid (Spanish) leader; Lord
Ciddie, Ciddy, Cyd, Sid

Cielo (Spanish) light

Cieran (Spanish) clarity

Cigler (Last name used as first name)

Cimarron (Place name) city in New Mexico; cowboy
Cimaronn

Cinco (Spanish) fifth child
Cinko, Sinko

Cione (Italian) last name used as first name

Ciprian (Latin) from the island of Cyprus
Cipriano

Ciriaco (Italian) Lordly

Ciriak (Spanish) believer

Ciriako (Italian) Lord's child

Cirill (English) form of Cyril: regal

Cirillo (Spanish) Lordly
Cirilo

Ciro (Italian) Lordly
Ciroh, Cirro, Cyro

Cirrus (Latin) thoughtful; cloud formation
Cerrus, Cirrey, Cirri, Cirrie, Cirry, Cirus, Serrus, Serus

Cisco (American) clever
Sisco, Sysco

Cisto (Spanish) form of Francisco: free spirit; from France

Citlalis (Spanish) star

Citronella (American) oil from fragrant grass; pungent
Cit, Citro, Cytronella, Sitronella

Cival (English) form of Percival: mysterious

Civille (American) form of Saville: willow town

Clady (French) form of Claude: slow-moving; lame

Claiborn (English) born of earth
Claiborne

Clair (English) renowned
Claire, Clare

Clairon (French) clear

Clamente (Spanish) form of Clemente: pleasant
Pleases

Clance (Irish) form of Clancy: lively; feisty redhead
Clancy, Clanse, Klance, Klancy

Clancy (Irish) lively; feisty redhead
Clance, Clancey, Clancie

Claney (American) form of Clancy: lively; feisty redhead

Clant (American) form of Clancy: lively; feisty redhead

Clanton (Last name used as first name)

Claran (Latin) bright
Clarance, Claransi, Claranse, Clare, Claren, Clarence, Clary, Klarense

Clarence (Latin) intelligent
Clarance, Clare, Clarens, Clarense, Clarons, Claronz, Clarrence, Klarence, Klarens

Clarinett (Invented) plays the clarinet
Clare, Clarinet, Clary, Klare, Klari

Clark (French) personable; scholar
Clarke

Clarkey (Last name used as first name) scholar

Clarson (American) clarity

Clary (English) clear

Clater (English) premier

Claude (Latin) slow-moving; lame
Claud, Claudey, Claudie, Claudy, Klaud, Klaude

Claudemir (Slavic) lame

Claudene (Italian) lame

Claudimir (Slavic) lame

Claudio-Clyde (Slavic) combo of Claudio and Claude

Claus (Greek) victorious
Klaas, Klaus

Clausen (English) form of Nicholas: the people's victory

Claven (English) endorsed
Klaven

Clavero (Spanish) lame

Clavey (Last name used as first name)

Clawdell (American) form of Claude: slow-moving; lame
Clawd

Claxton (English) townie
Clax, Klax

Clay (English) reliable
Claye, Klae, Klay

Claybey (American) southern; earthly
Claybie, Klaybee

Clayborne (English) earthly
Clabi, Claybie, Claybourne, Clayborn, Klay

Claybrook (English) sparkling smile
Claibrook, Clay, Claybrooke, Clayie

Clayeo (Spanish) form of Clay: reliable

Clayton (English) stodgy
Clay, Claytan, Clayten

Claywell (English) by the clay well

Cleadis (American) form of Cletus: creative; selected
Famed

Cleary (Irish) smart
Clear, Clearey, Clearie

Cleavon (English) daring
Cheavaughn, Cleavaughn, Cleave, Cleevaughan, Cleevon

Clegg (Last name used as first name)

Clem (Latin) casual
Cleme, Clemmey, Clemmie, Clemmy, Clim

Clemen (American) forgives

Clement (Scottish) gentle
Clem, Clemmyl

Clemente (Spanish) pleasant
Clemen, Clementay

Clements (Latin) forgiving man
Clem, Clement, Clemmants, Clemment

Clemer (Latin) mild
Clemmie, Clemmy, Klemer, Klemmie, Klemmye

Clemmie (Latin) mild
Clem, Klem, Klemmee, Klemmy

Clenzy (Spanish) forgiving; cleansed
Clense, Clensy, Klenzy

Cleofas (African American) brave lion

Cleofe (Greek) famed

Cleon (Greek) famed man
Clee, Cleone, Kleon

Cleophas (Greek) seeing glory; known
Cle, Cleofus, Cleoph, Klee, Kleofus, Kleophus

Clete (Greek) form of Cletus: creative; selected
Cleet, Cleete

Cletus (Greek) creative; selected
Clede, Cledus, Cletis

Cleve (English) precarious
Clive

Cleveland (English) daring
Cleavelan, Cleve, Clevon, Clevy, Cliveland

Clevis (Greek) prolific
Cleviss, Clevys, Clevyss

Cliff (English) form of Clifford: dashing
Clif, Cliffey, Cliffie, Cliffy

Cliffen (American)

Clifford (English) dashing
Cleford, Cliff, Cliffy, Clyford

Clift (American) cliff-dweller
Clifte

Clifton (English) risk-taker
Cliff, Clifftan, Clifften, Cliffy

Clim (American) form of Clem: casual

Cline (Last name as first name) musical

Clint (English) form of Clinton: town on a hill
Clent, Clynt, Klint

Clinton (English) town on a hill
Clenton, Clint, Clinten, Clynton, Klinten, Klinton

Clipper (American) boatsman

Clive (English) daring; living near a cliff
Cleve, Clyve

Clive-John (English) combo of Clive and John

Cliven (English) cliff boy

Clodagh (Scottish) winning

Clooney (American) dramatic
Cloone, Cloonie, Cloony, Clune, Cluney, Clunie, Cluny

Clotaire (French) famous
Clotie, Klotair, Klotie

Clovis (German) famed warrior
Clove, Cloves, Clovus, Klove, Kloves, Klovis

Clowry (Last name used as first name)

Cloyd (American) form of Floyd: practical; hair of gray
Cloy, Cloye, Kloy, Kloyd

Cloyd (American) form of Clyde: adventurer

Clske (Dutch) dark

Clue (Word as name)

Cluny (American) dramatic

Clwe (Dutch) face of a mountain

Clyde (Welsh) adventurer
Clide, Clydey, Clydie, Clydy, Clye, Klyde, Klye

Clydell (American) countrified
Clidell, Clydel

Clydenestra (Spanish) form of Clyde: adventurer
Clyde

Coad (English) form of Coady: comforted

Coady (English) comforted

Coal (American) word as a name
Coale, Koal

Coat (Native American) snake

Cobalt (Word as name) from the cottage

Cobb (English) cozy
Cob, Cobbe

Cobbie (American) form of
Jacob: he who supplants

Coben (Last name as first
name) creative
*Cob, Cobb, Cobe, Cobee, Cobey,
Cobi, Coby, Kob, Kobee, Koben,
Kobi, Koby*

Cobern (English) stream spot

Cobian (American) form of
Jacob: he who supplants

Coble (English) cobler

Cobo (American) friendly

Cobus (Dutch) friend

Coby (American) friendly
Cob, Cobe, Cobey, Cobie

Coca (American) excitable
Coka, Cokey, Cokie, Koca, Koka

Cochise (Native American)
warrior
Cocheece, Cochize

Cochran (Last name used as
first name)

Cocinero (Italian) slippery

Coco (French) brash
Coko, Koko

Coder (Last name used as
first name) form of Cody:
comforting

Codrington (Last name used
as first name) form of Cody:
comforting

Codryll (Last name used as
first name) form of Cody:
comforting

Cody ♥ (English) comforting
*Coday, Code, Codee, Codey,
Codi, Codie*

Coe (American) form of Cody:
comforting

Coenraad (Dutch) form of
Conrad: optimist

Coffey (English) Friday's child

Coffie (English) Friday's child

Coffman (Last name used as
first name)

Cog (American) form of
Cogdell: needed
Kog

Cogan (English) form of
Kegan: ball-of-fire

Cogdell (Last name as first
name) needed
Cogdale

Coggin (Last name used as
first name)

Cohn (American) winner
Kohn

Coil (Hebrew) giving

Coitlee (American) silver

Coitoine (French) silver

Cokie (American) bright
*Cokey, Coki, Cokie, Cokki,
Kokie*

Col (American) the colonel

Colak (Irish) bright

Colbert (English) cool and
calm
*Colbey, Colbi, Colbie, Colburt,
Colby, Cole*

Colborn (English)
intimidating; cold brook
*Colbey, Colborne, Colburn,
Colby, Cole*

Colby (English) bright;
secretive; dark farm
*Colbey, Colbi, Colbie, Cole,
Colie*

Colden (English) haunting
Coldan, Coldun, Cole

Cole ✪ (Greek) lively; winner
Coal, Coley, Colie, Kohl, Kole

Colee (American) victor

Coleman (English) lively;
peacemaker
*Cole, Colemann, Colman,
Kohlman*

Coley (American) victor

Colgate (English) passway
Colgait, Colgaite, Kolgate

Colier (Last name as first
name) sophisticated

Colin ✪ (Irish) young and
quiet; peaceful; the people's
victor
*Colan, Cole, Colen, Collin,
Collyn*

Colis (English) he who
delights others

Collan (Irish) farms

Coller (Irish) farms

Collett (English) black hair

Colley (English) dark-haired
Col, Colli, Collie

Collier (English)
hardworking; miner
Colier, Collie, Colly, Colyer

Collies (English) delights

Collin (Scottish) shy
Collen, Collie, Collon, Colly

Collins (Irish) shy; holly
*Collens, Collie, Collons, Colly,
Kolly*

Colm (Irish) dove; peaceful

Colorado (Place name) U.S.
state; multicolored

Coloss (Biblical) colossal

Colson (English) precocious;
son of Nicholas
Cole, Colsan, Colsen

Colster (English) colts

Colston (English) young
horse town

Colt (English) frisky; horse
trainer
Colty, Kolt, Koltt

Colten (English) dark town;
mysterious
*Cole, Collton, Colt, Coltan,
Coltawn, Colton, Kol*

Colter (English) keeping the
colts
Colt, Coltor, Colty

Colum (Latin) peaceful; dove
Colm, Kolm, Kolum

Colum (Latin) dove; calm

Columba (Latin) dove; calm

Columbus (Latin) peaceful
discovered America
Colom, Colombo, Columbe

Colvint (Spanish) river

Colwen (Irish) peaceful
Colwin, Colvin

Comanche (Native
American) tribe; wild-
spirited; industrious
Comanch, Komanche

Combs (English) last name
used as first name

Commander (Word as name)
leader

Commodore (French)
commander

Como (Spanish) similar
Comoh

Comus (Greek) humorous
*Comes, Comas, Commus,
Komus*

Con (Irish) form of Conan: worthy of praise

Conal (Irish) strong; wolflike

Conall (Scottish) highly regarded
Conal

Conall (Irish) wolflike

Conan (Irish) worthy of praise
Conen, Connie, Conny, Conon

Conant (Irish) top-notch
Conent, Connant

Concini (Italian) last name used as first name

Concord (English) agreeable
Con, Concor, Conny, Koncord, Konny

Conde (Last name as first name) driven

Cong (Chinese) bright

Conger (Irish) tall

Coniah (Irish) pure
Conias, Conah

Conk (Invented) from conch mollusk of the ocean; jazzy
Conch, Conkee, Conkee, Conkey, Conky, Konk, Kanch, Konkey, Konkey

Conkel (Last name used as first name)

Conkey (Last name used as first name)

Conklin (English) last name used as first name

Conlach (Irish) in accord

Conlan (Irish) winner
Con, Conland, Conlen, Conleth, Conlin, Connie, Conny

Conleth (Welsh) hero

Conley (Celtic) feminine form of Conley: hero

Connable (Last name used as first name)

Connaughton (American) sapient

Connell (Irish) strong
Con, Conal, Connall, Connel, Connelle, Connie, Conny

Connelly (Celtic/Gaelic) last name used as first name; friendship

Connery (Scottish) daring
Con, Conery, Connarie, Connary, Connie, Conny

Connie (Irish) form of Connor: brilliant; form of Conrad: optimist
Connery, Con, Conn, Connee, Conney, Connie, Conny

Connor ○ (Scottish) brilliant
Con, Conn, Conner, Conor, Kon, Konnor

Conra (Irish) wise

Conrad (German) optimist
Con, Connie, Conny, Conrade, Konrad

Conrado (Spanish) bright advisor
Conrad, Conrod, Conrodo

Conradt (Welsh) last name used as first name; bold in counsel

Conreed (Welsh) brave

Conridge (Last name as first name) advisor
Con, Conni, Connie, Conny, Ridge

Conroy (Irish) wise writer
Conrie, Conroye, Conry, Roy, Roye

Conrye (American) form of Conrad: optimist

Considine (Last name used as first name) considerate

Consis (Mythology) flourishing

Constant (French) devotee; loyal

Constantine (Latin) constant; steadfast
Con, Conn, Consta, Constance, Constant, Constantin Constantyne, Konstantin

Consydin (American) form of Considine: considerate

Conte (Italian) accountable

Conway (Irish) vigilant
Con, Connie, Kon, Konway

Cooke (Latin) cook
Cook, Cookie, Cooky

Cooker (English) cooks

Coolidge (Last name as first name) wary
Cooledge

Cooney (Last name as first name) giving

Cooper (English) handsome; maker of barrels
Coup, Couper, Koop, Kooper, Kouper

Coos (Dutch) friend

Cope (English) able
Cape

Coptos (Biblical) place name

Coral (Nature) from Hebrew goral; pebble

Corbell (Latin) raven; dark
Corbel

Corbet (Latin) dark
Corb, Corbett, Corbit, Corbitt, Korb, Korbet

Corbie (Latin) raven

Corbin (Latin) dark and brooding
Corban, Corben, Corby

Corbitt (Last name as first name) brooding
Corbet, Corbett, Corbie, Corbit, Corby

Corblee (American) dark

Corby (Latin) dark
Corbey, Korbee, Korby, Korry

Corcoran (Irish) ruddy-skinned
Corkie, Corky

Cord (Origin unknown) soap opera hunk
Corde, Kord

Cordaro (Italian) roped

Cordel (French) practical
Cordel, Cordell, Cordelle, Cordie, Cordill, Cordy

Cordell (Latin) bound; rope

Cordero (Spanish) gentle
Cordara, Cordaro, Cordarro, Kordarro, Kordero

Cordi (Spanish) makes ropes

Cordry (American) makes ropes

Corentin (French) stormy

Coret (French) stormy

Corey (Irish) laughing
Core, Corie, Corry, Cory, Korey, Korrie, Kory

Coril (American) coral

Corin (Latin) combative
Coren, Dorrin, Koren, Korrin

Corinth (Biblical) from Corinthians

Cork (Place name) county in
Ireland
*Corkee, Corkey, Corki, Corky,
Kork*

Corkeen (American) form of
Corky: casual

Corkel (American) form of
Corky: casual

Corkson (American) son of
Corky

Corky (American) casual
Corkee, Corkey, Korky

Corl (English) cheery

Corlan (English) of good
cheer

Corlon (American) tasteful

Cormac (Irish) the raven's
offspring; watchful
Cormack, Cormak

Cormic (Irish) raven

Cormick (Last name as first
name) old-fashioned
Cormac, Cormack

Corn (Latin) form of
Cornelius: horn; loquacious
Korn

Cornall (Irish) form of
Cornelius: horn; loquacious

Cornelio (Spanish) horn
blower

Cornelius (Greek) horn;
loquacious
*Coarn, Conny, Corn, Corni,
Cornie, Corny, Kornelius, Neel,
Neely, Neil, Neiley*

Cornell (French) fair
Corne, Cornelle, Corny, Kornell

Cornellian (Greek) horn color

Coro (Spanish) form of
Coronnel: colonel

Corodon (Greek) lark

Coronnel (Spanish) colonel

Corrado (Italian) worthy
advisor

Corrigan (Irish) aggressive
*Coregan, Corie, Correghan,
Corrie, Corry, Koregan,
Korrigan*

Cors (Spanish) from Corsica

Corso (Spanish) form of
Kyros: masterful
Sun

Cort (German) eloquent
Corte, Court, Kort

Cortal (Last name used as
first name) intellectual

Cortant (Spanish) bitter

Cortazar (Last name as first)
creative

Cortell (Spanish) cuts

Cortez (Spanish) victorious;
explorer
Cortes

Corum (English) form of
Corwin: heart's delight

Corvey (Greek) crest

Corvin (English) friend
*Corwin, Corwynn, Korry,
Korvin*

Corwen (English) delights the
heart

Corwin (English) heart's
delight
*Corrie, Corry, Corwan,
Corwann, Corwyn, Corwynne*

Cory (Latin) humorous
*Coarie, Core, Corey, Corrie,
Kohry, Kori*

Coryell (Greek) lark; devious

Cos (Biblical) place name; orderly

Cosell (French) outgoing

Cosgrove (Irish) winner
Cosgrave, Cossy, Kosgrove, Kossy

Cosimo (Greek) orderly

Cosma (Greek) universal
Cos, Kosma

Cosmas (Greek) universal
Cos, Kosmas, Koz

Cosmedin (Spanish) harmony

Cosmo (Greek) in harmony with life
Cos, Cosimo, Cosimon, Cosme, Cosmos, Kosmo

Cosner (English) organized; handsome
Cosnar, Kosner

Costas (Greek) constant
Costa, Costah

Coste (Greek) form of Constantine: constant; steadfast

Costel (Slavic) constant

Costello (Italian) form of Constantine: constant; steadfast

Cotledge (Last name used as first name) by the cottage ledge

Cotrer (Last name used as first name) contrary

Cotter (American) gregarious

Cottingham (Last name used as first name) day by day

Cottlings (English) in the cottage

Cotton (Botanical name) casual
Cottan

Cottrell (English) in the cottage

Coty (French) comforter
Cotey, Coti, Cotie, Koty

Coug (American) from cougar; fierce
Cougar, Koug, Kougar

Couland (French) from court land

Coulter (English) dealing in colts; horseman
Colter, Coult, Kolter, Koulter

Council (French) advisor

Counsel (Latin) advisor
Consel, Council, Kounse, Kounsell

Country (Word as name) cowboy

Court (English) royal

Courtland (English) born in the land of the court; dignitary

Courtnay (English) sophisticated
Cort, Corteney, Court, Courtney, Courtny

Covell (English) warm
Covele, Covelle

Covet (American) word as name; desires
Covett, Covette, Kovet

Covington (English) distinctive
Covey, Coving, Kovey, Kovington

Cowan (Irish) cozy
Cowen, Cowie, Cowy

Cowboy (American) western

Cowden (Irish) cave in the hill

Cowell (English) brash; frank
Kowell

Cowey (Irish) reclusive
Cowee, Cowie, Kowey

Coye (English) outdoorsman
Coy, Coyey, Coyie

Coyle (English) in the woods

Coylie (American) coy
Coyl, Koyl, Koylie

Coyne (French) demure

Coystal (American) bashful
Coy, Koy, Koystal

Crad (American) practical
Cradd, Krad, Kradd

Craddock (Last name as first name) practical

Crager (Scottish) from the crags

Crago (Last name as first name) macho
Crag, Craggy, Krago

Craig (Irish) brave climber
Crai, Craigie, Cray, Craye, Crayg, Creg, Cregge, Kraig

Crain (English) cranes

Crandal (English) open
Cran, Crandall, Crandell, Crane

Crandale (English) from the land of cranes
Crandall, Crandell

Crandan (English) from the cranes

Cranley (English) lives in a field of cranes

Cranston (English) from the town of cranes

Cranyon (English) from the cranes

Craon (Greek) leader

Crawford (English) flowing
Crafe, Craford, Craw, Fordy

Cray (English) place name

Crayton (English) substantial
Craeton, Cray, Creighton

Creach (Scottish) home-loving

Creasy (English) last name used as first name

Creed (American) believer
Crede, Creede, Creyd, Kreed

Creek (English) word as name

Creigh (English) lives near rocks

Creighton (English) sophisticated
Criton

Crenshaw (Last name as first name) good intentions

Crescin (Latin) expansive

Cresencio (Spanish) integrity

Creshaun (African American) inspired
Creshawn, Kreshaun

Cresp (Latin) man with curls
Crisp, Crispen, Crispun, Crispy, Cryspin, Kresp, Krisp, Krispin, Krispyn

Crever (Irish) sly fox

Crevin (Irish) sly fox

Crew (American) word as name; sailor
Krew

Crey (English) form of Creighton: sophisticated
Craedie, Cray, Creydie, Creigh

Crider (English) creek

Cris (Welsh) form of Crisiant: crystallike

Crisanto (Spanish) anoint

Crisiant (Welsh) crystallike

Crisman (Greek) golden

Crisoforo (Spanish) bearing Christ; form of Christopher

Crisoforo (Last name used as first name) gold clothing

Crispin (Latin) man with curls
Chrispy, Crespen, Crispo, Crispy, Krispin, Krispo

Crispo (Latin) curly-haired
Crisp, Krispo

Crist (Spanish) christian

Cristhian (Greek) christian

Cristian (Greek) form of Christian: follower of Christ
Kristian

Cristino (Greek) christian

Cristo (Spanish) mountain of Christ
Kristo

Cristobal (Spanish) bearing Christ

Cristovo (Greek) serves Christ

Criten (American) form ofm of Critendon: critical
Critan, Kriten

Critendon (Last name as first name) critical
Crit, Criten, Krit, Kritendon

Crofton (Irish) comforter
Croft, Croften

Crolley (English) last name used as first name

Cromaci (Greek) decorated

Cromer (English) adorned

Crompton (Last name as first name) giving

Cromwell (Irish) giving
Chromwell, Crom, Crommie

Cronin (German) timely

Cronus (Greek) reigning

Croom (American) giving

Crosby (Irish) easygoing
Crosbee, Crosbie, Cross, Krosbie, Krosby

Crosson (English) of the cross

Croston (English) by the cross
Cro, Croton, Kroston

Croswell (English) cross on the well

Crosy (American) of the cross

Crosz (American) of the cross

Crothers (Scottish) last name used as first name

Crow (English) crow

Crowson (English) son of Crow

Crue (American) form of Crew: word as name; sailor

Cruo (Spanish) cross

Crutcher (English) fighter

Cruz (Spanish) cross

Cruze (Spanish) cross
Cruise, Cruse, Kruise, Kruze

Cruzon (Spanish) cross

Csaba (Hungarian) shepherd

Ctirad (Czech) long-suffering

Cuauhtemoc (Spanish) eagle

Cuba (Place name)
distinctive; spicy
Cubah, Cueba, Kueba, Kuba

Cubbenah (African)
Wednesday

Cubby (American) child

Cucuta (Place name) city in
North Colombia; sharp
Cucu

Cudjo (Jamaican) Monday

Cuelly (American) wild spirit

Cuernavaca (Place name)
city in Mexico; cow horn
Vaca

Cuffy (Jamaican) Friday
Cuffee, Cuffey

Cuke (American) zany
Kook, Kooky, Kuke

Culber (American) woods
child

Culbert (Last name as first
name) practical

Culkin (American) child actor
Culki, Kulkin

Cull (American) selective
Cullee, Cullie, Cully, Kulley

Cullen (Irish) attractive
*Culen, Cull, Cullan, Cullen,
Cullie, Cully, Kullen, Kully*

Culley (Irish) secretive
Cull, Cullie, Cully, Kull, Kully

Cullom (American) wood

Culver (English) peaceful
*Colver, Cull, Culley, Culli,
Cully*

Culverado (American)
peaceful
*Cull, Cullan, Culver, Culvey,
Kull*

Cumal (Native American)
thunders

Cummings (Literature) for
the poet E.E. Cummings;
innovative
Cumming, Kummings

Cummings (Last name used
as first name)

Cuney (Last name as first
name) serious
Cune, Kune, Kuney

Cuneyt (Scandinavian)
warmth

Cunning (Irish) from
surname Cunningham;
wholesome
Cuning

Cunningham (Irish) milk-
pail town; practical
Cuningham

Cupid (Latin) heart's desire

Curb (American) dynamic
Kurb

Curbey (American) form of
Kirby: brilliant
Curby

Curbow (Last name used as
first name) stone

Curer (French) helps

Curgus (Greek) cunning

Curie (French) innovator

Curley (American) cowboy
Curly, Kurly

Curo (Spanish) sheltered

Curran (Irish) smiling hero
*Curan, Curr, Curren, Currey,
Currie, Curt*

Currere (French) sheltered

Currey (English) messenger;
calm

Currie (English) messenger;
courteous
Kurrie

Curro (Spanish) form of Curtis: gracious; kindhearted

Curt (French) form of Curtis: gracious; kindhearted
Kurt

Curtis (French) gracious; kindhearted
Curdi, Curdis, Curt, Curtey, Curtice, Curtie, Curtiss, Curty, Kurt

Cush (American) thrives

Custer (Last name as first name) watchful; stubborn
Cust, Kust, Kuster

Cuthah (Biblical) place name

Cuthbert (English) intelligent

Cutle (English) makes knives

Cutler (English) wily
Cutlar, Cutlur, Cuttie, Cutty

Cutlon (English) knife maker

Cutrer (French) knife dealer

Cutsy (English) form of Cutler: wily
Cutlar, Cutler, Cuttie, Cutty, Kutsee, Kutsi, Kutsy

Cutter (English) man who cuts gemstones

Cuttino (African American) athletic
Kuttino

Cuyler (American) form of Schuyler: protective
Kuyler

Cy (Greek) shining example
Cye, Si

Cybor (American) leader

Cygan (Last name used as first name) shines

Cyler (Irish) protective chapel
Cuyler, Cyle

Cyll (American) bright
Syll, Cyl

Cynric (Greek) thorn

Cyone (Greek) whirlwind

Cyprien (French) religious
Cyp, Cyprian

Cyprus (Place name) island south of Turkey; outgoing

Cyrano (Greek) shy heart
Cyranoh, Cyre, Cyrie, Cyrno, Cyry

Cyree (Greek) Lord

Cyril (Greek) regal
Ciril, Cyral, Cyrell, Cyrille

Cyrilon (Spanish) lofty

Cyrus (Persian) sunny
Cye, Syrus

Cyrx (American) conniving
Cyrxie

Czech (Slavic) czech

Czeslaw (Polish) honorable
Slav, Slavek

D

D'Artagnan (French) leader; ostentatious

D'Marques (American) form of Demarco: daring

Dablo (Spanish) form of Diablo: devil

Dabney (English) careful; funny
Dab, Dabnee, Dabnie, Dabny

Dabriel (American) teaches

Dacey (Irish) southerner
*Dace, Dacian, Dacius, Dacy,
Daicey, Daicy*

Dacga (Slavic) emotional

Dachary (English) form of
Dachry: stream

Dache (Latin) audacious

Dachry (English) stream

Dacias (Latin) brash
*Dace, Daceas, Dacey, Dacy,
Dayce, Daycie*

Dacko (American) zany

Dacosta (Italian) from the
coast

Dacus (Last name used as
first name)

Dada (African) curly-haired

Dade (Place name) county in
Florida; renegade
Daide, Dayde

Dadean (English) curly

Dadley (English) curly

Daedalus (Greek) father of
Icarus; inventor
Daidalos, Dedalus

Dag (Scandinavian) sunny
Dagg, Dagget, Daggett, Dagny

Dagan (Hebrew) earthy
Dagon

Dagfinn (Scandinavian)
sunshine

Daggan (Scandinavian) day

Daggs (Scandinavian) day

Dagny (Scandinavian) day
Dag

Dagoberto (Spanish) day
Dagbert, Dagobert

Dagwood (English) comic
Dag, Dawood, Woody

Dahryan (Indian)
compassionate

Dahy (Irish) lithe
Dahey

Dai (Japanese) great man

Daigle (Last name used as
first name) dark

Daiki (Japanese) shining

Dailey (English) form of
Dale: valley
Daley, Daly, Daily

Dain (Scandinavian) from
Denmark

Dainard (Irish) loved
*Danehard, Danehardt,
Dancard, Daneardt,
Dainehard, Dainhard,
Daynard*

Dairus (Invented) daring
Daras, Dares, Darus

Daithi (Irish) speedy

Daivat (Hindi) powerful man

Dakarai (African) happy
Dakarrai, Dakk

Dako (American) form of
Dakota: friendly

Dakota (Native American)
friendly
*Daccota, Dack, Dak, Dakoda,
Dakodah, Dakoetah, Dakotah,
Dekota, Dekohta, Dekowta,
Kota*

Dakote (Place name) from
the Dakotas
Dako

Dalai (Indian) peaceful
Dalee

Dalanee (Invented) form of Delaney: challenging
Dalaney, Dalani

Dalbert (English) man who lives in the valley
Del, Delbert

Dalcher (Last name used as first name) gathers

Dale (English) valley
Dail, Daile, Daley, Dallan, Dalle, Dallin, Day, Dayl, Dayle

Dalen (English) up-and-coming
Dalan, Dalin, Dallen, Dallin, Dalyn

Daley (Irish) organized
Dailey, Daily, Dale

Dalgienuz (Slavic) valor

Dalgus (American) loving the outdoors

Dalhart (Place name) city in Texas
Dal

Dalin (Spanish) proud

Dallard (English) proud

Dallas (Place name) good old boy; city in Texas
Dal, Dall, Dalles, Dallice, Dallis, Dallus, Delles

Dallin (English) valley-born; fine
Dal, Dallan, Dallen, Dallon

Dallin (American) form of Dylan: sea god; creative

Dalphy (French) dolphin

Dalsten (English) smart
Dal, Dalston

Dalt (English) abundant
Dall, Daltt, Daltey

Dalton (English) farmer
Daleton, Dall, Dallton, Daltan, Dalten

Daltrey (English) high river

Dalvis (Invented) form of Elvis: all-wise
Dal, Dalves, Dalvus, Dalvy

Daly (Irish) together
Daley, Dawley

Dalziel (Scottish) from the field

Damacio (Spanish) calm; tamed
Damas, Damasio, Damaso, Damazio

Damarcus (African American) confident
D'Marcus, Damarkes, Damarkus, Demarcus

Damare (Greek) form of Damario: tamer of wild things

Damari (Greek) gentle

Damario (Spanish) tamer of wild things
Damarios, Damarius, Damaro, Damero

Damarion (Greek) form of Damario: tamer of wild things

Damary (Greek) tame
Damaree, Damarie

Damascus (Place name) capital of Syria; dramatic
Damas, Damask

Damaskenos (Greek) form of Damascus: life-changing
Damascus, Damaskinos

Damaso (Spanish) taming
Damas

Damean (American) form of
Damian: fate
*Dama, Daman, Damas,
Damea*

Dameetre (Invented) form of
Dimitri: fertile; flourishing
Dimitri

Damek (Czech) earth
*Adamec, Adamek, Adamik,
Adamok, Adha, Damick,
Damicke*

Dameone (Greek) form of
Damian: fate

Dameron (American) form
of Cameron: mischievous;
crooked nose

Damian (Greek) fate
*Daemon, Daimen, Daimon,
Daman, Dame, Damean,
Damen, Dumeon, Damey,
Damiano, Damianos,
Damianus, Damien, Damion,
Damon, Damyan, Damyean,
Damyen, Damyon, Damyun,
Dayman, Daymian, Daymon,
Demyan*

Damiko (Slavic) gentle

Damin (Greek) comforts

Damon (Greek) dramatic;
spirited
Damonn, Damyn

Damron (Greek) comforts

Damyi (American) comforts

Dan (Hebrew) form of
Daniel: judged by God;
spiritual
Dahn, Dannie, Danny

Dana (Scandinavian)
light-haired
Danah, Dane, Danie, Dayna

Danar (English) from
Denmark; dry

Danaus (Mythology) king of
Argos
Denaus, Dinaus

Dand (Scottish) form of
Andrew: manly and brave

Dandin (Hindi) holy man

Dandre (American) light
*Dan, Dandrae, Dandray,
AeAndrae, DeAndray, Aiondrae*

Dandrer (French) form of
Dandre: light

Dandridge (English) last
name used as first name

Dandy (Hindi) form of
Dandin: holy man

Dane (English) man from
Denmark; light
*Dain, Daine, Dancy, Danie,
Danyn, Dayne, Dhane*

Daneck (American) well-
liked
*Danek, Danick, Danik,
Danike, Dannick*

Danel (Hebrew) God judges

Danely (Scandinavian) danish
Dainely, Daynelee

Danerin (Slavic) giving

Danez (English) helpful

Danfer (Slavic) faithful

Danford (English) place
name; "the way or ford of the
Danes"

Dang (Vietnamese) worthy

Dangelle (Italian) angelic

Dangelo (Italian) angelic
Danjelo

Danger (American)
dangerous
Dang, Dange, Dangery

Danial (Hebrew) form of
Daniel: judged by God;
spiritual

Daniel ○ ● (Hebrew) judged
by God; spiritual
Da, Danal, Dane, Daneal,
Danek, Dani, Danial, Daniele,
Danil, Danilo, Danko, Dann,
Dannel, Danney, Danni,
Dannie, Danniel, Danny,
Danyal, Danyel, Danyell,
Deiniol

Danilo (Slavic) form of
Daniel: judged by God;
spiritual

Danilon (Slavic) form of
Daniel: judged by God;
spiritual

Danne (Biblical) form of
Daniel: judged by God;
spiritual
Dann

Danner (Last name as first
name) rescued by God
Dan, Dann, Danny

Danno (Hebrew) kind
Dannoh, Dano

Danny (Hebrew) form of
Daniel: judged by God;
spiritual
Dan, Dann, Dannee, Danney,
Danni, Dannie

Danon (French) remembered
Danen, Danhann, Dannon,
Danton

Danron (American) combo of
Dan and Ron

Dante (Latin) enduring
Dan, Danne, Dantae, Dantay,
Dantey, Dauntay, Dayntay,
Dontae, Dontay, DontÈ

Danter (Latin) form of Dante:
enduring

Dantin (American) form of
Daniel: judged by God;
spiritual

Danton (Last name as first
name) Dan's town

Dantre (African American)
faithful
Dantray, Dantrae, Dontre,
Dantrey, Dantri, Dantry, Don,
Dont, Dontrey, Dontri

Dantrell (African American)
spunky
Dantrele, Dantrill, Dantrille

Dantzler (American) form of
Daniel: judged by God;
spiritual

Danube (Place name)
flowing; river
Dannube, Danuube, Donau

Danut (Slavic) form of Dan:
judged by God; spiritual

Danyo (Hebrew) form of
Daniel: judged by God;
spiritual

Danza (English) form of
Denzel: sensual

Daphnis (Greek) attractive

Daquan (African American)
rambunctious
Dakwan, Daquanne, Dequan,
Dequanne, Dekwan, Dekwohn,
Dekwohnne

Dar (English) deerlike

Darb (Irish) form of Darby:
free spirit

Darbrie (Irish) free man;
lighthearted
Dar, Darb, Darbree, Darbry

Darby (Irish) free spirit
Dar, Darb, Darbee, Darbey,
Darbie, Darre, Derby

Darce (Irish) dark
Darcy, Dars, Darsy, D'Arcy

Darcel (French) dark
Dar, Darce, Darcelle, Darcey, Darcy, Darsy

Darcell (Irish) dark hair

Darcus (Irish) dark hair

Darcy (French) slow-moving
Darce, Darse, Darsey, Darsy

Dard (Greek) clever

Dardanos (Greek) adored
Dar, Dardanio, Dardanios, Dardanus

Darhen (American) form of Darwin: dearest friend

Darian (American) inventive
Dari, Darien, Darion, Darrian, Darrien, Darrion, Derreynn

Darin (Irish) great
Daren, Darren, Darrie, Daryn

Dario (Spanish) rich
Darioh, Darrey

Darion (Irish) great potential
Dare, Darien, Darrion, Daryun

Daris (Greek) form of Darius: affluent

Darius (Greek) affluent
Dare, Dareas, Dareus, Darias, Ariess, Dario, Darious, Darrius, Derrius, Derry

Darji (American) rich

Dark (Slavic) form of Darko: macho
Dar, Darc

Darkell (English) brunette

Darko (Slavic) macho
Dark

Darko (English) brunette

Darlen (American) darling
Darlan, Darlun

Darman (English) hidden

Darnell (English) secretive
Dar, Darn, Darnall, Darnel, Darnie, Darny

Darnley (English) sly

Darold (American) clever
Dare, Darrold, Darroll, Derold

Daron (Irish) great
Darren, Dayron

Daros (Greek) loved

Darr (English) loved

Darrah (Irish) dark
Darach, Darragh

Darrel (Aboriginal) blue sky
Darral, Darrell, Darrill, Darrol, Darroll, Darry, Darryl, Darryll, Daryl, Derrel, Derrell, Derril, Derrill, Deryl, Deryll

Darrell (French) loved man
Darel, Darol, Darrel, Darrey, Daryl, Derrel, Derrell

Darren (Irish) great
Daren, Darin, Daron, Darran, Darrin, Darring, Darron, Darryn, Derrin, Derron, Derry

Darrett (American) form of Garrett: brave; watchful
Dare, Darry

Darrick (American) form of Derrick: bold heart

Darrien (Greek) with riches
Darian, Darion, Darrian, Darrion, Darryan, Darryen

Darrien (Irish) greatness

Darris (Greek) rich

Darrti (American) fast; deer
Dart, Darrt

Darryl (French) darling man
Darrie, Daryl, Derrie, Deryl, Deryll

Darshak (Sanskrit) insight

Darshan (African American) pious

Dart (English) decisive
Darte, Dartt

Darton (English) swift; deer

Darty (American) last name as first name

Darvin (English) friendship

Darwin (English) dearest friend
Dar, Darwen, Darwinne, Darwon, Darwyn, Derwin, Derwynn

Daryn (American) form of Darin: great
Darynn, Deryn

Darynth (English) form of Darren: great

Dash (American) speedy; dashing
Dashy

Dashawn (African American) unusual
D'Sean, D'Shawn, Dashaun, Deshaun, Deshawn

Dashell (African American) dashing
Dashiell

Dasher (American) dashing; fast
Dash

Dashiel (English) from author Dashiell Hammett

Dasno (Latin) royal

Dassinger (Last name as first name)

Dathan (Biblical) fountain of hope

Dauer (Last name as first name)

Daufen (French) dolphin

Dault (English) valley boy

Davao (Place name) city in the Philippines; exotic
Davo

Dave (Hebrew) form of David: beloved
Davey, Davi, Davie, Davy

Daven (American) dashing
Davan

Davender (Hebrew) form of David: beloved

Davenport (Last name as first name) of the old school; sea-loving

Davey (Hebrew) form of David: beloved
Dave, Davee, Davi, Davie, Davy

Davian (Hebrew) dear one
Daivian, Daivyan, Daveon, Davien, Davion, Davyan, Davyen, Davyon

David ✪ ✪ (Hebrew) beloved
Daffy, Daffyd, Dafydd, Dai, Davad, Dave, Daved, Davee, Daven, Davey, Davi, Davide, Davie, Davies, Davin, Davis, Davon, Davy, Davyd, Davydd

Davidpaul (American) beloved
David-Paul

Davidson (English) son of David
Davidsen, Davison

Davik (Slavic) form of David: beloved

Davin (Scandinavian) smart
Dave, Daven, Dayven

Davinal (American) form of David: beloved

Davinno (English) bright

Davins (American) form of David: beloved
Davion

Davion (American) form of David: beloved

Davis (Welsh) David's son; heart's child
Dave, Daves, Davidson, Davies, Davison, Daviss, Davy

Davon (American) sweet
Davaughan, Davaughn, Dave, Davone, Devon

Davonnae (African American) form of David: beloved
Davawnae, Davonae

Davonne (American) form of Davin: smart

Davonte (African American) energetic
D'Vontay, Davontay, Devonta

Daw (English) quiet
Dawe, Dawes

Dawber (Last name as first name) funny
Daw, Dawb, Dawbee, Dawbey, Dawby, Daws

Dawes (Last name used as first name) form of David: beloved

Dawk (American) spirited
Dawkins

Dawkins (Last name used as first name) form of David: beloved

Daws (English) dedicated
Daw, Dawsen, Dawz

Dawson (English) David's son; loved
Daw, Dawe, Dawes, Dawsan, Dawse, Dawsen, Dawsey, Dawsin

Dax (French) unique; water-loving
Dacks, Daxie

Day (English) calm
Daye

Dayanand (Hindi) a loving man

Dayman (Greek) form of Damon: dramatic; spirited

Daymond (Invented) compassionate

Dayt (Last name used as first name) day

Dayton (English) the town of David; planner
Daeton, Day, Daye, Daytan, Daytawn, Dayten, Deytawn, Deyton

Dazh (Slavic) giver

Dazo (American) form of David: beloved

Dazon (American) form of David: beloved

Deacon (Greek) giving
Deakin, Decon, Deecon, Deekon, Dekawn, Deke, Dekie, Dekon, Diakonos

Deadon (French) form of Dieudonne: loves a gracious God

Deagan (Last name as first name) capable
Degan

Deak (American) form of Richard: wealthy leader

Dean (English) leader
Deane, Deanie, Deany, Deen, Dene, Deyn, Dino

DeAndré (African American) very masculine
D'André, DeAndrae, DeAndray, Diandray, Diondrae, Diondray

Deangelo (Italian) sweet; personable
D'Angelo, Dang, Dange, DeAngelo, Deanjelo, Deeanjelo, DiAngelo, Di-Angelo

Deangelo (Italian) angelic

Deans (English) sylvan; valley
Dean, Deaney, Deanie

Deanthony (African American) rambunctious
Deanthe, Deanthoney, Deanthonie, Deeanthie, Dianth

Deanza (Spanish) smooth
Denza

Dearborn (Last name as first name) endearing; kind from birth
Dearbourn, Dearburne, Deerborn

Dearing (Last name as first name) endearing
Dear

Dearmon (Last name used as first name) man of deer

Dearon (American) dear one
Dear

Deason (Invented) cocky
Deace, Deas, Dease, Deasen, Deasun

Debdan (Indian) God's gift

Debonair (French) with a beautiful air; elegant and cultured
Debonaire, Debonnair, Debonnaire

Debrum (Czech) kindness

Debythis (African American) strange
Debiathes

Decatur (Place name) city in Illinois; special
Dec, Decatar, Decater, Deck

Deccan (Place name) region in India; scholar
Dec, Dek

Decimus (Latin) tenth child
Decio

Deck (Irish) form of Declan: strong; prayerful
Decky

Declan (Irish) strong; prayerful
Dec, Deck, Dek, Deklan, Deklon

Dedal (Greek) artistic

Dedan (Indian) form of Deodan: serving God

Deddrick (American) form of Dedric: leader
Dead, Dedric, Dedrick, Dedrik, Dietrich

Dedeaux (French) sweet
Dede, Dee

Dederic (American) substance

Dedlus (Greek) industrious

Dedric (German) leader
Dedrick, Deidrich

Dee (American) form of names that start with D
D, De

Deek (American) form of Deacon: giving
Deke

Deeley (Irish) assembly

Deems (English) merits

Deepak (Sanskrit) light of knowledge
Depak, Depakk, Dipak

Dees (Slavic) desires

Deeter (American) friendly
Deter

DeForest (French) of the forest
Defforest

DeFoy (French) child of Foy
Defoy, Defoye

Degner (Slavic) of the day

Degraf (French) child of Graf
DeGraf

Dehlin (American) form of Dylan: sea god; creative

Deicy (Latin) God-loving

Deidric (German) rules

Deldrich (German) leader
Dedric, Dedrick, Deed, Deide, Deidrick, Diedrich

Deinol (Greek) form of Daniel: judged by God; spiritual

Deinorus (African American) vigorous
Denorius, Denorus

Deion (Greek) form of Dion: joyous celebrant; god of wine
Dee

Dejanee (Slavic) action-oriented

Dejuan (African American) talkative
Dajuan, Dajuwan, Dejuane, Dejuwan, Dewaan, Dewan, Dewaughan, Dewon, Dewonn, Dewuan Dwon, Dwonn, Dwonne

Dejuon (American) form of Dejuan: talkative

Deke (Hebrew) form of Dekel: palm tree
Deek

Dekel (Hebrew) palm tree

Del (English) valley; laid-back and helpful
Dail, Dell, Delle

DeLane (Irish) form of Delaney: challenging

Delaney (Irish) challenging
Del, Delaine, Delainey, Delainie, Delane, Delanie, Delany, Dell

Delano (Irish) dark
Del, Delaynoh, Dell

Delanoy (Irish) darkness

Delayme (American) form of Delaney: challenging

Delber (English) daylight

Delbert (English) sunny
Bert, Bertie, Berty, Dalbert, Del, Delburt, Dell, Dilbert

Deleon (Spanish) last name used as first name

Delete (Origin unknown) ordinary
Delette

Delfino (Spanish) dolphin; sea-loving
Define, Fino

Delgado (Spanish) slim

Delin (English) of the sea

Delius (Greek) from the island Delos
Deli, Delia, Delios, Delos

Delk (American) celebrant

Dell (English) from the country; sparkles

Delley (Scandinavian) fascinates

Dellin (Scandinavian) fascinates

Delling (Norse) shines

Delm (Scandinavian) charismatic

Delman (French) from the mountain

Delmar (Last name as first name) friendly
Delm

Delmer (American) country
Del, Delmar, Delmir

Delmis (Spanish) friend
Del, Delms

Delmore (French) seagoing
Del, Delmar, Delmer, Delmor, Delmoor, Delmoore

Delmy (American) form of Delmore: seagoing
Delmi

Delp (Indian) form of Dilip: protests; royal

Delphin (French) dolphin
Delfin, Delfino, Delfinos, Delfinus, Delphino, Delphinos, Delphinus, Delvin

Delrin (English) of the dell

Delroy (French) royal; special
Del, Dell, Dellroy, Delroi, Roi, Roy

Delsen (Native American) of a just God

Delsi (American) easygoing
Delci, Delcie, Dels, Delsee, Delsey, Delsy

Delt (American) fraternity boy
Delta

Delton (English) friend
Delt, Deltan, Delten

DeLuca (Italian) lucky

Delvan (English) form of Delwin: companion
Del, Dell, Delly, Delven, Delvin, Delvun, Delvyn

Delvern (English) proud

Delvie (English) proud

Delwin (English) companion
Dalwin, Dalwyn, Delavan, Delevan, Dellwin, Delwins, Delwince, Delwen, Delwinse, Delwy, Delwyn

Deman (Dutch) man

Demarco (Italian) daring
D'Marco, Deemarko, Demarkoe, Demie, Demmy, Dimarco

Demarcus (American) zany; royal
Damarcus, DaMarkiss, DeMarco, DeMarcus, Demarkes, Demarkess, DeMarko, DeMarkus, Demarkus, DeMarquess, DeMarquez, Demarquiss, DeMarquiss

Demario (Italian) bold
D'Mareo, D'Mario, Demarioh, Demarrio, Demie, Demmy, Dimario

Demarion (American) combo of De and Marion

Demarques (African American) son of Marques; noble
Demark, Demarkes, Demarquis, Demmy

Demarris (American) combo of De and Marris
Loud

Demas (Greek) well-liked
Dimas

Dement (French) mountain

Demesio (Italian)
treacherous

Demete (American) form of
Demetrius: follower of
Demeter
Deme, Demetay

Demetrice (Greek) form of
Demetrius: follower of
Demeter

Demetrick (African
American) earthy
Demetrik, Demi, Demitrick

Demetrios (Greek) earth-
loving
*Demeetrius, Demetreus,
Demetri, Demetrious, Demetris,
Demi, Demie*

Demetrius (Greek) follower
of Demeter
*Dametrius, Dem, Demetri,
Demetrice, Demetris,
Demitrios, Demmy, Demos,
Dhimitrios, Dimetre, Dimitri,
Dimitrios, Dimitrious, Dimitry,
Dmitri, Dmitrios, Dmitry*

Demian (Slavic) form of
Damian: fate

Demin (Spanish) form of
Demos: of the people

Deming (English) form of
Demos: of the people

Demitree (American) form of
Dimitri: fertile; flourishing

Demitri (Greek) fertile; earthy
*Demetrie, Demetry, Demi,
Demie, Demitry, Dmitri*

Democri (Greek) judges

Demond (African American)
worldly
Demonde

Demondre (American) of the
world

Demos (Greek) of the people
Demas, Demmos

Demosthenes (Greek)
orator; eloquent
Demos

Demps (Irish) form of
Dempsey: respected; judge
Demps, Dempse, Dempz

Dempsey (Irish) respected;
judge
*Dem, Demi, Demps, Dempsie,
Dempsy*

Den (Greek) form of Dennis:
reveler

Denali (Hindi) great

Denard (Last name as first
name) envied
Den, Denar, Denarde, Denny

Denby (Scandinavian)
adventurous
*Danby, Denbee, Denbey,
Denbie, Denney, Dennie,
Denny*

Dene (Hungarian) reveler

Deneki (Slavic) star of the day

Denham (Scandinavian)
hamlet of Danes

Denholm (Scandinavian)
house of Danes

Deni (English) form of
Dionysius: joyous celebrant;
god of wine
Denni

Denim (French) cotton fabric

Denk (American) sporty
Denky, Dink

Denley (English) dark
Denlie, Denly

Denman (English) dark;
valley-dweller
*Den, Deni, Denmin, Denney,
Denni, Dennie, Dennman,
Denny, Dinman*

Denmark (Place name) from
Denmark

Dennar (English) valley boy

Dennard (English) valley boy

Dennell (English) valley boy

Dennis (Greek) reveler
*Den, Denes, Deni, Denies,
Denis, Deniss, Dennes, Dennet,
Denney, Denni, Dennie,
Dennies, Dennison, Denniz,
Denny, Dennys, Deno, Denys,
Deon, Dino, Dion, Dionisio,
Dionysius, Dionysus, Diot*

Dennisen (English) Dennis's
son; partier
*Den, Denison, Dennison,
Dennizon, Dennyson, Tennyson*

Denno (Greek) form of
Dennis: reveler

Denny (Greek) form of
Dennis: reveler
*Den, Denee, Deni, Denney,
Denni*

Denoy (Greek) form of
Dennis: reveler

Densey (English) place name

Dent (American) form of
Denzel: sensual

Denton (English) valley
settlement; happy
*Denny, Dent, Dentan, Denten,
Dentie, Dentin*

Denver (Place name) capital
of Colorado; climber
Den, Denny

Denzel (English) sensual
*Den, Denny, Densie, Denz,
Denze, Denzell, Denzelle,
Denziel, Denzil, Denzill,
Denzille, Denzyl, Denzylle,
Dinzie*

Denzie (English) place name

Deo (Sanskrit) God

Deodan (Latin) serving God

Deodar (Sanskrit) cedar

Deondray (African
American) romantic
*Deandre, Deeon, Deondrae,
Deondrey, Deone*

Deone (Greek) form of
Dionysius: joyous celebrant;
god of wine
Deion, Deonah, Deonne, Dion

Deonnetaye (American)
extrovert

Deonté (French) outgoing
*De'On, Deontae, Deontay,
Deontie, Diontay, Diontayye*

Deordre (African American)
outgoing
Deordray

Depp (American) dashing
Dep

Derby (Irish) guileless
Derbey, Derbie

Derek (German) ruler; bold
heart
*Darrick, Darriq, Derak, Dere,
Dereck, Deric, Derick, Derik,
Deriq, Deriqk, Derk, Derreck,
Derrek, Derrick, Derrik,
Derryck, Derryk, Deryk,
Deryke, Dirk, Dirke, Dyrk*

Derenzo (Italian) form of
Darren: great

Derett (American) form of
Derrick: bold heart

Derlam (American) form of Derlin; form of Derland: from the land of deer

Derland (English) from the land of deer
Durland

Derlin (English) form of Derland: from the land of deer
Derl, Derlan, Derland, Derlen, Derlyn, Durland, Durlin

Dermod (Irish) form of Dermot: unabashed; giving
Dermud

Dermond (Irish) unassuming
Dermon, Dermun, Dermund, Derr

Dermot (Irish) unabashed; giving
Der, Dermod, Dermott, Derree, Derrey, Derri, Diarmid, Diarmuid

Dern (Hebrew) form of Deron: smart

Deron (African American) form of on Darren: smart
Dare, Daron, DaRon, Darone, Darron, Dayron, Dere, DeRronn

Deronce (American) form of Direnc: resistance

Derrell (French) form of Darrell: loved
Dere, Derrel, Derrill

Derrence (American) form of Direnc: resistance

Derrett (French) form of Darren: great

Derri (American) breezy
Derree, Derry

Derrick (German) bold heart
Derak, Derick

Derry (Irish) red-haired
Dare, Darry, Derrey, Derri, Derrie

Dervando (Italian) friend

Derward (Last name as first name) clunky
Der, Derr, Derwy, Dur, Durr, Ward

Derwent (Last name as first name) of deer

Derwin (English) bookish
Darwin, Darwyn, Derwyn, Derwynn, Durwen, Durwin

Derya (Slavic) from the ocean

Des (Irish) form of Desmond: from Munster

Desaro (Spanish) desired

Deseo (Spanish) desire
Des, Desi, Dezi

Deshan (Hindi) patriot
Deshad, Deshal

Deshawn (African American) brassy
D'Sean, D'Shawn, Dashaun, Dashawn, Desean, Deshaun, Deshaune, Deshawnn, Deshon

Deshea (American) confident
Desh, DeShay, Deshay, Deshie

Deshon (African American) bold; open
Desh, Deshan, Deshann

Desi (Latin) form of Desmond: from Munster; form of Desiderio: yearning; sorrow; desired

Desiderio (Latin) yearning; sorrow; desired
Derito, Des, Desi, Desideratus, Desiderios, Desiderius, Desie, Diderot, Didier, Dizier, Deri

Desidoro (Spanish) desirable

Desire (American) desirable
Des, Desi, Desidero

Desley (American) form of
Lesley: strong-willed

Desmee (Irish) form of
Desmond: from Munster
*Desi, Dessy, Dezme, Dezmee,
Desmey, Dezmie, Dezmo,
Dezzy*

Desmond (Irish) from
Munster
*Des, Desi, Desmon, Desmund,
Dezmond, Dizmond*

Desmondae (Irish) loyal
Irishman

Desmun (Irish) form of
Desmond: from Munster
Dez, Dezmund

Desoto (Spanish) explores

Desperado (Spanish)
renegade
Des, Deseperado, Dessy, Dezzy

Dessles (African) happy

Destin (Place name) city in
Florida; destiny; fate
Desten, Destie, Deston, Destrie

Detleff (Germanic) decisive
Detlef, Detlev

Detler (German) decides

Detrick (German) rules

Detries (German) form of
Dedric: leader

Detroy (African American)
outgoing
Detroe

Detry (German) rules

Detton (Last name as first
name) determined
Deet, Dett

Deuce (American) two in
cards; second child
Doos, Duz

DeUndre (African American)
child of Undre
Deundrae, DeUndray, Deundry

Deuter (German) warrior

Dev (Irish) form of Devlin:
fearless
Deb, Deo

Deval (Hindi) godlike
Deven

Devann (American) divine
child
DeVanne, Deven

Devaughan (American)
bravado
Devan, Devaughn, Devonne

Devdan (Hindi) God's gift
Debdan, Deodan

Devend (Indian) from Hindu
god Indra Devendra

Devender (American) poetic
Devander, Deven, Devendar

Dever (American) generous

Deverell (American) special
*Dev, Devee, Deverel, Deverelle,
Devie, Devy*

Devereux (French surname)
divine
Deveraux

Deverges (French) diverges

Devin ◐ (Irish) poetic; writer
*Dev, Devan, Deven, Devinn,
Devon, Devvy, Devyn, Devynn*

Devine (Latin) divine
Dev, Devinne

Devinson (Irish) poetic
*Dev, Devan, Devee, Deven,
Davin, Devy*

Devland (Irish) courageous
Dev, Devlend, Devlind, Devvy

Devlin (Irish) fearless
*Devlan, Devlen, Devlon,
Devlyn, Devy*

Devo (American) quirky; fun
Divo

Devoe (French) last name
used as first name; lives near
beautiful valley

Devon (Irish) writer
*Deavon, Dev, Deven, Devin,
Devohne, Devond, Devonn,
Devy, Devyn*

Devonte (African American)
form of Devon: outgoing
Devontae, Devontay

Devroy (French) God as
royalty

Dew (English) word as name

Dewalt (Last name as first
name)

Dewan (American) form of
Dejuan: talkative
Dewey

Deward (Spanish) holy

Deway (American) invented

Dewayne (American) spirited
*Dewain, Dewaine, Duwain,
Dwain*

Dewell (Last name as first
name)

Dewey (Welsh) valued
Dew, Dewi, Dewie, Dewy, Duey

DeWhayne (American) form
of Dewayne: spirited

Dewitt (English) fair-haired
*Dewie, DeWitt, Dwight, Witt,
Wittie, Witty*

DeWittay (African American)
witty
Dewitt, De Witt, Witt, Witty

Dewon (African American)
clever
Dejuan, Dewan

Dex (Latin) form of Dexter:
skillful; right-handed
Dexe

Dexee (American) form of
Dexter: skillful; right-handed
Dex, Dexey, Dexi, Dexie

Dexter (Latin) skillful; right-
handed
*Decster, Dex, Dext, Dextah,
Dextar, Dextor*

Dezi (Irish) form of Desi:
from Munster; yearning;
sorrow; desired

Dhan (Indian) rich

Dhananjay (Indian) rich

Dhaval (Indian) purity

Dhiaa (African) winning

Dhillon (American) form of
Dillon: devoted

Dhrga (Indian) unreachable

Dhruv (Indian) star

Diablo (Spanish) devil

Dial (Word as name)

Diamon (American)
luminous
Dimon, Dimun, Diamund

Diamond (English)
bright; gem
*Dimah, Dime, Dimond,
Dimont*

Diante (English) form of
Deonte: outgoing

Diarmid (Irish) happy for
others' successes
Diarmaid, Diarmait, Diarmi

Diaz (Spanish) rowdy
Dias, Diazz

Dice (English) risk-taking
Dicey, Dies, Dize, Dyce, Dyse

Dick (German) form of Richard: wealthy leader
Dickey, Dicki, Dickie, Dicky, Dik

Dickens (Literature) for Charles Dickens; articulate

Dickinson (Last name as first name) poetic

Dickon (Last name as first name) strong king

Didier (French) desirable

Didionne (French) form of Didier: desirable

Diedrich (German) form of Dedric: leader
Dedric, Dedrick, Deed, Died, Dietrich

Diego ✪ (Spanish) form of James: he who supplants
Dago, Deago, Deagoh, Dee, Diago

Dierkes (Scandinavian) rules

Dierks (Scandinavian) rules

Diesel (American) rugged
Dees, Deez, Desel, Dezsel, Diezel

Diet (German) form of Dedric: leader

Dieter (German) prepared
Dedrick, Deke, Derek, Detah, Deter, Diederick, Dirk

Dietmar (German) famous

Dieudonne (French) loves a gracious God

Digby (Irish) man of simplicity

Diggory (French) lost
Diggery, Diggorey, Digory

Diggs (Last name as first name)

Digna (Scandinavian) worthwhile

Digneo (Latin) worthwhile

Dijon (Place name) city in France; refined
Dejawn

Dilean (Irish) loyal

Dilip (Hindi) protests; royal
Duleep

Dill (Irish) faithful
Dillard, Dilly

Dilley (Irish) loyal

Dillion (Irish) form of Dillon: devoted

Dillon (Irish) devoted
Dill, Dillan, Dillen, Dilly, Dilon, Dylan, Dylanne, Dyllon, Dylon

Dimas (Spanish) frank

Dimitri (Russian) fertile; flourishing
Demetry, Demi, Demitri, Demitry, Dmitri

Dimitrios (Greek) earth-loving

Dimter (Last name used as first name) form of Dimitri: fertile; flourishing

Dinesh (Hindi) day Lord

Dingo (Animal) wild spirit

Dink (American) from *Dink, the Little Dinosaur* television series

Dino (Italian) form of Dean: leader
Dean, Deanie, Deano, Deinoh, Dinoh

Dinos (Greek) form of
Constantine: proud
Dean, Dino, Dinohs, Dynos

Dinose (American) form of
Dino: leader
*Denoze, Dino, Dinoce, Dinoz,
Dinoze*

Dins (American) climber
Dinse, Dinz

Dinsdale (English) hill
protector; innovator

Dinsmore (Irish) guarded
*Dinnie, Dinnsmore, Dinny,
Dins*

Diogenes (Greek) honest
man
Dee, Dioge, Dioh

Diogo (Spanish) form of
Diego: untamed; wild
Rascal

Diohne (Greek) form of
Dion: joyous celebrant; god of
wine

Dion (Greek) form of
Dionysius: joyous celebrant;
god of wine
*Deion, Deon, Deonn, Deonys,
Deyon, Dio, Dionn*

Dionel (Welsh) form of
Daniel: judged by God;
spiritual
Deinel

Dionisio (Spanish) form of
Dionysius: joyous celebrant;
god of wine
Dionis, Dioniso, Dionysio

Dionysus (Greek) joyous
celebrant; god of wine
*Dee, Deonysios, Dion, Dionio,
Dioniso, Dionysios, Dionysius,
Dionysos, Dionysus*

Diosdado (Spanish) wise;
loves God

Direnc (Turkish) resistance

Direnzo (Italian) rules

Dirk (Scandinavian) leader
*Derk, Dierck, Dieric, Dierick,
Dirck, Dirke, Dirky, Durk,*

Diron (American) form of
Darin: great
Diran, Dirun, Dyronn

Dishan (Biblical) a threshing

Distan (American) invented

Diven (Last name as first
name)

Divina (Spanish) divine

Dix (American) energetic
Dex

Dixen (English) jovial

Dixie (American) southerner
Dix, Dixee, Dixey, Dixi

Dixon (English) Dick's son;
happy
Dickson, Dix, Dixie, Dixo

Dizon (Spanish) form of
Dixon: Dick's son; happy

Doak (Scottish) St. Cadoc's
servant

Doan (English) hills; quiet
Doane, Doe

Dobbs (English) fire

Dobes (American)
unassuming
Dobe, Doe

Dobie (American) reliable;
southern
Dobe, Dobee, Dobey, Dobi

Dobine (Slavic) goodness

Dobrin (Slavic) goodness

Dobro (Slavic) goodness

Dobromir (Polish) good
Dobe, Dobry, Doby

Dobry (Polish) good
Dobe, Dobree, Dobrey

Dobson (Slavic) goodness

Dodd (English) swaggering;
has a small-town sheriff feel
Dod

Dodge (English) swaggering
Dod, Dodds, Dodgson

Dodgen (English) last name
as first name; son of Dodd or
Dodda

Dodsworth (English) last
name as first name

Dody (Greek) God's gift
Doe

Dogan (English) last name as
first name

Doherty (Irish) rash
*Docherty, Doh, Doughertey,
Douherty*

Dolan (Irish) dark
Dolen

Dolbin (American) dark

Dolce (Italian) sweet

Dolek (American) doleful

Dolen (Irish) dark

Dolgen (American) tenacious
Dole, Dolg, Dolgan, Dolgin

Dollester (last name as first
name) dark

Dollus (American) dark

Dolon (Irish) brunette
Dole, Dolen, Dolton

Dolph (German) form of
Rudolph: wolf
*Dolf, Dollfus, Dollfuss,
Dollphus, Dolphus, Dolf, Dolfie*

Dolson (last name as first
name) son of Dolan; dark

Dom (Latin) form of
Dominic: child of the Lord;
saint
Dome, Dommie, Dommy

Domaneke (Latin) loves the
Lord; Dynamic

Domasz (Slavic) form of
Thomas: twin; look-a-like

Domenico (Italian) confident
Dom, Domeniko

Domero (Spanish)
courageous

Dominador (Latin) seeks
love

Domingo (Spanish) Sunday-
born boy
*Demingo, Dom, Domin,
Dominko*

Dominic ✪ (Latin) child of
the Lord; saint
*Demenico, Demingo, Dom,
Domenic, Domenico,
Domenique, Domingo, Domini,
Dominick, Dominie, Dominik,
Dominique, Domino, Dominy,
Nick*

Dominiel (American) form of
Dominic: child of the Lord;
saint

Dominique (French)
spiritual
*Dom, Dominick, Dominike,
Domminique*

Domino (Latin) winner
Domeno, Dominoh, Domuno

Domizio (Italian) form of
Dominic: child of the Lord;
saint

Dommond (Latin) form of Dominic: child of the Lord; saint

Domon (Latin) form of Dominic: child of the Lord; saint

Domy (Italian) of the Lord

Don (Scottish) form of Donald: world leader; powerful
Dahn, Doni, Donn, Donney, Donni, Donnie, Donny

Donaciano (Spanish) dark
Dona, Donace, Donae, Donase

Donahue (Irish) fighter
Don, Donahoe, Donohue, Donohue

Donald (Scottish) world leader; powerful
Don, Donal, Donaldo, Donall, Donalt, Donaugh, Donel, Doneld, Donelson, Donild, Donn, Donnel, Donnell, Donney, Donni, Donnie, Donny

Donat (French) gives

Donatello (Italian) giving
Don, Donatelo, Donetello, Donny, Tello

Donatien (French) generous
Don, Donatyen, Donn, Donnatyen

Donato (Italian) donates

Donato (Italian) giving

Donatus (Greek) giving

Donav (Irish) form of Donovan: combative

Donaway (last name as first name)

Donder (Dutch) thunder

Donegan (last name as first name)

Dong (Chinese) from the east

Donker (African) modest

Donley (American) generous

Donnan (Irish) brown-haired; popular

Donne (Irish) brave

Donnel (Irish) brave

Donnell (Irish) courageous
Dahn, Don, Donel, Donell, Donhelle, Donnie, Donny

Donnelly (Irish) righteous
Donalee, Donally, Donelli, Donely, Donn, Donnell, Donnellie, Donnie

Donnis (American) form of Donald: world leader; powerful
Don, Donnes, Donnus

Donny (Irish) fond leader
Donney, Donni, Donnie

Donovan (Irish) combative
Don, Donavan, Donavon, Donavaughn, Donavyn, Donevin, Donevon, Donivin, Donny, Donoven, Donovon

Dont (American) dark; giving
Don, Dontay

Dontae (African American) capricious
Dontay, Donté

Dontave (African American) wild spirit
Dontav, Donteve

Dontavious (African American) giving
Dantavius, Dawntavius, Dewontavius, Dontavious

Donté (Italian) lasting forever
Dantae, Dantay, Dohntae, Dontae, Dontay, Dontey

Donton (American) confident
Don, Donnee, Dont, Dontie

Dontrell (African American) jaded
Dontray, Dontree, Dontrel, Dontrelle, Dontrey, Dontrie, Dontrill

Donyale (African American) regal; dark
Donyel, Donyelle

Donyell (African American) loyal
Donny, Danyel, Donyal

Donzell (African American) form of Denzel: sensual
Dons, Donsell, Donz, Donzelle

Doocey (American) clever
Dooce, Doocee, Doocie, Doos

Dool (American) form of Dooley: shy hero

Dooley (Irish) shy hero
Doolee, Dooli, Dooly

Dop (American) form of Dophy: wise one

Dophy (French) wise one

Dor (Aboriginal) energetic
Doram, Doriel, Dorli

Doran (Irish) adventurer
Dore, Dorian, Doron, Dorran, Dorren

Dorcel (French) fleet

Dore (Greek) form of Isidore: special gift

Dorell (Scottish) brave

Dorgan (American) form of Dragan: dragon

Dorian (Greek) the sea's child; mysterious; youthful forever
Dora, Dore, Dorean, Dorey, Dorie, Dorien, Dorrian, Dorrien, Dorryen, Dory

Doriano (Spanish) thriving

Dorin (Romanian) form of Dorian: the sea's child; mysterious; youthful forever

Dorman (Last name as first name) practical
Dor, Dorm

Dorn (Slavic) form of Dorin: the sea's child; mysterious; youthful forever

Doro (Greek) God's gift

Doron (Greek) unlimited passion
Doran, Doroni

Dorral (Last name as first name) vain
Dorale, Dorry

Dorset (Place name) county in England
Dorsett, Dorzet

Dorsey (French) sturdy as a fortress
Dorsee, Dorsie

Dorum (American) form of Dorian: the sea's child; mysterious; youthful forever

Dorval (Irish) poet

Doss (Latin) wealthy

Dotan (African) hardworking
Dotann

Dothan (Biblical) obeys

Dotson (Last name as first name) loquacious; son of Dot
Dotsen, Dottson

Doug (Scottish) form of
Douglas: powerful; dark river
Dougie, Dougy, Dug, Dugy

Dougal (Irish) dark
*Doyle, Dougall, Dugal, Dugald,
Dugall*

Douglas (Scottish) powerful;
dark river
*Doug, Douggie, Dougie,
Douglace, Douglass, Douglis,
Dugaid*

Dougray (Irish) dwells by the
dark stream

Dov (Hebrew) bear

Dovan (Asian) village in
Himalayas (Nepal)

Dovie (American) peaceable
*Dove, Dovee, Dovey, Dovi,
Dovy*

Dow (Irish) brunette
Dowan, Dowe, Dowson

Dowd (American) serious
Doud, Dowdy, Dowed

Dowden (Irish) dark

Dowding (American) dark

Dowell (Welsh) last name as
first name; Dark

Dowen (Irish) dark

Downie (American) form of
surname Downey

Dowrick (last name as first
name)

Dox (American) form of Dax:
unique; waterloving

Doxey (American) form of
Dox: unique; water-loving

Doy (American) form of
Douglas: powerful; dark river

Doyal (American) form of
Doyle: deep; dark
Doile, Doyl, Doyle

Doyle (Irish) deep; dark
Doil, Doy, Doyal, Doye, Doyl

Doylton (Last name as first
name) pretentious
Doyl, Doyle

Dozier (German) last name
as first name

Draco (Italian) dragon

Dracy (American) form of
Stacey: hopeful
*Dra, Drace, Dracee, Dracey,
Draci, Drase, Drasee, Drasi*

Dradell (American) serious
Drade, Dray

Dragan (Slavic) dragon

Drake (English) dragonlike;
fire-breathing
Drago, Drakie, Drako

Draper (English) precise;
maker of drapes
Draiper, Drape

Draphus (English) draper

Draven (American) capable

Draven (American) cool

Dravey (American) groovy
Dravee, Dravie, Dravy

Dravis (American) form of
Travis: conflicted

Dray (Hindi) ambient light

Dren (Scandinavian) courage

Drew (Welsh) wise; well-liked
Dru, Druw

Drexel (American) thoughtful
Drex

Drexie (American) thinker

Dries (Dutch) brave
Dre

Drigger (English) last name as first name

Driscoll (Irish) pensive
Driscol, Drisk, Driskell

Driver (English) driver

Dru (English) wise; popular
Drew, Drue

Drulon (English) adoring

Drummar (English) drums

Drummon (English) drums

Drummond (Scottish) practical
Drum, Drumon, Drumond

Drurius (American) form of Darius: affluent

Drury (French) loving man
Drew, Drewry, Dru, Drure, Drurey, Drurie

Dryden (English) writer; calm
Driden, Drydan, Drydin

Drystan (Welsh) form of Tristan: sad; wistful
Drestan, Dristan, Drystyn

Dua (Arabic) prays

Dual (American) two

Duan (English) form of Dwayne: swarthy

Duane (Irish) dark man
Dewain, Dewayne, Duain, Duwain, Duwaine, Duwayne, Dwain, Dwaine, Dwayne

Duarte (Spanish) rich

Dub (Irish) form of Dublin: city in Ireland; trendy
Dubby

Dubai (Arabic) place name

Dubak (African) 11th child

Dubi (Slavic) dark

Duble (Slavic) dark

Dublin (Place name) city in Ireland; trendy

Dubray (English) dark

Duc (Vietnamese) honest

Ducio (Italian) docile

Ducy (Spanish) leads

Dude (American) cool guy

Dudley (English) compromiser; rich; stuffy
Dud, Dudd, Dudlee, Dudlie, Dudly

Dueart (American) kind
Art, Duart, Due, Duey

Duff (Scottish) dark
Duf, Duffey, Duffie, Duffy

Duffin (last name as first name) dark

DuFrane (French) of the frame

Dugal (Irish) dark

Dugan (Irish) dark man
Doogan, Dougan, Douggan, Duggan, Duggie, Duggy, Dugin

Dugar (French) dark

Dugas (French) dark

Duke (Latin) leader of the pack
Dook, Dukey, Dukie

Dulay (African) works cloth

Duleep (Indian) protects

Dulio (Italian) combative

Dulley (American) popular

Dumah (Biblical) in the mist

Dumas (French) last name as first name

Dumisani (African) leader

Dumont (French)
monumental
*Dummont, Dumon, Dumonde,
Dumonte, Dumontt*

Dunbar (Irish) castle-dweller
Dunbarr

Dunbaron (American) dark
Baron, Dunbar

Duncall (American) form of
Dunkle: handsome

Duncan (Scottish) spirited
fighter
*Dunc, Dunk, Dunkan, Dunn,
Dunne*

Dunce (English) hill

Dundee (Australian) spunky

Dune (English) word as name

Dunham (Last name as first
name) dark

Dunia (American) dark
Dunya

Dunk (Scottish) form of
Duncan: spirited fighter
Dunc, Dunk

Dunlap (Scottish) hill

Dunlavy (English) sylvan
Dunlave

Dunley (English) meadow-
loving
*Dunlea, Dunlee, Dunleigh,
Dunli, Dunlie, Dunly,
Dunnlea, Dunnleigh, Dunnley*

Dunley (English) meadow
with the hill

Dunlop (English) sylvan

Dunmore (Scottish) guarded
Dun, Dunmohr, Dunmoore

Dunn (Irish) neutral
Dun, Dunne

Dunney (Scottish) hill

Dunnigan (Scottish) hill

Dunning (Scottish) hill

Dunnson (Scottish) son of
Donald

Dunphy (American) dark;
serious
*Dun, Dunphe, Dunphee,
Dunphey*

Dunstan (English)
well-girded
*Dun, Duns, Dunse, Dunsten,
Dunstin, Dunston*

Dunstand (English) form of
Dunstan: well-girded
*Dunsce, Dunse, Dunst,
Dunsten, Dunstun*

Dupree (French) smooth

Durand (Latin) form of
Durant: lasting; alluring
Duran, Durayn

Durango (Spanish) place
name; Basque durango;
fertile lowland surrounded by
elevations

Durant (Latin) lasting;
alluring
*Dante, Duran, Durand,
Durante, Durr, Durrie, Durry*

Duray (American) endures

Durban (Place name) city in
South Africa
Durb, Durben

Durbon (last name as first
name)

Duren (Latin) lasts

Durg (Hindi) out of reach

Durham (Last name as first
name) supportive
Duram

Durke (American) form of
Dirk: leader

Durmot (French) has no malice

Durnford (English) last name as first name

Duro (Place name) palo Duro Canyon; enduring
Dure

Duron (American) form of Doran: adventurer

Durrell (English) protective
Durel, Durell, Durr, Durrel, Durry

Durward (English) gatekeeper

Durwin (English) dear friend
Derwin, Derwyn, Durwen, Durwinn, Durwyn

Durwood (English) vigilant; home-loving
Derrwood, Derwood, Durr, Durrwood, Durwould, Durward

Duryea (Hindi) invincible

Duskin (German) form of Dustin: bold and brave

Dusky (English) born at dusk

Dussen (Dutch) energetic

Duster (American) form of Dusty: bold and brave
Dust, Dustee, Dustey, Dusti, Dusty

Dustin (German) bold and brave
Dust, Dustan, Dusten, Duston, Dustie, Dusty, Dustyn

Dusty (German) form of Dustin: bold and brave
Dust, Dustee, Dustey, Dusti, Dustie

Dusty-Joe (American) cowboy
Dustee, Dusti, Dusty, Dustyjoe

Dutch (Dutch) from Holland; optimistic
Dutchie, Dutchy

Duth (Dutch) boy from the Netherlands

Duthrie (American) form of Guthrie: windy; heroic

Duval (French) valley; peaceful
Dovahl, Duv, Duvall, Duvalle

Duvin (French) of the wine

Dwain (American) form of Dwayne: swarthy
Dwaine

Dwan (African American) fresh
D'wan, D'Wan, Dewan, Dwawn, Dwon

Dwanae (African American) dark; small
Dwannay

Dwayne (Gaelic) swarthy
Duane, Duwain, Duwane, Duwayne, Dwain, Dwaine

Dweezel (American) creative
Dweez, Dweezil

Dwight (English) intelligent; white
Dwi, Dwite

Dwighton (English) Dwight's town

Dwyer (Irish) wise
Dwire, Dwyyer

Dwyke (American) form of Dwight: intelligent; white

Dyam (Native American) eagle

Dybry (Slavic) good

Dyer (English) creative
Di, Dier, Dyar, Dye

Dykins (English) near the dike

Dylan ○ ❶ (Welsh) sea god;
creative
*Dill, Dillan, Dillon, Dilloyn,
Dilon, Dyl, Dylahn, Dylen,
Dylin, Dyllan, Dylon, Dylonn*

Dyle (Welsh) form of Dylan:
sea god; creative

Dylion (Welsh) form of
Dylan: sea god; creative

Dym (Russian) form of
Dimitri: fertile; flourishing

Dynell (African American)
seaman; gambler
Dinell, Dyne

Dyre (Scandinavian) dearest

Dyron (African American)
mercurial; sea-loving
Diron, Dyronn, Dyronne

Dyron (Scandinavian) dearest

Dyson (English) sea-loving
*Dieson, Dison, Dysan, Dysen,
Dysun, Dyzon*

Dyvet (English) worker; dyes
Dye

Eagan (Irish) form of Egan:
spirited
Egan, Egon

Eagle (Native American)
sharp-eyed
Eagal, Egle

Eagul (American) eagle

Eamon (Irish) form of
Edmond: protective
Amon, Eamen, Emon

Ean (English) form of Ian:
believer; handsome

Earl (English) promising;
noble
*Earle, Earley, Earlie, Early, Eril,
Erl*

Earldon (English) noble

Earlen (Irish) form of Earl:
promising; noble

Early (English) punctual
Earl, Earlee, Earley

Earnest (English) genuine
Earn, Earnie, Ern, Ernie

Earon (American) form of
Aaron: revered; sharer
Earonn

Earvin (English) sea-loving
Dervin, Ervin

Easau (Biblical) equivocates

Easey (American) casygoing
Easy, Ezey

East (English) from the East
Easte

Easter (English) born on
Easter day

Eastland (English) boy from
the East

Easton (English) outdoorsy;
east town
Easten

Eaton (English) wealthy
Eaten, Etawn, Eton

Eaves (English) edges by

Eb (Hebrew) form of
Ebenezer: base of life; rock

Ebal (Biblical) merciful

Ebbe (Scandinavian) brave

Ebby (Hebrew) form of
Ebenezer: base of life; rock
Ebbey, Ebbi

Eben (Hebrew) helpful; loud
Eban

Ebenezer (Hebrew) base of life; rock
Eb, Ebbie, Ebby, Eben, Ebeneezer, Ebeneser

Eberhardt (German) brave
Eb, Eber, Eberhard

Ebert (French) bright

Ebo (African) Tuesday-born

Ebun (Hebrew) rock solid

Eckhardt (German) iron-willed
Eck, Eckhard, Eckhart, Ekhard

Ecklee (last name as first name) strong

Ector (Slavic) dedicated

Ed (English) form of Edward: prospering; defender
Edd, Eddie, Eddy, Edy

Eda (Scottish) fiery

Edan (Scottish) fiery
Edon

Eday (Irish) fiery

Edbert (German) courageous
Ediberto

Edcell (English) focused; wealthy
Ed, Edcelle, Eds, Edsel

Eddie (English) form of Edward: prospering; defender
Eddee, Eddey, Eddy

Edel (German) of noble birth
Adel, Edelmar, Edelweiss

Edeltraud (German) young

Eden (Hebrew) delight
Eadon, Edin, Edon, Edye, Edyn

Edenir (Hebrew) delights

Edenson (Hebrew) son of Eden; delight
Edence, Edens, Edensen

Edgar (English) success
Ed, Eddie, Edghur, Edgur

Edgard (English) spear thrower
Ed, Eddie, Edgarde

Edgardo (English) successful
Edgar, Edgard, Edgardoh

Edge (American) cutting edge; trendsetter
Eddge, Edgy

Edgin (last name as first name)

Edilberto (Spanish) noble
Edilbert

Edison (English) Edward's son; smart
Ed, Eddie, Edisen, Edyson

Ediwon (Slavic) form of Edward: prospering; defender

Edmond (English) protective
Ed, Edmon, Edmund

Edmun (Polish) rich

Edmundo (Spanish) wealthy protector
Ed, Eddie, Edmond

Edor (Spanish) snowy

Edrick (English) rich leader
Ed, Edri, Edrik, Edry

Edsel (English) rich
Ed, Eddie, Edsil, Edsyl

Edson (English) form of Edison: Edward's son; smart

Eduar (Spanish) form of Edward: prospering; defender

Eduardo (Spanish) flirtatious
Ed, Eddie, Edwardo

Eduviges (Italian) contentious

Edward (English) prospering;
defender
*Ed, Eddey, Eddi, Eddie, Eddy,
Edwar, Edwerd*

Edwards (English) last name
as first name; prospers

Edwiges (Spanish)
contentious

Edwin (English) prosperous
friend
Ed, Edwinn, Edwynn

Edzel (English) affluent

Efemy (Greek) eloquent

Efrain (Hebrew) form of
Ephraim: fertile
Efren

Efrat (Spanish) brave

Efremel (Russian) cheerful

Efrim (Hebrew) form of
Ephraim: fertile
Ef, Efrem, Efrum

Efton (American) form of
Ephraim: fertile
fruitful, Ef, Eft, Eften, Eftun

Egan (Irish) spirited
Eggie, Egin, Egon

Egbert (English) bright sword
Egber, Egburt, Eggie, Eggy

Egborn (English) ready; born
of Edgar
Eg, Egbornem, Egburn, Eggie

Eger (English) form of Edgar:
success

Egerton (English) town of a
spearman
*Edgarton, Edgartown, Edgerton,
Egeton*

Egeus (American) protective
Aegis, Egis

Eggleston (last name as first
name) town of Edgar

Eghert (German) smart
Eghertt, Eghurt

Egil (Scandinavian) the
sword's edge
Eigil

Egmon (German) protective
*Egmond, Egmont, Egmun,
Egmund, Egmunt*

Egon (Irish) passionate

Egypt (Place name)
mysterious; majestic

Ehab (Irish) vibrant

Ehren (Hebrew) form of
Aaron: revered; sharer

Ehrlich (last name as first
name) aware

Eikki (African) strong

Eilam (Hebrew) form of
Elam: eternal

Einar (Scandinavian) lone
fighter

Eirene (American) peaceful

Eiton (Hebrew) strong

Ejuan (Spanish) form of
Ewan: youthful spirit

Ekels (last name as first
name) echols variant

Eklund (last name as first
name) honored

Ekon (African) muscular

Ekul (last name as first name)
honored

El (English) old friend

El Fego (Spanish) bird;
articulate

El Mahdi (Spanish) loved

Elam (Hebrew) eternal

Elan (French) finesse
Elann, Elen, Elon, Elyn

Elbis (American) exalted
Elb, Elbace, Elbase, Elbus

Elbridge (American)
presidential
Elb, Elby

Elcim (Spanish) dignified

Eldaah (Biblical) battles

Eldan (Biblical) God loves

Eldemar (Slavic) old soul

Elder (English) older sibling
El, Eldor

Eldon (English) charitable
Edwin, El, Elden, Eldin

Eldorado (Place name) city in
Arkansas
El, Eld, Eldor

Eldread (English) wise
advisor
El, Eldred, Eldrid

Eldridge (English) supportive
Eldredge

Eleazar (Hebrew) helped by
God
*Elazar, Eleasar, Eliasar,
Eliazar, Elieser, Elizar*

Elegy (Spanish) memorable
Elegee, Elegie, Elgy

Elendor (Invented) special
Elen, Elend

Eleuter (Greek) freedom of
integrity

Eleuterio (Greek) freedom of
integrity

Elex (American) form of Alex:
great leader; helpful

Elger (German) of noble birth
Elger, Ellgar, Ellger

Elgin (English) elegant
Elgen

Elham (English) last name as
first name; place name

Eli (Hebrew) faithful man;
high priest
El, Elie, Eloy, Ely

Elian (Spanish) spirited
Eliann, Elyan

Elias (Greek) spiritual
El, Eli, Eliace, Elyas

Eliason (Greek) form of Elias:
spiritual

Eliazar (Hebrew) God assists
him

Elic (American) form of Alec:
high-minded

Eliel (Hebrew) religious

Eliett (Spanish) form of
Elliott: God-loving

Eliezer (Origin unknown) of
God
Elieser, Elyeser

Elige (Latin) God has chosen
him

Elighie (American) form of
Elijah: religious; Old
Testament prophet

Elihu (Hebrew) true believer
Elih, Eliu, Ellihu

Elijah ✪ ⚤ (Hebrew)
religious; Old Testament
prophet
El, Elie, Elija

Elik (Hawaiian) form of Eric:
powerful leader

Eliniod (American) God helps
him

Eliphaz (Biblical) the
endeavor of God

Elis (Hebrew) form of Eliseo:
darling

Eliseo (Spanish) daring
Elizeo

Elisha (Hebrew) of God's
salvation
Elishah, Elysha, Elyshah

Elkanah (Biblical) obedient to
God

Elkin (Hebrew) obedient to
God

Ellard (German) brave man
Ell, Ellarde, Ellee, Ellerd

Ellery (English) dominant
El, Ell, Ellary, Ellerie, Ellie

Ellezer (English) believer

Ellion (American) form of
Elliott: God-loving

Elliott (English) God-loving
Elie, Elio, Ell, Elliot

Ellis (English) form of Elias:
spiritual
Ellice, Ells

Ellison (English) circumspect
*Ell, Ellason, Ellisen, Ells,
Ellyson*

Ellkan (Hawaiian) saved by
God
Elkan, Elkin

Ellory (Cornish) graceful
swan
Elory, Elorey, Ellorey

Ellsha (Hebrew) saved by the
Lord
*Elljsha, Elisee, Elish, Elishia,
Elishua*

Elman (American) protective
El, Elle, Elmen, Elmon

Elmer (English) famed
*Ell, Elm, Elmar, Elmir, Elmo,
Elmoh*

Elmerre (English) form of
Elmer: famed

Elmito (Spanish) form of
Elmer: famed

Elmo (Greek) gregarious
Ellmo, Elmoh

Elmore (English) radiant
Elm, Elmie, Elmoor, Elmor

Elmore (Last name as first
name) sassy; royal

Elmot (American) lovable
Elm

Elof (Swedish) the one heir
Loff

Elohim (Hebrew) chosen

Eloi (French) chosen one
Eloie, Eloy

Elois (Spanish) chosen

Elonzo (Spanish) sturdy;
happy
El, Elon, Elonso

Elrad (Hebrew) God rules his
life

Elran (Spanish) God directs
him

Elreno (Spanish) God directs
him

Elrette (Spanish) God directs
him

Elrid (Hebrew) God directs
him

Elrin (American) God helps
him

Elroy (French) giving
Elroi, Elroye

Elsden (English) spiritual
Els, Elsdon

Elson (English) form of
Elston: sophisticated
Elsen

Elster (Scottish) form of
Alastair: strong leader

Elston (English) sophisticated
Els, Elstan, Elsten

Elsworth (Last name as first name) pretentious
Ells, Ellsworth

Elton (English) settlement; famous
Ell, Ellton, Elt, Eltan, Elten

Elusha (Slavic) treasured

Eluteria (Russian) believer

Eluye (Spanish) integrity

Elvie (Spanish) fair

Elvin (English) friend of elves
El, Elv, Elven

Elvind (American) form of Elvin: friend of elves
Elv

Elvis (Scandinavian) all-wise
El, Elvyse, The King

Elvy (English) elfin; small

Elwell (English) born in the old-well area

Elwen (English) friend of elves
Elwee, Elwin Elwy, Elwyn, Elwynn, Elwynt

Elwond (Last name as first name) steady
Ellwand, Elwon, Eldwund

Elwood (English) old wood; everlasting
Ell, Elwoode, Elwould, Woodie, Woody, Woodye

Elwyne (English) elf-friend

Ely (Hebrew) lifted up
Eli

Elyden (English) from the hill

Elyus (Hebrew) form of Elias: spiritual

Elzaphan (Biblical) God assists him

Emanuel (Hebrew) with God
Em, Eman, Emanuele

Embers (Spanish) fiery

Emberto (Italian) pushy
Berty, Embert, Emberte

Embree (American) fiery

Emerick (German) form of Emery: hardworking leader

Emerit (German) form of Emery: hardworking leader

Emeritus (Latin) having fully earned

Emerson (German) Emery's son; able
Emers, Emersen

Emery (German) hardworking leader
Em, Emeri, Emerie, Emmerie, Emory, Emrie

Emig (Greek) brown

Emigdio (Greek) brown

Emil (Latin) ingratiating
Em, Emel, Emele

Emiliano (Italian) charms

Emilio (Italian) competitive; Spanish
excelling, Emil, Emile, Emilioh, Emlo

Emjay (American) reliable
Em-J, Em-Jay, M.J., MJ

Emmanuel (Hebrew) with God
Em, Eman, Emmannuel, Emmanuele, Manny

Emmaus (Biblical) place name; safe in God

Emmett (Hebrew) truthful; sincere
Emit, Emmet, Emmit, Emmitt, Emmyt, Emmytt

Emory (German) industrious leader
Emery, Emmory, Emorey, Emori, Emorie

Emre (Turkish) bond of brothers
Emra, Emrah, Emreson

Emress (Spanish) proud

Emric (Slavic) form of Emery; perseveres

Emrick (Welsh) immortal
Emryk

Emser (American) hard worker

Emuel (Hebrew) form of Emmanuel: with God
Emanuel, Imuel

Enam (Biblical) place name

Enan (Welsh) hard

Encarnacion (Spanish) embodiment of life

Enda (Slavic) masculine

Ender (Slavic) form of Andrew: manly and brave

Eneas (Hebrew) much-praised
Ennes, Ennis

Engel (German) angel

Engelbert (German) angel-bright
Bert, Bertie, Berty, Engelber, Inglebert

Engen (American) smart

Enger (Scandinavian) angel

England (English) from England

Englun (American) from England

Engram (English) angelic

Engus (Irish) form of Angus: standout; important

Enlai (Chinese) thankful

Enlow (last name as first name)

Ennis (Irish) reliable

Enno (Hebrew) form of Enos: mortal

Enny (American) form of Enos: mortal

Enoch (Hebrew) dedicated instructor
En, Enoc, Enok

Enos (Hebrew) mortal
Enoes

Enosh (Biblical) man

Enrick (Spanish) cunning
Enric, Enrik

Enrico (Italian) ruler
Enrike, Enriko, Enryco

Enrique (Spanish) charismatic ruler
Enrika, Enrikae, Enriqué, Enryque, Quiqui

Enrsto (Spanish) form of Ernesto

Ensor (Slavic) form of Ernest: sincere

Enver (Turkish) brightest child

Enzi (African) strong boy

Enzo (Italian) fun-loving

Eodis (Biblical) good

Epher (Biblical) plenty

Ephesian (Biblical) gifted

Ephraim (Hebrew) fertile
Eff, Efraim, Efram, Efrem, Ephraime, Ephrame, Ephrayme

Epifanio (Spanish) showing intelligence

Eppey (Spanish) smart

Eran (Hebrew) watchful

Erasmus (Greek) beloved
Eras, Erasmas, Erasmis

Erastus (Greek) loved baby

Erazmo (Spanish) loved
Erasmo, Eraz, Ras, Raz

Erbert (German) form of Herbert: famed warrior
Ebert, Erberto

Erby (German) aggressive

Ercell (Italian) the gift

Ercole (Italian) glorious God's child

Ereb (Greek) dark

Erebus (Greek) nether darkness

Ergo (Latin) word as name; therefore; consequently

Erhardt (German) strong-willed
Erhar, Erhard, Erhart, Erheart

Eric ✪ (Scandinavian) powerful leader
Ehrick, Erek, Erick, Erik, Eryke

Erie (Place name) one of the Great Lakes; vast

Erikson (Scandinavian) Erik's son; bold man
Ericksen, Eriksen, Erycksen, Eryksen, Erykson

Erin (Irish) peace-loving
Aaron, Arin, Aron, Eryn

Eris (Greek) hard life

Erlan (English) aristocratic
Earlan, Earland, Erland, Erlen, Erlin

Erling (English) highborn

Ermitt (English) form of Kermit: droll

Ermot (French) form of Ernest: sincere

Ernest (English) sincere
Earnest, Ern, Ernie, Erno, Ernst, Erny, Ernye

Ernesto (Spanish) sincere
Ernie, Nesto, Nestoh

Ernie (English) form of Ernest: sincere
Ernee, Erney, Erny

Erno (Slavic) form of Ernest: sincere

Ernold (English) sincere

Ernst (Dutch) form of Ernest: sincere

Ernulfo (Spanish) sincere

Erol (American) noble
Eral, Eril, Errol

Erold (Welsh) form of Errol: noble

Erolden (English) wanders

Eronlon (American) form of Aaron: revered; sharer

Eros (Greek) sensual
Ero

Erose (Greek) form of Eros: sensual
Eroce

Errett (American) form of Aaron: revered; sharer

Errick (American) form of Eric: powerful leader

Errin (American) form of Aaron: revered; sharer

Errington (last name as first name) Aaron's town

Errol (German) noble
Erol, Erold, Erroll, Erryl

Ershcel (American) form of Herschel: deer; swift

Erskine (Scottish) high-minded
Ers, Ersk, Erskin

Erst (Scottish) cliff

Erv (English) good-looking

Ervin (English) sea-loving
Earvin, Erv, Ervan, Erven, Ervind, Ervyn

Ervine (English) sea-lover
Ervene, Ervin

Erving (Scottish) good-looking

Erwey (American) form of Irving: attractive

Erwin (English) friendly
Erwyn

Esau (Hebrew) rough-hewn
Es, Esa, Esauw, Esaw

Esau (Hebrew) raw

Escobar (Spanish) swept up

Escobedo (Spanish) last name as first name

Escoto (Spanish) shy

Esdras (Biblical) form of Ezra: helpful; strong

Eshban (Biblical) fire of discernment

Eshcol (Hebrew) the grapes

Eshter (Indian) form of Eshwar: Hindu god

Eskew (English) last name as first name

Eskil (Scandinavian) divine

Esmaeil (Spanish) loved

Esmaiel (Spanish) outcast son

Esmail (Indian) God listens

EsmÈ (French) beloved
Es, Esmae, Esmay

Esmer (Slavic) affluent

Esmond (French) handsome
Esmand, Esmon, Esmund

Esmun (American) kind
Es, Esman, Esmon

Esos (Irish) godlike

Espen (German) bear of God

Espen (Danish) the bear

Esperanza (Spanish) hopeful
Esper, Esperance, Esperence

Espie (Scandinavian) big

Espy (Scandinavian) of God

Esraa (Hebrew) form of Ezra: helpful; strong

Esser (Spanish) reassuring

Essex (English) dignified
Ess, Ez

Estanisiao (Spanish) glorified

Este (Spanish) form of Esteban: royal; friendly

Esteban (Spanish) royal; friendly
Estabon, Estebann, Estevan, Estiban, Estyban

Estel (American) from the East

Esterlin (last name as first name) Easterner

Estes (English) Eastern; open
Estas, Este, Estis

Estevan (Spanish) crowned
Estivan, Estyvan

Estridge (Last name as first name) fortified
Es, Estri, Estry

Esvin (English) friend of Esser

Etam (Biblical) place name

Etan (Irish) watchful

Etano (Italian) form of Ethan: firm will

Etereo (Spanish) heavenly; spiritual
Etero

Ethan ○ ❶ (Hebrew) firm will
Eth, Ethen, Ethin, Ethon

Ethaniel (Italian) form of Gaetano: from the city of Gaeta; Italian man

Etheal (English) of good birth
Ethal

Ethelbert (German) principled
Ethelburt, Ethylbert

Etren (American) form of Ethan: firm will
Resolved

Ettore (Italian) loyal
Etor, Etore

Ettore (Italian) steadfast

Etwin (American) friend of Ethan; resolved

Eual (Jewish) form of Eyal: deer-like

Euclid (Greek) brilliant
Euclide, Uclid

Eudin (Greek) leads

Eufronio (Greek) bright

Eugene (Greek) blue-blood
Eugean, Eugenie, Ugene

Eural (American) from Ural Mountains; upward
Eure, Ural, Ury

Eurby (Last name as first name) sea
Erby, Eurb

Eurskie (Invented) dorky
Ersky

Eurus (Greek) form of Eros: sensual

Eusebio (Spanish) devoted to God
Eucebio, Eusabio, Eusevio, Sebio, Usibo

Eustace (Latin) calming
Eustice, Eustis, Stace, Stacey, Ustace

Eustacio (Spanish) calm; visionary
Eustacio, Eustase, Eustasio, Eustazio, Eustes, Eustis

Eustorgio (Greek) beloved

Euxinus (Greek) highborn

Evagelos (Greek) form of Andrew: manly and brave
Evaggelos, Evangelo, Evangelos

Evan ○ ❶ (Irish) warrior
Ev, Evann, Evanne, Even, Evin

Evander (Greek) manly; champion
Evand, Evandar, Evandir

Evans (Welsh) believer in a gracious God
Evens, Evyns

Evanus (American) form of Evan: warrior
Evan, Evin, Evinas, Evinus

Evar (Scandinavian) courageous

Evaristo (Spanish) form of Evan: warrior
Evariso, Evaro

Eve (Invented) form of Yves: honest; handsome
Eeve

Evelle (American) vibrant

Evelyn (American) writer
Ev, Evlinn, Evlyn

Even (Latin) does well

Ever (German) strong wild board

Everard (German) tough
Ev, Evrard

Everest (Place name) highest mountain peak in the world

Everestin (American) everlasting

Everett (English) strong
Ev, Fveret, Everitt, Evret, Evrit

Everette (English) brave

Everhart (Scandinavian) vibrant
Evhart, Evert

Everly (American) singing
Everlee, Everley, Everlie, Evers

Evert (Dutch) of the wild boars

Everton (English) from the town of boars; fearless

Every (English) word as name

Evetier (French) good

Evett (American) bright
Ev, Evatt, Eve, Evidt, Evitt

Evince (American) invincible

Evitt (American) invincible

Evodio (Spanish) righteous

Evon (Welsh) form of Evan: warrior
Even, Evin, Evonne, Evonn, Evyn

Evre (American) form of Everett: strong

Evres (American) form of Everettt: strong

Evret (American) form of Everettt: strong

Evzek (Slavic) brave

Ewald (Polish) fair ruler

Ewan (Scottish) youthful spirit
Ewahn, Ewon

Ewand (Welsh) form of Evan: warrior
Ewen, Ewon

Ewanell (American) form of Ewan: youthful spirit
Ewanel, Ewenall

Ewart (English) shepherd; caring
Ewar, Eward, Ewert

Ewen (Scottish) form of Eugene: blue-blood

Ewing (English) law-abiding
Ewin, Ewyng

Excell (American) competitive
Excel, Exsel, Exsell

Exek (American) God gives strength

Exia (Spanish) demanding
Ex, Exy

Exios (Spanish) finds a way

Exiquio (Spanish) exacting

Exod (Spanish) his exodus

Exzel (American) form of Edsel: rich

Eyal (American) form of Eagle: sharp-eyed

Eydis (Scandinavian) island god

Eytin (American) form of
Ethan: firm will

Eza (Hebrew) form of Ezra:
helpful; strong
Esri

Ezekiel (Hebrew) God's
strength
*Eze, Ezek, Ezekhal, Ezekial,
Ezikiel, Ezkeil, Ezekyel, Ezikiel,
Ezikyel, Ezykiel, Zeke*

Ezequiel (Spanish) devout

Ezer (Hebrew) helpful boy

Ezion (Biblical) place name

Ezira (Hebrew) helpful
Ezirah, Ezyra, Ezyrah

Ezno (Spanish) humble

Ezra (Hebrew) helpful; strong
Esra, Ezrah

Ezri (Hebrew) my help
Ezrey, Ezry

Ezron (American) created

Ezzie (Hebrew) form of Ezra:
helpful; strong
Ez

F

Faakhir (Arabic) proud

Faber (German) grower
Fabar, Fabir, Fabyre

Faberto (Latin) form of
Fabian: grower
*Fabe, Fabey, Fabian, Fabien,
Fabre*

Fabian (Latin) grower
*Fab, Fabe, Fabean, Fabeone,
Fabie, Fabien, Fabiano*

Fabio (Italian) seductive;
handsome
Fab, Fabioh

Fabish (American) form of
Fabrice: skilled worker

Fable (American) storyteller
Fabal, Fabe, Fabel, Fabil

Fablo (American) form of
Fabio: seductive; handsome

Fabrice (French) skilled
worker
*Fabriano, Fabricius, Fabritius,
Fabrizio, Fabrizius*

Fabrizio (Italian) fabulous

Fabron (French) blacksmith

Fabryce (Latin) crafty
*Fab, Fabby, Fabreese, Fabrese,
Fabrice*

Fabulous (American) vain
Fab, Fabby, Fabu

Fachan (Last name as first
name) precocious

Factor (English) entrepreneur

Facundo (Last name as first
name) profound

Faddis (American) loner;
deals in beans
Faddes, Fadice, Fadis

Faddy (American) faddish
Fad, Faddey, Faddi

Fadi (Arabic) saved by grace

Fadil (Arabic) giving

Faeus (Biblical) form of
Alfeus: follower

Fagan (Irish) fiery
Fagane, Fagen, Fagin, Fegan

Fahd (Arabic) fierce; panther;
brave
Fahad

Faheem (Arabic) brilliant

Fahim (Arabic) intelligent

Fahren (American) form of Faran: sincere

Fahrer (French) leader

Faino (American) the start

Fair (English) blond

Fairbairn (Scottish) fair-haired child

Fairbanks (English) bank along the pathway
Farebanks, Fairbanx

Fairchild (English) fair-haired child

Fairfax (English) full of warmth
Fairfacks, Farefax, Fax, Faxy

Faisal (Arabic) authoritative
Faisel, Faizal, Fasel, Fayzelle

Faizon (Arabic) understanding

Fakhr (Arabic) proud

Faladrick (Origin unknown) form of Frederick: plainspoken leader; peaceful
Faldrick, Faldrik

Falcon (American) bird as name; dark; watchful
Falk, Falkon

Falcone (Latin) of the falcons

Faldo (Last name as first) brassy

Falguni (Indian) Hindi for month
Falgun

Faline (Hindi) fertile

Falk (Hebrew) falcon
Falke

Falkner (French) handles falcons
Fowler, Faulkner

Fallows (English) inactive
Fallow

Falvey (English) of the falcons

Fam (American) family-oriented
Fammy

Famous (American) ambitious
Fame

Fane (English) exuberant
Fain, Faine

Fanlie (American) free

Fannin (English) happy
Fane

Fant (Latin) guileless

Fantroy (French) naive, royal

Fany (Spanish) freedom

Faolan (Irish) wolf; sly
Felan, Phelan

Far (English) traveler
Farr

Faraji (African) he who comforts others

Faralito (Spanish) comforts

Faramond (English) protected
Faramund, Farrimond, Farrimund, Pharamond, Pharamund

Faran (American) sincere
Fahran, Faren, Faron, Feren, Ferren

Fardan (Arabic) unique

Fareed (Arabic) special

Fargo (American) jaunty
Fargouh

Farhad (Arabic) unusual

Faris (Arabic) knighted

Farkas (Last name as first name) strong man

Farley (English) open
Farl, Farlee, Farleigh, Farlie, Farly, Farlye

Farmer (English) he farms

Farnall (Last name as first name) strong man
Farnell, Fernald

Farnham (English) windblown; field
Farnhum, Farnie, Farnum, Farny

Farnley (English) from a place of ferns

Farno (Italian) in ferns

Farold (Invented) lively

Farolito (Spanish) little ferns

Farouk (Arabic) knowing what's true
Faruq, Faruqh

Farquar (French) masculine

Farr (English) adventurer
Far

Farrar (French) distinguished
Farr

Farre (English) wanders

Farrell (Irish) brave
Farel, Farell, Faryl

Farren (English) mover
Faran, Faron, Farrin, Farron

Farris (Arabic) rider; Irish rock; reliable, *Fare, Farice, Faris*

Farro (Italian) grain
Farron, Faro

Farrow (English) tends the pigs

Fasta (Spanish) offering

Fattah (Arabic) conqueror

Faughn (Italian) raven

Faulkner (English) disciplinarian
Falcon, Falconner, Falkner, Falkoner

Faunus (Latin) god of nature
Fawnus

Fausatino (Spanish) lucky

Faust (Latin) lucky
Fauston

Faustino (Italian) lucky

Favero (French) insightful

Favian (Latin) knowing
Fav, Favion

Favor (French) gives

Fawad (Arabic) victorious

Fawcett (American) audacious
Fawce, Fawcet, Fawcette, Fawcie, Fawsie, Fowcett

Faxan (Anglo-Saxon) outgoing
Faxen, Faxon

Faxon (German) lush hair

Fay (Irish) raven-haired
Faye, Fayette

Fayne (English) happy

Faysal (Arabic) judgmental

Fazio (Italian) diligent

Fe (Latin) shining

Fearon (American) keen

Febronio (Spanish) bright

Fedde (Dutch) ruler

Federico (Spanish) peaceful and affluent
Federik

Fedil (French) excellence

Fedor (German) form of Theodore: God's gift; a blessing
Faydor, Feodor, Fyodor

Fedrick (American) form of Cedric: leader
Fed, Fedric, Fedrik

Feeney (Irish) last name as first name; soldier

Feibush (Last name as first name) particular

Feivel (Hebrew) bright

Feixon (Hebrew) helped by God

Feldronio (Spanish) from the field

Felimy (Irish) good

Felipe (Spanish) horse-lover
Felepe, Filipe, Flippo

Felix (Latin) joyful
Felixce, Filix, Phelix, Philix

Felker (English) last name as first name

Fellini (Last name as first) carnivalesque

Felman (Last name as first name) smart
Fel, Fell

Felton (English) farming the field

Fenimore (Last name as first name) creative

Fenner (English) capable
Fen, Fenn, Fynner

Fennessey (English) form of Phineas: farsighted

Fenris (Scandinavian) fierce

Fenton (English) nature-loving
Fen, Fenn, Fennie, Fenny

Fentress (English) natural
Fentres, Fyntres

Fenwick (English) from the marsh village; able

Feo (Native American) confident
Feeo, Feoh

Ferdinand (German) adventurer
Ferdie, Ferdnand, Ferdy, Fernand

Ferenc (Hungarian) free

Ferg (Irish) strong

Fergall (Irish) bravest man
Fearghall, Forgael

Fergonn (French) strong

Fergus (Irish) feargus
Ferges, Fergie, Fergis, Fergy

Ferguson (Irish) bold; excellent
Fergie, Fergs, Fergus, Fergusahn, Fergusen, Fergy, Furgs, Furgus

Ferlin (American) countrified
Ferlan

Ferll (Irish) strong

Fermin (Spanish) strong-willed
Fer, Fermen, Fermun

Fernan (Spanish) risk-taker

Fernando (Spanish) bold leader
Ferd, Ferdie, Ferdinando, Ferdy, Fernand

Fernao (Spanish) form of Fernando: bold leader

Fernley (English) from the fern meadow; natural
Farnlea, Farnlee, Farnleigh, Farnley, Fernlea, Fernlee, Fernleigh

Feroza (Persian) lucky

Feroze (Persian) lucky

Ferrand (French) gray-haired
Ferrant, Farrand, Farrant

Ferraro (Italian) fiery

Ferrell (Irish) hero
Fere, Ferrel, Feryl

Ferret (English) star

Ferris (Irish) rock
Farris, Farrish, Ferriss

Ferylin (Irish) hero

Festatus (Irish) raven; dark

Festive (American) word as
name; joyful
Fest, Festas, Festes

Festus (Latin) happy
Festes

Feven (Russian) sees God

Fhoki (Japanese)
discriminating

Fiachra (Irish) raven;
watchful

Fico (Italian) form of
Frederick: plainspoken leader;
peaceful

Fidel (Latin) faithful
Fidele, Fidell, Fydel

Fideles (Latin) loyal

Fidencio (Spanish) fidence
Fidens, Fido

Fides (Greek) calms

Field (English) outdoorsman
Fields

Fielding (English)
outdoorsman; working the
fields

Fien (American) elegant
Fiene, Fine

Fiero (Spanish) fiery

Fierro (Spanish) fiery

Fife (Scottish) bright-eyed
Fyfe, Phyfe

Fifel (Scottish) form of Fife:
bright-eyed

Fiji (Place name) Fiji Islands;
islander
Fege, Fegee, Fijie

Fikry (American) industrious
Fike, Fikree, Fikrey

Filbert (English) genius
Fil, Filb, Bert, Phil

Filemon (Greek) loves horses

Filetus (Biblical) beloved

Filinto (Spanish) friendly

Filip (Greek) horse-lover;
Belgium
form of Philip, Fil, Fill

Filmer (English) form of
Filmore: famed
Fill, Filmar

Filmore (English) famed
*Fill, Fillie, Fillmore, Filly,
Fylmore*

Filomelo (Spanish) friend

Filson (last name as first
name) son of Phil; meanders

Fimy (African) loved by God

Finbar (Irish) blond

Finbarr (Irish) blond

Finch (Last name as first
name) birdlike

Fineas (Egyptian) dark

Finell (Irish) blond

Finesse (English) word as
name; extreme delicacy or
subtlety in action

Finian (Irish) fair
Fin, Finean, Finn, Fynian

Finis (Latin) finished

Finlan (Irish) blond

Finlay (Irish) blond soldier
Finley, Findlay, Findley

Finley (Irish) magical
Fin, Finny, Fynn, Fynnie

Finn (Scandinavian) fair-
haired; from Finland
Fin, Finnie, Finny

Finna (Scandinavian) blond

Finnegan (Irish) fair
Finegan, Finigan, Finn, Finny

Finnian (German) from
Finland

Finoch (Scottish) blond

Fintan (Irish) small blond
man

Finton (Irish) magical
Finn, Finny, Fynton

Fiorello (Italian) flowering

Firdaus (Arabic) from the
garden of paradise

Firman (French) loyal
*Firmin, Farman, Farmann,
Fermin*

Firoozeh (Arabic) succeeds

Fishel (Hebrew) fish
Fish, Fysh

Fisher (English) he fishes
Fish, Fischer, Fisscher, Visscher

Fisk (Scandinavian)
fisherman
Fiske

Fitch (French) throws spears

Fito (Spanish) little

Fitz (French) bright young
man; son
Fitzy

Fitzgerald (English) bright
young man; Gerald's son

Fitzhugh (French) Hugh's
son; big-hearted

Fitzmorris (Last name as first
name) son of Morris
Fitz, Morrey, Morris

Fitzpatrick (French) Patrick's
son; noble

Fitzroy (French) son of Roy;
lively

Fitzsimmons (English)
bright young man;
Simmons's son

Five (Word as name)

Fiven (American) five

Flabia (Spanish) light-haired
Flavia

Flag (American) patriotic
Flagg

Flame (last name as first
name) confident

Flaminio (Spanish) priest;
thoughtful
Flamino

Flann (Irish) red-haired
Flainn, Flannan, Flannery

Flannan (Irish) red-haired

Flannigan (last name as first
name) red-haired

Flappan (last name as first
name)

Flass (last name as first
name)

Flaubert (French) fame,
bright

Flavean (Flavian) form of Flavian: blond

Flavian (Greek) blond
Flovian

Flavio (Italian) shining
Flav, Flavioh

Fleada (American) introvert
Flayda

Fleetwood (English) from the woods

Flemmer (English) a native of Flanders

Flemming (English) a native of Flanders; confident
Fleming, Flyming

Fletcher (English) kindhearted; maker of arrows
Fletch, Fletchi, Fletchie, Fletchy

Flimmel (last name as first name)

Flint (English) stream; nature-lover
Flinn, Flintt, Flynt, Flynnt

Flintlee (English) of the stream

Flip (English) loves horses; wild movements

Flippin (Spanish) form of Felipe: horse-lover

Floan (American) form of Flynn: brash

Floran (Spanish) flourishing like a flower garden

Florante (Spanish) flowers

Florecio (Spanish) flowering

Florencione (Italian) flowering

Florentin (Italian) blooming
Florencio

Florian (Latin) flourishing
Florean, Florie

Floyd (English) practical; hair of gray
Floid

Flux (Middle English) flowing

Flynn (Irish) brash
Flin, Flinn, Flinnie, Flinny, Flyne

Flynt (English) flowing; stream
Flint, Flinte, Flinty, Flynte

Fobbs (last name as first name) flourishing

Fobo (Greek) fearful

Fogle (last name as first name)

Folan (last name as first name) of the folks

Foley (Last name as first name) creative
Folee, Folie

Folke (German) of the people

Folker (German) watchful
Folke, Folko

Follis (last name as first name) of the folks

Fonseca (Italian) fom Alphonso

Fontayne (French) giving; fountain
Font, Fontaine, Fontane, Fountaine

Fontenot (French) fountain

Fonzie (German) form of Alphonse: distinguished
Fons, Fonsi, Fonz, Fonzi

For (American) representative
Fore

Foran (American) derivative of foreign; exotic
Foren, Forun

Forbes (Irish) wealthy
Forb

Ford (English) strong
Feord, Forde, Fyord

Fordan (English) river crossing; inventive
Ford, Forday, Forden

Foreign (American) word as name; foreigner
Foran

Foreman (last name as first name) leader

Forend (American) forward
Fore, Foryn, Forynd

Forest (French) nature-loving
Forrest, Fory, Fourast

Forester (English) protective; of the forest
Forrester, Forry

Forge (English) crosses stream

Foros (Greek) carries forward

Forsey (Scottish) last name as first name; man of peace

Fortino (Spanish) fortune

Fortney (Latin) strength of character
Fortenay, Forteney, Forteny, Fortny, Fourtney

Fortune (French) fortunate man
Fortounay, Fortunae

Fortuno (Spanish) lucky man
Fortunio

Fost (Latin) form of Foster: worthy
Foste, Fostee, Fosty

Foster (Latin) worthy
Fauster, Fostay

Fotis (Greek) light

Fouad (Arabic) good heart
Fuad

Fowler (English) hunter; traps fowl
Fowller

Foy (American) foible

Frace (American) fragile

Fraime (Anglo-Saxon) newcomer

Fraine (English) ash tree; tall
Frayne, Freyne

Fralin (last name as first name) frail

Francesco (Italian) flirtatious
Fran, Francey, Frankie, Franky

Franchot (French) free

Francis (Latin) free spirit; from France
Fran, Frances, Franciss, Frank, Franky, Frannkie, Franny, Frans

Francisco (Spanish) form of Francis: free spirit; from France
Chuco, Cisco, Francisk, Franco, Frisco, Paco, Pancho

Francista (Spanish) frenchman; free
Cisco, Cisto, Francisco, Franciscus, Fransico

Franckie (German) dynamic

Franco (Spanish) defender; spear
Francoh, Franko

Francois (French) smooth; patriot; Frenchman
Frans, Franswaw, French, Frenchie, Frenchy

Frank (English) form of Franklin: outspoken; landowner
Franc, Franco, Frankee, Frankie, Frankey, Frankie, Franko, Franky

Frankel (German) free

Franklin (English) outspoken; landowner
Francklin, Franclin, Frank, Frankie, Franklinn, Franklyn, Franklynn, Franky

Franqueli (Italian) free

Frantisek (Czech) free man

Franz (German) man from France; free
Frans

Frasher (English) curls

Frasier (English) attractive; man with curls
Frase, Fraser, Fraze, Frazer

Frayley (English) of the ash meadow

Frayne (English) foreigner
Fraine, Frayn, Frean, Freen, Freyne

Fraze (English) curls

Fred (German) form of Frederick: plainspoken leader; peaceful
Fredde, Freddo, Freddy, Fredo

Fredder (German) form of Fred: plainspoken leader; peaceful

Freddie (German) form of Frederick: plainspoken leader; peaceful
Freddee, Freddey, Freddi, Freddy

Freddis (German) form of Frederick: plainspoken leader; peaceful
Freddus, Fredes, Fredis

Fredell (German) form of Frederick: plainspoken leader; peaceful

Frederic (French) peaceful king
Fred, Freddy

Frederick (German) plainspoken leader; peaceful
Fred, Freddy, Frederic, Fredrich, Fredrik, Fryderyk

Freeborn (English) born free

Freed (English) free boy
Fried

Freedom (American) loves freedom

Freedy (English) free

Freeman (English) free man
Free, Freedman, Freman

Fremont (German) protective; noble

Fren (Spanish) form of Francisco: free

French (English) boy from France

Francisco (Spanish) free

Fres (Spanish) fresh air

Fresco (Spanish) open

Freslev (American) freshness

Frewen (Anglo-Saxon) free
Frewin

Frey (Scandinavian) fertility god

Frick (English) brave man

Frid (German) peaceful

Fridmann (Last name as first name) free man

Fridolf (Scandinavian) relishes peace
Freydolf, Freydulf, Friedolf, Fridulf

Fridolin (German) free

Frieder (German) peaceful
leader
Frie, Fried, Friedrick

Friederich (German) form of
Frederick: plainspoken leader;
peaceful
Fridrich, Friedrich

Friedhelm (German)
peaceful helmet
Friedelm

Frisco (American) form of
Francisco: free spirit; from
France
Cisco, Frisko

Friso (Anglo-Saxon) best self

Fritz (German) form of
Frederick: plainspoken leader
*Firzie, Firzy, Frits, Fritts,
Fritzi, Fritzie, Fritzy*

Fritzie (German) peaceful

Fritzon (Norse) peacemaker

Frode (Scandinavian)
intellectual

Froilan (German) popular
leader

Fromel (Hebrew) outgoing

Frosino (Italian) merry

Frost (English) cold; freeze

Frosten (American) of the
winter

Froyim (Hebrew) kind

Fructuoso (Spanish) fruitful
Fru, Fructo

Fry (English) new sprout;
growing
Frye, Fryer

Fu (Japanese) form of Fudo:
the god of fire and wisdom

Fuddy (Origin unknown)
bright-eyed
Fuddie, Fudee, Fudi

Fudo (Japanese) the god of
fire and wisdom

Fukuda (Japanese) field

Fulbright (German) brilliant;
full of brightness
Fulbrite

Fulgentius (Latin) full of
kindness; shines
Fulgencio

Fulke (English) folksy
Fulk, Fawke, Fowke

Fuller (English) tough-willed
Fuler

Fullerton (English) strong
Fuller, Fullerten

Fulton (English) fresh mind;
field by the town

Funge (Last name as first
name) stodgy
Funje, Funny

Furlo (American) macho
Furl

Furman (German) form of
Firman: loyal
*Fuhrman, Fuhrmann,
Furmann*

Fursey (Irish) spiritual

Fyfe (Scottish) craftsman
Fife, Fyffe, Phyfe

Fyodor (Russian) divine
Feodor, Fyodr

G

Gabae (Biblical) loves God

Gabaldon (English) last name as first name

Gabata (Biblical) place name

Gabbana (Italian) creative
Gabi

Gabe (Hebrew) form of Gabriel: God's hero; devout
Gabbee, Gabbi, Gabbie, Gabby, Gabi, Gabie, Gaby

Gabino (Spanish) strong believer
Gabby, Gabi

Gable (French) dashing

Gablen (American) form of Gabriel: God's hero; devout

Gabor (Last name as first name) believer; colorful

Gabriel ❂ ❂ (Hebrew) God's hero; devout
Gabby, Gabe, Gabi, Gabreal, Gabrel, Gabriele, Gabrielle, Gabryel

Gad (Hebrew) lucky; audacious
Gadd

Gaddi (Arabic) loves God

Gaddiel (Hebrew) fortunate
Gadiel

Gaddiel (Biblical) loves God

Gaddis (American) hard to please; picky
Gad, Gaddes, Gadis

Gadi (Hebrew) form of Gaddiel: fortunate
Gadish

Gael (English) speaks Gaelic; independent

Gaetano (Italian) from the city of Gaeta; Italian man
Gaetan, Geitano, Guytano

Gaffar (Arabic) from the stream

Gagan (French) form of Gage: dedicated
Gage

Gage (French) dedicated

Gager (French) dedicated

Gaghe (American) jaunty

Gaham (Biblical) searches

Gahuj (African) hunts

Gailen (French) healer; physician
Galan, Galen, Galun

Gain (Word as name) gainful

Gaines (Last name as first name) rich
Ganes, Gaynes

Gaines (English) increase in wealth

Gair (Irish) little boy
Gaer, Geir

Gaither (French) victor

Gaius (Latin) joyful
Gal

Galatian (Biblical) bible book
Galatians

Galavis (Greek) white

Galax (Spanish) of the galaxy

Galbraith (Irish) sensible
Gal

Galbreath (Irish) practical man
Galbraith, Gall

Galdin (American) calm

Galdino (Spanish) calm

Gale (English) cheerful
Gael, Gail, Gaile, Gaille, Gayle

Galegina (Native American)
lithe; deer

Galen (Greek) calming;
intelligent
*Gaelin, Gailen, Gale, Galean,
Galey, Gaylen*

Galene (Spanish) shining

Galfrid (Last name as first
name) uplifted
Galfryd

Gali (Spanish) shining

Galileo (Italian) from Galilee
Galilayo

Gallagher (Irish) helpful
*Galagher, Gallager, Gallie,
Gally*

Gallant (American) savoir-
faire
Gael, Gail, Gaila, Gaile, Gayle

Gallman (Last name as first
name) lively
Galman, Gallway, Galway

Galloway (Irish) outgoing
Gallie, Gally, Galoway, Galway

Galo (Spanish) enthusiastic
Gallo

Galt (German) empowered

Galton (English) landowner;
reclusive

Galvin (Irish) sparrow; flighty
*Gallven, Gallvin, Galvan,
Galven, Galway*

Gamal (Arabic) camel; travels
long distances

Gamaliel (Hebrew) rewarded
by God
Gamaleel, Gamalyel

Gamba (African) warring

Gamberro (Spanish)
hooligan
Gami

Gamble (Scandinavian)
mature wisdom
*Gam, Gamb, Gambel, Gambie,
Gamby*

Gamel (Hebrew) God
rewards him

Gamliel (Arabic) camel;
wanders
Gamaliel

Gammon (Last name as first
name) game
Gamen, Gamon, Gamun

Gan (Chinese) wanders wide

Gandy (American)
adventurer

Ganesh (Hindi) Lord of all

Ganit (American) leader

Ganon (Irish) fair-skinned
Gannon, Ganny

Ganso (Spanish) goose; goofy
Gans, Ganz

Ganya (Russian) strong

Gar (English) form of Garbin:
pure

Garai (African) settled

Garbhan (Irish) rough boy

Garbin (Spanish) pure

Garbini (Spanish) pure

Garcia (Spanish) strong
Garce, Garcey, Garsey

Gard (English) guard
*Garde, Gardey, Gardi, Gardie,
Gardy, Guard*

Gardner (English) keeper of the garden
Gar, Gard, Gardener, Gardie, Gardiner, Gardnyr, Gardy

Garee (English) form of Gary: strong man

Garek (Polish) brave boy
Garreck, Garrik, Gerek

Gareth (Irish) kind
Gare

Garfiel (English) form of Garfield: armed

Garfield (English) armed
Gar, Garfeld

Gariana (Hindi) shout

Garin (American) form of Darin: great
Gare, Gary

Garis (Biblical) place name

Garl (French) form of Garland: adorned

Garland (French) adorned
Gar, Garlan, Garlend, Garlind, Garlynd

Garlando (Spanish) wreath

Garlon (French) wreath

Garmon (German) man who throws spears
Garmen

Garn (American) prepared
Gar, Garnie, Garny, Garr

Garner (French) guard
Gar, Garn, Garnar, Garnir

Garnett (English) armed; spear
Gar, Garn, Garnet, Garny

Garnock (Welsh) from the alder-tree place; outdoor spirit

Garoa (Spanish) morning dew

Garold (American) form of Harold: leader of an army

Garon (American) gentle
Garonn, Garonne

Garonzick (Last name as first name) secure
Gare, Garon, Garons, Garonz

Garr (English) form of Garrett: brave; watchful; form of Garth: sunny; gardener
Gar

Garrad (English) form of Gerard: brave

Garren (American) kind

Garreth (German) brave
Gareth, Garryth, Garyth

Garrett (Irish) brave; watchful
Gare, Garet, Garitt, Garret, Garritt, Gary, Gerrot

Garrick (English) ruler with a spear; brave
Garey, Garic, Garick, Garik, Garreck, Gary, Gerrick, Gerrieck

Garridan (English) form of Gary: strong man

Garrison (French) prepared
Garris, Garrish, Garry, Gary

Garrist (English) form of Garrison: prepared

Garroway (English) throws spears; physical presence
Garraway

Garson (English) son of Gar; fort home; industrious

Garth (Scandinavian) sunny; gardener
Gar, Gare, Garry, Gart, Garthe, Gary

Garthay (Irish) form of
Gareth: gentle
Garthae

Garton (English) place of
spear man; rowdy

Garv (English) peaceful
Garvey, Garvy

Garvan (English) throws
spears; athletic

Garver (English) friend

Garvy (Irish) peacemaker
Garvey

Garwin (English) friend who
struggles

Garwood (English) natural
*Garr, Garwode, Garwoode,
Woody*

Gary (English) strong man
Gare, Garrey, Garri

Garyle (German) form of
Gary: strong man
Strong

Gask (American) form of
Gaskill

Gaskill (last name as first
name)

Gasos (Greek) form of
Pegasus: horse; rider

Gaspard (French) holds
treasure
Gaspar, Gasper

Gaspare (Italian) treasure-
holder
Casper, Gasp, Gasparo

Gassia (Slavic) treasure

Gaston (French) native of
Gascony; stranger
Gastawn, Gastowyn

Gat (American) form of
Gatam: their lowing; their
touch

Gatam (Biblical) their lowing;
their touch

Gataz (Spanish) open-
minded

Gatch (American) jaunty

Gate (English) open
Gait, Gates

Gath (Biblical) place name

Gathen (American) form of
Gath: place name

Gathrir (American) form of
Gath: place name

Gatlin (last name as first
name)

Gatsby (Literature) from
Fitzgerald's *The Great Gatsby*;
ambitious; tragic

Gaudencio (Spanish) content

Gaudy (American) word as
name; colorful
Gaudin, Gaudy

Gauge (French) form of
Gage: dedicated

Gauran (French) form of
George: land-loving; farmer

Gaurav (Hindi) proud

Gauri (Indian) white

Gautier (French) form of
Walter: army leader
Gauther, Gauthier

Gavard (Last name as first
name) creative
Gav, Gaverd

Gavin ✪ (English) alert; hawk
*Gav, Gaven, Gavinn, Gavon,
Gavvin, Gavyn*

Gavine (French) hawk

Gavino (Italian) hawk

Gavra (Hebrew) dedicated to
God

Gavri (Hebrew) form of
Gavriel: filled by God's
strength

Gavriel (Herbew) filled by
God's strength
Gavryel

Gavril (Hebrew) strong
Gavrill, Gavryl, Gavryll

Gawain (Hebrew) archangel
Gawaine, Gawayne, Gwayne

Gawath (Welsh) form of
Gawain: archangel

Gawin (Scottish) watchful;
wise
Gawyn

Gayathri (Russian) God-
fearing

Gaylin (Greek) calm
Gaelin, Gayle, Gaylen, Gaylon

GayLord (French)
high-energy
*Gallerd, Galurd, Gaylar,
Gayllaird, Gaylor*

Gaynor (Irish) spunky
Gainer, Gaye, Gayner

Gayton (Irish) fair
Gayten, Gaytun

Gaza (Arabic) place name;
strong

Gazara (Biblical) place name

Gean (American) form of
Gene: noble

Gearld (English) changes

Gearn (English) changes

Geary (English) flexible
Gearey

Gebby (German) gifted

Gedaliah (Hebrew) great in
Jehovah's love
*Gedalia, Gedaliahu, Gedalya,
Gedalyahu*

Gedion (French) form of
Gideon: power-weilding

Gedor (Biblical) place name

Geer (German) spearman
Geere

Gefaniah (Hebrew) vineyard
of the Lord; grows
*Gefania, Gefanya, Gephania,
Gephaniah*

Geibe (American) bright

Geir (Biblical) shining

Geka (Scandinavian) armed

Gelo (Russian) nobility

Gemini (Astrology) zodiac
twins; intelligent

Gen (Slavic) family man

Genaro (Latin) dedicated
Genaroe, Genaroh

Gene (Greek) noble
Geno, Jene, Jeno

General (American) military
rank as name; leader

Genio (Spanish) blue blood

Gennaro (Latin) devout

Geno (Italian) spontaneous

Genoah (Place name) city in
Italy
Genoa, Jenoa, Jenoah

Genoris (Italian) giving

Genovese (Italian)
spontaneous; from Genoa
*Genno, Geno, Genovise,
Genovize*

Gent (American) from
gentleman; mannerly
Gynt, Jent, Jynt

Gentil (Spanish) charming
Gentilo

Gentry (American) high breeding
Genntrie, Gent, Gentree, Gentree, Gentrie

Genty (Irish) man of snow; changes

Geo (Greek) form of George: land-loving; farmer
Gee

Geoff (English) form of Geoffrey: peaceful
Jeff

Geoffrey (English) peaceful
Geffry, Geoff, Geoffie, Geoffry, Geoffy, Geofry, Jeff

Geordan (Scottish) from the hill

Georg (German) works with the earth

George (Greek) land-loving; farmer
Georg, Georgi, Georgie, Georgy, Jorg, Jorge

George-Hamilton (American) star quality

Georgio (Italian) earth-worker
Giorgio, Jorgio, Jorjeo, Jorjio

Georgios (Greek) land-loving

Georgy (Greek) form of George: land-loving; farmer
Georgee, Georgi, Georgie

Geraint (English) old

Gerald (German) strong; ruling with a spear
Geralde, Gerrald, Gerre, Gerry

Gerant (Welsh) eldest

Gerar (French) brave

Gerard (French) brave
Gerord, Gerr, Gerrard

Gerardus (American) brave

Gerben (Dutch) spear-wielder

Gerber (Last name as first name) particular
Gerb

Gerbold (German) bold with a spear
Gerbolde

Gerdano (Italian) descends

Gere (English) spear-wielding; dramatic
Gear

Gereon (German) old soul

Gerhard (German) forceful
Ger, Gerd

Gerhard (French) finds

Gerico (American) form of Jericho: nocturnal

Gerlach (German) athlete with spears; musical

Gerlie (Spanish) wins

Germain (French) growing; from Germany
Germa, Germaine, Germane, Germay, Germayne, Jermaine

German (German) from the country of Germany

Gerod (English) form of Gerard: brave
Garard, Geraldo, Gerard, Gerarde, Gere, Gererde, Gerry, Gerus, Giraud, Jerade, Jerard, Jere, Jerod, Jerott, Jerry

Gerodi (Italian) form of Gerod: brave

Gerold (Danish) rules with spears
Gerrold, Gerry

Geronimo (Italian) sacred name
Geronimoh

Gerrist (Slavic) strong

Gerrit (Dutch) protective

Gerry (English) form of
Gerald: strong; ruling with a
spear
*Gerr, Gerre, Gerree, Gerrey,
Gerri, Gerrie*

Gersh (Biblical) form of
Gershon: his banishment; the
change of pilgrimage
Gershe, Gursh, Gurshe

Gershom (Hebrew) exile

Gershon (Biblical) his
banishment; the change of
pilgrimage

Gerson (English) Gary's son

Gerton (English) town of
Gary

Gervaise (French) man of
honor
Gerv, Gervase, Gervay

Gervasio (Spanish)
aggressive
Gervase, Gervaso, Jervasio

Gervis (German) honored
*Jervis, Gerv, Gervace, Gervaise,
Gervey, Jervaise*

Gerwyn (Welsh) fair and
lovely

Geshem (Hebrew) raining

Geter (Origin unknown)
hopeful
Getterr, Getur

Gether (Biblical) in the dark

Gethin (Welsh) dark skin

Gevariah (Hebrew) strength
*Gevaria, Gevarya, Gevaryah,
Gevaryahu*

Ghalby (Origin unknown)
winning
Galby

Ghalib (Arabic) wins

Ghassan (Arabic) in the
prime of life

Ghayth (Arabic) victor
Ghaith

Gheorgh (Welsh) form of
George: land-loving; farmer

Ghorm (American) form of
Gorm: blue-eyed

Ghoshal (Hindi) the speaker
Ghoshil

Ghulam (Arabic) slave;
servant

Gi (Italian) form of Giann:
believer in a gracious God

Giacomo (Italian)
replacement; musical
Como, Gia

Giann (Italian) believer in a
gracious God
*Ghiann, Giahanni, Gian,
Gianni, Giannie, Gianny*

Gianni (Italian) calm; believer
in God's grace
Giannie, Gianny

Gibbon (Scottish) strong
Gibben, Gibbons

Gibbs (English) form of
Gibson: smiling
Gib, Gibb, Gibbes

Gibeah (Biblical) a hill

Gibeon (Biblical) place name

Giblen (English) last name as
first name

Gibor (Hebrew) strong one

Gibson (English) smiling
*Gib, Gibb, Gibbie, Gibbson,
Gibby, Gibsan, Gibsen, Gibsyn*

Gid (Hebrew) form of
Gideon: power-wielding
Gidd, Giddee, Giddi, Giddy

Gideon (Hebrew) power-
wielding
*Giddy, Gideone, Gidion,
Gidyun*

Gidney (English) strong
Gidnee, Gidni

Gidon (Biblical) form of
Gideon: power-wielding

Gif (English) giver
Giff

Giffin (English) giving
Giffyn

Gifford (English) generous-
hearted
Giford

Gifford (English) generous-
hearted
Giff, Gifferd, Giffie, Giffy

Gig (English) man in the
carriage

Giggs (English) carriage man

Gil (Hebrew) form of Gilam:
joyful people
Gill

Gilad (Hebrew) testimonial
hill; outspoken
Giladi, Gilead

Gilam (Hebrew) joyful people

Gilbert (English) intelligent
Gil, Gilber, Gilburt, Gill, Gilly

Gilberto (Spanish) bright
*Bertie, Berty, Gil, Gilb,
Gilburto, Gillberto, Gilly*

Gilboa (Biblical) place name

Gilbran (Spanish) thinker

Gilby (Irish) blond
Gilbie, Gill, Gillbi

Gilchrist (Irish) open
Gill

Gildardo (German) excellent

Gildea (Irish) God's servant

Gildo (Italian) macho
Gil, Gill, Gilly

Giles (French) protective
Gile, Gyles

Gilesp (Irish) form of
Gillespie: humble

Gilford (English) kindhearted
Gill, Gillford, Guilford

Gilgal (Biblical) place name

Gill (Hebrew) happy man
Gil, Gilli, Gillie, Gilly

Gillanders (Scottish) serves

Gillean (Scottish) able server
Gillan, Gillen, Gillian

Gillent (French) form of
Gilbert: intelligent

Gilles (French) miraculous
Geal, Zheal, Zheel

Gillespie (Irish) humble
Gilespie, Gill, Gilley, Gilli, Gilly

Gillett (French) hospitable
Gelett, Gelette, Gillette

Gilley (American) countrified
Gill, Gilleye, Gilli, Gilly

Gillian (Irish) devout
Gill, Gilley, Gilly, Gillyun

Gillor (American) serves well

Gilman (Irish) serving well
*Gilley, Gilli, Gillman,
Gillmand, Gilly, Gilmand,
Gilmon*

Gilmer (English) riveting
Gelmer, Gill, Gillmer, Gilly

Gilmi (Irish) devout

Gilmore (Irish) riveting
Gill, Gillmore, Gilmohr

Gilo (Hebrew) joyful

Gilon (Hebrew) joyful
Gill

Gilroy (Irish) king's devotee
Gilderoy, Gildray, Gildrey, Gildroy, Gillroy

Gilson (Irish) devoted son

Gilus (Scottish) Jesus's servant

Gimarrai (Biblical) place name

Gimzo (Biblical) place name

Ginnesar (Biblical) place name

Gino (Italian) of good breeding; outgoing
Geeno, Geino, Ginoh

Gins (Greek) life-giving

Ginton (Hebrew) garden

Giona (Italian) form of Giovanni: jovial; happy believer

Giordano (Italian) delivered
Giorgie, Jiordano

Giorgio (Italian) earthy; creative
George, Georgeeo, Georgo, Jorge, Jorgio

Giovanni (Italian) jovial; happy believer
Geovanni, Gio, Giovani, Giovannie, Giovanny, Vannie, Vanny, Vonny

Gipsy (English) travels widely

Girioel (Welsh) Lord

Girolamo (Italian) form of Jerome: holy name; blessed

Giron (American) form of Garon: gentle

Girvin (Irish) tough-minded

Girvan, Girven, Girvon

Gisbert (French) aggressor

Gisli (French) loyal

Gitel (Hebrew) good

Gittaim (Biblical) place name

Gitte (Scandinavian) celebrated

Gittel (Hebrew) good

Giulio (Italian) youth

Giuseppe (Italian) capable
Beppo, Giusepe, Gusepe

Given (Last name as first name) gift
Givens, Gyvan, Gyven, Gyvin

Givon (Hebrew) boy of heights

Gizmo (American) playful
Gis, Gismo, Giz

Gizon (Spanish) morning

Glad (American) happy
Gladd, Gladde, Gladdi, Gladdie, Gladdy

Gladspell (last name as first name) happy

Gladston (last name as first name) happy

Gladstone (English) cheering

Gladus (Welsh) lame; rueful

Gladwyn (English) friend who has a light heart
Glad, Gladdy, Gladwin, Gladwynn

Glaisne (Irish) serene
Glasny

Glancy (American) form of Clancy: lively; feisty redhead
Glance, Glancee, Glancey, Glanci

Glanville (French) serene

Glasgow (Place name) city in Scotland

Glasson (Scottish) from Glasgow, Scotland

Glause (Spanish) blue eyes

Glen (Irish) natural wonder
Glenn

Glenard (Irish) from a glen; nature-loving
*Glen, Glenerd, Glenn,
Glennard, Glenni, Glennie*

Glendon (Scottish) fortified in nature
*Glen, Glend, Glenden, Glenn,
Glynden*

Glendower (Welsh) water valley boy

Glenmore (English) valley boy

Glenn (Irish) natural wonder
*Glen, Glenni, Glennie, Glenny,
Glynn, Glynny*

Glennon (Last name as first name) living in a valley
Glenen, Glennen, Glenon

Glenward (last name as first name)

Gloster (Place name) from Gloucester

Glyndwr (Welsh) water valley life
Glyn, Glynn, Glynne

Glynn (Welsh) lives in a restful glen
Glyn, Glin, Glinn

Gobi (Place name) desert in Central Asia; audacious
Gobee, Gobie

Gobind (Sanskrit) the name of a Hindi deity

Govind

Gockley (Last name as first name) peaceful
Gocklee

Goddard (German) staunch in spirituality
Godard, Godderd, Goddird

Godfred (German) peaceful; God's child

Godfrey (Irish) peaceful
Godfree, Godfrie, Godfry

Godfried (German) imbued with God's peace
Godfreed

Godinez (Spanish) loves God

Godofredo (Spanish) form of Godfrey: peaceful

Godric (English) man of God
*Godrick, Godrik, Godryc,
Godryck, Godryk*

Godridge (Last name as first name) place of God

Godwin (English) close to God
Godwinn, Godwyn, Godwynn

Goel (Hebrew) redeemed

Goethe (Last name as first name) poet

Goforth (English) peace wish

Gofraidh (Irish) God's peace child
Gothfraidh, Gothraidh

Goger (last name as first name) paternal

Gohn (African American) spirited
Gon

Golan (Biblical) place name

Golding (English) golden boy

Goldo (English) golden
Golo

Goliath (Hebrew) large
Goliathe

Gombos (last name as first name) thorough

Gomda (Native American) wind's moods

Gomer (English) famed fighter
Gomar, Gomher, Gomor

Gomorr (Place name) the battle

Gong (American) forceful

Gonz (Spanish) form of Gonzalo: feisty wolf
Gons, Gonz, Gonza, Gonzales, Gonzalez

Gonzales (Spanish) feisty
Gonzalez

Gonzalo (Spanish) feisty wolf
Gonz, Gonzoloh

Goode (English) good
Good, Goodey, Goody

Goodman (Last name as first name) a good man
Goodeman

Goodreau (French) good

Goodrich (Last name as first name) giving; good
Goodriche

Gopin (Indian) cow song

Gor (last name as first name) hill

Goran (Croatian) good

Gordion (Biblical) place name

Gordo (American) jovial guy

Gordon (English) nature-lover; hill
Gord, Gordan, Gorden, Gordi, Gordie, Gordy

Gordy (English) form of Gordon: nature-lover; hill
Gordee, Gordi, Gordie

Gore (English) practical; pie-shaped land

Gorgey (Latin) gorge

Gorgonio (Greek) trouble

Gorham (English) sophisticated; name of a silver company
Goram

Gorky (Place name) Russian amusement park in the novel *Gorky Park*; mysterious
Gork, Gorkee, Gorkey, Gorki

Gorm (Irish) blue-eyed

Gorman (Irish) small man
Gormann, Gormen

Gormlee (Irish) blue-eyed

Goro (Japanese) fifth son

Goron (Welsh) handsome

Gosheven (Native American) leaps well; athletic

Goss (English/German) last name as first name

Gotam (Hindi) best cow; cherished
Gautam, Gautoma

Gottfried (German) form of Godfried: imbued with God's peace

Gotzon (German) angel

Goulet (French) last name as first name

Gouriet (French) charming

Govannon (Welsh) craftsman

Gower (Welsh) unblemished

Gowon (African) rainmaking

Gozal (Hebrew) baby bird; trying his wings

Gozan (Biblical) place name

Gradin (Irish) diligent

Grady (Irish) hardworking
Grade, Gradee, Gradey

Grae (Scottish) grand

Graem (Scottish) homebody
Graeme

Graffen (last name as first name) distinguished

Griffin (American) form of Griffin: unconventional

Graham (English) wealthy; grand house
Graeham, Graeme, Grame

Graig (American) form of Craig: brave climber

Grail (Word as name) desired; sought after
Grale, Grayle

Grajeda (Spanish) crow

Gram (American) form of Graham: wealthy; grand house

Granace (American) gray

Granados (Spanish) grand

Granbel (Last name as first name) grand and attractive
Granbell

Granberry (English) farms berries

Granderson (Last name as first name) grand
Grand, Grander

Grange (French) lonely; on the farm
Grainge, Granger, Grangher

Granicus (Biblical) place name

Granison (Last name as first name) son of Gran; grandiose
Gran, Grann

Granit (English) great

Granite (American) rock; hard
Granet

Grant (English) expansive
Grandt, Grann, Grannt

Grantland (French) tall

Grantly (French) tall; lithe •
Grantlea, Grantleigh, Grantley

Granvar (English) grand

Granville (French) grandiose
Grann, Granvel, Granvelle, Gravil

Grarol (English) gray

Grasshopper (American) lively

Gratton (last name as first name) God loved

Graven (English) gray

Gravette (Origin unknown) grave
Gravet

Gravitt (English) gray

Gray (English) hair of gray
Graye, Grey

Grayce (English) gray hair

Graydon (last name as first name) graceful

Grayer (English) gray

Graylon (English) gray-haired
Gray, Grayan, Graylan, Graylin

Grayson (English) son of man with gray hair
Gray, Grey, Greyson

Graz (Place name) city in Austria

Grazi (Italian) gracious

Graziano (Italian) dearest
Graciano, Graz

Greco (Italian) kind

Gredy (last name as first name)

Greek (American) Greek

Greeley (English) careful
Grealey, Greel, Greely

Greenlee (English) outdoorsy
Green, Greenlea, Greenly

Greenwood (English) untamed; forest
Greene, Greenwoode, Greenwude, Grenwood

Greer (Last name as first name) sly
Greere, Grier

Greerzen (American) son of Greer

Greg (Latin) form of Gregory: careful
Gregg, Greggie, Greggy

Greger (Scandinavian) form of Gregory: careful

Gregoire (French) watchful
Gregorie

Gregor (Greek) cautious
Greger, Gregors, Greig

Gregorio (Greek) careful

Gregory (Greek) careful
Greg, Greggory, Greggy, Gregori, Gregorie, Gregry

Gregson (Last name as first name) son of Greg; careful
Greggsen, Greggson, Gregsen

Grekel (American) vigilant

Grenville (New Zealand) outdoorsy
Granville, Gren

Gresham (English) of pasture village; sylvan
Grisham

Greville (English) thoughtful

Grey (Last name as first name) quiet; grey-haired
Greyson

Griden (Norse) peacemaker

Griffaw (Latin) ruddy

Griffin (Latin) unconventional
Greffen, Griff, Griffee, Griffen, Griffey, Griffie, Griffon, Griffy

Griffith (Welsh) able leader
Griff, Griffee, Griffey, Griffie, Griffy

Grigg (Welsh) vigilant

Grigori (Russian) watchful
Grig, Grigor

Grimbald (Last name as first name) dark
Grimbold

Grimes (English) spunky

Grimm (English) grim; dark
Grim, Grym

Grimshaw (English) from a dark forest; quiet

Grindon (last name as first name)

Gris (German) gray
Griz

Grischa (German) form of Gregory: careful

Griswald (German) bland
Greswold, Gris, Griswold

Grogan (last name as first name)

Grosvenor (French) hunts well

Grover (English) thriving
Grove

Gruver (Origin unknown) ambitious
Gruever

Gualberto (Spanish) believer

Gualter (Spanish) form of Walter: army leader

Guanjone (Spanish) strong

Guapo (Spanish) looker

Guard (American) protects

Guasparre (Italian) values

Gudy (German) good

Guenter (German) warrior

Guerdon (English) combative

Guerino (Italian) protects

Guerry (English) aggressive

Guido (Italian) form of Guy: wood
Guidoh, Gwedo, Gweedo

Guilford (English) from a ford with yellow flowers; nature-lover
Gilford, Guildford

Guillerm (German) form of William: staunch protector

Guillermo (Spanish) attentive
Guilermo, Gulermo

Gull (Scandinavian) godlike

Gullen (Scandinavian) godlike

Gullet (Latin) throat

Gulshan (Hindi) gardener; flourishes

Gultekin (Turkish) last name as first name

Gulzar (Arabic) thrives

Gumecindo (Spanish) excellent

Gunder (Scandinavian) form of Gunnar: bold

Gundy (American) friendly
Gundee

Gunion (last name as first name)

Gunn (Scandinavian) macho; gunman
Gun, Gunner

Gunnar (Scandinavian) bold
Gunn, Gunner, Gunnir

Guntersen (Scandinavian) macho; gunman
Gun, Gunth

Gunther (Scandinavian) able fighter
Funn, Gunnar, Gunner, Guntar, Gunthar, Gunthur

Gunvor (Scandinavian) watchful

Gunyon (American) tough; gunman
Gunn, Gunyun

Gur (Hindi) from guru; teacher

Gurd (Scandinavian) guards

Gurjeet (Indian) at the feet of the guru

Gurley (last name as first name) leads

Gurmot (German) speared

Gurpreet (Hindi) devoted follower

Guryon (Hebrew) lionlike
Garon, Gorion, Gurion

Gus (Scandinavian) form of Augustus: highly esteemed; form of Gustaf: armed; vital
Guss, Gussi, Gussy, Gussye

Gustachian (American) pretentious
Gus, Gussy, Gust

Gustaf (German) armed; vital
Gus, Gusstof, Gustav, Gustovo

Gustavo (Spanish) vital; gusto
Gus, Gustaffo, Gustav

Gustin (Spanish) serious

Gusto (Spanish) pleasure
Gusty

Gustus (Scandinavian) royal
Gus, Gustaf, Gustave, Gustavo

Guth (Irish) form of Guthrie: windy; heroic
Guthe, Guthry

Guthrie (Irish) windy; heroic
Guthree, Guthry

Gutierre (Spanish) form of Walter: army leader

Guto (Welsh) royal; tired

Guy (French) wood
leader, Guye

Guyon (French) leads

Guzet (American) bravado
Guzz, Guzzett, Guzzie

Gwandoya (African) miserable fate

Gweedo (Invented) form of Guido: wood

Gwent (Place name) city in Wales

Gwill (American) dark-eyed
Gewill, Guwill

Gwynedd (Welsh) fair-haired
Gwyn, Gwynfor, Gwynn, Gwynne

Gwynn (Welsh) fair
Gwen, Gwyn

Gyan (Hindi) knowledgeable
Gyani

Gyanee (Italian) form of Gianni: calm; believer in God's grace

Gyasi (African) terrific man

Gye (American) knowing

Gylfi (Scandinavian) king; stealthy

Gyllen (last name as first name) young

Gylmar (German) loyal

Gyorgy (Italian) form of George: land-loving; farmer

Gyronne (Hindi) wise

Gysen (Hindi) wise

Gysley (English) excellent

Gyth (American) capable
Gith, Gythe

Gyuri (Slavic) form of George: land-loving; farmer

H

Haadee (Arabic) leader

Haafiz (Arabic) protector

Haakon (Scandinavian) chosen son

Haaris (Arabic) good man

Haas (Last name as first name) good

Habakkuk (Hebrew) embrace

Habby (Hebrew) loved

Habib (Arabic) well loved
Habeeb

Habie (Origin unknown)
jovial
Hab

Habimama (African)
believer in God

Habor (Biblical) place name

Hachiro (Japanese) eighth
son

Hachman (Last name as first
name) chops
Hachmann, Hachmin

Hackett (Last name as first
name) chops

Hackman (German) fervent;
hacks wood
Hackmann

Hadad (Arabic) calm

Hadad (Arabic) blacksmith

Hadar (Hebrew) respected
Hadaram, Hadur, Heder

Hadaway (English) from the
heather hill

Hadden (American) bright;
natural
*Haddan, Haddon, Haddin,
Haden, Hadon*

Haddy (English) form of
Hadley: lover of nature;
meadow with heather
Had, Haddee, Haddey, Haddi

Hade (Arabic) leads in the
right way

Hades (Mythology) Greek
god of the dead

Hadi (Arabic) guide

Hadle (English) from the
meadow of heather

Hadley (English) lover of
nature; meadow with heather
*Haddleye, Hadlee, Hadlie,
Hadly*

Hadran (Latin) dark

Hadrian (Roman) from
Hadria

Hadriel (Hebrew) blessed

Hadwin (Last name as first
name) natural man
Hadwyn

Haffey (Indian) protects

Haffi (Indian) protects

Hafiz (Arabic) guards others
Hafeez, Hapheez, Haphiz

Hagan (German) defender
Hagen, Haggan, Haggin

Hagar (Hebrew) wanders

Hagen (German) chosen one
Hagan, Haggen

Haggai (Biblical) festive

Haggerty (Irish) last name as
first name; unjust

Hagins (German) strong

Hagit (last name as first
name) defends

Hagley (Last name as first
name) defensive

Hahn (last name as first
name) asks

Haidar (Hindi) lionlike
Haider, Haydar, Hyder

Haig (Last name as first
name) authoritative

Haig (Armenian) strong
ancestry

Haike (Asian) of the water

Hailen (Irish) clever

Haim (Hebrew) alive
Hayim, Hayyim

Haines (Last name as first name) confident
Hanus, Haynes

Hajile (Arabic) wanders

Hajir (Arabic) powerful

Hakan (Arabic) fair

Hakim (Arabic) brilliant
Hakeam, Hakeem, Hakym

Hako (Japanese) honorable

Hakon (Scandinavian) chosen son
Haaken, Haakin, Haakon, Hacon, Hagan, Hagen, Hakan, Hako

Hal (English) home ruler

Haland (Last name as first name) island
Halland

Halbert (Last name as first name) island
Hal, Bert

Haldane (German) fierce; person who is half Danish
Haldayn, Haldayne

Haldas (Last name as first name) dependable

Halden (German) man who is half Dane
Haldin, Haldane, Haldan, Halfdan

Haldin (Scandinavian) half-Danish

Haldor (Scandinavian) thunderous rock

Hale (English) heroic
Hal, Halee, Haley, Hali

Halen (Swedish) portal to life
Hailen, Hale, Haley, Hallen, Haylen, Haylin

Haley (Irish) innovative
Hail, Hailee, Hailey, Hale, Halee, Hayley

Halford (Last name as first name) kind

Hali (Greek) loves the sea

Hall (English) solemn

Hallahan (last name as first name)

Hallam (African) gentle

Hallberg (English) comes from a town of valleys
Halberg, Halburg, Hallburg

Halle (Scandinavian) rocklike dependability

Hallen (Scandinavian) from the hall

Halley (English) holy man

Halliwell (Last name as first name) sea-loving

Hallman (English) his hall

Hallmark (English) stalwart

Hallward (English) guards the hall; wily
Halward, Halwerd, Hawarden

Halmer (English) robust

Halos (Greek) halo

Halse (English) on the island
Halce, Halsi, Halsy, Halzee, Halzie

Halsey (English) isolated; island

Halstead (Last name as first name) home on the rock
Halsted

Halston (Origin unknown) fashionable

Halton (English) town on a hill; country boy
Halten, Hallton, Halton

Halvard (Scandinavian)
staunch
Halvor, Hallvard

Halver (Scandinavian)
protects

Halwell (English) special
Hallwell, Halwel, Halwelle

Halyna (Slavic) calm

Ham (Last name as first
name) praising

Hamaker (Last name as first
name) industrious
Ham

Hamal (Arabic) lamb

Hamar (Scandinavian)
hammer

Hamath (Biblical) place
name

Hamby (last name as first
name)

Hamid (Arabic) grateful
Hameed

Hamidi (Arabic) ham
*Hamedi, Hameedi, Hamm,
Hammad*

Hamil (English) rough-hewn
*Hamel, Hamell, Hamill,
Hamm*

Hamilton (English)
benefiting
Hamelton, Hamil, Hammilton

Hamish (Irish) form of
James: he who supplants

Hamlet (German) ham
Hamlette, Hamlit, Hamm

Hamlin (German) homebody
*Hamaline, Hamelin, Hamlen,
Hamlyn*

Hamm (English) last name as
first name; low-lying land by
a stream

Hammer (German) works
with a hammer; able
Hammar, Hammur

Hammond (English)
ingenious
*Ham, Hamm, Hammon,
Hamond*

Hamon (Scandinavian)
leader
Hamo

Hamor (Hebrew) organized

Hamp (American) fun-loving
Ham, Hampton

Hampden (English)
distinctive; valley home

Hampton (English)
distinctive
Ham, Hamm, Hamp, Hampt

Hamza (Arabic) endures

Han (Arabic) form of Hani:
happy

Hanan (Arabic) forgiving

Hanani (Arabic) merciful

Hancock (English) has a
farm; practical

Handel (German) form of
John: God is gracious

Haneef (Arabic) believer

Hanford (Last name as first
name) forgiving
Hamford

Hani (Arabic) happy

Hanif (Arabic) Islam believer

Hanisi (African) Thursday-
born

Hank (English) form of
Henry: leader
Hankey, Hanks, Hanky

Hanley (English) natural; meadow high
Han, Hanlee, Hanleigh, Hanly

Hannelore (Scandinavian) combo of Hanne and Lore

Hannes (Scandinavian) form of Johannes: God is gracious
Hahnes

Hannibal (Slavic) leader
Hanibal, Hanibel, Hann

Hannon (Hebrew) boy of gracefulness

Hanoch (Hebrew) loyal

Hanry (American) form of Henry: leader

Hans (Scandinavian) believer; warm
Hahns, Hanz, Hons

Hansa (Scandinavian) traditional; believer in a gracious Lord
Hans

Hansel (Scandinavian) gullible; open
Hans, Hansie, Hanzel

Hansen (Scandinavian) warm; Hans's son
Han, Handsen, Hans, Hansan, Hanson, Hanssen, Hansson, Hanz

Hans-Joachim (Scandinavian) combo

Hansonn (Scandinavian) son of Hans

Hansraj (Hindi) king of swans; smooth

Hany (Arabic) happy

Haon (Hawaiian) relaxed

Hap (American) form of Hapney

Hapney (English) happenstance

Haqq (Arabic) truth

Haran (Biblical) place name; Abraham's brother

Harbin (English) optimist

Harcourt (English) loves nature

Hardeep (Indian) God-loving

Hardell (German) bold

Hardeman (German) bold

Hardesty (German) brave

Hardin (English) lively; valley of hares
Hardee, Harden

Harding (English) fiery
Harden, Hardeng

Hardwick (English) castle boy
Harwyck

Hardwin (English) keeps hares

Hardy (American) fun-loving; substantial
Hardie, Hardey, Harday, Harding

Harean (African) aware

Harel (Scandinavian) ruler

Harence (English) swift

Harford (English) jolly
Harferd

Hargis (English) last name as first name; baptismal name of son of Agace

Hargrave (Saxon) last name as first name; provider or commissary of an army

Hargrove (English) fruitful

Hari (Hindi) brownish-orange

Harim (Arabic) above all

Harish (Indian) generous

Harjit (Indian) lights the way

Hark (American) word as name; behold
Harko

Harkin (Irish) red-faced
Harkan, Harken

Harlan (English) army land; athletic
Hal, Harl, Harlen, Harlon, Harlynn

Harland (English) strong fighter's land

Harld (Scandinavian) form of Harold: leader of an army

Harlemm (African American) dancer
Harl, Harlam, Harlem, Harlems, Harlum, Harly

Harley (English) wild-spirited
Harl, Harlee, Harly

Harlow (English) bold
Harlo, Harloh

Harmon (German) dependable
Harm, Harman, Harmen

Harmony (Mythology) from Harmonia; in harmony with life
Harmonio

Harness (English) word as name

Harod (Biblical) king
Harrod

Harold (Scandinavian) leader of an army
Hal, Harald, Hareld, Harry

Haron (Arabic) praiseworthy

Harper (English) artistic and musical; harpist
Harp

Harpo (American) jovial
Harpoh, Harrpo

Harpreet (Indian) God-loving

Harreal (Indian) happy

Harrell (Hebrew) likes the mountain of God; religious

Harrington (English) comes from the town of Harry; old-fashioned

Harris (English) dignified
Haris, Harriss

Harrison (English) Harry's son; adventurer
Harrey, Harrl, Harrie, Harris, Harrisan, Harrisen, Harry

Harrod (Hebrew) victor
Harod, Harry

Harry (English) home ruler
Harree, Harrey, Harri, Harrie, Harye

Harshad (Hindi) evokes joy

Harshal (Indian) delight

Harsho (Hindi) joy

Harshul (Indian) deer

Hart (English) giving
Harte

Hartley (English) wilderness wanderer
Hartlee, Hartleigh, Hartly

Hartly (English) boy from the deer field

Hartman (German) strong-willed
Hart, Hartmann, Harttman

Hartmut (German) strong

Hartsey (English) lazing on the meadow; sylvan
Harts, Hartz

Hartwell (English) good-hearted
Harwell, Harwill

Hartwig (German) strong

Haruki (Japanese) child of the spring

Harun (Arabic) highly regarded

Harv (German) able combatant
Har

Harve (French) strong fighter

Harvey (German) fighter
Harv, Harvi, Harvie, Harvy

Harwin (American) safe
Harwen, Harwon

Harwood (English) from the deer wood; artistic
Harewood

Hasan (Arabic) attractive

Hasani (African) good

Hasees (Arabic) good

Hashim (Arabic) force for good
Hasheem

Hashum (African) crushes
Heshum

Hasin (Arabic) handsome
Hassin, Hasen

Hask (Hebrew) form of Haskell: ingratiating
Haske

Haskell (Hebrew) ingratiating
Hask, Haskel, Haskie, Hasky

Haslett (English) land of hazel trees; worthy
Haslit, Haslitt, Hazel, Hazlett, Hazlitt

Hassan (Arabic) good-looking
Hasan

Hasso (German) sun
Hasson

Hastings (English) leader
Haste

Haswell (English) dignified
Has, Haz

Hattan (Place name) from Manhattan; sophisticate
Hatt

Hauran (Biblical) place name

Haval (Biblical) waste

Havard (Scandinavian) guardian of the home
Hav

Havelock (Czech) form of Paul: small; wise

Haven (English) sanctuary
Haiv, Hav

Haward (English) guards the hedge; border man
Hawarden

Hawes (English) stays by the hedges
Haws

Hawke (English) watchful; falcon
Hauk, Hawk

Hawley (English) boy from the hedge

Hawthorne (English) observer

Hay (English) hedge

Hayde (English) hedge

Hayden ✪ (English) respectful
Haden, Hadon, Hay, Haydon, Haydyn, Hayton

Haye (English) open

Hayes (English) open
Haies, Hay, Haye

Hayman (English) hedging
Hay

Haymo (Last name as first name) good-natured

Hayne (English) working outdoors
Haine, Haines, Haynes

Hayres (English) aware

Hayward (English) creative; good work ethic
Hay, Heyward

Hayword (English) open-minded
Haword, Hayward, Haywerd

Haz (Hebrew) sees God

Hazael (Old English) hazel tree

Hazaiah (Hebrew) believes God's decisions

Hazard (Origin Unknown) hazzard

Hazen (English) form of Hayes: open
Hazin

Hazleton (English) from woods of hazel trees

Hazlewood (English) from woods of hazel trees

Hearn (English) optimistic
Hearne, Hern

Heath (English) open space; natural
Heathe, Heith, Heth

Heathcliff (English) mysterious

Heaton (English) high-principled
Heat, Heatan, Heaten

Heber (Hebrew) partner; togetherness
Hebor

Hebron (Biblical) friend

Hector (Greek) loyal
Hec, Heck, Heco, Hect, Hectar, Hecter, Hekter, Tito

Heddwyn (Welsh) peaceful; fair-haired
Hedwin, Hedwyn, Hedwynn

Hedeon (Russian) woodsman

Hedgardo (Spanish) vigilant

Hedley (English) natural

Hedwig (German) combative

Hedwin (German) peaceful ally

Hefastus (Greek) clear

Heffington (last name as first name)

Heike (Welsh) peaceful

Heiko (Dutch) rowdy

Heimdall (Scandinavian) white god
Heiman, Heimann

Hein (German) advising
Heiiri, Heiner, Heini, Heinlich

Heinrich (German) form of Henry: leader
Hein, Heine, Heinrick, Heinrik

Heinz (German) advisor
Heinze

Heladio (Spanish) boy born in Greece; ingenious
Eladio, Elado, Helado

Heleph (Biblical) place name

Helger (Slavic) holy

Helgi (Scandinavian) happy
Helge

Helio (Hispanic) bright

Heliodor (Greek) sun's
adoration

Heliodoro (Greek) sun's
adoration

Helios (Greek) sun

Heller (German) brilliant

Hellerson (German) brilliant
one's son; smart
Helley

Helm (German) bravery

Helmand (German) helmet;
protected

Helmar (German) protected;
smart
Helm, Helmer, Helmet, Helmut

Helmut (German)
courageous

Helon (Biblical) window;
grief

Heman (Last name as first
name) direct

Hemant (Indian) season

Hemin (Hebrew) loyal
Heman

Hender (German) ruler;
illustrious
Hend

Henderson (English) reliable
Hender, Hendersen, Hendersyn

Hendrik (German) home
ruler
*Heinrich, Hendrick, Henrick,
Hindrick*

Hendtrax (Hebrew) gifted

Henech (Last name as first
name) leading the pack
Henach

Henley (English) surprising
Henlee, Henly, Henlye, Hinley

Henning (Scandinavian)
ruler

Henrik (Norwegian) leader
Henric, Henrick

Henry (German) leader
*Hal, Hank, Harry, Henny,
Henree, Henri*

Hensarling (last name as
first name)

Henshaw (last name as first
name)

Henson (Last name as first
name) son of Hen; quiet

Heraldo (Spanish) divine

Herb (German) energetic
Herbi, Herbie, Herby, Hurb

Herber (French) valiant

Herbert (German) famed
warrior
*Bert, Herb, Herbart, Herberto,
Herbie, Herbirt, Herby, Hurb,
Hurbert*

Herbertson (German) famed
soldier's son

Hercule (French) strong
Hercuel, Harekuel, Herkuel

Hercules (Greek) grand gift
Herc, Herk, Herkules

Heriberto (Spanish) form of
Herbert: famed warrior
Heribert

Herkamer (last name as first
name)

Herman (Latin) fair fighter
Heremon, Herm, Hermahn,
Hermann, Hermie, Hermon,
Hermy

Hermangildo (Spanish)
combative

Hermes (Greek) courier of
messages
Hermez

Hermod (Scandinavian)
greets and welcomes

Hermosillo (Spanish) fighter

Hernand (Spanish) form of
Hernando: bold

Hernando (Spanish) bold
Hernan

Herndon (English) nature-
loving
Hern, Hernd

Herne (English) from the
bird heron; inventive
Hearne, Hern

Hernley (English) from the
heron meadow; easygoing
Hernlea, Hernlee, Hernlie,
Hernly

Herodotus (Greek) the
father of history

Heroico (Spanish) hero

Herol (American) form of
Harold: leader of an army

Herrick (Last name as first
name) never alone

Herris (German) rules

Herrod (Biblical) king
Herod

Herron (Latin) heroic

Herschel (Hebrew) deer;
swift
Hersch, Hersh,
Hershel, Hershell, Hershelle,
Herzl, Hirchel, Hirsch, Hirshel

Hershall (Hebrew) deer;
swift
Hersch, Herschel, Hersh, Herzl,
Heshel, Hirschel, Hirsh,
Hirshel

Hertzel (Hebrew) form of
Herschel; deer; swift
Hert, Hertsel, Hyrt

Herve (French) ready for
battle

Hervey (American) form of
Harvey: fighter
Herv, Herve, Hervy

Herzon (American) fast
Herz, Herzan, Herzun

Hesed (Hebrew) sweet

Hesperos (Greek) evening
star
Hesperios, Hespers

Hess (Last name as first
name) bold
Hes, Hys

Hessel (Dutch) bold man

Heston (Last name as first
name) star quality

Hetrick (last name as first
name)

Hevel (Hebrew) alive

Hewis (German) smart

Hewitt (German) smart
Hew, Hewet, Hewett, Hewie,
Hewit, Hewy, Hugh

Hewney (Irish) smart
Owney

Hewson (Irish) son of Hugh;
smart; giving

Heywood (Last name as first name) thoughtful
Haywood

Hezekiah (Biblical) strong man
Hezeklah, Zeke

Hezron (Biblical) strength

Hiawatha (Native American) Iroquois chief
Hia

Hibah (Arabic) the gift

Hickam (English) last name as first name; enclosed dwelling

Hickok (American) wild Bill
Hickok

Hidalgo (American) westerner

Hidde (Japanese) excellent

Hideaki (Japanese) cautious

Hideo (Japanese) excellent
Hideyo

Hieremias (Greek) God lifts him up

Hieronymos (Greek) alternate of Jerome
Heronymous

Hifz (Arabic) memorable

Higinio (Hispanic) forceful

Hilaire (French) happy child

Hilarion (Greek) cheery; hilarious
Hilary, Hill

Hilary (Latin) joyful
Hilaire, Hill, Hillarie, Hillary, Hillery, Hilly, Hilorie

Hildebrand (German) combative; sword
Hill, Hilly

Hill (English) lives on a hill; dreamy

Hillard (German) wars; diligent
Hilliard, Hillier, Hillyer

Hillel (Hebrew) praised; devout
Hilel, Hill

Hillery (Latin) happy; cheerful
Hill

Hilliard (German) brave; settlement on the hill
Hill, Hillard, Hillierd, Hilly, Hillyerd, Hylliard

Hills (last name as first name) brave; from the hills

Hilton (English) sophisticated
Hillten, Hillton, Hiltan, Hiltawn, Hiltyn, Hylton

Himesh (Hindi) snow king

Hines (Last name as first name) strong
Hine, Hynes

Hipolito (Spanish) man who rides horses

Hippocrates (Greek) philosopher
Hipp

Hippolyte (Greek) frees horses
Hippolit, Hippolitos, Hippolytus, Ippolito

Hiram (Hebrew) most admired
Hi, Hirom, Hirym

Hiram (Hebrew) highly praised

Hiramatsu (Japanese) exalted

Hiranya (Indian) rich

Hiresh (Indian) treasured

Hiro (Japanese) giving

Hirsh (Hebrew) deer; swift
*Hersh, Hershel, Hirschel,
Hirshel*

Hirza (Hebrew) lithe; deer

Hisham (Arabic) generous
nature

Hitchcock (English) creative;
spooky
Hitch

Hixon (last name as first
name) high-energy

Hjalmar (Scandinavian)
protective warrior
Hjalamar, Hjallmar, Hjalmer

Ho (Chinese) good

Hoan (Asian) complete child

Hoashis (Japanese) God

Hobart (German) haughty
Hobb, Hobert, Hoebard

Hobbes (English) form of
Robert: brilliant; renowned
Hob, Hobbs

Hobe (German) hill child

Hobert (German) studious

Hobson (English) helpful
backer
*Hobb, Hobbie, Hobbson,
Hobby, Hobsen*

Hock (Asian) smart

Hockley (English) high
meadow boy
*Hocklea, Hocklee, Hocklie,
Hockly*

Hockney (English) from a
high island
Hockny

Hodge (English) form of
Roger: famed warrior
Hodges

Hodgie (English) short for
Hodge: famed warrior
Hodgy

Hodgson (English) boy born
to Roger; up-and-coming
Hodge, Hodges

Hoffman (Last name as first
name) sophisticated

Hogan (Irish) high-energy;
vibrant
Hogahn, Hoge, Hoghan

Hogue (Last name as first
name) youth
Hoge

Hojar (American) wild spirit
Hobar, Hogar

Hoke (Origin unknown)
popular

Hoken (American) liked

Holbert (German) capable
Hilbert

Holbrook (English) educated
*Brooke, Brookie, Brooky, Holb,
Holbrooke*

Holcomb (Last name as first
name) bright

Holday (American) form of
Holiday: born on a holy day

Holden (English) quiet;
gracious
Holdan, Holdin, Holldun

Holder (English) musical
Hold, Holdher, Holdyer

Holdern (last name as first
name)

Holegario (Spanish)
superfluous
Holegard

Holger (Last name as first
name) devoted

Holiday (English) born on a holy day
Holliday

Holling (English) holly

Hollis (English) flourishing
Holl, Hollace, Hollice, Hollie, Holly

Holloway (Last name as first name) jovial
Hollo, Hollway, Holoway

Hollywood (Place name) city in California; showoff
Holly, Wood

Holm (English) natural; woodsy
Holms

Holmes (English) safe haven
Holmm, Holmmes

Holmes (English) from the river; natural home

Holmfrid (Last name as first name) prefers home-and-hearth

Holon (Biblical) place name

Holt (English) shaded view
Holte, Holyte

Homain (Last name as first name) homebody
Holman, Holmen

Homarl (Greek) form of Homer: secure

Homaros (Greek) form of Homer: secure

Homer (Greek) secure
Hohmer, Home, Homere, Homero

Honda (African) form of Hondo: warrior

Hondo (African) warrior

Honesto (Spanish) truthful
Honesta, Honestoh

Hong (Vietnamese) pink; tasteful

Honorato (Spanish) full of honor
Honor, Honoratoh

HonorÈ (Latin) man who is honored
Honor, Honoray

Hood (Last name as first name) easygoing; player
Hoode, Hoodey

Hooker (English) shepherd

Hoolihan (American) hooligan
Hool, Hoole, Hooli

Hoop (American) ball player
Hooper, Hoopy

Hoover (last name as first name)

Hopkins (Welsh) robert's son; famous
Hopkin, Hopkinson, Hopkyns, Hopper, Hoppner

Hopper (Last name as first name) creative

Hoppy (American) lively

Horace (Latin) poetic
Horaace, Horase, Horice

Horatio (Latin) poetic; dashing
Horate, Horaysho

Horeb (Biblical) place name

Horgan (last name as first name)

Hori (Biblical) prince; freeborn

Hornal (German) gardens

Horsley (English) calm field of horses; keeper
Horslea, Horsleigh, Horslie, Horsly

Horst (German) deep; thicket
Hurst

Horstman (German)
profound
Horst, Horstmen, Horstmun

Horstmar (German) from
the thicket; emphatic

Horston (German) thicket;
sturdy
Horst

Horton (English) brash
Horten, Hortun

Horus (Egyptian) kind

Hosa (Native American) crow

Hosaam (Arabic) handsome

Hosea (Hebrew) prophet

Hoshea (Hebrew) saved

Hosie (Hebrew) form of
Hosea: prophet
Hosaya, Hose

Hosni (Arabic) excellent

Houchan (English) spirited

Houghton (Last name as
first name) bravado

Houghton (English) boy
from the town on high

Houston (English) Texas city;
rogue; hill town
Houst, Hust, Huston

Hovannes (Hebrew) form of
Johannes: God is gracious

How (American) word as a
name
Howe, Howey, Howie

Howard (English) well-liked
*How, Howerd, Howie, Howurd,
Howy*

Howart (Origin unknown)
admired
Howar

Howden (English) careful

Howe (German) high-minded
How, Howey, Howie

Howell (Welsh) outstanding
Howel, Howey, Howie, Howill

Howent (English) distinctive

Howerd (English) form of
Howard: well-liked

Howlan (English) living on a
hill; high

Howland (American) well-
known
Howlend, Howlond, Howlyn

Howze (American) form of
Howard: well-liked

Hoyt (Irish) spirited
Hoit, Hoye

Hrothgar (Literature) king

Huang (Chinese) rich

Hubbard (German) fine
Hubberd, Hubert, Hubie

Huber (German) intelligent

Hubert (German) intellectual
*Bert, Bertie, Burt, Hubart,
Huberd, Hue, Huebert, Hugh*

Hubie (English) form of
Hubert: intellectual
Hube, Hubee, Hubey, Hubi

Huck (Literature) from
Huckleberry Finn

Huckleberry (American)
glossy black berry; from
Huckleberry Finn;
mischevious

Hud (English) charismatic
cowboy
Hudd

Hudson (English) Hugh's
son; charismatic adventurer
Hud, Hudsan, Hudsen

Hudspeth (English) form of Hud: charismatic cowboy
Special

Hudya (Arabic) going the right way

Huelett (American) bright; southern
Hu, Hue, Huel, Hugh, Hulette

Huey (French) hearty

Hugh (English) intelligent
Hue, Huey, Hughey, Hughi, Hughie, Hughy

Hughes (English) smart

Hughie (English) intelligent; lucky in parentage
Hughee, Hughi, Hughy

Hugo (Latin) spirited heart

Huitt (English) smart

Hul (Biblical) pain; infirmity

Huland (English) bright
Hue, Huel, Huey, Hugh

Hulbard (Last name as first name) singing; bright
Hulbert, Hulburt

Hull (English) spirited; confident

Hulsey (English) wise eye

Humbert (German) famous giant; renowned warrior

Humberto (Spanish) brilliant
Hum, Humb, Humbie

Hume (Last name as first name) daunting

Humphrey (German) strong peacemaker
Hum, Humfry, Hump, Humphry, Humprey

Hundy (last name as first name)

Hunghui (Asian)

Hunn (German) combative
Hun

Hunt (English) active

Hunter ♂ (English) hunter; adventurer
Hunt

Hunting (English) hunter
Huntyng

Huntington (Last name as first name) town of hunters

Huntler (English) hunter
Huntt

Huntley (English) hunter
Hunt, Hunter, Huntlea, Huntlee, Huntlie, Huntly

Huon (Hebrew) form of John: God is gracious

Hur (Biblical) liberty; whiteness; hole

Hurd (Last name as first name) tends the herd

Hurlbert (English) shining army man
Hulbert, Hurlburt, Hurlbutt

Hurley (Irish) the tide; flowing
Hurlea, Hurlee, Hurli, Hurly

Hurst (Last name as first name) entrepreneurial

Hurston (English) boy from town of thickets

Husham (Biblical) good-looking

Husky (American) big
Husk, Huskee, Huskey, Huski

Huss (American) small

Hussein (Arabic) attractive man
Husain, Husane, Husein, Hussain

Hussein (Arabic) handsome

Hust (American) form of Houston: Texas city; rogue; hill town

Huston (English) form of Houston: Texas city; rogue; hill town

Hutch (American) safe haven; unique
Hut, Hutchey, Hutchie, Hutchy

Hutner (last name as first name) child of the house

Hutter (Last name as first name) tough
Hut, Hutt, Huttey, Huttie, Hutty

Hutton (English) sophisticated
Hutt, Huttan, Hutten, Hutts

Huxford (Last name as first name) outdoorsman

Huxley (English) outdoorsman
Hux, Huxel, Huxle, Huxlee, Huxlie

Hwang (Japanese) yellow

Hyacinthe (French) flowering
Hyacinthos, Hyacinthus, Hyakinthos

Hyatt (English) secure
Hy, Hye, Hyett, Hyut

Hyde (English) special; a hyde is 120 acres
Hide, Hy

Hyden (English) tans hides

Hyghner (Last name as first name) lofty goals
High, Highner, Hygh

Hylan (Asian) hopeful

Hyll (Origin unknown) open-minded
Hy, Hye, Hyell

Hyman (Hebrew) life
Hy, Hymen, Hymie

Hyo (Vietnamese) optimist

I

Iagan (Scottish) fire

Iago (Spanish) feisty villain
Iagoh, Jago

Iah (Egyptian) moonlike

Iain (Scottish) believer

Ian (Scottish) believer; handsome
Iain, Ean, Eon, Eyon

Iathan (Spanish) form of Nathan: God's gift to mankind

Ib (Arabic) joy

Ibrahim (Arabic) fathering many
Ibraham, Ibrahem

Ibu (Japanese) creative

Icarus (Mythology) ill-fated
Ikarus

Ich (Hebrew) form of Ichabod: glory in the past; slim
Ick, Ickee, Ickie, Icky

Ichabod (Hebrew) glory in the past; slim
Ich, Icha, Ickabod, Ika, Ikabod, Ikie

Idelfonso (Spanish) ready

Idi (Swahili) born during the Idd festival

Idris (Welsh) impulse-driven
Idriss, Idriys

Idwal (Welsh) known

Iefan (Welsh) form of John: God is gracious

Ieuan (Welsh) form of Ivan: believer in a gracious God; reliable one

Ifan (Welsh) form of John: God is gracious

Ifor (Welsh) archer

Igal (Biblical) redeemed; defiled

Iggy (Latin) form of Ignatius: firebrand
Iggee, Iggey, Iggi, Iggie

Ignace (French) fiery
Iggy, Ignase

Ignash (Latin) form of Ignatius: firebrand

Ignasha (Latin) form of Ignatius: firebrand

Ignatius (Latin) firebrand
Ig, Iggie, Iggy, Ignacius, Ignashus, Ignatious, Ignnatius

Igor (Russian) warrior

Igoran (Russian) army boy

Ihsan (Arabic) charitable

Ijon (Biblical) place name

Ike (Hebrew) form of Isaac: laughter
Ika, Ikee, Ikey, Ikie

Ilan (Hebrew) tree
Illan

Ilesh (Indian) earth king

Illtyd (Welsh) from the well-populated homeland
Illtud

Ilmar (Scandinavian) airy

Ilom (Welsh) happy

Immanuel (Hebrew) with God
Emmanuel, Imanuel

Imran (Arabic) host

Imre (Slavic) form of Emery: hardworking leader

Inder (Hindi) the Lord of sky gods is Indra; ethereal
Inderjeet, Inderjit, Inderpal, Indervir, Indra, Indrajit

Indiana (Place name) U.S. state; rowdy; dashing
Indio, Indy

Indore (Place name) city in India
Indor

Indra (Hindi) Lord of sky gods

Ing (Scandinavian) he who is foremost
Inge

Ingan (Scandinavian) prolific

Ingeborg (Scandinavian) fertile

Ingelbert (German) combative
Ing, Inge, Ingelbart, Ingelburt, Inglebert

Inger (Scandinavian) fertile
Ingemar, Ingmar

Ingmar (Scandinavian) famous son
Ing, Ingamar, Ingamur, Inge, Ingemar, Ingmer

Ingra (English) form of Ingram: angelic; kind
Ingie, Ingrah, Ingrie

Ingram (English) angelic; kind
Ing, Ingraham, Ingre, Ingrie, Ingry

Ingvar (Scandinavian) fertility god
Ingevar

Inigo (Spanish) form of Ignatius: firebrand

Iniko (Japanese) serves

Innis (Irish) isolated
Ines, Inis, Innes, Inness, Inniss

Innocencio (Spanish) innocent

Inteus (Native American) proud

Into (Scandinavian) excitable

Ioan (Slavic) believer

Ionel (Slavic) believer

Ior (Welsh) form of Iorwerth: worthy Lord

Iorgos (Greek) outgoing

Iorwerth (Welsh) worthy Lord

Ira (Hebrew) cautious
Irae, Irah

Irakli (Slavic) athletic

Iram (English) smart
Irem, Irham, Irum

Iranga (Sri Lankan) special

Irfan (Arabic) grateful child

Irind (American) peaceful

Irineo (Spanish) peaceful

Irish (English) boy from Ireland

Irmtraud (German) strong soldier

Irv (English) form of Irving: attractive

Irvin (English) attractive
Irv, Irvine

Irving (English) attractive
Irv, Irve, Irveng, Irvy

Irwin (English) practical
Irwen, Irwhen, Irwie, Irwinn, Irwy, Irwynn

Isa (African) saved

Isaac ✪ ✟ (Hebrew) laughter
Isaak, Isack, Izak, Ize, Izek, Izzy

Isadore (Greek) special gift
Isador, Isedore, Isidore, Issy, Izzie, Izzy

Isai (Hebrew) believer

Isaiah ✪ ✟ (Hebrew) saved by God
Isa, Isay, Isayah, Isey, Izaiah, Izey

Isak (Scandinavian) laughter
Isac

Isam (Arabic) protector

Isamu (Japanese) bravery

Isas (Japanese) worthwhile

Isham (Last name as first name) athletic

Ishan (Hindi) sun

Ishan (Indian) sun

Ishbak (Biblical) protector

Ishmael (Hebrew) God hears
Hish, Ish, Ishmel, Ismael

Ishtar (Mythology) goddess of fertility and love

Isidore (Greek) gift of Isis
Izzie

Isidoro (Spanish) gift
Cedro, Cidro, Doro, Izidro, Sidro, Ysidor

Isidro (Greek) gift
Isydro

Israel (Hebrew) God's prince; conflicted
Israyel, Issy, Izzy

Israj (Hindi) king of gods

Issa (Hebrew) laughing

Issachar (Biblical) reward

Isser (Slavic) creative

Ithamar (Biblical) island of the palm tree

Ithiel (Biblical) with God beside him

Itil (Welsh) has a giving nature

Itlus (Roman) from Italy

Itsik (Hebrew) form of Isaac: laughter

Itzak (Hebrew) form of Isaac: laughter
Itzik

Iuri (Slavic) form of Yuri: dashing

Ivan (Russian) believer in a gracious God; reliable one
Ivahn, Ive, Ivey, Ivie

Ivanore (Scandinavian) child of God

Ivar (Scandinavian) norse god

Ive (English) able
Ivee, Ives, Ivey, Ivie

Ives (American) musical
Ive

Ivo (Polish) yew tree; sturdy
Ivar, Ives, Ivon, Ivonnie, Yvo

Ivon (Slavic) believer

Ivor (Scandinavian) outgoing; ready
Ifot, Ivar, Ive, Iver, Ivy

Izaak (Polish) full of mirth

Izacz (Slavic) spicy; happy
Isaac, Izak, Izie, Izze, Izzee

Izador (Spanish) gift
Dorrie, Dory, Isa, Isador, Isadoro, Isidoros, Isodore, Iza, Izadoro

Izaiah (Czech) form of Isaiah: saved by God

Izaith (Spanish) form of Isaiah: saved by God

Izan (Slavic) asks

Izedin (Spanish) gives

Izhar (Indian) serves well

Izrail (American) form of Isaiah: saved by God

Izzy (Hebrew) friendly
Issie, Issy, Izi, Izzee, Izzie

J

Ja (Korean) gorgeous

Jaak (Scandinavian) form of Jack: God is gracious

Jaan (Scandinavian) form of John: God is gracious

Jabal (Place name) form of Japalpur, a city in India: attractive

Jabari (African American) brave

Jabbar (Arabic) comforting

Jaber (American) form of Jabir: supportive
Jabar, Jabe, Jabir

Jabez (Hebrew) sorrow
Jabezz

Jabin (Hebrew) God's own

Jabir (Arabic) supportive
Jabbar

Jabon (American) wild
Jabonne

Jabot (French) shirt ruffle

Jace (American) audacious
Jase, Jhace

Jacek (Polish) hyacinth;
growing
Jack, Yahcik

Jacen (Greek) form of Jason:
healer; the Lord is salvation

Jacett (Invented) jaunty
Jaycett

Jachin (Biblical) ready

Jachym (Hebrew) form of
Jacob: he who supplants
Jach

Jacinto (Spanish) hyacinth;
fragrant
Jacint

Jack ♀ (Hebrew) form of
John: God is gracious
Jackee, Jackie, Jacko, Jacky, Jax

Jackal (Sanskrit) wild dog;
betrays
Jackel, Jackell, Jackyl, Jackyll

Jackie (English) personable
Jackee, Jackey, Jacki, Jacky, Jaki

Jackie-Lee (American) combo
of Jackie and Lee

Jackson ♀ (English) Jack's
son; full of personality
*Jackee, Jackie, Jacks, Jacsen,
Jakson, Jax, Jaxon*

Jacksonville (Last name as
first name) town of Jack's
son; sturdy
Jacsonville, Jaksonville

Jaclo (Spanish) combo of Jack
and Lo

Jacob ♀ ♂ (Hebrew) he who
supplants
*Jaccob, Jacobe, Jacobee, Jake,
Jakes, Jakey, Jakob*

Jacoben (American) replaces;
friend

Jacobo (Spanish) warm
Jake, Jakey

Jacobs (Biblical) replacing
Jakobs, Jakey

Jacobus (Latin) form of
Jacob: he who supplants
Jakobus

Jacobus (American) replaces;
friend

Jacoby (Hebrew) form of
Jacob: he who supplants
Jacobey, Jakobey, Jukoby

Jacoby (Hebrew) form of
Jacob: he who supplants

Jacquard (French) class act
*Jackard, Jackarde, Jacquarde,
Jaqard, Jaquard, Jaquarde*

Jacques (French) romantic;
ingenious
Jacquie, Jacue, Jaques, Jock, Jok

Jacy (American) form of
Jacob: he who supplants

Jadaan (Last name as first
name) content

Jadall (Invented) punctual
Jada, Jade

Jade (Spanish) valued jade
stone
Jadee, Jadie, Jayde

Jaden ♀ ♂ (Hebrew) Jehovah
has heard
*Jade, Jadon, Jadin, Jadun,
Jadyn, Jaiden, Jaydie, Jaydon*

Jadney (Last name as first
name) pleased
Jad

Jadran (Slavic) form of Adrian: wealthy; dark-skinned

Jae (French) form of Jay: colorful

Jaegel (English) salesman
Jaeg, Jaeger, Jael

Jaeger (German) outdoorsman
Jaegir, Jagher, Jagur

Jael (Hebrew) climber

Jaewon (African American) form of Juwon: devout; lively
Jaewan, Jaywan, Jaywon

Jaeyel (Hebrew) form of Jael: salesman

Jafar (Arabic) from the stream
Gafar, Jafari

Jafeth (Hebrew) handsome

Jaffar (Arabic) directs

Jaffey (Hebrew) beautiful

Jaffey (English) form of Jaffe: beautiful
Jaff

Jaffiel (Spanish) loves the water

Jafon (Dutch) growth

Jagan (English) confident
Jagen, Jagun, Jago

Jagannath (Indian) Hindi god Vishna; world leader

Jagger (English) brash
Jagar, Jager, Jaggar, Jagir

Jaggerton (English) brash
Jag, Jagg

Jagit (Invented) brisk
Jaggett, Jaggit, Jagitt

Jago (English) self-assured

Jaguar (Spanish) fast
Jag, Jagg, Jaggy, Jagwar, Jagwhar

Jahan (Sanskrit) worldly

Jaheim (Hindi) worldly

Jahi (African) runs well; dignity

Jahlel (Biblical) God helps

Jahmal (Arabic) beautiful
Jahmaal, Jahmall

Jahmil (Arabic) beautiful
Jahmeel, Jahmyl

Jai (American) adventurer
Jay

Jaidev (Hindi) God's victory

Jaidov (Indian) winning

Jailo (Hindi) worldwise

Jaime (Spanish) follower
Jaimey, Jaimie, Jamee, Jaymie

Jaimini (Hindi) winner

Jaimo (Asian) form of James: he who supplants

Jair (Hebrew) teacher
Jairo

Jairaj (Hindi) Lord's victor

Jairam (Slavic) God informs him

Jaircineo (Spanish) enlightened

Jairemaine (French) form of Germain: growing; from Germany

Jairo (Spanish) God enlightens
Jaero, Jairoh

Jairus (Biblical) faithful

Jaison (American) form of Jason: healer; the Lord is salvation
Jaizon

Jaja (African) praise-worthy

Jakar (Place name) from
Jakarta
Jakart, Jakarta, Jakarte

Jake ❶ (Hebrew) form of
Jacob: he who supplants
Jaik, Jakee, Jakey, Jakie, Jayke

Jakeem (Arabic) has been
lifted

Jakey (American) nickname
for Jake; friendly
Jaky

Jakin (Biblical) form of
Jachin: ready

Jakiren (American) playful

Jakob (Hebrew) form of
Jacob: he who supplants
*Jakab, Jake, Jakeb, Jakey, Jakie,
Jakobe, Jakub*

Jal (English) wanderer

Jalal (Hindi) glory

Jalam (Biblical) victor

Jaleel (Arabic) handsome
Jalil

Jalen (American) vivacious
Jalon, Jaylen, Jaylin, Jaylon

Jalenal (American) wins

Jaliseo (Spanish) modest

Jallen (American) winner

Jalmar (Scandinavian) soldier

Jamail (Arabic) good-looking
*Jahmil, Jam, Jamaal, Jamahal,
Jamal, Jamil, Jamile, Jamy*

Jamaine (Arabic) good-
looking

Jaman (American) wonder

Jamar (American) form of
Jamail: good-looking
Jamarr, Jemar, Jimar

Jamari (African American)
attractive

Jamarr (African American)
attractive; formidable
*Jam, Jamaar, Jamar, Jammy
Jamel, Arabic, form of Jamal*

Jamerson (English) son of
James

James ✚ ❶ (English) form of
Jacob: he who supplants
*Jaimes, Jamsey, Jamze, Jaymes,
Jim, Jimmy*

James-Bolton (American)
musical

Jameson (English) able;
James's son
*Jamesan, Jamesen, Jamesey,
Jamison, Jamsie*

Jamie (English) form of
James: he who supplants
*Jaimey, Jaimie, Jamee, Jamey,
Jay, Jaymey, Jaymsey*

Jamil (Arabic) beautiful
Jameel, Jamyl

Jamile (Arabic) handsome

Jamin (Hebrew) favored son
*Jamen, James, Jamie, Jamon,
Jaymon*

Jamisen (American) form of
James: he who supplants
Jami, Jamie, Jamis, Jamison

Jan (Dutch) form of John:
God is gracious
Jaan, Jann, Janne

Janardan (Indian) helper

Jance (Scandinavian) form of
John: God is gracious
Devout

Janesh (Hindi) thankful

Janier (French) form of John:
God is gracious

Janis (Slavic) devout

Janko (Slavic) happy

Janon (Hebrew) chosen

Janson (Scandinavian) Jan's son; hardworking
Jan, Janne, Janny, Jansahn, Jansen, Jansey

Jantz (Scandinavian) form of Jantzen: God is gracious
Janson, Janssen, Jantzon, Janz, Janzon

Jantzen (Scandinavian) form of John: God is gracious

Janus (Latin) Roman god of beginnings and endings; optimistic; born in January
Jan, Janis

Januson (Scandinavian) son of Janus; year's gateway

Japheth (Hebrew) grows
Japhet

Jaquanace (American) growth

Jaquawn (African American) rock
Jacquon, Jakka, Jaquan, Jaquan, Jaquie, Jaqwen, Jequon, Jock

Jaquier (French) form of Jacques: romantic; ingenious

Jarah (Hebrew) sweet

Jarat (American) form of Jared: descendant; giving

Jaraus (American) form of Jaran: sings

Jard (American) form of Jared: descendant; giving
Jarra, Jarrd, Jarri, Jerd, Jord

Jareb (Hebrew) contender
Jarib, Yarev, Yariv

Jared (Hebrew) descendant; giving
Jarad, Jarod, Jarode, Jarret, Jarrett, Jerod, Jerrad, Jerrod

Jarek (Slavic) fresh
Jarec

Jarell (Scandinavian) giving
Jare, Jarelle, Jarey, Jarrell, Jerrell

Jaren (Hebrew) vocal
Jaron, Jayrone, J'ron

Jarenal (American) form of Jaren: vocal
Jaranall, Jaret, Jarn, Jaronal, Jarry, Jerry

Jarenn (American) form of Jaran: sings

Jarent (French) sings

Jares (Biblical) form of Jairus: generous

Jareth (American) open to adventure
Jarey, Jarith, Jarth, Jary

Jariath (American) sings

Jarib (Hebrew) competes

Jaribon (American) laughs

Jario (Hebrew) believer

Jarius (Spanish) generous

Jarkko (Finnish) form of George: land-loving; farmer

Jarl (Scandinavian) noble

Jarles (Scandinavian) noble

Jarman (German) stoic
Jerman

Jarmuth (Biblical) place name

Jarnigan (German) German boy

Jaro (Polish) spring child

Jaroe (American) form of Gerald: strong; ruling with a spear

Jarol (English) form of Gerald: strong; ruling with a spear

Jarold (Polish) form of Gerald: strong; ruling with a spear

Jaromil (Czech) spring love
Jarmil

Jaron (Hebrew) spirited singer

Jarons (Hebrew) spirited singer

Jarred (Hebrew) form of Jared: descendant; giving
Jared, Jere, Jerod, Jerred, Jerud

Jarrell (English) jaunty
Jare, Jarell, Jarrel, Jarry, Jerele, Jerrell

Jarrett (English) confident
Jare, Jaret, Jaritt, Jarret, Jarrit, Jarritt, Jarry, Jarryt, Jarrytt, Jerot, Jerret, Jerrett, Jurett, Jurette

Jarrod (Hebrew) form of Jared: descendant; giving
Jare, Jarod, Jarry, Jerod

Jarvett (American) form of Jarrett: descendant; giving

Jarvey (German) celebrated
Garvey, Garvy, Jarvee, Jarvi, Jarvy

Jarvis (German) athletic
Jarv, Jarvee, Jarves, Jarvey, Jarvhus, Jarvie, Jarvus, Jarvy

Jary (Spanish) form of Jerry: strong; ruling with a spear
Jaree

Jaryn (Hebrew) sings

Jasdeep (Indian) bright light

Jase (American) hip

Jaskarn (Indian) praises

Jason ✪ ❂ (Greek) healer; the Lord is salvation

Jaspal (Pakistani) pure

Jasper (English) guard
Jasp, Jaspur, Jaspy, Jaspyr

Jasraj (Indian) famous

Jassel (Spanish) form of Jason: healer; the Lord is salvation

Jasson (American) form of Jason: healer; the Lord is salvation

Jaster (English) form of Jasper: guard
Jast

Jasvir (Indian) famous

Jatauan (American) joker

Jatin (American) form of Gaetano: from the city of Gaeta; Italian man

Jattir (Biblical) place name

Jaumet (French) foremost

Jaun (American) form of John: God is gracious

Javan (Biblical) righteous
Javin, Javon

Javaris (African American) prepared
Javares, Javarez

Javas (Sanskrit) bright eyes

Jave (American) form of Jove: Roman sky god

Javed (American) form of Jove: Roman sky god

Javen (Hebrew) form of Javan: righteous

Javier (Spanish) affluent;
homeowner
Havyaire, Javey, Javiar

Javion (American) form of
Javan: righteous

Javon (Hebrew) hopeful
*Javan, Javaughn, Javen,
Javonn, Javonte*

Javonte (African American)
jaunty
*Javaughantay, Javawnte, Ja-
Vonnetay, Ja-Vontae*

Javor (Slavic) sturdy tree

Javy (American) form of
Javaris; prepared
Javey, Javie

Jawahir (Arabic) gems

Jawdat (Arabic) excellent
Gawdat

Jawhar (Arabic) gem

Jawon (African American)
shy
*Jawan, Jawaughn, Jawaun,
Jawuane, Jewan, Jewon, Jowon*

Jax (American) form of
Jackson: Jack's son; full of
personality
Jacks, Jaxx

Jaxon (English) form of
Jackson: Jack's son; full of
personality

Jaxson (English) form of
Jackson: Jack's son; full of
personality

Jay (English) form of a name
starting with J; colorful
Jai, Jaye

Jaya (American) jazzy
Jay, Jayah

Jayan (Indian) wins

Jayant (Hindi) winner

Jayant (Indian) victor

Jayashree (Indian) victor

JayC (American) combo of Jay
and C

Jayden ✪ ⊕ (American)
bright-eyed
*Jayde, Jaydon, Jaydey, Jaydi,
Jaydie, Jaydun, Jaydy*

Jayes (English) form of Jay:
form of a name starting with
J; colorful

Jayesh (Indian) victor

Jaylon (American) combo of
Jay and Lon

Jayme (English) form of
Jamie: he who supplants

Jaymee (English) form of
Jamie: he who supplants

Jaymes (American) form of
James: he who supplants
Jaimes, James

Jaymz (American) form of
James: he who supplants

Jayson (Greek) form of Jason:
healer; the Lord is salvation

Jaz (American) form of Jazz:
jazzy

Jazeps (Latvian) God will
increase

Jazer (American) form of
Jazz: jazzy

Jazon (Polish) heals

Jazz (American) jazzy
Jazze, Jazzee, Jazzy

Jean (French) form of John:
God is gracious
Jeanne, Jeannie, Jene

Jeanis (French) form of John:
God is gracious

Jean-Marc (French) combo of Jean and Marc

Jean-Pierr (French) combo of Jean and Pierr

Jean-Sebastien (French) combo of Jean and Sebastian

Jeardo (Polish) form of Jerard: confident

Jearoslav (Polish) glory

Jeb (Hebrew) jolly
Jebb, Jebby

Jebben (Hebrew) form of Jebediah: close to God

Jebediah (Hebrew) close to God
Jeb, Jebadiah, Jebby, Jebedyah

Jebus (Biblical) place name

Jecori (American) exuberant
Jekori

Jed (Hebrew) helpful
Jedd, Jeddy, Jede

Jediah (Hebrew) God's help
Jedi, Jedyah

Jedidiah (Hebrew) close to God
Jed, Jeddy, Jeddyah, Jedidyah

Jedrek (Polish) virile
Jedrick, Jedrus

Jedwog (Polish) manly

Jeeps (French) jaunty

Jeevan (African American) form of Jevan: spirited
Jevaughn, Jevaun

Jeevan (Hebrew) religious

Jeevik (Indian) water

Jeff (English) form of Jeffrey: peaceful; form of Jefferson: dignified
Geoff, Jeffie, Jeffy

Jeffers (English) form of Jeffrey: peaceful

Jefferson (English) dignified
Jeff, Jeffarson, Jeffersen, Jeffursen, Jeffy

Jeffery (English) form of Jeffrey: peaceful
Jeffrey, Jeffrie, Jeffry, Jefry

Jeffrey (English) peaceful
Geoffrey, Jeff, Jeffree, Jeffrie, Jeffry, Jeffy, Jefree

Jehan (French) form of John: God is gracious

Jehu (Hebrew) true believer

Jela (African) honors

Jelani (African American) trendy
Jelanee, Jeluney, Jelanne

Jem (English) form of James: he who supplants
Jemmi, Jemmy, Jemmye, Jemy

Jemarr (African American) worldly
Jemahr

Jemonde (French) man of the world
Jemond

Jenda (Czech) form of John: God is gracious

Jenkins (Last name as first name) God is gracious
Jenkin, Jenks, Jenky, Jenkyns, Jenx, Jinx

Jennett (Hindi) heavenly
Jennet, Jennit, Jennitt, Jennyt, Jennytt, Jinnat

Jennings (Last name as first name) attractive
Jennyngs

Jensi (Hungarian) noble
Jenci, Jens

Jenson (English) son of Jen;
blessed
Jensen, Jenssen, Jensson

Jep (American) easygoing
Jepp

Jephtha (Biblical) judges
others; outgoing

Jerald (English) form of
Gerald: strong; ruling with a
spear
Jere, Jereld, Jerold, Jerrie, Jerry

Jeramy (Hebrew) exciting
Jeramah, Jeramie, Jere, Jeremy

Jerard (French) confident
Jerrard

Jere (Hebrew) form of
Jeremy: talkative
Jeree, Jerey

Jeremiah ✪ ✿ (Hebrew)
prophet uplifted by God;
farsighted
*Jeramiah, Jere, Jeremyah,
Jerome, Jerry*

Jeremie (Hebrew) loquacious
Jeremee, Jeremy

Jeremy ✿ (English) talkative
*Jaramie, Jere, Jeremah, Jereme,
Jeremey, Jerrey, Jerry*

Jeriah (Hebrew) form of
Jeremiah: prophet uplifted by
God; farsighted

Jericho (Arabic) nocturnal
*Jerako, Jere, Jerico, Jeriko,
Jerycho, Jerycko, Jeryco, Jeryko*

Jerick (American) form of
Jericho: nocturnal
*Gericho, Jereck, Jerik, Jero,
Jerok, Jerrico*

Jeril (American) form of
Jarrell: leader
Jerill, Jerl, Jerry

Jerma (American) form of
Germaine: growing; from
Germany
Jermah, Jermane, Jermayne

Jermain (French) from
Germany
*German, Germane, Germanes,
Germano, Germanus,
Jermaine, Jerman, Jermane,
Jermayn, Jermayne*

Jermaine (German) form of
Germaine: growing; from
Germany
*Germain, Germaine, Jere,
Jermain, Jermane, Jermene,
Jerry*

Jermey (American) form of
Jermaine: growing; from
Germany
Jermy

Jermon (African American)
dependable
Jermonn

Jerney (Hebrew) exalted of
the Lord

Jernigan (Last name as first
name) spontaneous
Jerni, Jerny

Jero (American) jaunty
Jeroh, Jerree, Jerri, Jerro, Jerry

Jerod (Hebrew) form of Jared:
descendant; giving

Jerold (English) merry
Jerrold, Jerry

Jerome (Latin) holy name;
blessed
*Jarome, Jere, Jerohm, Jeromy,
Jerree, Jerrome, Jerry, Jirome*

Jerone (English) hopeful
Jere, Jerohn, Jeron, Jerrone

Jeronimo (Italian) form of
Geronimo: sacred name
Gerry, Jero, Jerry

Jerral (American) form of Jerald: strong; ruling with a spear
Jeral, Jere, Jerry

Jerram (Hebrew) God has uplifted
Jeram, Jerem, Jerrem, Jerrym, Jerym

Jerrell (American) exciting
Jarell, Jerre, Jerrel, Jerrie, Jerry

Jerrett (Hebrew) form of Jarrett: confident
Jeret, Jerete, Jerod, Jerot, Jerret

Jerry (German) form of Gerald: strong; ruling with a spear
Gerry, Gery, Jerre, Jerri, Jerrie, Jerrye

Jerse (Place name) calm; rural
Jerce, Jercey, Jersey, Jersy, Jerzy

Jervis (Greek) honorable
Gervase

Jesmar (American) form of Jesse: wealthy
Jess, Jessie, Jezz, Jezzie

Jesper (American) easygoing
Jesp, Jess

Jess (Hebrew) wealthy
Jes

Jesse ♥ (Hebrew) wealthy
Jess, Jessee, Jessey, Jessi, Jessye

Jessup (Last name as first name) rich
Jesop, Jesopp, Jess, Jessa, Jessie, Jessopp, Jessy, Jesup, Jesupp, Jessupp

Jesuan (Spanish) devout

Jesus ♥ (Hebrew) saved by God
Hesus, Jesu, Jesuso, Jezus

Jet (English) black gem

Jetal (American) zany
Jetahl, Jetil, Jett, Jettale, Jetty

Jethro (Hebrew) fertile
Jeto, Jett, Jetty

Jeton (French) a chip for gamblers; wild spirit
Jet, Jetawn, Jets, Jett, Jetty

Jett (American) free
Jet, Jets, Jetty, The Jet

Jettie (American) form of Jett: free
Jette, Jettee, Jetti

Jetty (American) form of Jett: free
Jettey

Jevan (African American) spirited
Jevaughn, Jevaun, Jevin, Jevon

Jex (American) form of Jack: God is gracious

Jhonatan (African) spiritual
Jhon, Jon

Ji (Chinese) organized; orderly

Jibben (American) form of Jivon: living; vibrant
alive

Jibri (Arabic) angel

Jie (Chinese) wonderful

Jiggins (English) lost

Jiles (American) form of Giles: protective

Jilve (American) form of Jiles: protective

Jim (Hebrew) form of James: he who supplants
Jem, Jihm, Jimi, Jimmee, Jimmy

Jimbo (American) cowhand; endearment for Jim
Jim, Jimb, Jimbee, Jimbey, Jimby

Jimbob (American) countrified
Gembob, Jim Bob, Jim-Bob, Jymbob

Jimere (Biblical) from Gemar

Jimmy (English) form of James: he who supplants
Jim, Jimi, Jimmey, Jimmi, Jimmye, Jimy

Jimmy-John (American) country boy
Jimmiejon, Jimmyjohn, Jimmy-Jon, Jymmejon

Jimoh (African) Friday's child

Jin (Chinese) golden

Jinan (Place name) city in China
Jin

Jindrich (Czech) ruling
Jindra, Jindrik, Jindrisek, Jindrousek

Jing (Chinese) unblemished; capital

Jinghua (Asian) ruler

Jinkon (American) vibrant

Jiri (Czech) working the earth
Jira, Jiricek

Jiri (Czech) form of George: land-loving; farmer

Jiro (Japanese) second boy born

Jiten (Indian) conquers

Jivon (Hindi) living; vibrant
Jivan

Joab (Hebrew) praising God; hovering
Joabb

Joachim (Hebrew) a king of Judah; powerful; believer
Akim, Jakim, Yachim, Yakim

Joah (Greek) form of Jonah: peacemaker

Joanus (German) form of Johann: God is gracious

Joao (Spanish) form of John: God is gracious

Joaquin (Spanish) bold; hip
Joakeen, Joaquim, Joaquin, Juakeen, Jwaqueen

Joar (Biblical) form of Jair: teacher

Job (Hebrew) patient
Jobb, Jobe, Jobi, Joby

Jobab (Biblical) sorrowful

Jobin (Biblical) perceives

Jobo (Hebrew) patient

Jobse (American) patient

Jobson (English) son of Job; patient

Joby (Hebrew) patient; tested
Job, Jobee, Jobi

Jochen (German) established

Jock (Hebrew) grace in God; athlete
Jockie, Jocky

Joda (Hebrew) devout

Jodbin (Hebrew) combo of Jod and Bin

Jody (Hebrew) believer in Jehovah; American combo of Joe and Dee, *Jodee, Jodey, Jodie, Jodye, Joe*

Joe (Hebrew) form of Joel: prophet in the Bible; form of Joseph: He will add
Jo, Joey, Joeye, Joie

JoeGee (American) combo of Joe and Gee

Joel (Hebrew) Jehovah is the Lord
Joelie, Joell, Jole, Joly

Joerd (Dutch) guards

Joergen (Scandinavian) earth worker

Joest (Scandinavian) just

Joey (Hebrew) form of Joel: prophet in the Bible; form of Joseph: He will add
Joee, Joie

Joffre (German) form of Jeffrey: peaceful

Johann (German) form of John: God is gracious
Johan, Johane, Yohann, Yohanne, Yohon

Johannes (Hebrew) form of John: God is gracious
Johan, Jon

Johar (Hindi) gem

John ✪ ✿ (Hebrew) God is gracious
Jahn, Jhan, Johne, Johnne, Johnni, Johnnie, Johnny, Johnnye, Jon

Johnny (Hebrew) form of John: God is gracious
Gianni, Johnie, Johnnie, Jonni, Jonny

Johnny-Dodd (American) country sheriff
Johnniedodd, Johnny Dodd

Johnny-Ramon (Spanish) renegade
Johnnyramon, Johnny Ramon

Johnson (English) John's son; credible
Johnsen, Johnsonne, Jonsen, Jonson

Joji (Japanese) form of John: God is gracious

JoJo (American) friendly; popular
Jo-Jo

Jokel (American) form of Joachim: king of Judah; powerful; believer

Jokshan (American) form of Jackson: Jack's son; full of personality

Joktan (Biblical) small

Jole (American) jolly

Jolly (American) jolly

Jolon (Native American) oak valley dweller

Joloyd (American) combo of Jo and Lloyd

Jomar (African American) helpful
Joemar, Jomarr

Jomei (Japanese) lightens

Jomo (American) grows crops

Jon (Hebrew) alternative for John
Jonni, Jonnie, Jonny, Jony

Jonah (Hebrew) peacemaker
Joneh

Jonald (Hebrew) combo of Jon and Ronald

Jonas (Hebrew) capable; active
Jon

Jonathan ✪ ✿ (Hebrew) gift of God
Johnathan, Johnathon, Jonathon

Jonavon (Hebrew) calm

Jonaz (Hebrew) form of Jonas: capable; active

Jones (American) saucy

Jonnie (Hebrew) form of John: God is gracious

Jonnley (American) form of John: God is gracious
Jonn, Jonnie

Jonte (American) form of John: God is gracious
Johatay, Johate, Jontae

Jonte (French) form of John: God is gracious

Jools (English) form of Julius: attractive

Joplin (Place name) city in Montana; sings
Joplyn

Joppa (Biblical) place name

Joram (Biblical) giving

Joran (Scandinavian) dependable

Jord (Scandinavian) strong

Jordahno (Invented) form of Giordano: delivered

Jordan ○ ● (Hebrew) downflowing river
Jorden, Jordon, Jordun, Jordy, Jordyn

Jordane (Hebrew) form of Jordan: downflowing river

Jordan-Michael (American) athletic

Jordison (American) son of Jordy; glowing
Jordisen, Jordysen, Jordyson

Jordy (Hebrew) form of Jordan: downflowing river
Jordie, Jordey, Jordi

Jorge (Spanish) form of George: land-loving; farmer
Jorje, Quiqui

Jorgen (Scandinavian) farmer
Jorgan

Jorger (Scandinavian) form of George: land-loving; farmer

Jorget (French) mutinous

Jorine (French) form of George: land-loving; farmer

Joris (Dutch) form of George: land-loving; farmer

Jory (Hebrew) descendant
Jorey

Jos (Place name) city in Nigeria

Josa (Hebrew) God judges him

José ○ (Spanish) asset; favored
Joesay, Jose, Pepe, Pepito

Joseph ○ ● (Hebrew) He will add
Jodie, Joe, Joey, Josep, Josef, Josephe, Jozef, Yusif

Josh (Hebrew) form of Joshua: devout
Joshua, Joshuam, Joshyam, Josue, Jozua

Josha (Hebrew) form of Joshua: devout

Joshua ○ ● (Hebrew) devout

Josia (Hebrew) form of Josiah: supported by the Lord
Josea

Josiah (Hebrew) supported by the Lord
Josyah

Joson (English) form of Jason: healer; the Lord is salvation

Joss (English) form of Joseph: He will add
Josslin, Jossly

Josue (Spanish) devout

Jotham (Biblical) a king of
Judah; believer in perfect
Jehovah
Jothem, Jothym

Jour (French) form of
Jourdain: flowing

Jourdain (French) flowing
Jordane, Jorden

Jourdyun (Slavic) form of
Jourdain: flowing

Jovan (Slavic) gifted
Jovahn, Jovohn

Jovani (Italian) form of Jove:
Roman sky god
*Jovani, Jovanni, Jovanny,
Jovany*

Jove (Mythology) Roman sky
god

Jovi (American) sky

Jovito (Spanish) jubilant

Joza (Czech) form of Joseph:
He will add

Jozef (Polish) supported by
Jehovah; asset
Joe, Joze

Jozo (Slavic) little Joe

Juan ☻ (Spanish) devout;
lively
Juann, Juwon

Juanie (Spanish) form of
John: God is gracious

Jubal (Hebrew) celebrant

Jubilo (Spanish) rejoicing;
jubilant
Jube

Judah (Biblical) praised
Juda

Judas (Latin) praised

Judd (Latin) secretive
Jud

Jude (Latin) form of Judas:
praised
Judah

Judge (English) judgmental
Judg

Judges (Biblical) judgmental

Judson (Last name as first
name) mercurial
*Juddsen, Juddson, Judsen,
Judssen*

Judule (American) form of
Judah: praised
Jud, Judsen, Judsun

Juhi (Indian) flowers

Julan (American) attractive

Jules (Greek) young Adonis
Jewels, Jule

Julian ☻ (Greek) gorgeous
Juliane, Julien, Julyon, Julyun

Julias (Biblical) place name

Julio (Spanish) handsome;
youthful
Huleeo, Hulie, Julie

Julius (Greek) attractive
Juleus, Jul-yus, Jul-yuz

Ju-Long (Chinese) powerful

Jumaane (African) Tuesday-
born

Jumah (African) born on
Friday
Juma

Jumahl (African) form of
Jumah: born on Friday

Jumbe (African) strong
Jumbey, Jumby

Jumble (American) awry

Jumoke (African) beloved

Jun (Japanese) follows the
rules

Jund (Arabic) soldier

Juneau (Place name) capital of Alaska
Juno, Junoe

Junior (Latin) young son of the father
Junnie, Junny, Junyer

Junius (Latin) youngster
Junie, Junnie, Junny

Junny (Asian) honest

Juper (German) form of Joseph: He will add

Jupiter (Roman) god of thunder and lightning; guardian
Jupe

Jur (Czech) form of George: land-loving; farmer

Jura (Place name) mountain range between France and Switzerland
Jurah

Juraj (Slavic) form of George: land-loving; farmer

Jurass (American) from Jurassic period of dinosaurs; daunting
Jurases, Jurassic

Jurate (Slavic) forgives

Jurg (Dutch) form of Jurgen: working the earth

Jurgen (Scandinavian) working the earth

Jurgin (Dutch) form of Jurgen: working the earth

Jurgs (Dutch) form of Jurgen: working the earth

Juri (Slavic) farms

Juric (Slavic) form of George: land-loving; farmer

Jus (French) just
Just, Justice, Justis

Juste (French) law-abiding
Just, Zhuste

Juster (American) fair and honest

Justice (Latin) just
Jusees, Just, Justice, Justiz, Justus, Juztice

Justie (Latin) honest; fair
Jus, Justee, Justey, Justi

Justin ☼ ☻ (Latin) fair
Just, Justan, Justen, Justun, Justyn, Justyne

Justinian (Latin) ruler; Roman emperor
Justinyan

Justino (Spanish) fair
Justyno

Justiz (American) judging; fair
Justice, Justis

Justo (Scandinavian) handsome

Justus (German) fair

Jute (Botanical) practical

Juven (Latin) youthful

Juvenal (Latin) young
Juve

Juventino (Spanish) young
Juve, Juven, Juvey, Tino, Tito

Juventino (Spanish) youthful

Juver (Spanish) form of Javor: sturdy tree

Juwon (African American) form of Juan: devout; lively
Jujuane, Juwan, Juwonne

Jvon (American) form of Juan: devout; lively

Jyles (American) form of
Giles: protective

Jyree (Scandinavian) form of
George: land-loving; farmer

Kaar (American) form of Kar:
bold; Michael's follower

Kaarlo (American) form of
Carlo: sensual; manly

Kabir (Hindi) spiritual leader
Kabar

Kabonero (African) symbol

Kabonesa (African) born in
hard times

Kacancu (Rukonjo) firstborn

Kacy (American) happy
*K.C., Kace, Kacee, Kase, Kasee,
Kasy, Kaycee*

Kadar (Arabic) empowered
Kader

Kade (American) exciting
*Cade, Caden, K.D. Kadey,
Kaid, Kayde, Kydee*

Kadeem (Arabic) servant
Kadim

Kaden (American) exciting
*Cade, Caden, Caiden, Caidin,
Caidon, Caydan, Cayden,
Caydin, Caydon, Kadan,
Kadon, Kadyn, Kaiden*

Kading (last name as first
name) powerful

Kadir (Hindi) talented
Kadeer, Qadeer, Qadir

Kadjaly (African) born from
God

Kadmiel (Hebrew) God-
loving

Kado (Japanese) through
life's gate

Kaelan (Irish) strong
Kael, Kaelen, Kaelin, Kaelyn

Kaemon (Japanese) happy

Kaeto (American) cato
Cayto, Caytoe, Kato

Kafele (African) supreme

Kafus (American) laughing
boy

Kaha (Hawaiian)
domesticated

Kahale (Hawaiian) homebody

Kahane (Egyptian) brave

Kahil (Turkish) ingenue;
Arabic
*friend; Greek, handsome,
Cahill, Kaleel, Kalil, Kayhil,
Khalil*

Kaholo (Hawaiian) boy who
runs

Kai (Hawaiian) kay
Keh

Kaid (English) round; happy
*Caiden, Cayde, Caydin, Kaden,
Kadin, Kayd*

Kaihe (Hawaiian) spear

Kailey (Hawaiian) religious

Kailin (Irish) sporty
*Kailyn, Kale, Kalen, Kaley,
Kalin, Kallen, Kaylen*

Kaine (Irish) handsome

Kainen (Irish) handsome

Kaipo (Hawaiian) embraces

Kairo (Arabic) from Cairo;
exotic

Kaiser (German) title that means emperor

Kaiyan (Indian) place name

Kaj (Scandinavian) earthy

Kajah (Biblical) form of Caja: close proximity

Kal (Hawaiian) born of the sun

Kala (Hawaiian) sun boy

Kalama (Hawaiian) source of light
Kalam

Kalani (Hawaiian) of one sky
Kalan

Kalb (Hawaiian) studies

Kale (American) healthy; vegetable
Kail, Kayle, Kaylee, Kayley, Kaylie

Kaleb (American) form of Caleb: faithful; brave
Caleb

Kalebbe (Hebrew) form of Kaleb: faithful; brave

Kalen (Hawaiian) young

Kalgan (Place name) city in China
Kal

Kali (Polynesian) comforts

Kalidas (Indian) creative

Kalil (Arabic) best friend
Kahil, Kahleel, Kahlil, Kaleel, Khaleel, Khalil

Kalin (Arabic) young

Kalkin (Hindi) tenth child

Kallahan (American) form of Callahan: spiritual

Kallen (Greek) handsome
Kallan, Kallin, Kallon, Kallun, Kalon, Kalun, Kalyn

Kalman (Irish) slim

Kalogeros (Greek) beautiful in aging

Kalonn (Irish) strong

Kalunga (African) watchful; the personal god of the Mbunda of Angola

Kalvim (Latin) form of Calvin: bald

Kalvin (Latin) form of Calvin: bald
Kal

Kalyan (Indian) handsome

Kama (Sanskrit) perfection

Kamaka (Hawaiian) pretty face

Kamal (Arabic) perfect
Kameel, Kamil

Kamal (African) lotus child

Kamari (African) moonlight child

Kamau (African) quiet soldier
Kamall

Kamden (Scottish) form of Camden: conflicted

Kameron (Scottish) form of Cameron: mischievous; crooked nose
Kameren, Kammeron, Kammi, Kammie, Kammy, Kamran, Kamrin, Kamron

Kammer (African) moon; pained

Kamon (American) alligator
Cayman, Caymun, Kame, Kammy, Kayman, Kaymon

Kamon (Biblical) place name

Kamran (American) form of Cameron: mischievous; crooked nose

Kamrino (Italian) form of Cameron: mischievous; crooked nose

Kamyar (Indian) handsome

Kan (American) good-looking

Kana (Japanese) strength of character

Kanah (Biblical) form of Elkanah: obedient to God

Kanak (Indian) golden child

Kanan (Hindi) forest

Kandall (American) form of Kendall: shy

Kane (Gaelic) warlike; honor; tribute
Cahan, Cahane, Cain, Kaince, Kaine, Kaney, Kanie, Kayne

Kang (Korean) healthy

Kaniel (Hebrew) confident; supported by the Lord; hopeful
Kane, Kan-El, Kanel, Kanelle, Kaney

Kano (Place name) city in Nigeria
Kan, Kanoh

Kant (German) philosopher
Cant

Kantu (Hindi) joyous

Kany (Australian) stone

Kanye (American) unbreakable

Kanzler (German) last name as first name

Kaori (Japanese) scented

Kaper (American) capricious
Cape, Caper, Kahper, Kape

Kapila (Hindi) foresees
Kapil

Kapono (Hawaiian) anointed one

Kapp (Greek) form of the surname Kaparos
Kap, Kappy

Kapple (English) last name as first name; From Cable; Son of Cabel

Kar (American) form of Carr: outdoorsy

Karan (Hindi) listens

Karau (English) loyal

Karcher (German) beautiful blond boy

Kare (Scandinavian) large
Karee

Kareem (Arabic) generous
Karehm, Karem, Karim, Karreem, Krehm

Kareem (Arabic) generous
Karam, Karim

Karekin (Scandinavian) large

Karel (Slavic) form of Carl: kingly

Karey (Greek) form of Cary: pretty brook; charming; form of Carey: masculine; by the castle
Karee, Kari, Karrey, Karry

Kari (Scandinavian) hair curls

Kariah (Biblical) form of Zechariah: Lord remembers

Karif (Arabic) fall-born
Kareef

Karime (Arabic) distinctive

Karimen (Scandinavian) big

Karkor (Biblical) place name

Karl (German) manly; forceful
Carl, Kale, Karel, Karll, Karlie, Karol, Karoly

Karlen (Slavic) form of Carl: kingly

Karmel (Hebrew) red-haired
Carmel, Carmelo, Karmeli, Karmelli, Karmelo, Karmello, Karmi

Karmmer (Hebrew) form of Carmel: growing; garden

Karnaim (Biblical) place name

Karney (Irish) wins
Carney

Karolek (Polish) form of Charles: manly; well-loved
Karol

Karp (Russian) abundant

Karp (Greek) fruitful

Karr (Scandinavian) curly hair
Carr

Karst (Greek) anointed

Karstell (last name as first name)

Karsten (Greek) chosen one

Kartik (Indian) hopes

Karu (Hindi) cousin
Karun

Karyim (Arabic) divisive

Kaseem (Arabic) divides
Kasceem, Kaseym, Kasim, Kazeem

Kaseko (African) ridiculed

Kasem (Asian) joyful

Kasen (Spanish) helmet; protected

Kasey (Irish) form of Casey: courageous
Kasi, Kasie

Kasi (Egyptian) form of Kasiya: leaving
Kasee, Kasey, Kasie

Kasim (Hindi) shining

Kasimir (Arabic) serene
Kasim Kazimir, Kazmer

Kasin (Slavic) wolf; safety

Kasiya (Egyptian) leaving

Kason (Spanish) safe

Kasper (German) reliable
Caspar, Casper, Kasp, Kaspar, Kaspy

Kass (German) standout among men
Cass, Kasse

Kassidy (Irish) form of Cassidy: humorous
Kass, Kassidi, Kassidie, Kassie

Kastor (Greek) wins

Katell (Scandinavian) pure

Kato (African) second of twins

Katzir (Hebrew) reaping
Katzeer

Kauai (Place name) Hawaiian island; breezy spirit
Kawai

Kaufman (Last name as first name) serious
Kauffmann, Kaufmann

Kauri (Scandinavian) blessed

Kaushal (Indian) smart

Kavan (Irish) good-looking
Cavan, Kaven, Kavin

Kavi (Hindi) poetic

Kavin (Irish) form of Kevin: handsome; gentle

Kawai (Hawaiian) form of Kauai: Hawaiian island; breezy spirit

Kay (Greek) joyful
Kai, Kaye, Kaysie, Kaysy, Keh

Kayin (African) desired baby

Kayle (Hebrew) faithful
Kail, Kayl

Kaylen (Irish) form of Kellen:
strong-willed
Kaylan, Kaylin, Kaylon, Kaylyn

Kayo (Sanskrit) wordsmith

Kayode (African) joy-giver

Kayven (Irish) handsome
Cavan, Kavan, Kave

Kaz (Greek) creative

Kazan (Greek) creative
Kazann

Kazar (Slavic) kind

Kazimierz (Polish) practical
Kaz

Kazuo (Japanese) peace-
loving

Kazuo (Asian) good son

Kealoha (Hawaiian) bright
path

Keane (German) attractive
Kean, Keen, Keene, Kiene

Keanu (Hawaiian) cool breeze
over mountains
Keahnu

Kearn (Irish) outspoken
Kearny, Kern, Kerne, Kerney

Kearney (Irish) sparkling
*Karney, Karny, Kearns, Kerney,
Kirney*

Kearon (Irish) form of
Kieran: handsome brunette

Keary (Irish) form of Kerry:
dark

Keat (English) hawk

Keatal (English) hawk

Keaton (English) nature-lover
Keaten, Keatt, Keatun, Keton

Keats (Literature) for poet
John Keats; melancholy
Keatz

Keawe (Hawaiian) lovable

Keb (Egyptian) loves the earth

Kecalf (American) inventive
Keecalf

Kechel (African American)
kach
Kachelle

Keda (Hindi) form of Kedar:
powerful

Kedar (Hindi) powerful
Kadar, Keder

Kedding (English) last name
as first name

Kedem (Hebrew) old soul

Kedemah (Biblical) old

Kedrick (American) form of
Kendrick: heroic
Ked, Keddy, Kedric, Kedrik

Kedron (Biblical) place name;
King

Kee (Irish) from Keefe:
handsome

Kee-Bun (Taiwanese) good
news
Keebun

Keefa (Irish) loved and lovely

Keefe (Irish) handsome
Keaf, Keafe, Keef, Keeffe, Kief

Keegan (Irish) ball-of-fire
*Keagan, Keagin, Kegan, Kege,
Keghun*

Keelan (Irish) slim
*Kealan, Keallan, Keallin,
Keilan, Keillan, Kelan*

Keeley (Irish) handsome
*Kealey, Kealy, Keelee, Keelie,
Keely, Keilie*

Keen (German) smart
*Kean, Keane, Keene, Keeney,
Kene*

Keenan (Irish) bright-eyed
Kenan

Keeney (American) incisive
*Kean, Keane, Keaney, Keene,
Kene*

Keesen (Dutch) adored

Keever (Irish) form of Kevin:
handsome; gentle

Keevin (Irish) form of Kevin:
handsome; gentle

Keffry (American) form of
Jeffrey: peaceful

Kefil (African) given by God

Kefir (Hebrew) young lion;
high spirits

Kefiwy (African) loyal

Kehlor (American) friend

Keir (Irish) brunette

Keirer (Irish) dark
Kerer

Keiron (Irish) dark
Keiren, Keronn

Keitaro (Japanese) blessed
baby
Keita

Keith (English) witty
Keath, Keeth, Keithe

Keithen (Scottish) gentle
Keith

Keizo (American) spice

Keko (Hawaiian) bold

Kekoa (Hawaiian) one
warrior

Kekoa (Asian) brave

Kel (Irish) fighter; energetic
Kell

Kelby (English) snappy;
charming
*Kel, Kelbey, Kelbi, Kelbie,
Kelbye, Kell, Kellby, Kelly*

Kelcy (English) helpful
Kelci, Kelcie, Kelcye, Kelsie

Kele (Hawaiian) watches like
a hawk

Kelemen (Hungarian) soft-
spoken

Kell (English) fresh-faced
Kel, Kelly

Kellagh (Irish) hardworking
Kellach

Kellam (Scottish) calm

Kelle (Scandinavian)
springlike

Kellen (Irish) strong-willed
*Kel, Kelen, Kelin, Kell, Kellan,
Kellin, Kelly, Kelyn*

Keller (Last name as first
name) bountiful
Kel, Keler, Kelher, Kell, Kylher

Kellins (Irish) strong

Kelly (Irish) able combatant
Keli, Kellee, Kelley, Kelli, Kellie

Kelmen (Hungarian) form of
Kelemen: soft-spoken

Kelsen (English) port town
child

Kelsey (Scandinavian) unique
among men
*Kel, Kells, Kelly, Kels, Kelsi,
Kelsie, Kelsy, Kelsye, Kelzie,
Kelzy*

Kelto (Greek) unrequited love

Kelton (Irish) energetic
Keldon, Kelltin, Kellton, Kelten, Kelti, Keltonn

Kelts (Origin unknown) energetic
Kel, Kelly, Kelse, Kelsey, Keltz

Kelvin (English) goal-oriented
Kelvan, Kelven, Kellven, Kelvon, Kelvun, Kelvynn, Kilvin

Kemal (Turkish) honored infant; generous

Kemmer (American) ethical

Kemp (English) champion

Kemper (American) high-minded
Kemp, Kempar

Kempton (American) takes the high road

Kemuel (Hebrew) God's advocate

Ken (Scottish) form of Kenneth: good-looking
Kenn, Kenny, Kinn

Kenan (Irish) strong

Kenaz (Hebrew) bright

Kendall (English) shy
Ken, Kend, Kendahl, Kendal, Kendoll, Kendy, Kenney, Kennie, Kenny, Kindal

Kendan (English) strong; serious
Ken, Kend, Kenden

Kendrick (English) heroic
Kendricks, Kendrik, Kendryck, Kenric, Kenrick, Kenricks, Kenrik

Kenel (Invented) form of Kendall: shy
Kenele

Kenelm (English) handsome boy
Kenhelm, Kennelm

Kenitsu (Asian) many summers

Kenix (American) form of Kenneth: good-looking

Kenji (Asian) careful

Kenley (English) distinguished
Kenlea, Kenlee, Kenleigh, Kenlie, Kenly

Kenn (English) river; flowing

Kennard (English) courageous; selfless
Ken, Kenard, Kennaird, Kennar, Kenny

Kennard (Irish) bold leader

Kennavy (Irish) brave

Kennean (Scottish) little Ken

Kennedy (Irish) leader
Canaday, Canady, Kennedey, Kennedie, Kennidy

Kenner (English) capable
Kennard

Kennern (American) able

Kennet (Scandinavian) form of Kenneth: good-looking
Kenet, Kennete

Kenneth (Scottish) good-looking
good-looking, Ken, Keneth, Kenith, Kennath, Kennie, Kenny

Kenny (Scottish) form of Kenneth: good-looking
Kennee, Kenney, Kenni, Kennie

Kenric (English) bold

Kenrick (English) heroic boy

Kensil (English) form of Kenneth: good-looking

Kent (English) fair-skinned
Kennt, Kentt

Kentaro (Japanese) large baby boy

Kentlee (Last name as first name) dignified
Ken, Kenny, Kent, Kentlea, Kentleigh, Kently

Kentley (English) meadow boy

Kenton (English) form of Kent: fair-skinned
Kentan, Kentin, Kenton

Kentos (American) form of Quintus: fifth child

Kentrell (English) white

Kenward (Last name as first name) bold

Kenway (Last name as first name) bold

Kenyatta (African) from Kenya; patriotic

Kenyon (Irish) dear blond boy
Ken, Kenjon, Kenny, Kenyawn, Kenyun

Kenzel (Scottish) wise

Kenzie (Scottish) form of Kinsey: affectionate; winning
Kensie

Kenzo (American) form of Ken: good-looking

Keola (Hawaiian) vibrant

Keon (American) unbridled enthusiasm
Keion, Keonne, Keyon, Kion, Kionn

Keontay (African American) outrageous
Keon, Keontae, Keontee

Kepler (German) loves astrology; starry-eyed
Kappler, Keppel, Keppeler, Keppler

Kepner (German) last name as first name

Kerbie (American) form of Kirby: brilliant

Kerel (African) forever young

Kerem (Hebrew) works in vineyard

Keren (Hebrew) of the horns

Kerey (Irish) dark

Kerm (Irish) form of Kermit: droll
Kurm

Kermit (German) droll
Kerm, Kermee, Kermet, Kermey, Kermi, Kermie, Kermy

Kern (Irish) dark; musically inclined
Curran, Kearn, Kearne, Kearns

Kernaghan (Last name as first name) dark
Carnahan, Kernohan

Kernis (Invented) dark; different
Kernes

Kerr (Scandinavian) serious
Karr, Kerre, Kurr

Kerr (Scottish) surname

Kerrick (English) rules

Kerrins (English) of the horns

Kerry (Irish) dark
Keary, Kere, Keri, Kerrey, Kerrie

Kers (Todas) an Indian plant

Kersen (Indonesian) cherry bright

Kerstie (American) spunky
Kerstee, Kersty

Kert (American) form of Curt/Curtis: gracious; kindhearted

Kerwyn (Irish) energetic
Kerwen, Kerwin, Kerwun, Kir, Kirs, Kirwin

Keshawn (African American) friendly
Kesh, Keshaun, Keyshawn, Shawn

Keshet (Hebrew) rainbow; bright hopes

Keshon (African American) sociable
Kesh

Kesin (Hindi) needy

Kesley (American) derivative of Lesley: active
Keslee, Kesli, Kezley

Kesse (American) attractive
Kessee, Kessey, Kessi, Kessie

Kester (Scottish) form of Christopher: the bearer of Christ

Kestrel (English) soars

Ketchum (Place name) city in Idaho
Catch, Ketch, Ketcham, Ketchim

Keth (Irish) form of Keith: witty

Kettil (Scandinavian) self-sacrificing
Keld, Kjeld, Ketil, Ketti

Keung (Chinese) universal spirit

Kevann (Irish) good-looking

Kevin ○ (Irish) handsome; gentle
Kev, Kevahngn, Kevan, Keven, Kevvie, Kevvy

Kevis (Irish) form of Kevin: handsome; gentle
Handsome

Kevontay (American) combo of Kevon and Tay

Kevork (English) noble

Key (English) key
Keye, Keyes

Keylor (Irish) friend

Keyon (Irish) form of Ewan: youthful spirit

Keyshawn (African American) clever; believer

Keyth (Welsh) form of Keith: witty

Keyvan (American) form of Kevin: handsome; gentle

Khaalis (Greek) beauty

Khadijah (Arabic) premature baby

Khadim (Hindi) forever
Kadeem, Kadeen, Kahdeem, Khadeem

Khak (American) form of Khaki: laughing

Khaldoun (Arabic) everlasting

Khaldun (Arabic) everlasting

Khalid (Arabic) everlasting
Khalead, Khaled, Khaleed

Khalil (Arabic) good friend

Khaliq (Arabic) ingenious
Kaliq, Khalique

Khambrel (American)
articulate
*Kambrel, Kham, Khambrell,
Khambrelle, Khambryll,
Khamme, Khammie, Khammy*

Khan (Turkish) shares; prince

Khayrat (Arabic) good

Khayru (Arabic) giving
Khiri, Khiry, Kiry

Khevin (American) form of
Kevin: handsome; gentle
Khev

Khiam (American) old

Khosrow (Slavic) denies

Khouri (Arabic) spiritual
Couri, Khory, Khourae, Kori

Khyber (Place name) pass on
border of Pakistan and
Afghanistan
Kibe, Kiber, Kyber

Kibbe (Nayas) nocturnal bird

Kibo (Place name) mountain
peak highest peak of
Kilimanjaro; spectacular
Kib

Kibwy (African) God blesses

Kidd (Last name as first
name) adventurous

Kidder (Last name as first
name) brash; confident

Kidron (English) youthful

Kiefer (Irish) loving
*Keefer, Kieffer, Kiefner, Kieffner,
Kiefert, Kuefer, Kueffner*

Kiel (Place name) city in
North Germany

Kiel (Irish) form of Kyle:
serene

Kien (Irish) form of Keenan:
bright-eyed

Kier (Icelandic) large vat or
tub

Kieran (Scottish) dark-haired
*Keiran, Keiren, Keiron, Kern,
Kernan, Kiernan, Kieron,
Kyran*

Kieran (Irish) handsome
brunette
*Keiran, Kier, Kieren, Kierin,
Kiers, Kyran*

Kiet (Asian) respected

Kiev (Place name) capital city
of Ukraine

Kiho (Hawaiian) moves
carefully

Kilbane (English) last name
as first name

Kilgore (Scottish) last name
as first name

Killam (Irish) slim

Killi (Irish) form of Killian:
effervescent
Killean, Killee, Killey, Killyun

Killian (Irish) effervescent
*Kilean, Kilian, Killean, Killee,
Killi, Killie, Killyun, Kylian*

Killion (Irish) slim

Kilroy (Irish) royal

Kilyun (American) form of
Killion: slim

Kim (Vietnamese) gold
Kimmie, Kimmy, Kimy, Kym

Kimball (Greek) inviting
*Kim, Kimb, Kimbal, Kimbie,
Kimble, Kymball*

Kimberly (English) bold
*Kim, Kimbo, Kimberleigh,
Kimberley*

Kin (Japanese) gold

Kin (Japanese) golden

Kincaid (Scottish) vigorous
Kincaide, Kinkaid

Kincannon (Scottish) last name as first name; I'll defend

Kinch (Last name as first name) knife blade

King (English) royal leader

Kingman (Last name as first name) gracious man

Kingsley (English) royal nature
King, Kings, Kingslea, Kingslee, Kingsleigh, Kingsly, Kins

Kingston (English) gracious
King, Kingstan, Kingsten

Kingswell (English) royal; king

Kinnard (Last name as first name) leaning
Kinnaird

Kinnel (Gaelic) dweller at the head of the cliff

Kinney (English) simplifies

Kinsey (English) affectionate; winning
Kensey, Kinsie

Kinton (Hindi) adorned

Kioshi (Japanese) thoughtful silence

Kip (English) focused
Kipp, Kippi, Kippie, Kippy

Kipling (Literature) for writer Rudyard; adventurous
Kiplen, Kippling

Kipp (American) hill; upward bound
Kip, Kyp

Kipster (English) boy from the hill

Kirabo (African) treasured

Kiral (Greek) Lord

Kiran (Hindi) light

Kirann (American) purehearted

Kirby (English) brilliant
Kerb, Kirb, Kirbee, Kirbey, Kirbie, Kyrbee, Kyrby

Kiri (Vietnamese) like mountains

Kiril (Russian) Lord
Cyril, Cyrill, Kirill, Kirillos, Kyril, Kyrill

Kirk (Scandinavian) believer
Kerk, Kirke, Kurk

Kirkan (Scandinavian) of the church

Kirkland (Last name as first name) church land

Kirkley (Last name as first name) church wood
Kirklea, Kirklee, Kirklie, Kirkly

Kirkor (English) of the church

Kirkson (English) church son

Kirkwell (Last name as first name) wood; giving of faith

Kirkwood (English) heavenly
Kirkwoode, Kurkwood

Kirton (English) from the town of churches

Kirvin (American) form of Kevin: handsome; gentle
Kerven, Kervin, Kirv, Kirvan, Kirven

Kishore (Indian) little colt

Kit (Greek) mischievous
Kitt

Kitchell (American) form of Mitchell: optimistic

Kito (African) precious

Kiva (Hebrew) form of Akiva: cunning

Kizza (African) child born after twins' birth

Kjeld (Scandinavian) form of Carl: kingly

Kjell-Ake (Scandinavian) form of Carl: kingly

Kjetil (Scandinavian) form of Carl: kingly

Klaus (German) wealthy
Klaas, Klaes, Klas, Klass

Klausen (German) victor

Klay (English) form of Clay: reliable
Klaie, Klaye

Kleber (Last name as first name) serious
Klebe

Kleef (Dutch) boy from the cliff; daring

Kleigh (American) form of Clay: reliable

Klein (Last name as first name) bright
Kleiner, Kleinert, Kline

Klemens (Latin) gentle
Klemenis, Klement, Kliment

Kleng (Scandinavian) claw; struggles

Klev (Invented) form of Cleve: precarious
Kleve

Knight (English) protector
Knighte, Nighte

Knightley (English) protects
Knight, Knightlea, Knightlee, Knightlie, Knightly, Knights

Knoll (American) flamboyant
Noll

Knollie (English) form of Knowles: outdoorsman

Knossos (Biblical) place name

Knoten (Native American) windy

Knowah (American) form of Noah: peacemaker

Knowles (English) outdoorsman
Knowlie, Knowls, Nowles

Knowlton (English) from the grassy knoll

Knox (English) bold

Knud (Scandinavian) ruler

Knut (Scandinavian) aggressive
Canute, Cnut, Knute

Kobe (Hebrew) cunning
Kobee, Kobey, Kobi, Koby

Kobi (Hebrew) cunning; smart
Cobe, Cobey, Cobi, Cobie, Coby, Kobe, Kobey, Kobie, Koby

Kobin (African) Tuesday's child

Kobus (Dutch) form of Jacob: he who supplants

Kodiak (American) bear; daunting

Kody (English) brash
Kodee, Kodey, Kodi, Kodie, Kodye

Kofi (African) friday-born

Kohana (Hawaiian) best

Kohath (Biblical) congregation

Kohl (English) form of Cole: lively; winner

Kohler (German) coal

Koji (African) Monday's baby

Kojo (African) Monday-born

Koka (Hawaiian) man from Scotland; strategist

Kolby (American) form of Colby: bright; secretive; dark farm
Kelby, Kole, Kollby

Kole (English) form of Cole: lively; winner

Kolen (Irish) beautiful; light

Kolibar (American) form of Colbert: cool and calm

Kolton (English) coal town

Kombs (American) from catacombs

Komic (Invented) funny
Com, Comic, Kom

Konane (Hawaiian) spot of moonlight

Kondo (African) fights

Kone (Word as name) cone

Kong (Chinese) heavenly

Konnor (Irish) another spelling of Connor; brilliant
Konnar, Konner

Kono (African) industrious

Konrad (German) bold advisor
Khonred, Kon, Konn, Konny, Konraad, Konradd, Konrade, Kord, Kort

Konsa (American) form of Constantine: constant; steadfast

Konstandin (Slavic) steadfast

Konstantin (Greek) loyal
Kon, Konny, Kons, Konstance, Konstantine, Konstantyne

Konstantinos (Greek) loyal
Constance, Konstance, Konstant, Tino, Tinos

Koralion (Greek) coral

Korb (German) form of Korbel: black raven

Korbel (German) black raven

Kore (Greek) pure

Koren (Greek) strong-willed

Korent (English) form of Corentin: stormy

Koresh (Hebrew) farms
Choresh

Korey (Irish) lovable
Kori, Korrey, Korrie

Korling (American) bold

Kornel (Czech) horn; communicator
Kornelisz, Kornelius, Kornell

Kornelius (Latin) form of Cornelius
Korne, Kornellius, Kornelyus, Korney, Kornnelyus

Korrigan (Irish) form of Corrigan
Koregan, Korigan, Korre, Korreghan, Korri, Korrigon

Kort (German) talkative

Korten (German) of the court

Kory (Irish) hollow
Kori, Korre, Korrey, Korrye

Kosana (African) prince

Kosey (African) temperamental; lionlike

Koshua (American) form of Joshua: devout

Koshy (American) jolly
Koshee, Koshey, Koshi

Kosmo (Greek) likes order
Kosmy, Cosmos

Kostas (Russian) form of
Konstantin: loyal

Koster (American) spiritual
Kost, Kostar, Koste, Koster

Kosumi (Native American)
fishes with a spear; smart

Kosyantyn (Slavic) leader

Kovit (Asian) talented

Krael (Slavic) form of Kyryl:
Lord's child

Kraig (Irish) another spelling
for Craig
Krag, Kragg, Kraggy

Kramer (German)
shopkeeper; humorous

Krater (American) form of the
word crater

Krause (German) outdoorsy

Krayton (Russian) kind

Kreig (Irish) form of Craig:
brave climber

Kres (Slavic) peaceful

Kreso (Slavic) peaceful

Kricker (Last name as first
name) reliable
Krick

Krikor (Armenian) form of
Gregory: careful

Kris (Greek) form of Kristian:
follower of Christ; form of
Kristopher: the bearer of
Christ
Krissy, Krys

Krishna (Hindu) pleasant
Krishnah

Krispin (Irish) form of
Crispin: man with curls

Krissel (German) curly-haired

Krister (Scandinavian)
religious

Kristian (Greek) form of
Christian: follower of Christ
Kris, Krist, Kristyan

Kristiyan (Slavic) christian

Kristo (Greek) form of
Kristopher: the bearer of
Christ

Kristoffer (Scandinavian)
form of Christopher: the
bearer of Christ

Kristopher (Greek) form of
Christopher: the bearer of
Christ
Kris, Krist, Kristo, Kristofer

Kroenen (Polish) form of
Cronin: timely

Kronos (Greek) black

Kruz (Spanish) delight

Krystyn (Polish) christian
Krys, Krystian

Krzysztof (Polish) bearing
Christ
Kreestof

Kubrick (Last name as first
name) creative
Kubrik

Kueng (Chinese) of the
universe; fine

Kugonza (African) in love

Kumar (Hindi) boy

Kundayo (African) joy

Kunig (Dutch) clever

Kuno (German) courageous

Kunyo (African) brave

Kuper (Hebrew) copper

Kurt (Latin) wise advisor
Curt, Kurty

Kurtis (Latin) form of Curtis:
gracious; kindhearted
*Kurt, Kurtes, Kurtey, Kurtie,
Kurts, Kurtus, Kurty*

Kuster (American) form of
Custer: watchful; stubborn

Kutrer (last name as first
name) form of Cutrer: knife
dealer

Kutter (American) form of
Cutter: man who cuts
gemstones

Kutty (English) knife-wielding
Cutty

Kwadjo (African) monday-
born

Kwako (African) wednesday-
born

Kwame (African) saturday's
child
Kwamee, Kwami

Kwan (Korean) bold character

Kwasi (African) born on
Sunday
Kweisi, Kwesi

Kwintyn (Polish) fifth child
Kwint, Kwintin, Kwynt

Ky (Irish) form of Kyle: serene

Kyan (Place name) village in
Japan
Kyann

Kylan (Irish) form of Kyle:
serene

Kyland (Irish) calm

Kyle ❂ ✝ (Irish) serene
*Kiel, Kiyle, Kye, Kyl, Kyley,
Kylie, Kyly*

Kyler (English) peaceful
Cuyler, Kieler, Kiler, Kye, Kylor

Kylerly (English) unusual

Kylerton (American) form of
Kyle: serene
Kylten

Kymond (American) brave

Kynan (Welsh) leads

Kynaston (English) serene

Kyne (English) blue-blooded

Kyran (Irish) form of Kieran:
handsome brunette

Kyriacos (Greek) masterful

Kyriak (Greek) loves God

Kyros (Greek) masterful

Kyryl (Slavic) Lord's child

Kyston (American) form of
Constantine: constant;
steadfast
Loyal

Kyzer (American) wild spirit
Kaizer, Kizer, Kyze

L

La Var (American) combo of
La and Var

Laasch (Scandinavian)
forward-thinking

Laban (Hebrew) white
Lavan

Labarne (American) form of
Laban: white
white, Labarn

Labaron (French) the baron
LaBaron, LaBaronne

Labhras (Irish) form of
Lawrence: honored
Lubhras

LaBryant (African American)
son of Bryant; brash
*Bryant, La Brian, La Bryan,
Labryan, Labryant*

Lachean (Scottish) from
place of lakes

Lachlan (Scottish) feisty
*Lachlann, Lacklan, Lackland,
Laughlin, Lock, Locklan*

Lachman (Scottish) prospers

Lachtna (Irish) gray; aging
with grace

Lacido (Spanish) bright

Lacy (Scottish) warlike
Lacey

Ladan (Hebrew) having seen;
aware

Ladd (English) helper; smart
*Lad, Laddee, Laddey, Laddie,
Laddy*

Ladden (American) athletic

Laddie (English) youthful
*Lad, Ladd, Laddee, Laddey,
Laddy*

Laden (English) from Layton:
musical

Ladisiao (Spanish) helpful
Laddy

Ladislav (Czech) form of
Walter: army leader

Lado (Spanish) artistic

Lael (Hebrew) belonging to
Jehovah
Lale

Laertes (Literature) from
Shakespeare's Hamlet;
action-oriented

Lafaye (American) cheerful
Lafay, Lafayye, Laphay, Laphe

Lafayetta (Spanish) form of
Lafayette: ambitious
Lafay

Lafayette (French) ambitious
Lafayet, Lafayett

Lafe (American) punctual
Laafe, Laife, Laiffe

Lafen (English) dearest friend

Lafett (French) form of
Lafayette: ambitious

Lafi (Polynesian) shy

Lagos (Place name) city in
Nigeria
Lago

Lagrand (African American)
the grand
Grand, Grandy, Lagrande

Lahahana (Hawaiian) warm
as sunshine

Laionela (Hawaiian) lion
boldness

Laird (Scottish) rich
Layrd, Layrde

Lais (Indian) leonine

Laish (Biblical) place name

Laizer (French) form of
Lazarus: helped by God

Lajos (Hungarian) famed

Lake (English) tranquil water

Lakista (African American)
bold man

Laksen (Scandinavian) lucky
son

Lakshman (Hindi)
promising; (Indian) rich

Lal (Hindi) beloved

Lalit (Indian) handsome

Lalo (Latin) singer of a lullaby
Laloh

Lam (African) picks lemons

Lamalcom (African
American) son of Malcolm;
kingly
*LaMalcolm, LaMalcom, Mal,
Malcolm, Malcom*

Lamar (Latin) renowned
*Lamahr, Lamarr, Lemar,
Lemarr*

Lamber (German) form of
Lambert: bright
Lambur

Lambert (German) bright
*Lamb, Lamber, Lambie,
Lamburt, Lammie, Lammy*

Lamberto (Spanish) bright

Lamech (Biblical) to lower

Lamek (Biblical) form of
Lamech: to lower

Lament (Biblical) from
Lamentations

Lamis (Arabic) speaks softly

Lamond (French) worldly
*Lammond, Lamon, Lamonde,
Lemond*

Lamont (Scandinavian)
lawman
Lamon

Lamonte (French) mountain

Lan (Chinese) orchid

Lance (German) confident
Lanse, Lantz, Lanz

Lancelot (French) romantic
*Lance, Lancelott, Launcelot,
Launcey*

Land (English) form of
Landon: plain; old-fashioned

Landan (English) from the
plains; quiet

Lander (English) landed
Land, Landor

Landers (English) wealthy
Land, Landar, Lander, Landor

Landis (English) owning
land; earthy
*Land, Landes, Landice,
Landise, Landly, Landus*

Lando (American) masculine
Land

Landon ○ ❶ (English) plain;
old-fashioned
Land, Landan, Landen

Landry (French) entrepreneur
Landré, Landree

Lane (English) secure
*Laine, Laney, Lanie, Lanni,
Layne*

Lang (English) top
Lange

Langdon (English) long-
winded
Lang, Langden, Langdun

Langen (English) tall

Langerson (Scandinavian)
long

Langford (English) healthy
Lanford, Langferd

Langham (Last name as first
name) long
Lang

Langilea (Polynesian) loud as
thunder

Langiloa (Polynesian)
stormy; moody

Langley (English) natural
Lang, Langlee, Langli, Langly

Langston (English) long-suffering
Lang, Langstan, Langsten

Langton (English) long
Lange

Langundo (Polynesian) graceful

Langward (Last name as first name) long

Langworth (Last name as first name) of long worth

Lani (Hawaiian) lithe

Lanie (Scandinavian) son of tall man

Laning (last name as first name)

Lanndson (English) last name as first name

Lanny (American) popular
Lann, Lanney, Lanni, Lannie

Lansing (Place name) city in Michigan
Lance, Lans

Lanty (Irish) lively
Laughun, Leachlainn, Lochlainn, Lochlann

Lantz (American) form of Lance: confident

Lanu (Native American) circular

Lanzo (Italian) lance

Laoghaire (Irish) caretaker of cows

Laoiseach (Place name) from the county Leix in Ireland

Lap (Vietnamese) independent

Laphonso (African American) prepared; centered

Lapidos (Greek) cologne
Lapidus

Laramie (French) pensive
Laramee

Lare (American) wealthy
Larre, Layr

Laredo (Spanish) place name

Larence (English) form of Lorenzo: honored

Largel (American) intrepid
Large

Lari (American) form of Larry: extrovert

Lariat (American) roper
Lare, Lari

Larios (Spanish) form of Lawrence: honored

Larkin (Irish) brash
Lark, Larkan, Larken, Larkie, Larky

Larndell (American) generous
Larn, Larndelle, Larndey, Larne

Larne (Place name) district in Northern Ireland
Larn, Larney, Larny

Larnell (American) giving
Larne

Laron (American) outgoing
Larron, Larrone

Laroyce (French) royal

Larrimore (Last name as first name) loud
Larimore, Larmer, Larmor

Larrmyne (American) boisterous
Larmie, Larmine, Larmy, Larmyne

Larry (Latin) extrovert
Lare, Larrey, Larri, Larrie, Lary

Lars (Scandinavian) form of
Lawrence: honored
Larrs, Larse, Larsy

Larsa (Biblical) ancient
Babylonian city

Larson (Scandinavian) son of
Lars

Lasha (Biblical) place name
(east of the Dead Sea);
Fissure

Lashaun (African American)
enthusiastic
*Lashawn, La-Shawn, Lashon,
Lashond*

Lashe (Scandinavian) form of
Lasse: winner; the people's
victory

Laskey (Last name as first
name) jovial
Lask, Laski

Lasse (Scandinavian) form of
Nicholas

Lassen (Place name) a peak
in California in the Cascade
Range
Lase, Lasen, Lassan, Lassun

Lassit (American) broad-
minded
Lasset, Lassitte

Lassiter (American) witty
Lassater, Lasseter, Lassie, Lassy

Laszlo (Hungarian) famous
leader
Laslo, Lazuli

Lateef (Arabic) a gentle man

Lath (Scandinavian) boy from
the barn

Latham (Scandinavian)
farmer; knowing
Lathe, Lay

Lathrop (English) home-
loving
*Lathe, Lathrap, Latrope, Lay,
Laye, Laythrep*

Latif (Arabic) nice

Latimer (English) interprets;
philanthropic
Latymer

Latorris (African American)
notorious
LaTorris

Latoure (French) torn

Latravious (African
American) healthy
Latrave

Latty (English) giving
Lat, Latti, Lattie

Laughlin (Irish) servant

Laurence (Latin) form of
Lawrence: honored
*Larence, Laurance, Laurans,
Laure, Lorence*

Laurens (German) brilliant
*Larrie, Larry, Laure, Laurins,
Lorens, Lors*

Laurent (French) martyred
Laurynt

Laurie (Latin) form of
Lawrence: honored

Lavan (Latin) pure

Lavaughn (African
American) perky
*Lavan, Lavon, Lavonn, Levan,
Levaughn*

Lavaughor (African
American) laughing
Lavaugher, Lavawnar

Lavay (Italian) form of Livia:
place name

Lavega (French) eagle star

Laven (Hebrew) white

Lavesh (Hindi) little piece; calm

Lavi (Hebrew) uniter

Lavunn (American) form of Levon: forward-thinking

Law (American) feisty

Lawerence (Latin) form of Lawrence: honored

Lawford (English) dignified
Laford, Lauford, Lawferd

Lawler (Last name as first name) honoring; teacher
Lawlor, Lollar, Loller

Lawrence (Latin) honored
Larrie, Larry, Laurence, Lawrance, Lawrunce

Lawrie (Latin) form of Lawrence: honored
Lowrie

Lawson (English) lawrence's son; special
Law, Laws, Lawsan, Lawsen

Lawton (Last name as first name) honored town

Laylan (English) from land of Leigh

Layneln (English) form of Lane: secure

Layshaun (African American) merry
Laysh, Layshawn

Laysy (Last name as first name) sophisticated
Lay, Laycie, Laysee

Layt (American) fascinating
Lait, Laite, Late, Layte

Layte (English) meadow boy

Layton (English) musical
Laytan, Laytawn, Layten

Laz (Spanish) form of Lazarus: helped by God

Lazar (Hebrew) form of Lazarus: helped by God
Lazare, Lazaro, Lazear, Lazer

Lazaro (Italian) form of Lazarus: helped by God

Lazarus (Greek) helped by God
Eleazer, Lasarus, Lazerus, Lazoros

Lazo (Spanish) form of Lazarus: helped by God

Leal (Greek) self-assured

Leal (Spanish) form of Lael: belonging to Jehovah

Leamon (American) powerful
Leamm, Leamond, Leemon

Leand (Greek) form of Leander: ferocious; lionlike
Leander

Leander (Greek) ferocious; lionlike
Anders, Leann, Leannder

Leandro (Spanish) of Leander

Lear (Greek) royal
Leare, Leere

Learly (Last name as first name) terrific
Learley

Leary (Irish) herds; high goals

Leather (American) word as name; tough
Leath

Leavery (American) giving
Leautree, Leautri, Leautry, Levry, Lo, Lotree, Lotrey, Lotri, Lotry

Leben (Last name as first name) small; hopeful

Lebna (African) soulful

Lebrun (French) brown-haired
Lebron, Labron

Lechoslaw (Polish) glorious Pole; envied
Lech, Leslaw, Leszek

Lecil (American) form of Cecil: unseeing; hard-headed; blind

Leckto (Greek) everlasting

Lectoy (American) form of Leroy: king; loyal
Lec, Lecto, Lek

Lee (English) loving
Lea, Lee, Leigh

Leeander (Invented) form of Leander: ferocious; lionlike

Legario (Spanish) cheerful

Leger (French) sent to earth

Leggett (Last name as first name) able
Legate, Leggitt, Liggett

Lei (Hawaiian) wreath; decorative

Leibel (Hebrew) lion

Leif (Scandinavian) loved one
Laif, Leaf, Leife

Leigh (English) smooth

Leighton (Last name as first name) hearty
Laytan, Layton, Leighten, Leightun

Leith (Scottish) broad

Lel (Gypsy) taker

Leland (English) protective
Leeland, Leighlon, Leiland, Lelan, Lelond

Leldon (American) form of Eldon: charitable
Leldun

Lem (Hebrew) form of Lemuel: loves God

Lemar (American) form of Lamar: renowned
Lemarr

Lemmy (Hebrew) loves God

Lemon (American) fruit; tart
Lemonn, Lemun, Limon

Lemuel (Hebrew) loves God
Lem, Lemmie, Lemmy, Lemy

Lemus (Spanish) loves God

Len (German) form of Leonard: courageous
Lennie, Lynn

Lenard (American) form of Leonard: courageous
Lenerd

Lencio (Spanish) valiant; gentle

Leni (Polynesian) lives for today

Lenjun (Dutch) helps

Lennan (Irish) gentle

Lennart (Scandinavian) brave
Lenn, Lenne

Lenno (Italian) brave

Lennon (Irish) renowned; caped
Lenn, Lennan, Lennen, Lenin

Lennor (Last name as first name) brave

Lennox (Scottish) authoritative
Lennix, Lenocks, Lenox, Linnox

Lenny (German) form of Leonard: courageous
Lenn, Lenney, Lenni, Lennie, Leny, Linn

Lensar (English) stays with parents

Lentin (English) summery

Lenton (American) religious
Lent, Lenten, Lentun

Lenvil (Invented) typical
Lenval, Level

Leny (German) form of
Leonard: courageous

Leo (Latin) lionlike; fierce

Leobardo (Italian) lionlike

Leocadio (Spanish)
lionhearted
Leo

Leolin (Polynesian) watchful
Leoline, Llewelyn

Leon (Greek) tenacious
Lee, Leo, Leone, Leonn

Leonard (German)
courageous
*Lee, Leo, Leonar, Leonerd,
Leonord, Lynar, Lynard, Lynerd*

LeOnarda (Spanish) form of
Leonardo: lion-hearted

Leonardo (Italian)
lionhearted
Leo

Leoncio (Spanish)
lionhearted
Leon, Leonce, Leonse

Leondras (African American)
lionine
*Leon, Leondre, Leondrus,
Leonid*

Leondus (Spanish) lion

Leone (Spanish) lion

Leonel (American) form of
Lionel: fierce

Leonidus (Latin) strong
*Leon, Leone, Leonidas,
Leonydus*

Leontes (German) lion's
courage

Leonzo (Spanish) lion's
courage

Leopold (German) brave
Lee, Leo

Leor (Latin) listens

Leoti (American) outdoorsy
Lee, Leo

Leovardo (Spanish) form of
Leonardo: lionhearted
Leo, Leovard

Leovigildo (Spanish) lion
heart

Lepern (Italian) lionine

Lepoldo (Spanish) form of
Leopold: brave
Lee, Lepold, Poldo

Lepolo (Polynesian)
handsome

Lerby (French) circular life

Lerett (last name as first
name) gentle

Lerey (American) form of
Larry: extrovert
Lerrie, Lery

Leroy (French) king; royal
Leeroy, Leroi, Le-Roy, Roy, Roye

Leroye (French) royal

Les (English) form of Leslie:
fortified
Lez, Lezli

Leshawn (African American)
cheery
Lashawn, Leshaun, Le-Shawn

Leslie (Scottish) fortified
*Lee, Les, Lesley, Lesli, Lezlie,
Lezly*

Lesner (Last name as first
name) serious
Les, Lez, Lezner

Lester (American) large
persona
Les, Lestor

Letian (Spanish) happy

Leto (Latin) happy

Letrae (French) joyful

Letushim (Biblical)
hammermen; filemen

Leuk (Irish) form of Lake:
tranquil water

Leumas (Biblical) name
spelled backward

Leummim (Biblical)
countries, without water.

Lev (Russian) lionine

Levar (American) soft-spoken
Levarr

Levega (French) star

Leven (Hebrew) heart's child

Leveratto (Italian) organized

Leverett (Last name as first
name) planner
Lev, Leveret, Leverit, Leveritt

Leverton (Last name as first
name) town of Lever;
organized

Levesque (French)
gatekeeper

Levi (Hebrew) harmonious
Lev, Levey, Levie, Levy

Levonne (African American)
forward-thinking
Lavonne, Leevon, Levon

Lew (Polish) form of Louis:
famous warrior
Leu

Leward (French) contentious
Lewar, Lewerd

Lewie (French) form of Louis:
famous warrior
Lew, Lewee, Lewey, Lewy

Lewin (Last name as first
name) lionlike

Lewis (German) form of
Louis: famous warrior
Lewey, Lewie, Lewus, Lewy

Lewy (Irish) giving

Lex (English) form of
Alexander: great leader;
helpful
Lexa, Lexe, Lexi, Lexie, Lexy

Lexonne (American) form of
Alexander: great leader;
helpful

Leyland (Last name as first
name) protective

Leyth (Scottish) river

Li (Chinese) strong man

Liam (Irish) protective;
handsome
Leam, Leeam, Leeum

Liang (Chinese) good man

Libardo (Spanish) free

Liber (Roman) freedom

Liberio (Spanish) liberated
Libere, Lyberio

Liberty (American) freedom-
loving
Lib

Libni (Slavic) love

Libor (Czech) free

Licien (French) form of
Lucian: soothing

Lidio (Greek) pleasant man

Lidon (Hebrew) judge

Liem (Vietnamese) truthful

Lienad (Biblical) name
spelled backward

Lif (Scandinavian) full of life

Lifen (Dutch) beloved

Lige (Spanish) form of Ligia: clear

Ligi (Spanish) form of Ligia: clear

Ligia (Spanish) clear

Lihau (Hawaiian) cool; fresh

Like (Asian) soft-spoken

Liko (Hawaiian) budding; flourishing

Lillo (American) triple-threat talent
Lilo

Limo (Invented) from limousine; sporty
Lim

Limu (Polynesian) seaweed; natural

Linc (English) form of Lincoln: leader; lake colony
Link, Links

Lincoln (English) leader; lake colony
Link

Lindberg (German) linden-tree mountain
Lin, Lind, Lindburg, Lindie, Lindy, Lyndberg, Lyndburg

Lindell (Last name as first name) in harmony with nature
Lindall, Lindel, Lyndall, Lyndell

Linden (Botanical) tree
Lindun

Lindoh (American) sturdy
Lindo, Lindy

Lindsay (English) natural
Lind, Lindsee, Lindsey, Linz, Linzee, Lyndsey, Lyndzie, Lynz, Lynzie

Lindy (German) form of Lindberg: linden-tree mountain
Lind

Linford (Last name as first name) bold man
Lynford

Linfred (Last name as first name) proactive

Linley (English) open-minded
Lin, Linlee, Linleigh, Lynlie

Linnard (German) form of Leonard: courageous
Linard, Lynard

Lino (American) form of Linus: blond
Linus

Linos (Spanish) praised

Linton (English) lives near lime trees
Lintonn, Lynton, Lyntonn

Linus (Greek) blond
Linas, Line, Lines

Linvel (English) from flax town

Linwood (American) open

Lionel (French) fierce
Li, Lion, Lionell, Lye, Lyon, Lyonel, Lyonell

Liron (Hebrew) my song
Lyron

Lisiate (Polynesian) courageous

Lisimba (African) attacked by lion; victim

Lister (Origin unknown) intelligent

Littlejoe (Spanish) small

Litton (English) centered
Lyten, Lyton, Lytton

Liu (Asian) quiet

Liuz (Polish) light

Livias (Biblical) place name

Livingston (English) comforting
Liv, Livey, Livingstone

Liwanu (Asian) released

Llano (Place name) river in Texas; flowing
Lano

Llewellyn (English) fiery; fast
Lew, Lewellen, Lewellyn

Lleyton (Slavic) of the garden

Lloy (Welsh) holy

Lloyd (English) spiritual; joyful
Loy, Loyd, Loydde, Loye

Lobo (Spanish) wolf
Loboe, Lobow

Loc (English) of the forest

Lochan (Irish) lively

Lochlain (Irish) assertive
Lochlaine, Lochlane, Locklain

Lock (English) natural
Locke

Lod (Biblical) place name

Lodewuk (Scandinavian) warrior
Ladewijk, Ludovic

Lodge (English) safe haven

Lodi (American) place name

Lodovico (Italian) famous

Lodur (Scandinavian) vivid

Loey (American) daring
Loie, Lowee, Lowi

Lofton (Last name as first name) lofty
Loften

Logan ✪ ❶ (Irish) eloquent
Logen, Loggy, Logun

Lohan (Last name as first name) capable

Lokela (Hawaiian) famed spear-thrower

Lokene (Hawaiian) form of Rodney: open-minded

Lokesh (Indian) hindu god Brahma

Lokie (Mythology) chaotic

Loknath (Indian) world leader

Lokni (Hawaiian) red rose

Loman (Irish) bare

Lomas (Spanish) good man

Lomax (English) last name as first name

Lombain (French) peaceful (from the name Colombain)

Lombard (Teutonic) long-Beard

Lombardi (Italian) winner
Bardi, Bardy, Lom, Lombard, Lombardy

Lon (Irish) intense

Lonata (Spanish) bravery

Lonato (Native American) flint stone; calm

Loncel (French) gentle

Lond (English) form of London: ethereal; capital of great Britain

London (English) ethereal; capital of great Britain
Londen

Long (Last name as first name) chinese dragon; methodical

Lonnie (Spanish) form of Alonzo: enthusiastic
Lonney, Lonni, Lonny

Lono (Hawaiian) god of peace and agriculture

Loocho (Invented) form of Lucho: lucky; light

Loomis (American) young

Loramie (American) form of Laramie: pensive

Loran (American) form of Lauren: laurel-crowned

Lorance (Latin) form of Lawrence: honored
Lorans, Lorence

Lorca (Last name as first) poet

Lorcan (Irish) fiery

Lord (English) regal
Lorde

Lordlee (English) regal
Lordly, Lords

Lordson (English) Lord's son

Loredo (Spanish) smart; cowboy
Lorado, Loredoh, Lorre, Lorrey

Loren (Latin) hopeful; winning
Lorin, Lorrin

Lorens (Scandinavian) form of Lawrence: honored

Lorenzo (Spanish) form of Lawrence: honored
Larenzo, Loranzo, Lore, Lorence, Lorenso, Lorentz, Lorenz, Lorrie, Lorry

Loreto (Italian) form of Lawrence: honored

Loriano (Italian) form of Lorenzo; form of Lawrence: honored

Lorimer (Last name as first name) brash
Lorrimer

Loring (German) brash
Looring, Lorrie, Louring

Loring (Greek) son of soldier

Lorl (English) laurel plant

Lorne (Latin) grounded
Lorn, Lorny

Lorry (English) form of Laurie: honored
Lore, Lorri, Lorrie, Lorry, Lory 🌐

Loryn (Latin) praised

Lot (Hebrew) furtive
Lott

Lotan (Biblical) secret

Lothario (German) lover
Lotario, Lothaire, Lotherio, Lothurio

Lou (German) form of Louis: famous warrior
Lew

Loudin (German) from low valley; blessed child

Loudon (American) enthusiastic
Louden, Lowden, Lowdon

Louie (German) form of Louis: famous warrior
Louey

Louis (German) famous warrior
Lewis, Lou, Louie, Lue, Luie, Luis

Louks (Dutch) mysterious

Loundis (American) visionary
Lound, Loundas, Loundes, Lowndis

Louvain (English) city in Belgium; wanderer

Love (Swedish) form of Louis: famous warrior

Lovell (English) brilliant
Lovall, Love, Lovelle, Lovie

Lovett (Last name as first name) loving
Lovat, Lovet

Low (American) word as a name; low-key
Lowey

Lowell (English) loved
Lowall, Lowel

Lowry (Last name as first name) leader
Lowree, Lowrey

Loy (English) loyal

Loyal (English) true to the word
Loy

Loyal (English) loyal

Loys (American) loyal
Loyce, Loyse

Loza (Spanish) form of Louis: famous warrior

Lozano (Spanish) last name as first name

Luas (Slavic) combative

Lubin (Slavic) loving

Lubomil (Polish) loves grace

Lubomir (Slavic) loves peace

Lubos (Slavic) loving

Luboslaw (Polish) loves glory

Luc (French) light; laidback
Lucca, Luke

Luca (Italian) lighthearted
Louca, Louka, Luka

Lucan (Irish) light

Lucas ✪ ✆ (Greek) patron saint of doctors/artists; creative
Lucca, Luces, Luka, Lukas, Luke, Lukes, Lukus

Lucason (German) son of Lucas; Light

Lucho (Spanish) lucky; light

Lucian (Latin) soothing
Lew, Luciyan, Lushun

Luciano (Italian) lighthearted
Luca, Lucas, Luke

Lucious (African American) light; delicious
Luceous, Lushus

Lucius (Latin) sunny
Lucca, Luchious, Lushus

Lucky (American) lucky
Luckee, Luckey, Luckie

Lud (Biblical) warring

Luddey (Scandinavian) warring

Ludger (Scandinavian) wielding spears

Ludie (English) glorious
Ludd

Ludim (Biblical) warring

Luding (English) warrior

Ludington (English) warrior

Ludlow (German) respected
Ludlo, Ludloe

Ludolf (English) form of Rudolf: wolf

Ludomir (Polish) of well-known ancestry

Ludoslav (Polish) of glorified people

Ludovic (Slavic) smart; spiritual
Luddovik, Lude, Ludovik, Ludvic, Vick

Ludrie (last name as first name) respected

Ludwig (German) talented
Ludvig, Ludweg, Ludwige

Ludwin (English) friend of Ludwig

Lugus (Irish) shining

Luigi (Italian) famed warrior
Lui, Louie

Luis ☼ (Spanish) outspoken
Luez, Luise, Luiz

Luisito (Spanish) form of Louis: famous warrior

Luister (Irish) form of Louis: famous warrior

Lujo (Spanish) luxurious
Luj

Luka (Italian) form of Luca: lighthearted
Luke

Lukae (Slavic) form of Luke: worshipful

Lukah (Invented) form of Luca: lighthearted

Lukas (Greek) lighthearted; creative
Lucus

Luke ☼ ☾ (Latin) worshipful
Luc, Lucc, Luk, Lukus

Lukman (Last name as first name) vivacious

Lulani (Hawaiian) light sky

Lullo (American) form of Luke: worshipful

Lumer (American) light
Lumar, Lume, Lumur

Luna (Spanish) moon

Lund (Scottish) island grove child

Lundy (Scandinavian) island-lover

Lunell (Irish) light

Lunn (Irish) smart and brave
Lun, Lunne

Lunt (Scandinavian) grove-dweller

Luo (Hawaiian) light

Luong (Vietnamese) from the land of bamboo

Lusk (Last name as first name) hearty
Lus, Luske, Luskee, Luskey, Luski, Lusky

Lussier (French) last name as first name

Lutalo (African) bold fighter

Lute (Polynesian) pigeon; inconspicuous

Luther (German) reformer
Luthar, Luth, Luthur

Luthus (American) form of Luther: reformer
Luth, Luthas

Luto (Greek) from Pluto

Lux (English) light

Lyal (English) form of Lyle: unique
Lye

Lyall (Scottish) faithful

Lycur (Greek) sly

Lydan (Irish) gray

Lyfe (American) life

Lyle (French) unique
Lile, Ly, Lyle

Lyleon (Scottish) of the isles

Lyles (English) of the isles

Lyman (English)
meadow-man; sportsman
Leaman, Leyman

Lyndall (English)
nature-lover
Lynd, Lyndal, Lyndell

Lyndles (English) of nature

Lyndon (English) verbose
Lindon, Lyn, Lynd, Lyndonn

Lynge (Scandinavian) sylvan
nature

Lynn (English) water-loving
Lin, Linn, Lyn, Lynne

Lynton (English) town of
nature lovers
Linton

Lynus (Greek) flax

Lynusse (American) form of
Lynus: flax

Lynwood (English) forest

Lyon (Place name) city in
France
Lyone

Lyr (Welsh) sea god

Lyron (Hebrew) my song

Lysande (Greek)
freewheeling
Lyse

Lysander (Greek) lover
Lysand

Lyulf (German) haughty;
combative
Lyulfe, Lyulff

M

Maarten (Welsh) form of
Martin: warlike; god of war

Mablevi (African) do not
deceive

Mac (Irish) mack
Mackee, Macki, Mackie, Macky

Macabee (Biblical/Hebrew)
hammer

MacAdam (Scottish) son of
Adam; first

Macadee (Scandinavian)
headstrong

Macaffie (Scottish) charming
*Mac, Mack, Mackey, McAfee,
McAffee, McAffie*

Macario (Spanish) blessed
Macareo, Makario

Macarlos (Spanish) manly
Carlos

Macarthur (Irish) arthur's
son

Macaru (Spanish)

Macaul (Scottish) form of
Macaulley: devout son

Macauley (Scottish)
righteous; dramatic
Mac, Macaulay, McCauley

Macauliffe (Last name as
first name) bookish
Macaulif, Macauliff

Macaulley (Scottish) devout
son

Macbey (American) form of
Mackie: friendly
Mackbey, Makbee, Makbi

Macdowell (Last name as first name) giving
Macdowl

Mace (French) club

Macedonio (Spanish) from Macedonia; travels

MacEgan (Last name as first name) son of Egan; capable

Maceo (Spanish) form of Macedonio: from Macedonia; travels

Maceson (French) son of Mace

Macgowan (Irish) able; gallant
Macgowen, Macgowyn

Machen (Slavic) winner

Mackay (Scottish) form of Mackie: friendly

Mackeane (Last name as first name) attractive
Mackeene

Macken (Scottish) from Mackay

Mackenna (Irish) giving; leader
Mackena

Mackenzie (Irish) giving
Mack, Mackenzy, Mackinsey, Makinzie, McKenzie

Mackeon (Last name as first name) smiling

Mackie (Irish) friendly
Mackey

MacKinley (Irish) son of Kinley; educated

Mackinney (Last name as first name) good-looking
Mackinny

Macklin (Irish) good-humored

Maclain (Irish) natural wonder
McLain, McLaine, McLean

Maclean (Irish) dependable
Macleen

MacMurray (Irish) loves the sea

Macnair (Scottish) practical

Macon (Place name) city in Georgia; creative
Makon

Macy (French) lasting; wealthy
Mace, Macee, Macey, Macye

Madai (Biblical) of the Medes (ancient Persians)

Madan (Hindi) god of love; loving

Madan (Indian) cupid

Madden (Pakistani) planner
Maddin, Maddyn, Maden, Madin, Madyn

Maddock (Welsh) generous
Maddoc, Madocock, Maddox, Madox

Maddok (Welsh) form of Maddock: generous

Maddox (English) giving
Maddocks, Maddy, Madox

Madeo (Italian) form of Mateo: God's gift

Madhav (Hindi) sweet
Madhu

Madhavi (Indian) sweet as honey

Madison (English) good
Maddison, Maddy, Madisan, Madisen, Son

Madock (American) giving
Maddock, Maddy, Madoc

Madon (Irish) giving

Madras (Place name) city in India

Madu (African) manly

Madzimoyo (African) nourished by water; simple

Magaidi (African) last

Magalirio (Spanish) charming

Magee (Irish) practical; lively *Mackie, Maggy, McGee*

Magellan (Spanish) explorer

Magene (Latin) creative

Magglio (Hispanic) athletic

Magic (American) magical *Majic*

Magick (American) magical

Magli (Icelandic) magnanimous

Magne (Latin) great

Magni (Latin) greatness

Magno (Latin) greatness

Magnus (Latin) outstanding *Maggy, Magnes*

Magog (Biblical) son of Gog; place name

Maguire (Irish) subtle *Macky, Maggy, McGuire*

Mahadev (Indian) omnipotent

Mahali (Biblical) unhealthy

Mahan (American) cowboy *Mahahn, Mahand, Mahen, Mayhan*

Maharba (Biblical) name spelled backward

Mahatma (Sanskrit) spiritually elevated

Maheshkumar (Indian) son of Lord Shiva

Mahir (Arabic) skilled

Mahler (Last name as first) famous composer; sweeping

Mahli (Hebrew) brilliant

Mahlon (English) astute

Mahluli (African) conqueror

Mahmud (Arabic) remarkable

Maikan (Welsh) calm

Maimon (Arabic) of good fortune

Main (Place name) river in Germany; leader *Mainess, Mane, Maness*

Maisel (Persian) warrior *Meisel*

Maitland (English) of the meadow; fresh ideas

Maj (Arabic) form of Majid: glorious

Majeed (Arabic) majestic *Majid*

Majid (Arabic) glorious

Major (Latin) leading *Mage, Magy, Majar, Maje, Majer*

Makale (Invented) form of Mikhail: godlike

Makaz (Biblical) place name

Makhi (American) form of Mikhail: godlike

Makio (Hawaiian) great

Makoto (Japanese) sincere; honest

Makoto (Japanese) earnest

Maks (Russian) form of Maksimilian: competitor

Maksimilian (Russian) competitor
Maksim

Makya (Native American) hunter

Mal (Hindi) gardens; flourishes

Mala (Indian) necklace

Malachi (Hebrew) angelic; magnanimous
Malachy, Malakai, Malaki, Maleki

Malachil (Hawaiian) angel

Malack (American) form of Malakai: God's angel

Malakai (Hebrew) God's angel

Malaki (Hebrew) God's angel

Malakinn (African) Lordly

Malawa (African) flowering

Malcolm (Scottish) peaceful
Mal, Malkalm, Malkelm, Malkolm

Maldon (French) strong and combative
Maldan, Malden

Malfred (German) feisty
Malfrid, Mann

Malidan (English) meets

Malik (Arabic) angelic
Malic

Malik (Arabic) masterful

Malikah (Hindi) royalty

Malise (French) masterful

Malk (Hindi) royal

Malla-Ki (Invented) form of Malachi: angelic; magnanimous

Malley (German) form of Mallory: wild spirit

Mallin (English) rowdy; warrior
Malen, Malin, Mallan, Mallen, Mallie, Mally

Mallory (French) wild spirit
Mal, Mallie, Malloree, Mallorie, Mally, Malory

Mallun (English) soldier's strength

Maloney (Irish) religious
Mal, Malone, Malonie, Malony

Malta (Biblical) place name

Malvin (English) open-minded
Mal, Malv, Malven, Malvyne

Mamre (Biblical) rebellious; bitter; set with trees

Mamun (Arabic) trustworthy

Manahath (Biblical) among men

Manasseh (Hebrew) cannot remember
Manases

Manchester (English) dignity; Place name
city in England

Manchu (Chinese) unflawed

Mandar (Indian) flower

Mandell (German) tough; almond
Mandee, Mandel, Mandela, Mandie, Mandy

Mandla (African) powerful

Mandy (Latin) lovable
Mandey

Manfred (English) peaceful
Manferd, Manford, Mannfred, Mannie, Manny, Mannye

Manfredo (Italian) strong
peacefulness

Mani (Spanish) God's gift

Manila (Place name) capital
of Philippines
Manilla

Maninder (Hindi)
masculine; potent

Manish (Indian) mind god

Manjuk (Arabic) lightness

Manley (English) virile;
haven
Man, Manlee, Manlie, Manly

Mann (German) masculine
Mannes, Manning

Manning (English) heroic
Man, Maning, Mann

Mannis (Irish) great
Manish, Manus

Mannix (Irish) spiritual
Manix, Mann, Mannicks

Mannon (French) exciting

Manny (Spanish) form of
Manuel: with God
Manney, Manni, Mannie

Manoj (Sanskrit) cupid

Manolito (Spanish) God
loves

Manolo (Spanish) from
Spanish shoe designer
Manolo Blahnik; cutting-edge

Manpreet (Indian) beloved;
calm

Manriquez (German) brave

Manse (English) winning

Mansfield (English)
outdoorsman
Manesfeld, Mans, Mansfeld, Mansfielde

Manshel (English) of the
house; domestic
Mansel

Mantel (English) formidable
Mantell, Mantle

Manton (English) man's
town; special

Manu (Hindi) father of
people; masculine

Manuel (Hebrew) form of
Emmanuel: with God
Mannuel, Manny, Manual, Manuelle

Manus (American)
strong-willed
Manes, Mann, Mannas, Mannes, Mannis, Mannus

Manus (Slavic) daybreak

Manvel (French) great town;
hardworking
Mann, Manny, Manvil, Manville

Manzo (Japanese) third-born

Mao (Chinese) hair

Maquinn (Native American)
generous

Marat (Russian) desirable

Marathon (Biblical) place
name

Marathus (Biblical) place
name

Marble (English) word as
name

Marc (French) combative
Markee, Markey, Markeye, Markie Mark, Markie, Marko, Marky

Marcel (French) singing
God's praises
Marcell, Mars, Marsel

Marceli (French) form of
Marcellus: romantic;
persevering

Marcellin (French) combative

Marc-Elliott (French)
combination of Marc and
Elliott

Marcellus (Latin) romantic;
persevering
*Marcel, Marcelis, Marcey,
Marsellus, Marsey*

Marcelno (Slavic) combative

Marcelo (Italian) combative

March (English) fruitful
month
Marche

Marchand (French)
merchant

Marchell (English) has limits

Marcial (Spanish) martial;
combative
Mars

Marciano (Italian) manly;
macho
Marcyano

Marciel (French) warring

Marcin (Polish) form of
Martin: warlike; god of war

Marcio (Italian) warring

Marcion (Italian) warring

Marcionne (Italian) form of
Martin: combative

Marco (Italian) tender
*Marc, Mark, Markie, Marko,
Marky*

Marconi (Italian) inventive;
tough

Marcos (Spanish) outgoing
Marco, Marko, Markos, Marky

Marco-Tulio (Spanish)
fighter; substantial
Marco Tulio, Marcotulio

Marcoux (French) aggressive;
manly
Marce, Mars

Marcus (Latin) combative
Marc, Mark, Markus, Marky

Marcus-Anthony (Spanish)
valuable; aggressive
*Marc Anthony, Marc-Antonito,
Marcus-Antoneo,
Marcusantonio, Markanthony,
Taco, Tonio, Tono*

Marduk (Hindi) bothered

Mardy (Jewish) competitive

Marek (Polish) masculine

Marekel (Slavic) form of
Marcus: combative

Marett (Greek) pearl

Margarito (Italian) pearl

Marguez (Spanish) noble
Marguiz

Mariano (Italian) combative;
manly
Mario

Marico (Italian) reasonable

Marin (French) ocean-loving
Maren, Marino, Maryn

Mariner (Greek) form of
Myron: aromatic oil

Mario (Italian) masculine
Marioh, Marius, Marrio, Morio

Marion (Latin) suspicious
Mareon, Marionn

Marios (Italian) combative

Marius (German) masculine; virile
Marrius

Marjuan (Spanish) contentious
Marhwon, Marwon, Marwond

Mark ♂ (Latin) form of Marcus: combative

Markan (Latin) form of Marcus: combative

Markay (American) manly

Markee (Polish) warring

Markel (Latin) form of Mark: combative

Markell (African American) personable
Markelle

Marker (American) form of Mark: combative

Markham (English) homebody
Marcum, Markhum, Markum

Markos (Greek) warring; masculine

Markys (French) form of Marcus: combative

Marl (English) rebel
Marley, Marli

Marley (English) secretive
Marlee, Marleigh, Marly

Marley (English) boy of the woods

Marlin (English) opportunistic; fish
Marllin

Marlo (English) hill by a lake; optimistic
Mar, Marl, Marlow, Marlowe

Marlon (French) wizard; strange
Marlan, Marlen, Marlin, Marly

Marlones (French) form of Marlon: wizard; strange

Marlous (English) boy from lake

Marlowes (English) boy from lake

Marmaduke (English) haughty
Duke, Marmadook, Marmahduke

Marmion (French) famed
Marmeonne, Marmyon

Marnin (Hebrew) ebullient

Maroulis (Greek) dark

Marq (French) noble
Mark, Marque, Marquie

Marque (French) noble; smart
Marcqe, Marcque, Marqe

Marquel (French) nobleman

Marques (African American) noble
Marqes, Marqis, Marquez, Marquis

Marquise (French) noble
Mark, Markese, Marky, Marq, Marquese, Marquie, Marquis

Marquison (last name as first name) capable

Mars (Latin) warlike; god of war
Marrs, Marz

Marsdon (English) comforting
Marr, Mars, Marsden, Marsdyn

Marsh (English) handsome
Marr, Mars, Marsch, Marsey, Marsy

Marshall (French) giving care
Marsh, Marshal, Marshel, Marshell, Marsy

Marson (English) mark's son

Marston (English)
personable
Mars, Marst, Marstan, Marsten

Martand (Indian) sunny

Marte (English) warring

Martial (French) form of
Mark: combative

Martim (Latin) form of
Martin: warlike; god of war

Martin (Latin) form of Mars:
warlike; god of war
Mart, Marten, Marti, Martie, Marton, Marty

Martone (French) form of
Martin: warlike; god of war

Marty (Latin) form of Martin:
warlike; god of war
Mart, Martee, Martey, Marti, Martie, Martye

Martyn (French) form of
Martin: warlike; god of war

Marv (English) form of
Marvin: steadfast friend
Marve, Marvy

Marvell (French) marvelous
man
Marvel, Marvil, Marvill, Marvyl, Marvyll

Marvie (English) form of
Marvin: steadfast friend

Marvin (English) steadfast
friend
Marv, Marven, Marvy

Marvous (American)
marvelous

Marwood (English) forest man

Masa (African) centered

Masaaki (Japanese) correct
brightness

Masada (Hebrew) stronghold

Masajiro (Japanese) integrity
Masahiro, Masaji

Masamba (African) departs

Masamitsu (Japanese)
feeling

Masanao (Japanese) good

Masayuki (Japanese)
problematic

Mash (African) delights

Mashael (Invented) form of
Michael: like the Lord

Mashane (English) form of
Maxime: greatest

Mashawn (African
American) vivacious
Masean, Mashaun, Mayshawn

Maslen (American)
promising
Mas, Masline, Maslyn

Mason ○ ○ (French)
ingenious; reliable; stone
mason
Mace, Mase

Masood (Iranian) helpful

Massa (Biblical) a burden;
prophecy

Massey (English) doubly
excellent
Maccey, Masey, Massi

Massiel (Slavic) best; from
Massimo

Massim (Italian) best; from
Massimo

Massimo (Italian) great
Masimo, Massey, Massimmo

Masson (French) stone
mason

Master (English) masterful

Masura (Japanese) fated for good life

Mate (Spanish) form of Mateo: God's gift

Matej (Polish) form of Matthew: God's gift

Mateo (Italian) God's gift

Mateus (Italian) God's gift

Mathan (Hebrew) fine gift

Mathau (American) spunky
Mathou, Mathow, Mathoy

Mather (English) leader; army; strong
Mathar

Matheson (English) son of God's gift
Mathesen, Mathisen, Mathison, Mathysen, Mathyson

Matheu (French) form of Matthew: God's gift
Matt, Matty

Mathias (German) form of Matthew: God's gift
Mathies, Mathyes, Matt, Matthias, Matty

Mathieson (German) son of Mathias

Mathieu (French) form of Matthew: God's gift

Matias (Spanish) form of Matthew: God's gift
Mathias, Matios, Mattias

Matin (Hebrew) gift

Matine (French) kind

Matisse (French) gifted

Matland (English) mat's land; homesteader

Matlock (American) rancher
Lock, Mat, Matt

Mato (Native American) bear; brawler

Matson (Hebrew) son of Matthew
Matsan, Matsen, Matt, Matty

Matt (Hebrew) form of Matthew: God's gift
Mat, Matte

Matteo (Spanish) God's gift

Matteson (English) son of Matt; God's gift

Matthew ✪ ✆ (Hebrew) God's gift
Math, Matheu, Mathieu, Matt, Mattie, Mattsy, Matty

Matthewson (Last name as first name) son of Matthew; devout
Mathewsen, Mathewson, Matthewsen

Matthias (Scandinavian) form of Matthew: God's gift

Matti (Scandinavian) form of Mathias: God's gift
Mat, Mats

Mattison (Last name as first name) son of Matti; worldly
Matisen, Matison, Matisen, Mattysen, Mattyson, Matysen, Matyson

Matts (Swedish) form of Matthew: God's gift

Matty (Hebrew) form of Matthew: God's gift
Mattey, Matti

Matun (Biblical) treasure

Matunde (African) form of Matthew: God's gift

Matus (Czech) form of Matthew: God's gift

Mauli (Hawaiian) spirited

Maurice (Latin) dark
*Maur, Maurie, Maurise,
Maury, Moorice, Morice,
Morrie, Morry*

Mauricio (Italian) dark
Mari, Mauri, Maurizio

Mauricion (Latin) dark

Maurizio (Italian) dark
*Marits, Miritza, Moritz,
Moritza, Moritzio*

Mauro (Latin) form of
Maurice: dark

Maury (Latin) form of
Maurice: dark
Mauree, Maurey, Mauri

Maven (American) dramatic

Maverick (American)
unconventional
*Mav, Mavarick, Mavereck,
Mavreck, Mavvy*

Mavis (French) bird; thrush;
free
Mavas, Mavus

Mawali (African) vibrant

Mawulol (African) thanks
God

Max (Latin) best
*Mac, Mack, Macks, Maxey,
Maxie, Maxx, Maxy*

Maxcy (Slavic) form of
Maximilian: most wonderful

Maxence (French) excellent

Maxfield (English) of the
great field; lives large

Maxime (French) greatest
Max, Maxeem, Maxim

Maximeen (French) best

Maximilian (Latin) most
wonderful
*Max, Maxemillion, Maxie,
Maxima, Maximillion,
Maxmyllyun, Maxy*

Maximino (Spanish)
maximum; tops
*Max, Maxem, Maxey, Maxi,
Maxim, Maxy*

Maximinole (Italian) best

Maximus (Greek) best

Maxinen (Spanish)
maximum
Max, Maxanen, Maxi

Maxwell (English) full of
excellence
*Maxe, Maxie, Maxwel,
Maxwill, Maxy*

Mayer (Hebrew) smart
Mayar, Maye, Mayor, Mayur

Mayfield (English) grace

Maynard (English) reliable
Mayne, Maynerd

Mayne (English) power figure

Mayner (English) form of
Maynard: reliable

Mayo (Irish) nature-loving
*Maio, Maioh, May, Mayes,
Mayoh, Mays*

Mayon (Place name) volcano
in the Philippines
May, Mayan, Mays, Mayun

Mays (English) of the field;
athlete

Mayz (Arabic) form of Mazin:
mannered

Maz (Hebrew) aid
*Maise, Maiz, Mazey, Mazi,
Mazie, Mazy*

Mazaca (Biblical) place name

Mazal (Arabic) sedate

Mazin (Arabic) mannered

McCoy (Irish) jaunty; coy
Coye, MacCoy

McDonald (Scottish) open-
minded
Mac-D, Macdonald

McFarlin (Last name as first
name) son of Farlin;
confident
Far, Farr

McGill (Irish) tricky

McGowan (Irish) feisty
Mac-G, Mcgowan

McGregor (Irish)
philanthropic
Macgregor

McKay (Scottish) connives

McKinley (Last name as first
name) son of Kinley; holding
his own
Kin, Kinley, McKinlee

McLean (Scottish) stays lithe

McLin (Irish) careful
Mac, Mack

Mead (English) outdoorsman
Meade, Meede

Meadey (English) child of the
meadow

Meallan (Irish) sweet
Maylan, Meall

Meant (American) closed

Mearl (French) form of
Merlin: clever

Mechell (French) strong
ancestry

Medad (Hebrew) loves

Medan (Biblical) judgment;
process

Medardo (Spanish) power
figure

Medford (French) natural;
comical
Med, Medfor

Medgar (German) strong

Medina (Spanish) place
name

Medwin (German) friendly

Megiddo (Biblical) place
name

Mehmet (Sanskrit) royal

Mehrdad (Persian) sun

Mehul (Indian) rainy

Meindert (German) hearty
boy
Meinhard, Meinrad

Meir (Hebrew) teacher
Mayer, Myer

Mek (Scandinavian) spiritual

Mekhi (Asian) vision

Mel (Irish) form of Melvin:
friendly
Mell

Melanio (Spanish) royal

Melar (English) mill man;
pleases

Melbourne (Place name) city
in Australia; serene
*Mel, Melborn, Melbourn,
Melburn, Melburne*

Melbourne (English) from
the mill stream

Melburn (English) sylvan;
outdoorsy
*Mel, Melbourn, Melburne,
Milbourn, Milburn*

Melch (Hebrew) royalty

Melchor (Polish) city's king

Meldon (English) destined
for fame
Melden, Meldin, Meldyn

Meldric (English) leader
Mel, Meldrik

Melech (Jewish) king

Melecio (Spanish) cautious
Melesio, Melezio, Mesio

Meletius (Greek) ultra-
cautious
Meletios, Meletus

Melford (English) boy from
mill ford

Melito (Spanish) small and
calm

Meliton (Greek) malta child

Melle (English) masculine
form of Mary: star of the sea;
sea of bitterness

Melos (Greek) favorite
Milos

Melquiades (Spanish) gypsy

Melroy (American) form of
Elroy: giving
Mel

Melroy (Irish)

Melton (English) nature;
natural
Mel, Meltan

Melvan (Irish) form of
Melvin: friendly

Melville (French) mill town
Mel, Mell, Melvil, Melvill

Melvin (English) friendly
*Mel, Melvine, Melvon, Melvyn,
Milvin*

Melvis (American) form of
Elvis: all-wise
Mel, Melv

Melvo (American) form of
Melvin: friendly

Memphis (Place name) city
in Tennessee
Memphus

Menas (Hebrew) forgets

Mendel (English) methodical
*Mendl, Menka, Menke, Mela,
Menlin*

Menes (Egyptian) first king
of the 1st Egyptian Dynasty

Menlus (Greek) endures

Menno (Dutch) strong

Mensa (African) third son;
genius
Mensah

Ment (Greek) teaches

Menter (Greek) helper;
Mentor

Merari (Biblical/Hebrew)
bitter

Merce (English) merchant

Mercer (English) affluent
Merce, Mercur, Murcer

Merch (English) merchant

Merchant (English)
merchant

Mercury (Latin) mercurial

Mercutio (Literature) from
Shakespeare's Romeo and
Juliet; mercurial

Merdyth (Welsh) form of
Meredith: protector

Meredith (Welsh) protector
*Merdith, Mere, Meredyth,
Meridith, Merrey*

Mereld (Irish) form of
Merrill: renowned

Merika (Slavic) sea child

Merlin (English) clever
*Merl, Merlan, Merle, Merlinn,
Merlun, Murlin*

Merlot (Word as name) wine

Merrical (American) miracle

Merrick (English) bountiful
seaman
*Mere, Meric, Merik, Merrack,
Merrik*

Merrie (English) giving
Merey, Meri, Merri

Merrill (French) renowned
*Mere, Merell, Merill, Merrell,
Merril, Meryll*

Merritt (Latin) worthy
Merid, Merit, Merret, Merrid

Merson (Irish) son of the sea

Merv (Irish) form of Mervin:
bold
Murv

Mervin (Irish) bold
*Merv, Merven, Mervun, Mervy,
Mervyn, Murv, Murvin*

Merwin (Irish) friend of the
sea

Merzian (American) sea child

Meshach (Hebrew) fortunate
Meeshak, Meshack, Meshak

Meson (Spanish) of the
house

Mesquite (American)
rancher; spiny shrub
Meskeet

Messiah (Biblical) delivered
the Jews

Metheus (Greek) form of
Prometheus: friend of man;
bringer of fire

Methuse (Biblical) from
Methuselah

Metin (Turkish) dominant

Metzger (last name as first
name)

Meyer (Hebrew) brilliant
Maye, Meier, Mye, Myer

Meyshaun (African
American) searching
*Maysh, Mayshaun, Mayshawn,
Meyshawn*

Mibsam (Biblical) smelling
sweet

Micah (Hebrew) prophet;
sees all
Mica, Micha, Michah

Mican (Hebrew) form of
Michael: like the Lord

Michael ✪ ☎ (Hebrew) like
the Lord
*Mical, Michaelle, Mickey,
Mikael, Mike, Mikey, Mikiee,
Miko*

Michel (French) fond
Mich, Michelle, Mike, Mikey

Michelangelo (Italian) God's
angel/messenger; artistic
*Michel, Michelanjelo,
Mikalangelo, Mike, Mikel,
Mikelangelo*

Michitt (American) form of
Michael: like the Lord

Michon (French) form of
Michel: fond
Mich, Michonn, Mish, Mishon

Mick (Hebrew) closest to God
Mic, Mik

Mickel (American) form of
Michael: like the Lord
Mick, Mikel

Mickey (American)
enthusiastic
*Mick, Micki, Mickie, Micky,
Miki, Myck*

Mickey-Lee (American)
friendly
*Mickey Lee, Mickeylee,
Mickie-Lee*

Miga (Spanish) persona; essence

Migdol (Biblical) place name

Migio (Spanish) form of Remigio: from Rheims

Migron (Biblical) place name

Miguel ○ (Spanish) form of Michael: like the Lord
Megel, Migel, Migelle

Miguelangel (Spanish) angelic
Miguelanjel

Mihir (Hindi) sunny

Mihir (Indian) sun

Mika (Hebrew) form of Micah: prophet; sees all
Mikah, Mikie, Myka, Mykie, Myky

Mikael (Scandinavian) warrior
Michael, Mikel, Mikkel

Mikahael (Slavic) form of Michael: like the Lord

Mikaile (Scandinavian) form of Michael: like the Lord

Mikas (Russian) form of Mikhail: godlike

Mike (Hebrew) form of Michael: like the Lord
Meik, Miik, Myke

Mikel (Slavic) form of Mikhail: godlike

Mikelis (Slavic) form of Michael: like the Lord

Mikhail (Russian) godlike
Mika, Mikey, Mikkail, Mykhey

Mikolaj (Polish) form of Michael: like the Lord

Mikolas (Greek) form of Nicholas: winner; the people's victory
Mick, Mickey, Mickolas, Mik, Miko, Mikolus, Miky

Mil (Slavic) loved

Milagros (Spanish) miracle
Milagro

Milam (Last name as first name) uncomplicated
Mylam

Milan (Place name) city in Italy; smooth
Milano

Milburn (Scottish) volatile
Milbyrn, Milbyrne, Millburn

Miles (German) forgiving
Mile, Miley, Myles, Myyles

Miletus (Biblical) loved

Miley (American) reliable; forgiving
Mile, Miles, Mili, Mily, Myles, Myley

Milford (English) from a calm mill
setting; country, Milferd, Milfor

Milid (Biblical) place name

Milko (Czech) form of Michael: like the Lord

Millard (Latin) old-fashioned
Milard, Mill, Millerd, Millurd, Milly

Miller (English) practical
Mille, Myller

Milli (English) miller

Millian (English) miller

Millo (German) form of Miles: forgiving

Mills (English) safe
Mill, Milly, Mylls

Milo (German) soft-hearted
Miles, Milos, Mye, Mylo

Milos (Slavic) kind
Mile, Miles, Myle, Mylos

Milou (French) mill man

Milton (English) innovative
*Melton, Milt, Miltey, Milti,
Miltie, Milty, Mylt, Mylton*

Mimi (Greek) outspoken
Mims

Miner (Last name as first
name) hardworking; miner
Mine, Miney

Mingo (American) flirtatious
Ming-O, Myngo

Minnow (American)
beachcomber

Minter (Last name as first
name) dull

Mirko (Slavic) glory in peace

Mirlam (American) great
Mir, Mirsam, Mirtam

Mirsab (Arabic) judicious

Misa (Slavic) form of
Michael: like the Lord

Misael (Hebrew) godlike

Misha (Russian) form of
Mikhail: godlike; graceful

Mishael (Hebrew) form of
Michael: like the Lord

Mishma (Biblical) hearing;
obeying

Mitch (English) form of
Mitchell: optimistic

Mitchell (English) optimistic
*Mitch, Mitchel, Mitchelle,
Mitchie, Mitchill, Mitchy,
Mitshell, Mytchil*

Mitchum (Last name as first
name) dramatic; known
Mitchem

Mithun (Indian) Gemini;
couple; soft

Mitul (Indian) basic

Mizzah (Biblical/Hebrew)
despair

Moab (Biblical) of his father;
Son of Lot; Place name (east
of Dead Sea)

Modein (Biblical) place name

Modesto (Spanish) modest
Modysto

Modi (Norse) son of Thor

Modred (Greek) unafraid
Modrede, Modrid

Moc (American) form of
names beginning with Mo or
Moe; easygoing
Mo

Moey (Hebrew) easygoing
Moe, Moeye

Moges (Dutch) power

Mohammad (Arabic)
praiseworthy
*Mohamad, Mohamid,
Mohamud, Muhammad,
Mohammed*

Mohan (Hindi) compelling

Mohan (Hindi) riveting

Mohana (Sanskrit)
handsome
Mohann

Mohawk (Place name) river
in New York

Mohit (Indian) seeks beauty

Mohsen (Persian) one who
does good deeds
Mosen

Mois (Hebrew) humble

Moises (Hebrew) drawn
from the water
Moe

Mojave (Place name) desert
in California; towering man
Mohave, Mohavey

Mokei (Hawaiian) moses
child

Molim (African) softspoken

Moline (American) narrow
Moleen, Molene

Momo (American) rascal

Monaco (Place name)
unique, alone

Monahan (Irish) believer
*Mon, Monaghan, Monehan,
Monnahan*

Mondo (Spanish) world

Money (American) word as
name; popular
Muney

Monico (Spanish) player
Mon

Monroe (Irish) delightful;
presidential
Mon, Monro, Munro, Munroe

Montague (French) forward-
thinking
*Mont, Montagew, Montagu,
Montegue, Monty*

Montana (Spanish)
mountain; Place name
*U.S. state; American, sports
icon, Mont, Montane,
Montayna, Monty*

Monte (Spanish) form of
Montgomery: wealthy; form
of Montague: forward-
thinking
*Mont, Montee, Monti, Monts,
Monty*

Montero (Spanish) mountain

Montes (French)
discriminating

Montford (English) of the
mount

Montgomery (English)
wealthy
*Mongomerey, Monte,
Montgomry, Monty*

Montoi (French) mountain

Montrae (French)
ostentatious

Montraie (African American)
fussy
*Mont, Montray, Montraye,
Monty*

Montrel (African American)
popular
Montrell, Montrelle, Monty

Montrese (American) form
of Montgomery: wealthy

Montrose (French) high and
mighty
*Mont, Montroce, Montros,
Monty*

Monty (English) form of
Montgomery: wealthy; form
of Montague: forward-
thinking
Monte, Montee, Montey, Monti

Moody (American) expansive
Moodee, Moodey, Moodie

Moon (African) dreamer

Mooney (American) dreamer
Moon, Moonee, Moonie

Moore (French) dark-haired
Mohr, Moores, More

Mooring (Last name as first
name) centered
Moring

Moose (American) large guy
Moos, Mooz, Mooze

Moray (Place name) scottish

Mordchai (Hebrew) combative

Mordecai (Hebrew) combative
Mord, Morde, Mordekai, Morducai, Mordy

Mordechay (American) form of Mordecai: combative

Moreland (Last name as first name) of wealth
Mooreland, Moorland, Moorlande, Morland, Morlande

Morell (French) secretive
More, Morelle, Morey, Morrell, Mourell, Murell

Moretti (Italian) desired child

Morey (Latin) dark
Morrie, Morry

Morgan (Celtic) confident; seaman
Morg, Morgen, Morghan

Moriah (Hebrew) jehovah is my teacher

Moric (Slavic) form of Maurice: dark

Morland (English) from the land of moors

Morlen (English) outdoorsy
Morlan, Morlie, Morly

Morones (Spanish) joyful

Moroni (Place name) city in Comoros; joyful
Maroney, Maroni, Marony, Moroney, Morony

Morph (Greek) changing

Morpheus (Greek) god of dreams; shapes

Morrell (French) dark

Morris (Latin) dark
Maurice, Moris, Morse, Mouris

Morrison (Last name as first name) son of Morris; dark
Morrisen, Morrysen, Morryson

Morrley (English) outdoors-loving
More, Morlee, Morley, Morly, Morrs

Morrow (Last name as first name) follower
Morrowe

Morry (Hebrew) taught by God; old friend
Morey, Morrey, Mory

Morse (English) bright; code-maker
Morce, Morcey, Morry, Morsey

Mortimer (French) deep
Mort, Mortemer, Mortie, Morty, Mortymer

Morton (English) town of moors; dark
Mort, Mortan, Mortun, Morty

Mos (American) special

Moschi (Jewish) form of Moses: appointed for special things

Moses (Hebrew) appointed for special things
Mosa, Mose, Mosesh, Mosie, Mozes, Mozie

Moshe (Hebrew) special
Mosh, Moshie

Mosi (African) firstborn

Moss (Irish) giving
Mossy

Mostin (Welsh) settler

Mostyn (Welsh) mossy

Motaz (Slavic) form of Matthew: God's gift

Motor (American) word as name; speedy; active
Mote

Mottel (Hebrew) form of Max: best

Moushegh (Welsh) form of Moses: appointed for special things

Moylan (American) lights in the sky

Mozam (Place name) from Mozambique
Moze

Mudge (Last name as first name) friendly
Mud, Mudj

Muhammad (Arabic) form of Mohammad: praiseworthy
Muhamed, Muhammed

Mukul (Hindi) bird; beginnings

Mulder (American) of the dark

Muldoon (Last name as first name) different
Muldoone, Muldune

Muna (Arabic) wished for

Munday (English) monday's child

Mundo (Spanish) form of Edmundo: wealthy protector
Mun, Mund

Mungo (Scottish) loved; congenial
Mongo, Mongoh, Munge, Mungoh

Munir (Arabic) shines strongly

Munnin (Scandinavian) memorable

Murcia (Place name) region in Spain
Mursea

Murdoch (Scottish) rich
Merdock, Merdok, Murd, Murdock, Murdok, Murdy

Murfain (American) bold spirit
Merfaine, Murf, Murfee, Murfy, Murphy

Murff (Irish) form of Murphy: fighter
Merf, Murf

Murk (Slavic) content

Murl (English) nature-lover; sea

Murli (Hindi) flute

Murlie (Hindi) form of Murli: flute

Murphy (Irish) fighter
Merph, Merphy, Murfie, Murph

Murray (Scottish) sea-loving; sailor
Mur, Muray, Murrey, Murry

Murrell (English) nature-lover; sea

Murrill (English) Nature-loving

Murt (American) happy

Murthy (American) form of Murphy: fighter

Murtough (Irish) of the sea
Murtagh, Murrough

Murugan (last name as first name)

Musa (African) forgiving

Mushi (Biblical) giving

Mushki (Biblical) place name

Muslim (Arabic) religious

Musri (Biblical) place name

Mustafa (Arabic) chosen one; Turkish *ingenious*

Mustapha (Arabic) the right one

Mutka (African) new Year's baby

Mycheal (African American) devoted
Mysheal

Myle (Latin) soldier

Myles (German) form of Miles: forgiving

Mylie (German) form of Miles: forgiving

Mylik (Slavic) form of Miles: forgiving

Mylos (Slavic) kind
Milos

Mynor (Latin) form of Miner: hardworking; miner

Mynton (English) town of miners

Myrden (Irish) fragrant

Myren (Greek) form of Myron: aromatic oil

Myreon (Greek) aromatic oil
Myron

Myrle (American) able
Merl, Merle, Myrie, Myryee

Myron (Greek) aromatic oil
Mi, Miron, My, Myrayn

Myrzon (American) humorous
Merzon, Myrs, Myrz

Mystikal (American) musician; mystical

Mystry (American) mysterious

N

Nabil (Arabic) of noble birth; honored
Nabeel, Nobila

Nabor (Hebrew) light of the future

Nachman (Last name as first name) unique
Menachem, Menahem, Nacham, Nachmann, Nahum

Nachson (Last name as first name) son of Nach; up-and-coming

Nachum (Hebrew) comforts others

Nad (Biblical) name spelled backward

Nada (Arabic) morning dew; giver
Nadah

Nadab (Biblical) free and voluntary gift; prince

Nader (Arabic) dearest

Nadim (Arabic) fellow celebrant
Nadeem

Nadir (Arabic) rare man
Nadeer, Nadeir

Naeem (Arabic) happy

Nafis (Hebrew) struggles

Naftali (African) runs in woods
Naphtali, Naphtali, Neftali, Nefthali, Nephtali, Nephthali

Nag (Indian) form of Nagesh: Hindi serpent god

Nagel (English) smooth
Naegel, Nageler, Nagelle, Nagle, Nagler

Nagesh (Indian) hindi serpent god

Nagid (Arabic) regal

Nahath (Biblical) rest; a leader

Nahbi (Biblical) very secret

Nahir (Hebrew) light
Naheer, Nahor

Nahshon (Biblical) that foretells; that conjectures

Nahum (Arabic) content
Nemo

Nahum (Biblical) comforter; penitent

Naim (Arabic) content
Naeem

Naima (arabic) comforting

Nain (Biblical) place name

Nairi (Biblical) place name

Nairn (Last name as first name) born again
Nairne

Nairobi (Place name) city in Kenya; starting out

Naissus (Biblical) place name

Najib (Arabic) noble
Nageeb, Nagib, Najeeb

Naldo (Italian) form of Reynaldo: knowledgeable tutor

Nalin (Hindi) lotus; pretty boy
Naleen

Nalin (Indian) lotus child

Namir (Hebrew) leopard; fast
Nameer

Nana (African) king

Nanda (Indian) achiever

Nando (Spanish) form of Fernando: bold leader

Nandor (Hungarian) form of Ferdinand: adventurer

Nandy (Hindi) from the god Nandin; destructs

Nano (Hawaiian) springtime

Nanson (American) spunky
Nance, Nanse, Nansen, Nansson

Nansor (Indian) defiant

Napier (French) mover
Neper

Napoleon (German) lion of Naples; domineering
Nap, Napo, Napoleone, Napolion, Napolleon, Nappy

Narayana (Indian) secure

Narciso (Latin) lily; daffodil
Narcis

Narcissus (Greek) self-loving; vain
Narciss, Narcissah, Narcisse, Nars

Nardino (Spanish) kind

Naren (Hindi) best

Narendar (Indian) king

Narendra (Indian) king

Narithier (Indian) king

Narjis (Indian) Lord

Narmad (Indian) delights

Nartan (Indian) dancing

Nasario (Spanish) dedicated to God
Nasar, Nasareo, Nassario, Nazareo, Nazarlo, Nazaro, Nazor

Nash (Last name as first name) exciting
Nashe, Nashey

Nashe (Arabic) soothing advisor

Nashua (Native American) thunderous

Nasir (Arabic) wins

Nason (Biblical) perseveres

Nasser (Arabic) winning
Naser, Nasir, Nasr, Nassar, Nasse, Nassee, Nassor

Nat (Hebrew) form of Nathaniel: God's gift to mankind
Natt, Natte, Nattie, Natty

Natal (Hebrew) gift of God
Natale, Natalino, Natalio, Nataly

Natan (Hebrew) magnanimous

Natchio (Spanish) form of Nathan: God's gift to mankind

Nate (Hebrew) form of Nathan and Nathaniel: God's gift to mankind
Natey

Nath (Hebrew) form of Nathan: God's gift to mankind

Nathan ○ ❶ (Hebrew) form of Nathaniel: God's gift to mankind
Nat, Nate, Nathen, Nathin, Natthaen, Natthan, Natthen, Natty

Nathaniel ○ ❶ (Hebrew) God's gift to mankind
Nat, Nate, Nathan, Nathaneal, Nathanial, Nathe, Nathenial

Nation (American) patriotic

Natividad (Spanish) a child born at Christmastime

Nato (American) gentle
Nate, Natoe, Natoh

Navarro (Spanish) wild spirit
Navaro, Navarroh, Naverro

Naveed (Hindi) wishing you well
Navid

Naveen (Hindi) new

Navnit (Indian) smooth

Nayan (Hebrew) form of Nathan: God's gift to mankind

Naylor (English) likes order
Nailer, Nailor

Nazaire (Biblical) from Nazareth; religious boy
Nasareo, Nasarrio, Nazario, Nazarius, Nazaro, Nazor

Neal (Irish) winner
Neale, Nealey, Neall, Nealy, Neel, Neelee, Neely, Nele

Nebaioth (Biblical) firstborn

Nebo (Mythology) babylonian god of wisdom

Nebraska (Place name) U.S. state
Neb

Nebulous (Word as name)

Nectarios (Greek) sweet nectar; immortal man
Nectaire, Nectarius, Nektario, Nektarios, Nektarius

Ned (English) form of Edward: prospering; defender
Neddee, Neddie, Neddy

Nedrun (American) difficult
Ned, Nedd, Neddy, Nedran, Nedro

Neely (Scottish) winning
Neel, Neels

Negasi (African) destined for royalty

Negeb (Arabic) well-known

Nehemiah (Hebrew) compassionate
Nechemia, Nechemiah, Nechemya, Nehemyah, Nemo

Neiel (Biblical) place name

Neil (Scottish) victor
Neal, Neale, Neall, Nealle, Nealon, Neel, Neile, Neill, Neille, Neils, Nels, Nial, Niall, Niel, Niles

Neirin (Irish) light

Nekane (Spanish) saddened

Nellie (English) form of Nelson: broad-minded
Nell, Nellee, Nelli, Nells, Nelly

Nelo (Spanish) form of Daniel: judged by God; spiritual

Nels (Scandinavian) victor

Nelson (English) broad-minded
Nell, Nels, Nelsen, Nelsun, Nilsson

Nemesio (Spanish) justice
Nemo

Nemo (Literature) from Herman Melville's *Moby Dick*; courageous

Neo (Greek) new

Nepheg (Biblical) weak; slacked

Neptune (Latin) god of the sea
Neptoon, Neptoone, Neptunne

Ner (Hebrew) light

Neral (Greek) of the sea

Nereus (Greek) of the sea
Nereo

Neris (Greek) of the sea

Nero (Latin) unyielding
Neroh

Nery (Spanish) daring
Neree, Nerey, Nerrie, Nerry

Nesbit (Last name as first name) man who wanders
Naisbit, Naisbitt, Nesbitt, Nisbet, Nisbett

Ness (English) form of Nesbit: man who wanders

Nesto (Greek) adventurer
Nestoh, Nestoro

Nestor (Greek) wanderer
Nest, Nester, Nestir, Nesto, Nesty

Netar (African American) bright
Netardas

Nethanel (Hebrew) form of Nathaniel: God's gift to mankind

Nets (American) athletic

Netuno (Spanish) form of Neptune: god of the sea

Netzer (American) form of Nestor: wanderer
Net

Nevada (Place name) U.S. state
Nev, Nevadah

Nevardo (Spanish) masculine

Never (English) word as name

Neville (French) innovator
Nev, Nevil, Nevile, Nevvy, Nevyle, Niville

Nevin (Irish) small holy man
Nev, Nevan, Neven, Nevins,
Nevon, Niven

Nevins (Irish) devout

Newbie (American) novice
New, Newb

Newbury (Last name as first
name) renewal
Newbery, Newberry

Newcomb (Last name as first
name) renewal
Newcombe

Newell (English) new hall
New, Newall, Newel, Newy,
Nywell

Newland (Last name as first
name) of a new land

Newlin (Welsh) able; new
pond
Newl, Newlynn, Nule

Newman (English) attractive
young man
Neuman, Neumann, New,
Newmann

Newport (Last name as first
name) from a new seaport

Newt (English) new

Newton (English) bright;
new mind
New, Newt

Neyman (American) son of
Ney; bookish
Ney, Neymann, Neysa

Nezer (Arabic) winning boy

Nezib (Biblical) place name

Nga (Asian) herb

Niall (Irish) winner
Nial

Niambi (African (Swahili))
melody

Niaz (Hindi) gift

Nibshan (Biblical) place
name

Nicah (Greek) victorious
Nik, Nike

Nicandro (Spanish) a man
who excels
Nicandreo, Nicandrios,
Nicandros, Nikander,
Nikandreo, Nikandrios

Nicasio (Spanish) winning

Nicholas ☼ ☻ (Greek)
winner; the people's victory
Nichelas, Nicholus, Nick,
Nickee, Nickie, Nicklus,
Nickolas, Nicky, Nikolas, Nyck,
Nykolas

Nichols (English)
kindhearted
Nicholes, Nick, Nicky, Nikols

Nick (English) form of
Nicholas: victorious
Nic, Nik

Nickel (English) word as
name

Nicklaus (Greek) form of
Nicholas: winner; the
people's victory
Nicklaws, Niklus

Nickleby (Last name as first
name) betting on the odds

Nickler (American) fleet-
footed; perspicacious

Nicko (Greek) form of Nico:
victors

Nicky (Greek) form of
Nicholas: victorious
Nick, Nickee, Nickey, Nicki,
Nik, Nikee, Nikki

Nico (Italian) victor
Nicos, Niko, Nikos

Nicodemus (Greek) people's victory
Nicodemo, Nikodema

Nicol (Scottish) form of Nicholas: winner; the people's victory

Nicolas (Italian) form of Nicholas: winner; the people's victory
Nic, Nico, Nicolus

Nicomedes (Greek) thinking of victory
Nicomedo, Nikomedes

Nieblas (Spanish) winner

Niels (Scandinavian) victorious
Neels

Nigel (English) champion
Nigie, Nigil, Nygelle

Night (American) nocturnal

Nike (Greek) winning
Nykee, Nykie, Nyke

Nikhil (Russian) form of Nicholas: winner; the people's victory

Nikita (Russian) not yet won
Nika

Niklas (Scandinavian) winner
Niklaas, Nils, Klaas

Nikolai (Russian) winning
Nika

Nikolas (Greek) form of Nicholas: winner; the people's victory
Nik, Nike, Niko, Nikos, Nyloas

Nikolaus (Greek) form of Nicholas: winner, the people's victory

Nikom (Greek) winning

Nikon (Greek) victorious

Nikos (Greek) victor
Nicos, Niko, Nikolos

Nikostratos (Greek) the army's victory
Nicostrato, Nicostratos, Nicostratus

Niles (English) smooth
Ni, Nile, Niley, Nyles, Nyley

Nimro (American) form of Nimrod: renegade

Nimrod (Hebrew) renegade
Nimrodd, Nymrod

Ninad (Indian) gentle noise

Ninian (Gaelic) name given in honor of a fifth-century Irish saint

Nino (Spanish) child; young boy

Ninus (Biblical) place name

Ninyun (American) spirited
Ninian, Ninion, Ninyan, Nynyun

Niran (Indian) everlasting

Nissan (Hebrew) omen
Nisan, Nissyn

Nissim (Hebrew) nisan is seventh Jewish month; believer

Nitin (Indian) attractive

Nito (Italian) form of Benito: blessed

Nivea (Spanish) reborn

Niven (Last name as first name) smooth

Nix (American) negative
Nicks, Nixy

Nixon (English) audacious
Nickson, Nixen, Nixun

Nizam (Arabic) leader

Njord (Scandinavian) man of the north
Njorth

Noah ✪ ✪ (Hebrew) peacemaker
Noa, Noe, Nouh

Noam (Hebrew) sweet man
Noahm, Noe

Noam (Jewish) pleases others

Nob (Biblical) place name

Noble (Latin) regal
Nobe, Nobee, Nobel, Nobie, Noby

Noblen (American) protected

Nocona (Native American) leads man

Nod (Biblical) vagabond; fugitive

Noden (Native American) windy day

Noe (Spanish) quiet;
Noeh, Noey

Noean (Spanish) calm

Noel (French) born on Christmas
Noelle, Noelly, Nole, Nollie

Noey (Spanish) form of Noah: peacemaker
Noe, Noie

Nofri (Italian) ancestor

Nolan (Irish) outstanding; noble
Nole, Nolen, Nolline, Nolun, Nolyn

Nolden (American) noble
Nold

Noll (Scandinavian) form of Oliver; loving nature

Nolly (Scandinavian) hopeful
Nole, Noli, Noll, Nolley, Nolleye, Nolli, Nollie

Nonan (Latin) superb

Noon (English) word as name, from Latin nona: ninth hour

Noor (Hindi) light
Nour, Nur

Noph (Biblical) place name

Norb (Scandinavian) innovative
Noberto, Norbie, Norbs, Norby

Norberito (Spanish) form of Norbert: bright north

Norbert (German) bright north
Norb, Norbie, Norby

Norberto (Spanish) form of Norberto: bright north

Nordin (Nordic) handsome
Nord, Nordan, Norde, Nordee, Nordeen, Nordi, Nordun, Nordy

Noriel (Spanish) hero

Norin (French) from the north

Norka (Scandinavian) charming

Norman (English) sincere; man of the North
Norm, Normen, Normey, Normi, Normie, Normon, Normun, Normy

Norrell (French) from the north

Norris (English) from the north

Norrison (French) northerner

Norriston (French) northern town

Norse (English) scandinavian boy

Norshell (African American) brash
Norshel, Norshelle

North (American) directional
Norf, Northe

Northcliff (English) from the north cliff
Northcliffe, Northclyff, Northclyffe

Northrop (English) northerner
Northrup

Norton (English) dignified man of the north
Nort, Nortan, Norten

Norval (English) from the north
Norvan

Norvell (French) northern town

Norville (French) resident of a northern village; warmhearted
Norval, Norvel, Norvil, Norvill, Norvyl

Norward (English) going north
Norwerd

Norwell (English) northward bound

Norwin (English) friendly
Norvin, Norwen, Norwind, Norwinn

Norwood (English) of the north woods

Novae (Biblical) place name

Novak (Slavic) last name as first name

Novio (Spanish) boyfriend

Nowell (Last name as first name) dependable
Nowe

Nowey (American) knowing
Nowee, Nowie

Nuad (Welsh) tolerant

Nueces (Place name) river in Texas

Nuell (American) form of Newell: new hall
Nuel

Numa (Arabic) nice

Nun (Biblical) from the ocean

Nuncio (Spanish) messenger; informant
Nunzio

Nunry (Last name as first name) giving
Nunri

Nuri (Arabic) light
Noori, Nur, Nuriel, Nuris

Nuriel (Hebrew) light of God
Nooriel, Nuriya, Nuriyah, Nurya

Nuys (Place name) from Van Nuys
Nies, Nyes, Nys

Nye (Welsh) focused
Ni, Nie, Nyee

Nyle (American) form of Niles: smooth
Nyl, Nyles

Nyron (English) form of Neil: victor

Nyx (American) humorous

O

Oak (English) sturdy
Oake, Oakes, Oakie

Oakes (English) sturdy oak

Oakley (English) sturdy;
strong
*Oak, Oakie, Oaklee, Oakleigh,
Oakly, Oklie*

Oakley (English) sturdy oak

Oat (English) word as name

Oba (Hebrew) form of
Obadiah: serving God

Obadiah (Hebrew) serving
God
*Obadyah, Obediah, Obee,
Obie, Oby*

Obadiah (Hebrew) serves
God

Obal (Biblical) leader

Obasi (African) God-loving

Obataiye (African) world
leader

Obayana (African) king by
the fire

Obba (African) form of Obi:
big heart

Obbie (Biblical) form of
Obadiah: serving God
Obey, Obi, Obie

Obed (Hebrew) serves

Obedience (American) strict
Obie

Ober (Scandinavian) famed

Oberon (German) strong-
bearing
*Auberon, Auberron, Obaron,
Oberahn, Oberone, Oburon*

Obert (German) rich man

Obey (American) form of
Obadiah: serving God
Obe, Obee, Obie, Oby

Obi (African) big heart

Obie (Hebrew) form of
Obadiah: serving God
Obbie, Obe, Oby

Obie (English) form of
Obadiah; Serves God

Obike (African) loved by his
family

Oboth (Biblical) place name

Ocean (Greek) ocean; child
born under a water sign
Oceane, Oceanus

Ocie (Greek) form of Ocean:
ocean; child born under a
water sign
Osie

O'Connor (Irish) son of
Connor

Octavio (Latin) eight; able
*Octave, Octavian, Octavien,
Octavioh, Octavo, Ottavio*

Oda (Scandinavian) precise

Odakota (Native American)
has many friends

Ode (Greek) poetry as a
name; poetic
Odee, Odie

Oded (Hebrew) supportive

Odegard (Scandinavian)
powerful guard

Odell (American) musical
Dell, Odall, Ode, Odey, Odyll

Oder (Place name) river in
Europe
Ode

Odessus (Biblical) place
name

Odhran (Irish) green;
creative
Odran, Oran

Odie (English) form of Odell:
musical

Odilon (German) rich

Odin (Scandinavian) norse
god of magic; soulful
Odan, Oden

Odinan (Hungarian) rich;
powerful

Odion (African) the first twin

Odisoose (Invented) form of
Odysseus: wanderer
Ode

Odissan (African) wanderer

Odolf (Japanese) from the
field of deer; lithe

Odom (African) the oak;
strong

Odysseus (Greek) wanderer
Ode, Odey, Odie

Oelen (Spanish) giving

Oescus (Biblical) place name

Ofer (Hebrew) deer

Ofer (Hebrew) deer

Og (Aramaic) king

Ogano (Japanese) wise

Ogdon (English) literate
Og, Ogdan, Ogden

Ogen (German) invincible

Oghe (Irish) horse rider
Oghie, Oho

Ogle (American) word as
name; leer; stare
Ogal, Ogel, Ogll, Ogul

Ogun (Japanese) undaunted

Ohad (Biblical) praising;
confessing

Ohanko (Japanese) invincible

Ohanzee (Native American)
shadowy figure

Ohin (Japanese) wanted child

Oisin (Irish) fawn; gentle

Oistin (Latin) much revered

Ojas (Indian) shiny

Ojay (American) brash
O.J., Oojai

Ojo (African) he came of a
hard birth

Okan (Turkish) horse
Oke

Okapi (African) graceful

Okechuku (African) God's
blessing

Okello (African) child after
twins were born

Okemos (African) advises

Okie (American) man from
Oklahoma
Okey, Okeydokey

Oko (Japanese) evoker;
charming

Okon (Japanese) from the
darkness

Okoth (African) sad child;
born during rainfall

Okpara (African) first son

Oktawian (African) eighth
child

Ola (African) child much
honored

Olabisi (African) rich

Oladele (African) honored at home

Olaf (Scandinavian) watchful
Olay, Ole, Olef, Olev, Oluf

Olafemi (African) lucky child

Olafur (Scandinavian) forunate

Olajuwon (Arabic) honorable
Olajuwan, Olujuwon

Olakeakua (Hawaiian) living for God

Olamina (African) rich of spirit

Olan (Scandinavian) royal ancestor
Olin, Ollee

Olaniyan (African) honored all around

Olav (Scandinavian) traditional
Ola, Olov, Oluf

Oldrich (Czech) leader; strong
Olda, Oldra, Oldrisek, Olecek, Olik, Olin, Olouvsek

Ole (Scandinavian) watchful
Olay

Oleg (Russian) holy; religious
Olag, Ole, Olig

Olegario (Spanish) aggressor

Olek (Scandinavian) holy

Olin (English) holly; jubilant
Olen, Olney, Olyn

Olindo (Latin) sweet fragrance

Oliver (Latin) loving nature
Olaver, Olive, Ollie, Olliver, Olly, Oluvor

Olivier (French) eloquent
Oliveay

Oliwa (Hawaiian) from an army of elves

Ollie (English) form of Oliver: loving nature
Olie, Ollee, Olley, Olly

Ollie (English) form of Oliver: loving nature

Olliem (Scandinavian) form of William: staunch protector

Olmos (Spanish) altruistic

Olney (English) lonely field

Olo (Spanish) form of Orlando: famed; distinctive

Olorun (African) blessed; counsels others

Olsen (Scandinavian) last name as first name

Olubayo (African) full of happiness

Olufemi (African) God's loved child
Olviemi

Olugbala (African) the people's God

Olujimi (African) hand in hand with God

Olumide (African) God has come

Olumoi (African) blessed by God

Olushegun (African) marches with God

Olushola (African) blessed

Oluwa (African) believer

Oluyemi (African) man full of God

Olvera (Spanish) form of Oliver: loving nature

Olvery (English) draws others near

Omaha (Place name) city in Nebraska

Omanand (Hindi) joyful thinker

Omar (Arabic) spiritual
Omahr, Omarr

Omari (African) in high esteem

Ombre (Spanish) man

Omedes (Greek) ponders

Omer (Arabic) form of Omar: spiritual

Omie (Italian) homebody
Omey, Omi, Omye

Omri (Hebrew) jehovah's servant; giving

On (African) desirable

Onacona (Native American) white owl; watchful

Onam (Biblical) success

Onan (Turkish) rich

Onaney (African) sees all

Onani (Asian) sweet

Onaona (Hawaiian) fragrant

Onder (Scandinavian) form of Andrew: manly and brave

Ondraze (Scandinavian) form of Andrew: manly and brave

Ondrej (Czech) masculine
Ondra, Ondravsek, Ondrejek, Ondrousek

Onesimo (Spanish) number one
Onie

Onesimo (Spanish) important

Onkar (Hindi) purest one

Ono (Biblical) place name

Onofrio (German) smart
Ono, Onofreeo, Onofrioh

Onorato (Spanish) honored

Onslow (Arabic) climbing passion's hill
Ounslow

Onur (Turkish) promising boy

Onwoachi (African) God's world

Ophel (Biblical) place name

Ophir (Hebrew) loyal

Ophlas (Biblical) place name

Oqwapi (Native American) red cloud

Oracio (Spanish) oracle

Oral (Latin) eloquent

Oran (Irish) pale
Orin, Orran, Orren, Orrin

Orangel (Greek) angel of truth

Oranos (Greek) universal

Orban (Hungarian) city man; sophisticated

Orbie (Slavic) sophisticated

Orchard (English) botanical name

Ordell (Latin) the start

Oregon (Place name) state

Oren (Hebrew) form of Owen: wellborn; high-principled

Orenthiel (American) sturdy as a pine
Ore, Oren

Orenthiem (American) sturdy as a pine
Orenth, Orenthe

Orest (Greek) form of Orestes: leader

Orestes (Greek) leader
Oresta, Oreste, Restie, Resty

Orestis (Greek) form of Orestes: leader

Orev (Hebrew) raven; observing

Orford (Last name as first name) noble

Ori (Hebrew) flame of truth

Orie (English) form of Orrin: river boy

Oriol (Spanish) best
Orioll

Orion (Greek) fiery hunter
Oreon, Ori, Orie, Ory

Orji (African) sturdy tree

Orlando (Spanish) famed; distinctive
Orl, Orland, Orlie, Orlondo, Orly

Orlay (Spanish) famed

Orlean (Latin) gold

Orleans (Latin) the golden boy
Orlins

Orlis (English) bearlike

Orman (Latin) noble
Ormand, Ormond, Ormonde

Orme (English) kind
Orm

Ormond (English) kindhearted
Ormand, Ormande, Orme, Ormon, Ormonde, Ormund, Ormunde

Orn (Latin) form of Oren: well-born; high principled

Oro (Spanish) golden child

Oron (Hebrew) light spirit

Orontes (Biblical) place name

Orpheus (Greek) darkness of night; mythological musician

Orr (English) form of Orrick: sturdy as an oak

Orran (Irish) green-eyed
Ore, Oren, Orin

Orrent (Greek) excites

Orrial (Latin) form of Uriel: light; God-inspired

Orrick (English) sturdy as an oak
Oric, Orick, Orreck, Orrik

Orrie (American) form of Orson: strong as a bear
Orry

Orrin (English) river boy

Orris (Latin) form of Horatio: poetic; dashing
Oris, Orriss

Orry (Latin) oriental; exotic
Oarrie, Orrey, Orrie

Orso (Latin) form of Orson: strong as a bear

Orson (Latin) strong as a bear
Orsan, Orsen, Orsey, Orsun

Orth (English) honest
Orthe

Orton (English) town on the shore; reaching

Orturo (Spanish) form of Arturo: talented

Ortwin (English) shore friend

Orunjan (African) god of the noon-time sun

Orval (American) form of Orville: brave
Orvale

Orval (Scandinavian) eagle-eyed

Orven (English) spears

Orville (French) brave
Orv, Orvelle, Orvie, Orvil

Orvin (Last name as first name) fated for success
Orwin, Orwynn

Orway (American) kind
Orwaye

Osai (Afghanistan) deerlike

Osakwe (Japanese) good destiny

Osanmwesr (Japanese) leaving

Osayaba (Japanese) wonders

Osbert (English) smart

Osborne (English) strong-spirited
Osborn, Osbourne, Osburn, Osburne, Ossie, Oz, Ozzie, Ozzy

Osburt (English) smart
Osbart, Osbert, Ozbert, Ozburt

Oscar (Scandinavian) divine
Ozkar

Oscard (Greek) fighter
Oscar, Oskard

Osceola (Native American) black drink

Osciel (Spanish) gracious

Osei (African) gracious

Osgood (English) good man
Osgude, Ozgood

Oshea (Hebrew) kind spirit

Osileani (Polynesian) talking forever

Osin (Irish) small deer

Osk (Scandinavian) spears

Oslo (Place name) capital of Norway
Os, Oz

Osman (Spanish) verbose
Os, Osmen, Osmin, Ossie, Oz, Ozzie

Osmar (English) amazing; divine

Osmenio (Spanish) talkative

Osmond (English) singing to the world
Os, Osmonde, Osmund, Ossie, Oz, Ozzy

Ospe (Russian) form of Joseph: He will add

Osrec (Scandinavian) leader
Os, Ossie

Osred (Scandinavian) leads mankind

Osric (Scandinavian) leader
Osrick

Ossie (Hebrew) powerful
Os, Oz, Ozzy

Osten (Last name as first name) religious leader
Ostin, Ostyn

Osval (Slavic) form of Oswald: divine power

Osvaldo (German) divine power
Osvald, Oswaldo

Oswald (English) divine power
Oswalde, Oswold, Oswuld, Oszie, Oz

Oswin (English) God's ally
Osvin, Oswinn, Oswyn,
Oswynn

Ota (Czech) affluent

Otadan (Native American)
abundance

Otey (Slavic) wealthy

Othar (Slavic) leader

Othell (African American)
thriving
Oth, Othey, Otho

Othello (Spanish) bold
Otello, Othell

Othman (Last name as first
name) man of bravery

Othnel (Biblical) God's lion

Othniel (Hebrew) rendered
brave by God's love

Othon (German) rich

Otik (German) lucky

Otis (Greek) intuitive
Oates, Odis, Otes, Ottes, Ottis

Otokar (Czech) prudent in
wealth

Otoniel (Spanish)
fashionable
Otonel

Otskai (Native American)
leaving

Ottah (African) thin boy

Ottar (Scandinavian) warring
Otomars, Ottomar

Otto (German) wealthy
Oto, Ott, Ottoh

Ottokar (German) can-do
spirit; fighter
Otokars, Ottocar

Ottway (German) fortunate
Otwae, Otway

Otu (Native American)
industrious

Oukounaka (Asian) from the
surf

Ouray (Native American)
arrow man

Oved (Hebrew) serving
Obed

Overton (Last name as first
name) leader
Ove, Overten

Ovidio (Spanish) from
Roman poet Ovid; creative
Ovido

Ovido (Spanish) tends sheep

Owen ○ (Welsh) wellborn;
high-principled
Owan, Owin, Owwen

Owney (Irish) old one
Oney

Ox (American) animal; strong
Oxy

Oxford (English) scholar; ox
crossing
Fordy, Oxferd, Oxfor

Oya (African) vocal

Oz (Hebrew) courageous;
unusual

Ozais (Hebrew) strong in
God

Ozden (Hebrew) good in God

Ozeas (Italian) strong

Ozell (English) strong
Ozel

Oziel (Spanish) strong

Ozni (Hebrew) knows God

Ozuru (Japanese) stork; lively
hope

Ozzie (English) form of
Oswald: divine power
Oz, Ozzee, Ozzey, Ozzy

P

Paal (Scandinavian) form of
Paul: small; wise

Pablo (Spanish) strong;
creative
Pabel, Pabo, Paublo

Pace (English) peace

Pacian (Spanish) peaceful
Pacien, Pace

Packer (Last name as first
name) orderly
Pack

Paco (Spanish) energetic
Pak, Pakkoh, Pako, Paquito

Padden (English) form of
Patton: warrior's town
Paddin, Paddyn

Paddy (Irish) form of Patrick:
noble
Paddey, Paddi, Paddie, Padee

Paden (English) form of
Patrick: noble

Padget (French) learning;
growing
Padgett, Pagas

Padraic (Irish) form of
Patrick: noble
*Padraick, Padraik, Padrayc,
Padrayck, Padrayk*

Padre (Spanish) father;
cajoles
Padrae, Padray

Paeter (Scandinavian) form
of Peter: dependable; rock

Page (French) helpful
Pagey, Paige, Payg

Pageman (Last name as first
name) sharp

Pagiel (Hebrew) worships

Pago (Place name) for Pago
Pago
Pay

Pagolo (Italian) placid

Pahan (Native American)
summons

Paine (Latin) countryman
Payne

Paki (African) has seen the
truth

Palani (Slavic) long-suffering

Pall (Scandinavian) form of
Paul: small; wise

Palladin (Greek)
confrontational; wise
*Palidin, Palladyn, Palleden,
Pallie, Pally*

Pallaton (Native American)
tough; fighter
Palladin

Pallav (Indian) new growth

Pallu (Biblical) distinct

Palma (Latin) successful

Palmer (English) open
*Pallmar, Pallmer, Palmar,
Palmur*

Palmer (English) grows
palms

Palti (Hebrew) getaway

Pampa (Place name) city in
Texas

Pan (Greek mythology) god of
forest and shepherds
Pann

Panama (Place name) canal connecting North and South America; rounder
Pan

Pancho (Spanish) form of Francisco: free spirit; from France
Panchoh, Ponchito

Pancrazio (Italian) all-powerful
Pankraz

Pandy (English) from Panda

Panfilo (Spanish) loving all nature

Pankaj (Hindi) lotus flower

Panos (Greek) rock; sturdy

Pantaleon (Spanish) pants; trousers; manly
Pant, Pantalon

Pantias (Greek) philosophical

Pao (Italian) form of Paul: small; wise

Paolo (Italian) form of Paul: small; wise
Paoloh, Paulo

Paphos (Biblical) place name

Papillion (French) butterfly

Paquito (Spanish) dear Paco

Parah (Biblical) place name

Paran (Biblical) place name

Parindra (Indian) lion

Paris (English) lover; France's capital
Pare, Paree, Parris

Parish (French) priest's place; lovely boy
Parrish, Parrysh, Parysh

Park (English) calming
Parke, Parkey, Parks

Parker ✪ (English) manager
Park, Parks

Parley (Scottish) reluctant
Parly

Parnell (French) ribald
Parne, Parnel, Parnelle, Perne, Parle

Parnelli (Italian) frisky
Parnell

Parnes (French) form of Peter: dependable; rock

Paros (Place name) Greek island; charming
Par, Paro

Parr (English) protective
Par, Parre

Parris (French) priest's place; lovely boy
Paris, Pariss, Parriss, Parrys, Parryss

Parrish (French) separate and unique; district

Parry (Welsh) young son
Parrie, Pary

Parryth (American) up-and-coming
Pareth, Parre, Parry, Parythe

Parson (English) clergyman
Parsen

Parthik (Greek) virginal

Partholon (Irish) form of Bartholomew: friendly; earthy
Parlan

Parvati (Indian) best

Pascal (French) boy born on Easter or Passover; spiritual
Pascalle, Paschal, Pasco, Pascual, Paskalle, Pasky

Pascasio (Spanish) easter baby

Pasko (English) form of Pascal: boy born on Easter or Passover; spiritual

Pasquale (Italian) spiritual
Pask, Paskwoll, Pasq, Pasquell, Posquel

Pass (Russian) form of Paul: small; wise

Pastor (English) clergyman
Pastar, Paster

Pat (English) form of Patrick: noble
Pattey, Patti, Patty, Pattye, Pattee

Patcher (American) unusual

Pate (Latin) form of Patrick: noble
Pait, Payte

Patek (Latin) form of Patrick: noble
Patec, Pateck

Pater (Greek) father

Paterno (Spanish) fatherly

Paterson (Last name as first name) intelligent father

Patricio (Spanish) form of Patrick: noble
Patricyo

Patricius (Latin) noble

Patrick (Irish) noble
Paddy, Partric, Patric, Patrik, Patriquek, Patryk, Pats, Patsy

Patriot (American) patriotic

Patterson (English) intellectual
Paterson, Pattersen, Pattersun, Pattersund

Pattison (English) son of Pat; noble
Pattisen, Pattysen, Pattyson, Patysen, Patyson

Patton (English) warrior's town
Patten, Pattun, Patun, Peyton

Paul (Latin) small; wise
Pauley, Paulie, Pauly

Paul-Erik (Scandinavian) combination of Paul and Erik

Pauli (Italian) dear Paul
Paulee, Pauley, Paulie, Pauly

Paulin (German) form of Paul: small; wise
Paulyn

Paulis (Latin) form of Paul: small; wise
Pauliss, Paulys, Paulyss

Paulo (Spanish) form of Paul: small; wise

Paulos (Greek) form of Paul: small; wise

Paulus (Latin) small
Paul, Paulie, Paulis, Pauly

Paun (American) form of Paul: small; wise

Pavan (Indian) wind

Pavel (Russian) inspired
Pasha

Paviter (Indian) pure

Pavlof (Last name as first name) reactive; small
Pavel

Pavol (Slavic) form of Paul: small; wise

Pavun (Indian) belonging to the middle

Pawel (Polish) believer
Pawl

Pax (Latin) peace-loving
Paks, Paxy

Paxon (German) peaceful
Packston, Packton

Paxton (English) from a town of peace; gentle boy
Paxten

Payam (Slavic) message

Payan (Indian) ornamented

Payne (Latin) countryman
Paine, Payn

Payton ♥ (English) soldier's town
Pate, Paton, Payten, Paytun, Peyton

Peabo (Irish) rock

Peader (Scottish) rock or stone; reliable
Peder, Peter

Peak (English) word as name

Peale (English) bell-ringer in a church; religious
Peal, Peel, Peele

Pearson (English) dark-eyed
Pearse, Pearsen, Pearsun, Peerson

Peat (English) form of Pete: dependable; rock

Peck (American) peaceful

Pecos (Place name) texas river; cowboy
Peck, Pekos

Pedaias (Biblical) God loves
Pedaiah

Peder (Scandinavian) form of Peter: dependable; rock

Pederson (Scandinavian) form of Peterson: son of Peter
Pedersen

Pedram (Indian)

Pedro (Spanish) form of Peter: dependable; rock
Pedra, Pedrin, Pedroh

Peer (Scandinavian) rock

Peerson (English) son of Peter; smart
Peersen

Pegasus (Mythology) horse; rider

Peili (Spanish) joyful

Peirano (Italian) form of Peter: dependable; rock

Peleg (Greek) the sea

Pelle (Swedish) for Peter; rock
Pele, Pelee

Pelly (English) happy
Peli, Pelley, Pelli

Pelon (Spanish) joyful

Pelton (Last name as first name) town of Pel; respectful

Pembroke (French) sophisticated
Brookie, Pemb, Pembrooke, Pimbroke

Pender (Last name as first name) loves music

Penley (Last name as first name) strong

Penn (German) strong-willed
Pen, Pennee, Penney, Pennie, Penny

Penrod (German) respected leader

Penrose (Last name as first name) liked

Pentecost (Religion) pious person
Penticost, Pentycost

Pentige (Last name as first name) worthy

Pentz (Last name as first name) visionary

Penuel (Hebrew) face of God

Pepic (German) perseveres

Pepin (German) ardent
*Pepen, Pepi, Pepp, Peppi,
Peppy, Pepun*

Pepper (Botanical) live wire
Pep, Pepp, Peppy

Peppino (Spanish) energetic

Per (Scandinavian) secretive

Peralta (Italian) pearl

Percival (French) mysterious
*Parsival, Perc, Perce, Perceval,
Percey, Percy, Perseval,
Purcival, Purcy*

Percy (French) form of
Percival: mysterious
Percee, Percey, Perci, Percie

Peregrino (Italian) bird;
ordinary

Perfecto (Spanish) perfect
Perfek

Peri (English) form of Perry:
tough-minded

Perick (French) form of Peter:
dependable; rock

Pericles (Greek) fair leader
Periklees, Perikles, Perry

Perine (Latin) adventurer
Perrin, Perrine, Perry, Peryne

Perk (American) perky
Perkey, Perki, Perky

Perkin (English) opinionated
Parkin

Perkins (English) political
Perk, Perkens, Perkey

Pernell (French) form of
Parnell: ribald; form of Peter:
dependable; rock
Pernel

Peron (Last name as first
name) leader

Perre (English) form of Peter:
dependable; rock

Perrin (Latin) traveler
Perrine, Pero, Per

Perrince (American) form of
Terrence: calm

Perris (Greek) legendary
kidnapper of Helen of Troy;
daring
*Paris, Peris, Periss, Perrys,
Perys*

Perry (English) tough-minded
Parry, Perr, Perrey, Perri, Perrie

Perryman (Last name as first
name) nature-lover
Perry

Perseus (Greek) destroyer;
mythological hero

Persis (Biblical) place name

Perth (Place name) capital of
Western Australia
Purth

Perun (Slavic) thunder; god
of lightning

Pete (English) form of Peter:
dependable; rock
Petey, Petie

Peter (Greek) dependable;
rock
*Per, Petar, Pete, Petee, Petey,
Petie, Petur, Pyotr*

Peterson (Scandinavian) son
of Peter
Petersen

Pethuel (Aramaic) God's
vision

Petra (Place name) city in
Arabia; dashing

Petre (Slavic) form of Peter:
dependable; rock

Petru (Slavic) form of Peter:
dependable; rock

Petrus (Scandinavian)
dependable

Petter (Scandinavian) form of
Peter: dependable; rock
Petya

Petter (Scandinavian) form of
Peter: dependable; rock

Peverel (Latin) peverell
Peveril

Peyman (English) form of
Peyten: soldier's town

Peyton (English) form of
Payton: soldier's town
Pey, Peyt

Pharaton (Biblical) place
name

Pharis (Irish) heroic
Farres, Farrus, Pharris

Pharo (Latin) ruler

Pharpar (Biblical) place name

Pharrington (last name as
first name)

Phasael (Biblical) place name

Phelan (Irish) the small wolf;
fierce

Phelgen (Last name as first
name) stylish
Phelgon

Phelim (Irish) wolfish; fierce
Phelym

Phelps (English) droll
Felps, Filps

Phex (American) kind
Fex

Phil (Greek) form of Philip:
outdoorsman; horse-lover
Fill, Phill

Philander (Greek) lover of
many; infidel
*Filander, Phil, Philandyr,
Philender*

Philemon (Greek) showing
affection
Filemon, Philamon, Philo

Philemon (Biblical) loves
others

Philetus (Greek) collector

Philip (Greek) outdoorsman;
horse-lover
*Felipe, Filipp, Flippo, Phil,
Phillie, Phillip, Phillippe, Philly*

Philippe (French) form of
Philip: outdoorsman; horse-
lover
Felipe, Filippe, Philipe

Philo (Greek) lover
Filo

Phineas (English) farsighted
*Fineas, Finny, Pheneas,
Phineus, Phinny*

Phoenix (Greek) bird of
immortality; everlasting
Fee, Feenix, Fenix, Nix

Photius (Greek) scholarly

Picardus (Hispanic)
adventurous

Pickford (Last name as first
name) old-fashioned

Pico (Spanish) the epitome;
peak

Pier (Dutch) for Peter

Pierce (English) insightful;
piercing
*Pearce, Peerce, Peers, Peersey,
Percy, Piercy, Piers*

Piero (Italian) form of Peter:
dependable; rock
Pierro

Pierre (French) socially adroit
Piere

Pierrepont (French) social
Pierpont

Pierre-Yves (French) combination of Pierre and Yves

Pierrick (English) form of Pier: for Peter

Piers (English) form of Philip: outdoorsman; horse-lover

Pierson (English) son of Pier; rock
Peirsen, Pearson

Pietro (Italian) reliable
Pete

Pike (English) word as name

Pilar (Spanish) basic
Pilarr

Pildash (Biblical) biblical relative of Abraham

Pilgrim (English) a traveler
Pilgrym

Pillion (French) excellence
Pilion, Pillyon, Pilyon

Pilot (French) excellence

Pim (Dutch) precise

Pin (Vietnamese) joyful

Pincus (American) dark
Pincas, Pinchas, Pinchus, Pinkus

Pinechas (Hebrew) form of Paul: small; wise

Pineda (Spanish) last name as first name

Pinero (Spanish) springtime

Piney (American) living among pines; comfortable
Pine, Pyney

Pinkston (Last name as first name) different
Pink, Pinky

Pinky (American) familiar form of Pinchas

Pinya (Hebrew) loyal

Pio (Italian) pious

Piotr (Slavic) form of Peter: dependable; rock

Pip (German) ingenious
Pipp, Pippin, Pippo, Pippy

Pippin (English) shy

Pippo (Italian) gift

Pirney (Scottish) from the island

Pirro (Greek) red hair

Pitch (American) musical

Pithom (Biblical) place name

Piton (Spanish) form of Felix: joyful

Pitt (English) swerving dramatically

Pittman (English) blue-collar worker

Pius (Polish) pious

Placid (Latin) calm
Plasid

Placido (Italian) serene songster
Placeedo, Placidoh, Placydo

Placidon (Spanish) serene

Plan (American) word as name; organized

Plash (American) splashy; zany

Plat (French) from the flatlands; landowner
Platt

Platinum (English) worthwhile

Plato (Greek) broad-minded
Plata, Platoh

Playtoh (Invented) form of Plato: broad-minded

Plicerio (Spanish) capable

Plinio (Spanish) talented

Pluck (American) audacious; plucky

Plutarco (Greek) nefarious

Po (Biblical) place name

Poe (Last name as first name) dark spirit

Poet (American) writer
Poe

Pola (Biblical) place name

Polemos (Greek) warlike

Policarpo (Greek) with much fruit

Polja (Russian) creative

Polk (Last name as first name) political

Pollard (German) closed-minded
Polard, Pollar, Pollerd, Polley

Pollock (Last name as first name) creative

Pollux (Last name as first name) underdog

Polo (Greek) adventurer
Poloe, Poloh

Polonice (Polish) respects

Polygnotos (Greek) lover of many

Pomeroy (Last name as first name) polite

Pomposo (Spanish) pompous

Ponce (Spanish) fifth; wanderer
Poncey, Ponciano, Ponse

Ponciano (Spanish) of the sea

Poncio (Spanish) of the sea

Ponipake (Hawaiian) good luck

Pons (Spanish) fifth; explores
Ponse

Pontius (Latin) the fifth
Pontias, Pontus

Pontos (Greek) sea

Pony (Scottish) dashing
Poney, Ponie

Poogie (American) snuggly
Poog, Poogee, Poogi, Poogs, Pookie

Poole (Place name) area in England
Pool

Pope (Greek) father
Po

Porfirio (Spanish) audacious

Port (Latin) gatekeeper
Porte

Porter (Latin) decisive
Poart, Port, Portur, Porty

Portnoy (Latin) gate

Potiphar (Biblical) bull of Africa; a fat bull

Poul (Scandinavian) small

Powder (American) cowboy
Powd, Powe

Powell (English) ready

Powers (English) wields power

Pragedis (Spanish) prays

Prairie (American) rural man or rancher
Prair, Prairey, Prairi, Prairy

Prakash (Indian) light

Pramad (Indian) happy

Pranav (Indian) om (syllable)

Prasanna (Indian) happy

Prashant (Indian) calm

Pratt (Last name as first name) talkative

Pravat (Indian) leads

Pravin (Indian) talented

Praxedes (Last name as first name) prayerful

Preemoh (Invented) form of Primo: top-notch

Prentice (English) learning
Prenticce, Prentis, Prentiss, Printiss

Prescott (Last name as first name) sophisticated

Presley (English) songbird; meadow of the priest
Preslee, Preslie, Presly

Prest (English) priest

Preston (English) spiritual
Prestyn

Preston (Last name as first name) village of a priest; religious home

Pretio (Spanish) prays

Pretivo (Spanish) prays

Preto (Latin) important

Priamos (Greek) saved

Price (Welsh) vigorous
Pricey, Pryce

Priestley (English) cottage of the priest
Priestlea, Priestlee, Priestly

Primerica (American) from America; patriotic
Prime

Primitivo (Spanish) primitive
Primi, Tito, Tivo

Primitivus (Spanish) first

Primo (Italian) top-notch
Preemo, Primoh, Prymo

Prince (Latin) regal leader
Preenz, Prins, Prinz, Prinze

Prine (English) prime

Priore (Italian) first

Prisciliano (Spanish) wise old man

Procopio (Greek) progressive

Procter (Last name as first name) leads
Proctor

Prometheus (Mythology) friend of man; bringer of fire

Promiz (Slavic) first

Prop (American) word as name; fun-loving
Propp

Prospen (French) prospers

Prosper (Italian) having good fortune
Pros

Proteus (Greek) first

Prudencio (Spanish) wise

Prusa (Biblical) place name

Pry (Latin) before

Pryor (Latin) spiritual director
Pry, Prye

Publias (Greek) thinker
Publius

Puck (Literature) vibrant

Pullman (English) train man; motivator
Pulman, Pulmann, Pullmann

Pullum (Greek) song

Puneet (Indian) purest

Punon (Biblical) place name

Pura (Spanish) pure of heart

Pureza (Spanish) pure

Purley (Welsh) caring

Pursey (American) form of Percy: mysterious

Purvin (English) helpful
Pervin

Purvis (French) provider
Pervis, Purviss

Pushkin (Last name as first) poet; playful

Puskar (Indian) fountain

Putiel (English) inquiring mind

Putnam (English) fond of water
Puddy, Putnum, Puttie, Putty

Pyke (English) a spear

Pynchon (Last name as first) brilliant; inventive

Pyre (Latin) fire; excitable

Q

Qabil (Arabic) capable

Qadim (Arabic) able

Qadir (Arabic) talented
Qadar, Qadeer, Quadeer, Quadir

Qamar (Arabic) moon; dreamy

Qasim (Arabic) generous

Qidri (Biblical) place name

Qimat (Hindi) valued

Quaashie (African American) ambitious

Quaddus (African American) bright

Quadrees (Latin) fourth
Kwadrees, Quadrhys

Quais (American) form of Qusay: rough hewn

Quan (Vietnamese) dignified

Quanah (Native American) good-smelling
Quan

Quannell (African American) strong-willed
Kwan, Kwanell, Kwanelle, Quan, Quanelle, Quannel

Quant (Latin) knowing his worth
Quanta, Quantae, Quantal, Quantay, Quantea, Quantey, Quantez

Quanza (Spanish) giving

Quaronne (African American) haughty
Kwarohn, Kwaronne, Quaronn

Quashawn (African American) tenacious
Kwashan, Kwashaun, Kwashawn, Quasha, Quashie, Quashy

Qudamah (Arabic) courage

Quebrado (Spanish) broken

Qued (Native American) decorated robe

Quelatikan (Native American) blue horn

Quenby (English) giving
Quenbee, Quenbie, Quenbey

Quennell (French) strength of an oak
Quenell, Quennel

Quentel (Latin) fifth

Quentin (Latin) fifth
Kwent, Qeuntin, Quantin, Quent, Quenten, Quenton, Quientin, Quienton, Quint, Quintin, Quinton, Qwent, Qwentin, Qwenton

Quention (Latin) fifth

Querubin (Hebrew) fast bull

Quick (American) fast; remarkable

Quico (Spanish) stands by his friends
Paco

Quidem (American) believer

Quiessencia (Spanish) essential; essence
Quiess, Quiessence

Quigley (Irish) loving nature
Quiglee, Quigly, Quiggly, Quiggy

Quilaq (Native American) seal

Quillan (Irish) club; joined
Quill, Quillen, Quillon

Quimby (Norse) woman's house

Quincy (French) fifth; patient
Quensie, Quincee, Quincey, Quinci, Quincie, Quinnsy, Quinsey

Quinlan (Irish) fit physique
Quindlen, Quinlen, Quinlin, Quinn, Quinnlan

Quinlin (Irish) strong

Quinn (Irish) form of Quintin: planner
Kwen, Kwene, Quenn, Quin

Quinnton (Latin) fifth

Quinntone (Latin) fifth

Quintavius (African American) fifth child
Quint

Quintin (Latin) planner
Quenten, Quint, Quinton

Quinto (Spanish) fifth
Quiqui

Quintus (Spanish) fifth child
Quin, Quinn, Quint

Quiqui (Spanish) friend; form of Enrique
Kaka, Keke, Quinto, Quiquin

Quirin (English) a magic spell

Quirinus (Latin) spear; Roman god of war

Quito (Spanish) lively
Kito

Qumran (Biblical) place name

Qunnoune (Native American) tall

Quoitrel (African American) equalizer
Kwotrel, Quoitrelle

Quon (Chinese) bright; light

Qusay (Arabic) rough hewn
Qussay

R

Raamah (Hebrew) thunders

Raashid (Arabic) form of
Rashad: wise

Rab (Scottish) form of
Raibeart: brilliant; renowned
Rabbie

Rabbaanee (African)
easygoing

Rabbi (Hebrew) master

Rabbit (Literature) for John
Updike's novels; fast
Rab

Rabul (Hispanic) rich

Race (English) one who races

Racelis (Spanish) of the sky

Racey (English) form of Race:
one who races

Rachins (Hebrew) merciful

Racine (French) last name as
first name; root

Racqueab (Arabic)
homebody

Rad (Scandinavian) helpful;
confident
Radd

Radbert (English) intelligent
Rad

Radborne (English) born
happy
Radbourne, Radburn

Radcliff (English) from the
bright cliff; able

Radcliff (English) child from
the cliff

Raddy (Slavic) cheerful
Rad, Radde, Raddie, Radey

Radford (English) helpful
*Rad, Raddey, Raddie, Raddy,
Radferd*

Radimir (Polish) joyful

Radko (Slavic) happy child

Radley (English) sways with
the wind
Radlea, Radlee, Radleigh

Radnor (English) boy of the
bright shore; natural

Radolf (Anglo-Saxon) warrior

Radomir (Slavic) delightful

Radonir (Polish) form of
Radomir: delightful

Radovan (Czech) delighted

Rady (Filipino) happy

Raekwon (African American)
proud
Raykwonn

Raenn (American) form of
Rain: helpful; smart

Raeshawn (American) brainy

Raeshon (American) form of
Raeshawn; brainy
Rayshawn, Rashone, Reshawn

Raf (Spanish) healed by God

Rafael (Hebrew) rafaelle
*Rafayel, Rafayelle, Rafe,
Raphael, Raphaele*

Rafe (Irish) tough
Raff, Raffe, Raif

Rafeeq (Arabic) gregarious

Rafferty (Irish) wealthy
Rafarty, Rafe, Raff, Raferty, Raffarty, Raffertie, Raffety

Raffin (Hebrew) form of Raphael: God has healed

Rafi (Arabic) musical; friend
Rafee, Raffy

Rafik (Arabic) friendly

Rage (American) trendsetter

Raghib (Arabic) rapturous

Ragin (Biblical) in God's circle

Ragnar (Scandinavian) power fighter

Ragu (Indian) fast

Ragul (Scandinavian) advises

Raheem (Arabic) having empathy
Rahim

Rahime (Arabic) sweet

Rahman (Arabic) full of compassion
Raman, Rahmahn

Rahn (American) form of Ron: kind
Rahnney, Rahnnie, Rahnny

Rahn (American) form of Ron: kind

Rahsaan (Arabic) organized

Rai (Japanese) next child

Raibeart (Gaelic) form of Robert: brilliant; renowned

Raiden (Japanese) storm; thunder god

Railee (American) gregarious

Raimund (German) wise

Rain (English) helpful; smart
Raine, Rainey, Rainey, Raini, Rains, Raney, Rayne

Rainer (German) advisor
Rainor, Rayner, Raynor

Rainey (German) generous
Rain, Raine, Raney, Raynie

Rainier (Place name) distinguished

Rainy (German) advises

Raj (Sanskrit) with stripes
Rajiv

Raja (Sanskrit) king
Raj

Rajab (Arabic) glorified

Rajan (Pakistani) kingly

Rajendra (Hindi) strong king

Rajendran (Indian) indra is the king

Rajesh (Hindi) king rules

Rajnish (Indian) night rules

Rake (American) mischief

Rakesh (Hindi) king

Raleigh (English) jovial
Ralea, Ralee, Raleighe, Rawlee, Rawley, Rawlie

Ralf (American) form of Ralph: advisor to all
Raulf

Ralik (Hindi) purified

Ralis (Latin) thin
Rallus

Ralph (English) advisor to all
Ralf, Ralphie, Ralphy, Raulf, Rolf

Ralpheal (American) form of Raphael: God has healed

Ralphie (English) form of Ralph: advisor to all
Ralphee, Ralphi

Ralston (English) ralph's town; quirky boy
Ralfston, Rolfston

Ralton (last name as first name) from the rail town

Ram (Sanskrit) compelling; pleasant
Rama, Ramm

Ramah (Indian) pleases

Rambert (German) pleasant kid
Ramburt

Rambo (American) daring; action-oriented
Ram

Ramel (Hindi) godlike
Raymel

Rameshwar (Indian) rama Lord

Rami (Spanish) form of Ramiro: judicious
Ramiah

Raminz (Indian) charms

Ramiro (Spanish) judicious
Rameero, Ramero, Ramey, Rami

Ramjee (Indian) pleasing

Ramman (Biblical) form of Ram: compelling; pleasant

Rammy (Spanish) charming

Ramone (Spanish) wise advocate; romantic
Ramond, Raymond, Romon

Ramono (Spanish) form of Raymond: strong

Ramp (American) word as name; hyper
Ram, Rams

Rams (English) form of Ramsey: savvy
Ramm, Ramz

Ramsden (English) born in ram valley; loves the outdoors

Ramsey (English) savvy
Rams, Ramsay, Ramsy, Ramz, Ramzee, Ramzy

Ramsis (Egyptian) born

Ramzan (Indian) pleases

Ramzey (American) form of Ramsey: savvy

Ran (Scottish) form of Ronald: kind
Ranald

Rance (American) renegade
Rans, Ranse

Ranceford (English) from the ford of Laurence; rooted in reality

Rancye (American) form of Rance: renegade
Rancel, Rancy

Rand (Place name) ridge of gold-bearing rock in South Africa

Randall (English) secretive
Randahl, Randel, Randey, Randull, Randy, Randal

Randic (American) form of Randall: secretive

Randolph (English) protective
Rand, Randolf, Randolphe, Randy

Randy (English) form of Randall: secretive; form of Randolph: protective
Randee, Randey, Randi, Randie

Ranean (Biblical) from Mediterranean

Ranen (Hebrew) joyful

Rangarajan (Hindi) charming

Ranger (French) vigilant
Rainge, Range, Rangur

Rangini (Polynesian) celestial

Rani (Hebrew) joyful
Ran, Ranie, Rannie

Ranien (American) counsels

Ranjan (Hindi) delightful

Rank (American) top
Ran

Rankin (English) shielded

Rankin (English) shielded

Rannon (Jewish) renewed

Ransell (English) form of Lawrence: honored; form of Ransom: wealthy
Rancell

Ransford (English) the raven's ford; watchful

Ransley (English) the raven's field; watchful

Ransom (Latin) wealthy
Rance, Ranse, Ransome, Ransum, Ransym

Ranson (English) form of Ransom: wealthy

Rant (English) word as name; from Dutch ranten: to talk foolishly

Rante (American) form of Randy: secretive; protective

Ranteen (Italian) prudent

Ranuel (Hebrew) God's own

Ranulf (English) a Lord chancellor; regal

Rao (French) form of Raoul: advisor to all

Raoul (Spanish) form of Raul: advisor to all
Raul, Raulio

Raous (French) form of Raoul: advisor to all

Raphael (Hebrew) God has healed
Rafael, Rafe, Rapfaele

Raphon (Biblical) place name

Raqib (Arabic) glorified

Rascheed (Arabic) giving

Rashad (Arabic) wise
Rachad, Rashaud, Rashid, Rashod, Roshad

Rashard (American) good

Rasheed (Arabic) intelligent

Rashid (Arabic) focused

Rasmus (Greek) form of Erasmus: beloved

Rasool (Arabic) herald

Rasputin (Russian) a Russian mystic
Rasp

Rastus (Greek) form of Erastus: loved baby
Rastas

Rasul (Arabic) brings message

Rathik (Slavic) vengeful

Raudel (African American) rowdy
Raudell, Rowdel

Rauf (Arabic) compassionate

Raul (Spanish) form of Ralph: advisor to all
Rauly, Rawl

Raven (American) bird; dark and mysterious
Rave, Ravey, Ravy, Rayven

Ravenel (English) darkness of ravens

Ravi (Hindi) sun god
Ravee

Ravid (Hebrew) searching

Ravin (Indian) sun

Ravindra (Hindi) a strong sun

Ravis (Sanskrit) sunny

Rawdan (English) hilly; adventurous
Rawden, Rawdin, Rawdon

Rawle (American) form of Raul: advisor to all

Rawleigh (American) jovial
Rawlee, Rawli

Rawleigh (English) from the deer meadow

Rawlins (French) form of Roland: renowned

Ray (French) royal; king
Rae, Raye, Rayray

Rayal (Irish) form of Ray: royal; king

Rayan (Irish) form of Ryan: royal; good-looking

Raybourne (English) from the deer brook; sylvan
Rayburn, Raybin

Rayce (American) form of Raymond: strong
Rays, Rayse

Rayfield (English) woodsy; capable
Rafe, Ray, Rayfe

Rayk (American) form of Rake: mischief

Rayland (English) streamland boy

Rayman (English) form of Raymond: strong

Raymond (English) strong
Rai, Ramand, Ramond, Ray, Raymie, Raymonde, Raymun, Raymund, Raymy

Raynard (French) judge; sly
Ray, Raynaud, Renard, Renaud, Rey, Reynard, Reynaud

Rayner (French) form of Raymond: strong
Ray, Rayne

Rayon (English) word as name; fabric from "ray" as in "ray of light"

Raypheon (American) form of Raphael: God has healed

Raysh (American) form of Rayshan: inventive

Rayshan (African American) inventive
Ray, Raysh, Raysha, Rayshun

Rayson (American) son of Ray

Razi (Aramaic) secretive

Razus (American) happy

Reace (Welsh) passionate
Reece, Rees, Rees, Reese

Read (English) red-haired
Reade, Reed, Reid

Reagan (Irish) kingly
Ragan, Raghan, Reagen, Reegan, Regan

Reaman (Irish) prolific

Reaner (Last name as first name) even-tempered
Rean, Rener

Rearden (Irish) creative

Reaser (Welsh) excitable

Reavis (American) enthusiastic

Rebal (American) variant on Rebel: outlaw

Rebel (American) outlaw
Reb, Rebbe, Rebele

Red (English) man with red hair
Redd, Reddy

Redford (English) handsome man with ruddy skin
Readford, Red, Reddy, Redferd, Redfor

Redin (last name as first name) red-haired

Redmon (German) protective
Redd, Reddy, Redmond, Redmun, Redmund

Redney (American) form of Rodney: open minded

Reece (Welsh) vivacious
Rees, Reese, Reez

Reed (English) red-haired
Read, Reede, Reid

Reed-Kanan (Scandinavian)

Reef (Nature) water-loving boy

Reem (Hebrew) horned animal or unicorn

Rees (Welsh) form of Rhys: loving
Reece, Reese, Reez, Rez

Reese (Welsh) vivacious
Reis, Rhys

Reesey (Welsh) form of Reese: vivacious

Reeves (English) giving
Reave, Reaves, Reeve

Reez (American) form of Reese: vivacious

Reg (Scandinavian) form of Reginald: wise advisor

Regal (American) debonair
Regall

Regane (Scandinavian) decides

Regen (English) leader

Regent (Latin) royal; grand

Reggie (English) form of Reginald: wise advisor
Reg, Reggey, Reggi, Reggye

Reginald (English) wise advisor
Reg, Reggie, Reginal, Regineld

Reginaldo (Spanish) leader

Regine (French) artistic
Regeen

Regis (Latin) kingly
Reggis

Regney (Slavic) leader

Regulo (Italian) form of Reginald: wise advisor

Rehob (Biblical) place name

Rehoboam (Biblical) son of Solomon

Reid (English) red-haired
Reide

Reidar (Scandinavian) soldier

Reider (Scottish) red-skinned

Reillon (Spanish) realm

Reilly (Irish) daring
Rilee, Riley, Rilie

Rein (German) advises

Reinald (French) judges

Reinder (German) wins

Reine (Scandinavian) victor

Reinhart (German) brave-hearted
Reinhar, Reinhardt, Rhinehard, Rhinehart

Reith (American) shy

Relio (Spanish) gold

Rema (English) form of Remus: fast

Remberto (Spanish) pious

Remeth (Biblical) place name

Remi (French) fun-loving
Remee, Remey, Remmy, Remy

Remiel (Hebrew) saved by God

Remigio (Italian) from Rheims

Remigio (Italian) religious

Reming (English) raven

Remington (Last name as first name) intellectual
Rem, Remmy

Remko (last name as first name) believes

Remo (Italian) confident

Remuda (Spanish) herd of horses
Rem, Remmie, Remmy

Remus (Latin) fast
Reemus, Remes, Remous

Renaloza (Spanish) reborn

Renard (French) smart
Renardt

Renard (French) brave; fox

Renato (Italian) born again
Renata, Renate

Renaud (English) powerful
Renny

Renba (Biblical) name spelled backward

Render (Dutch) draws

RenÈ (French) born again
Renee, Rennie, Renny, Re-Re

Renferd (English) peace-loving
Renfred

Renfro (Welsh) calm
Renfroe, Renfrow, Renphro, Rinfro

Renji (Japanese) truthful

Rennell (Irish) advises

Renny (French) able
Renney, Renni, Rennye

Rennye (Irish) advises

Reno (Place name) city in Nevada
Reen, Reenie, Renoh

Renshaw (English) born in the raven wood

Renson (last name as first name) son of Ren

Renton (English) born in the town of deer

Renwick (English) born in the village of deer

Renze (Italian) excellence

Renzo (Italian) form of Lorenzo: honored

ReShard (African American) rough
Reshar, Reshard

Reshma (Indian) sun

Resk (American) variant on Rex: kingly

Reslie (American) form of Leslie: fiesty; beautiful and smart

Restes (Greek) form of Orestes: leader

Reston (English) form of Royston: town of Royce

Reth (American) form of Seth: chosen

Reto (German) resides

Rett (Literature) form of Rhett: romantic

Reuben (Hebrew) behold, a son
creative, Rube, Rubey, Rubie, Rubin, Ruby, Rubyn

Rev (Invented) ramped up
Revv

Revera (Spanish) values God

Revin (American) distinctive
Revan, Revinn, Revun

Rex (Latin) kingly
Rexe

Rexel (Latin) king

Rexford (American) form of Rex: kingly
Rex, Rexferd, Rexfor, Rexy

Rey (Spanish) form of Reynaldo: knowledgable tutor
Ray, Reye, Reyes

Reymund (French) honored

Reymundo (Spanish) form of Raymond: strong

Reynaldo (Spanish) knowledgeable tutor

Reynard (French) brilliant
Raynard, Rayne, Renardo

Reynaud (French) advisor; judge

Reynold (English) knowledgeable tutor
Ranald, Ranold, Reinold, Renald, Renalde, Rey, Reye, Reynolds

Reza (Iranian) content

Rezeile (Biblical) name spelled backward

Rezeph (Biblical) place name

Rhagae (Biblical) place name

Rhegium (Biblical) place name

Rhene (American) smiley
Reen, Rheen

Rhett (American) romantic
Rhet, Rhette

Rho (Welsh) rose

Rhoden (Greek) rose

Rhodes (Greek) lovely
Rhoades, Rodes

Rhodree (Welsh) ruler
Rodree, Rodrey, Rodry

Rhondel (English) form of Rondel: poetic

Rhoris (Irish) red hair

Rhymen (American) form of Ryan: royal; good-looking

Rhyon (American) form of Ryan: royal; good-looking
Rhyan, Rhyen

Rhyon (Irish) form of Ryan: royal; good-looking

Rhyph (Welsh) jovial

Rhys (Welsh) loving
Reece, Reese

Rian (Irish) little king

Riano (Italian) king

Riao (Spanish) form of Rio: water-loving

Ribal (American) from ribald; revels

Ribog (Slavic) of God

Ricardo (Spanish) snappy
Recardo, Ric, Riccardo, Ricky

Ricardoph (Spanish) energetic

Riccardio (Italian) brave

Rice (English) rich
Ryes

Rich (English) affluent
Richie, Ritchie

Richard ✪ (English) wealthy leader
Rich, Richerd, Richey, Richi, Richie, Rickie, Ricky, Ritchie

Richey (German) ruler
Rich, Richee, Richie, Ritch, Ritchee, Ritchee, Ritchey

Richie (English) form of Richard: wealthy leader
Richey, Richi, Ritchey, Ritchie

Richman (German) has power

Richmond (German) rich and protective
Rich, Richie, Richmon, Richmun, Ricky, Ritchmun

Richshae (English) form of Richard: wealthy leader

Richter (Last name as first name) hopeful
Rick, Ricky, Rik, Rikter

Rick (German) form of Richard: wealthy leader
Ric, Rickey, Ricki, Rickie, Ricky, Rik

Rickard (Scandinavian) form of Richard: wealthy leader
Rick, Rickert, Rickward, Rikkert

Rico (Italian) spirited; ruler
Reco, Reko, Ricko, Rikko, Riko

Ricod (American) form of Rico: spirited; ruler

Ricsi (American) form of Richie: wealthy leader

Riddle (Word as name) perplexes

Riddock (Irish) man of the field

Rider (American) horse rider
Ryder

Ridge (English) on the ridge; risk-taker

Ridglee (English) man of the ridge
Ridgley, Ridglea

Ridhaa (Arabic) delight

Ridley (English) ingenious
Redley, Rid, Ridley, Ridlie, Ridly, Rydley

Riemer (English) from Rheims

Rien (Dutch) mariner

Rigby (English) high-energy
Rigbie, Rigbye, Rygby

Rigel (Arabic) foot; star in constellation Orion

Rigney (Greek) power

Rigo (Spanish) ridge boy

Rigoberto (Spanish) strong
Bert, Berto, Rigo

Rigoberto (Spanish) ridge boy

Rike (American) form of Nike: winning
Rikee, Rykee, Rykie, Ryky

Rikken (Slavic) form of Rik: hopeful

Rilan (English) land of rye

Rilee (American) form of Riley: brave
Rilea, Rileigh

Rileigh (American) form of Riley: brave
Ryleigh

Riley (Irish) brave
Reilly, Rylee, Ryley, Rylie, Ryly

Rimme (French) form of Remi: fun-loving

Rimmon (Biblical) place name

Rimon (Hebrew)
pomegranate

Ringo (English) funny
Ring, Ringgoh, Ryngo

Rinus (American) form of
Ryan: royal; good-looking

Rinzel (American) thinker

Rio (Spanish) water-loving
Reeo

Rio Grande (Spanish) a river
in Texas
Rio, Riogrande

Rion (American) form of
Ryan/Rian: royal; good-
looking; little king

Rione (Spanish) flowing
Reo, Reone, Rio

Rionn (Greek) form of Orion:
fiery hunter

Riordan (Irish) Lordly
Rearden

Riordene (Irish) poetic

Rip (English) serene
Ripp, Rippe

Ripley (English) serene
Riplee

Ris (English) outdoorsman;
smart
*Rislea, Rislee, Risleigh, Riz,
Rizlee*

Rise (Welsh) form of Rhys:
loving

Rishab (American) form of
Rashad: wise

Rishi (Arabic) first

Rishi (Indian) wise man

Rishon (Hebrew) first

Risley (English) smart and
quiet
Rislee, Risleye, Rizlee, Rizley

Risto (Scandinavian) bears
Christ

Ristoffer (American) form of
Christopher: the bearer of
Christ

Ristoph (German) form of
Christopher: the bearer of
Christ

Ritch (American) leader
*Rich, Richee, Richey, Ritch,
Ritchal, Ritchee, Ritchi*

Ritchell (English) controller

Ritchie (English) form of
Richie: wealthy leader
Ritchee, Ritchey, Ritchy

Rito (American) spunky
Reit

Ritt (German) debonair
Rit, Rittie, Rittly

Ritter (German) debonair
Riter, Rittyr

Rivan (Literature) from
Eddings's The Rivan Codex;
esoteric

River (English) flowing water;
hip
Riv, Ryver

Rivers (English) flowing river

Riverson (English) son of
River

Rixus (Greek) excites

Rizal (Spanish) athletic

Rizalino (Spanish) pleased

Rizo (Italian) lively

Roald (Scandinavian) famous
ruler

Roam (American) wanderer
Roamey, Roamy, Roma, Rome

Roan (English) form of
Rogan: spirited redhead

Roar (Irish) form of Roarke:
ruler

Roarke (Irish) ruler
Roark, Rork, Rourke

Rob (English) form of Robert:
brilliant; renowned
Robb

Robbie (English) form of
Robert: brilliant; renowned
Robbee, Robbey, Robbi, Robby

Robert ✪ (English) brilliant;
renowned
*Bob, Bobbie, Bobby, Rob,
Robart, Robbie, Robby, Roberto,
Robs, Roburt*

Robert-Lee (American)
patriotic
*Bobbylee, Robby Lee, Robert
Lee, Robert-E-Lee, Robertlee*

Roberto (Spanish) form of
Robert: brilliant; renowned
Berto, Rob, Robert, Tito

Roberts (Last name as first
name) luminous
Rob, Robards, Robarts, Roburts

Robeson (English) rob's son;
bright
Roberson, Robison

Robhert (Welsh) form of
Robert: brilliant; renowned

Robin (English) gregarious
Robb, Robbin, Robby, Robyn

Roble (Last name as first
name) divine
Robel, Robl, Robley

Roblee (American) patriot

Robles (English) royal

Robson (English) sterling
character
Robb, Robbson, Robsen

Roc (Italian) form of Rocco:
tough

Rocal (American) form of
Rocco: tough

Rocco (Italian) tough
*Roc, Rock, Rockie, Rocko,
Rocky, Rok, Rokee, Rokko, Roko*

Roch (English) form of Rock:
hardy

Rochester (English) guarded
Roche

Rocio (Spanish) form of
Rocco: tough

Rock (American) hardy
Roc, Rocky, Rok

Rocket (American) word as a
name; snappy
Rokket

Rockleigh (English)
dependable; outdoorsy
*Rocco, Rock, Rocklee, Rockley,
Rocky, Roklee*

Rockmun (English) man who
rests

Rockne (English) form of
Rocco/Rock: tough; hardy

Rockney (American) brash

Rockwell (American) spring
of strength
Rock, Rockwelle, Rocky

Rocky (English) hardy; tough
*Rocco, Rock, Rockee, Rockey,
Rocki, Rockie*

Rocquin (Spanish) form of
Joaquin: bold; hip

Rod (English) brash
Rodd, Roddy

Rodalfo (Spanish) form of
Rudolph: wolf

Rodas (Spanish) spanish
name for the Rhone River in
France
Rod, Roda

Rodas (Spanish) of Rhodes;
Place

Rodden (English) powerful

Roddick (Last name as first
name) goes far

Roddy (German) form of
Roderick: effective leader
Roddee, Roddi, Roddie

Rodel (American) generous
Rodell, Rodey, Rodie

Rodeo (Spanish) roundup;
cowboy
Rodayo, Roddy, Rodyo

Roderick (German) effective
leader
*Roddy, Roddyrke, Roderic,
Roderik, Rodreck, Rodrick,
Rodrik*

Rodger (German) form of
Roger: famed warrior
Rodge, Roge

Rodion (Biblical) form of
Herodion: heroic

Rodman (German) hero
Rodmin, Rodmun

Rodney (English)
open-minded
*Rod, Roddy, Rodnee, Rodni,
Rodnie*

Rodo (French) wolflike

Rodolfo (Spanish) spark
Rod, Rudolfo, Rudolpho

Rodree (American) leader
Rodrey, Rodri, Rodry

Rodrigo (Spanish) feisty
leader
Rod, Roddy, Rodrego, Rodriko

Rodriguez (Spanish) hot-
blooded
*Rod, Roddy, Rodreguez,
Rodrigues*

Rodwell (German) renowned

Roe (English) deer

Roel (Dutch) famed hero

Roemello (Italian) form of
Romulus: presumptuous

Rogan (Irish) spirited
redhead

Rogasiano (Spanish) red hair

Rogelio (Spanish) aggressive
Rojel, Rojelio

Rogell (Dutch) strong

Roger (German) famed
warrior
*Rodge, Rodger, Roge, Rogie,
Rogyer, Rogers*

Rognan (Slavic) upward

Rohan (Hindi) going higher

Rohanee (Indian) comes
down to earth

Rohit (Hindi) he fishes

Roi (French) form of Roy:
king

Roisin (Irish) the rose

Rokee (Slavic) peaceful boy

Rokel (Scandinavian) a ewe

Roland (German) renowned
*Rolend, Rollan, Rolland, Rollie,
Rollo, Rolund*

Rolando (Spanish) famous
Rolan

Roldan (Spanish) leader

Role (American) brash
Roel, Roll

Rolf (German) kind advisor
Rolfee, Rolfie, Rolfy, Rolph

Rolfon (Norwegian)
overbearing

Rollan (Russian) from
Roland: renowned

Rollie (English) form of
Roland: renowned
Rollee, Rolley, Rolli, Rolly

Rollins (German) form of
Roland: renowned
Rolin, Rolins, Rollin, Rolyn

Rollo (German) famous

Rolly (English) famous

Rolt (Latin) wolfish

Roly (English) form of
Roland: renowned

Roman (Latin) fun-loving
*Romen, Romey, Romi, Romun,
Romy, Romain*

Romano (Italian) from Rome

Romar (English) from Rome

Rombert (Latin) from Rome

Rome (Place name) city in
Italy
Romeo

Romedios (Spanish) roman

Romeo (Italian) romantic
lover
*Romah, Rome, Romeoh,
Romero, Romey, Romi, Romy*

Romer (American) form of
Rome: city in Italy
Roamar, Roamer

Rommel (Latin) from Rome

Romney (Welsh) roamer
Rom, Romnie

Romo (French) boy from
Rome

Romulo (Spanish) man from
Rome
Romo

Romulo (Spanish) of Rome

Romulon (Mythology) of
Rome

Romulus (Latin)
presumptuous
Rom, Romules, Romulo

Romy (German) form of
Romulus: presumptuous

Ron (English) form of Ronald:
kind
Ronn

Ronak (Scandinavian)
powerful

Ronald (English) kind
*Ron, Ronal, Ronel, Ronney,
Ronni, Ronnie, Ronuld*

Ronalk (Slavic) form of
Ronald: kind

Ronan (Irish) seal; playful

Rond (American) from the
word round

Rondel (French) poetic
*Ron, Rondal, Rondell, Rondie,
Rondy*

Ronen (Jewish) joyful

Ronford (English)
distinguished
Ronferd, Ronnforde

Rong (Chinese) warring

Roni (Hebrew) joyful
Rone, Ronee

Ronicle (American) form of
Ron: kind

Ronit (Jewish) sings

Ronneal (American) leaving

Ronnie (English) form of
Ronald: kind
Ronnee, Ronney, Ronni, Ronny

Ronomy (Biblical) from
Deuteronomy

Ronson (Scottish) ron's son; likable

Rook (Spanish) form of Roque: rock

Roon (Scandinavian) form of Rune: secretive

Roone (Irish) distinctive; bright face
Rooney, Roune

Rooney (Irish) man with red hair
Rooni, Roony

Roose (Last name as first name) high-energy
Rooce, Roos, Rooz, Ruz

Roosevelt (Dutch) strong leader
Rooseveldt, Rosevelt, Rosy, Velte

Rooster (American) loud
Roos, Rooz

Roper (American) roper
Rope

Roque (Portuguese) rock

Rorden (Irish) creative

Rorelle (English) red-haired

Rorick (French) red-haired

Rorin (American) form of Rory: strong

Rory (German) strong
Roree, Rorey, Roreye, Rorie

Rosalio (Spanish) rose; charmer

Rosano (Italian) rosy prospects; romantic

Roscoe (English) woods; nature-loving
Rosco, Roskie, Rosko, Rosky

Rosembelt (Spanish) beauty of roses

Rosendo (Italian) rose

Roser (American) redhead; outgoing
Rozer

Roshanek (Slavic) bright flower

Roshaun (African American) loyal
Roshawn

Roshni (Indian) brightness

Rosk (American) swift
Roske

Rosley (English) of the rosary

Rosling (Scottish) redhead; explosive
Roslin, Rosy, Rozling

Ross (Latin) attractive
Rossey, Rossie, Rossy

Rossa (American) exuberant
Ross, Rosz

Rossain (American) hopeful
Rossane

Rossan (French) rose

Rossano (Italian) handsome

Rossell (French) rose

Rossi (Italian) rose red

Roston (English) rusting

Roswell (English) fascinating
Roswel, Roswelle, Rosy, Rozwell, Well

Roteus (Greek) form of Proteus: first

Roteus (Greek) form of Proteus: first

Roth (German) man with red hair
Rothe, Rauth

Rouel (French) form of Rule: emphatic

Roumen (Slavic) roman

Roupen (American) quiet
Ropan, Ropen, Ropun

Roven (English) wanders

Rover (English) wanderer
Rovar, Rovey, Rovur, Rovy

Roverb (Invented) from
Proverb

Rovere (French) travels

Rovonte (French) roving

Rowan (English) red-haired;
adorned
Rowe, Rowen

Rowand (Last name as first)
reliable

Rowdy (English) athletic;
loud
Roudy, Rowdee, Rowdi, Rowdie

Rowe (English) outgoing
Roe, Row, Rowie

Rowel (English) famed

Rowell (English) rocker
Roll, Rowl

Rowenam (English) red-
haired

Rowland (Scandinavian)
form of Roland: renowned

Rowley (English) from the
rough meadow; spirited

Rown (English) form of
Rowan: red-haired; adorned

Roxen (English) precise

Roy (French) king
Roi

Royal (French) king
Roy, Royall, Royalle, Roye

Royalton (French) king
Royal, Royallton

Royce (German) famous
Roy, Royse

Roycell (French) form of
Royce: famous

Roycie (American) form of
Royce: famous
Rory, Roy, Royce, Royse, Roysie

Royd (English) good humor

Roydean (American) combo
of Roy and Dean

Roydee (English) natural

Royden (English) outdoors;
regal
Roy, Roydin

Royderrick (English) form of
Roderick: effective leader

Royelio (Spanish) royal

Royle (English) kingly

Roysell (American) form of
Royce: famous

Royst (American) form of
Royce: famous

Royston (English) town of
Royce

Ruadhan (Hindi) brash

Ruari (Irish) red-haired
Ruairi, Ruaridh

Rube (Spanish) form of
Ruben: behold, a son
Rubino

Ruben (Spanish) form of
Reuben: behold, a son
Rube, Ruby

Rubens (Dutch) son

Rubi (Hebrew) form of
Rubin: behold, a son

Ruchirat (French) rich

Rudder (English) ruddy skin

Ruddy (English) ruddy skin

Rudeger (German) friendly
*Rudger, Rudgyr, Rudigar,
Rudiger, Rudy*

Rudo (African) loving

Rudolf (German) wolf
Rodolf, Rudy

Rudolph (German) wolf
*Rodolf, Rodolph, Rud, Rudee,
Rudey, Rudi, Rudolpho, Rudy*

Rudow (German) lovable

Rudy (German) form of
Rudolph: wolf
Rude, Rudee, Rudey, Rudi

Rudyard (English) closed off
Rud, Rudd, Ruddy

Rueban (American) form of
Reuben: behold, a son
Ruban

Rued (Spanish) dishonest

Ruel (French) variant on Rule:
emphatic

Ruelas (Spanish) ambitious

Rufaro (African) gives
happiness

Ruffo (Spanish) form of
Rufus: redhead

Rufine (French) red hair

Rufino (Spanish) redhead

Rufino (Italian) red hair

Rufus (Latin) redhead
*Fue, Rufas, Rufes, Ruffie,
Ruffis, Ruffy, Rufous*

Rugby (English) braced for
contact
Rug, Rugbee, Rugbie, Ruggy

Rugerd (Slavic) famed

Ruggier (French) form of
Roger: famed warrior

Rugo (Italian) famed

Rui (Spanish) powerful fighter

Ruiden (Irish) red-haired

Ruiz (Spanish) chummy

Rujul (Indian) truthful

Rule (English) emphatic

Rulei (French) unit

Rulon (Native American)
spirited
Rulonn

Rumford (English) lives at
river crossing; grounded

Rummel (American) form of
Rommel: from Rome

Rumont (French) red
mountain

Runa (German) keeps score

Runako (African) attractive

Rune (German) secretive
Roone, Runes

Rupad (Hindi) secretive
Rupesh

Rupchand (Sanskrit) as
beautiful as the moon

Rupert (English) prince
Rupe

Rupin (Indian) handsome

Rurik (Russian) famous

Rush (English) loquacious
Rusch

Rushford (English) from the
ford of rushes; found

Rushon (French) red hair

Rusi (English) red-haired

Rusim (Biblical) traditional

Rusk (Spanish) innovator
Rusck, Ruske, Ruskk

Ruskin (French) red-haired

Ruslan (English) rusty hair

Russ (French) form of
Russell: man with red hair;
charmer

Russell (French) man with red hair; charmer
Russ, Russel, Russy, Rusty

Russo (Italian) russet

Russon (French) red hair

Rustice (French) rusty hair

Rustin (English) redhead
Rustan, Ruston, Rusty

Rusty (French) form of Russell: man with red hair; charmer
Rustee, Rustey, Rusti

Rutherford (English) dignified
Ruthe, Rutherfurd, Rutherfyrd

Rutil (Spanish) faithful

Rutilio (Spanish) faithful

Rutland (Norse) red land

Rutledge (English) substantial
Rutlidge

Rutley (English) from red country; fertile

Ruud (Dutch) like a wolf

Ruud (Dutch) well-known

Ruvim (Hebrew) meaningful

Ryall (American) capable

Ryan ✪ ✆ (Irish) royal; good-looking
Rhine, Rhyan, Rhyne, Ry, Ryane, Ryann, Ryanne, Ryen, Ryun

Ryander (American) competitive; obstinate

Ryden (English) form of Ryder: outdoorsy; man who rides horses

Ryder (English) outdoorsy; man who rides horses
Rider, Rye

Ryderin (Welsh) caring

Rye (Botanical) grain; basic

Ryerson (English) fit outdoorsman
Rye

Rygel (Spanish) regal

Ryk (American) form of Rick: wealthy leader

Ryke (Slavic) form of Richard: wealthy leader

Ryken (Slavic) form of Richard: wealthy leader

Ryker (English) of the rye land; farms

Rykey (American) easygoing

Ryland (English) excellent
Rilan, Riland, Rye, Rylan

Rylandar (English) farmer
Rye, Rylan, Ryland

Rylant (American) form of Ryland: excellent

Ryle (American) form of Kyle: serene

Ryman (English) man of rye; fundamental

Rymmy (Spanish) form of Romy: presumptuous

Ryne (Irish) form of Ryan: royal; good-looking
Rine, Ryn, Rynn

Ryoun (American) form of Ryan: royal; good-looking

Ryston (English) form of Royston: town of Royce

Ryszard (Polish) courageous leader
Reshard

Ryton (English) from the town of rye; fundamental

Ryvers (American) form of
Rivers: flowing river

S

Saad (Aramaic) helping
others

Saahdia (Aramaic) helped by
the Lord
Saadya, Seadya

Saarik (Hindi) sings like a
bird
Saariq, Sareek, Sareeq, Sariq

Sabene (Latin) optimist
Sabe, Sabeen, Sabin, Sabyn,
Sabyne

Saber (French) armed; sword
Sabar, Sabe, Sabre

Sabin (Latin) sabine
Sabeeno, Sabino, Savin, Savino

Sable (French) animal;
brown-haired child

Sacha (Russian) defends;
charms
Sascha, Sasha

Sachar (Hebrew) well-
rewarded
Sacar

Sachetan (Indian) logical

Saddam (Arabic) powerful
ruler
Saddum

Sadiki (African) loyal
Sadeeki

Sadler (English) practical
Sadd, Saddle, Sadlar, Sadlur

Sae (American) talkative
Saye

Saeed (African) lucky

Safford (English) boy from
the river of willows

Saffron (Botanical)
spice/plant; orange-haired
Saffran, Saffren, Saphron

Sagar (Indian) ocean

Sagaz (Spanish) clever
Saga, Sago

Sage (Botanical) wise
Saje

Sageal (Spanish) smart

Sagel (Indian) ocean

Sager (American) rewarded;
short
Sayger

Sagi (Hebrew) best

Saginaw (Place name) city in
Michigan; Native American
bold, *Sag, Saggy*

Sagiv (Hebrew) the best
Segev

Saguaro (Botanical) cactus;
prickly
Seguaro

Sahak (Slavic) jovial

Sahil (Hindi) leader
Sahel

Sahn (Hindi) held high

Sai (Arabic) sword

Saied (Arabic) fortunate

Sail (American) water; natural

Sailan (American) of the sea

Sainsbury (English) from the
home of saints; religious
Sainsberry

Saint (Latin) holy man

Saith (English) to speak
Saithe, Saythe

Sajan (Hindi) beloved

Sakar (Biblical) form of Issachar: reward

Sal (Italian) form of Salvador: savior; spirited; form of Salvatore: rescuer; spirited
Sall, Sallie, Sally

Saladin (Arabic) devout
Saladdin

Salado (Spanish) funny
Sal

Salath (Biblical) generous

Salehe (African) good

Salem (Hebrew) peaceful

Salford (Place name) city in England

Salim (Arabic) safe; peaceful
Saleem

Salisbury (English) born in the willows
Salisbery, Salisberry, Saulsberry, Saulsbery, Saulsbury, Saulisbury

Salm (Biblical) from Psalms

Salman (Arabic) protected

Salom (Biblical) form of Absalom: my father is peace

Salomaa (Spanish) ideal

Salt (American) salt-of-the-earth
Salty

Salustia (Spanish) healthy

Salute (American) patriotic

Salvacion (Spanish) salvation

Salvador (Spanish) savior; spirited
Sal, Sally, Salvadore

Salvatore (Italian) rescuer; spirited
Sal, Sallie, Sally, Salvatori, Salvatorre

Salvio (Latin) saved
Salvian, Salviano, Salviatus

Salvoterre (Spanish) salvation

Sam (Hebrew) form of Samuel: man who heard God; prophet
Samm, Sammey, Sammi, Sammy

Samaga (Biblical) place name

Samal (Biblical) place name

Saman (Hebrew) hears all

Samce (Biblical) form of Samson: strong man

Samed (Arabic) everlasting

Sami (Lebanese) high

Samilo (Italian) upward

Samir (Arabic) special
Sameer, Samere, Samyr

Sammon (Arabic) grocer
Sammen

Sammy (Hebrew) wise
Samie, Sammee, Sammey, Sammi, Sammie, Samy

Samos (Place name) casual

Samrat (Indian) of the emperor

Samson (Hebrew) strong man
Sam, Sampson

Samuel ○ ◐ (Hebrew) man who heard God; prophet
Sam, Samael, Sammeul, Sammie, Sammo, Sammuel, Sammy, Samual

Samvel (Hebrew) know the name of God
Samvell, Samvelle

Sanborn (English) one with nature
Sanborne, Sanbourn, Sandy

Sancho (Latin) genuine
Sanch, Sanchoh

Sandage (English) form of Sander: savior of mankind; nice

Sandalio (Spanish) wolflike

Sandberg (Last name as first name) writer
Sandburg

Sander (Greek) savior of mankind; nice
Sandor

Sanders (English) kind
Sandars, Sandors, Saunders

Sanderson (Last name as first name) defender
Sandersen

Sandhurst (English) from the sandy thicket; undaunted
Sandhirst

Sandiego (Spanish) place name

Sanditon (English) from the sandy town; perseveres

Sandro (Italian) form of Alexander: great leader; helpful

Sandy (English) personable
Sandee, Sandey, Sandi

Sanford (English) negotiator
Sandford, Sandy, Sanferd, Sanfor

Sangarius (Biblical) place name

Sango (Asian) coral

Sanjay (Sanskrit) wins every time

Sanjiv (Hindi) longlasting

Sanjog (Indian) lucky chance

Sanogo (Spanish) brave

Sanorelle (African American) honest
Sanny, Sano, Sanorel, Sanorell

Sansone (Italian) strong

Santana (Spanish) saintly
Santa, Santanah, Santanna, Santee

Santiago (Spanish) sainted; valuable
Sandiago, Santego, Santiagoh, Santy, Tago

Santino (Italian) sacred
Santeeno, Santyno

Santon (English) sandy home

Santos (Italian) holy; blessed
Sant, Santo

Santosh (Hindi) happy

Sapir (Hebrew) sapphire; jewel
Safir, Saphir, Saphiros

Saral (Indian) straightforward

Sarang (Indian) deer

Sarday (American) extrovert
Sardae, Sardaye

Sardica (Biblical) place name

Sardis (Biblical) place name

Sargent (French) officer/leader
Sarge, Sergeant

Sargis (Slavic) serves

Sargon (Persian) sun king

Sarid (Biblical) place name

Sarkis (Greek) the Lord

Sasan (Hebrew) happy

Sasha (Russian) helpful
Sacha, Sash, Sasha

Sassacus (Native American) wild soul

Sasso (Hebrew) happy

Sasson (Hebrew) happy

Sastry (Indian) safe

Satchel (American) unique
Satch, Satchell

Saturnin (Spanish) from planet Saturn; melancholy
Saturnino

Satya (Indian) honesty

Saul (Hebrew) gift
Sawl, Saulie, Sol, Solly

Saunder (English) defensive; focused
Saunders

Sava (Slavic) aware

Savage (Last name as first name) wild
Sav

Saverio (Spanish) bright

Saviero (Spanish) form of Xavier: home; shining

Saville (French) willow town
Savelle, Savile, Savill, Seville

Savini (Italian) bright

Savio (Italian) smart

Savone (Italian) form of Savino: sabine

Savoy (Place name) region in France
Savoe

Savyon (Spanish) great attitude

Sawyer (English) hardworking
Saw, Sawyrr

Saxe (English) form of Saxon: sword-fighter; feisty
Sax, Saxee, Saxey, Saxie

Saxon (English) sword-fighter; feisty
Sackson, Sax, Saxan, Saxe, Saxen

Saxton (Place name) stern
Saxten

Sayan (Asian) standing

Sayre (Welsh) skilled
Saye, Sayer, Sayers

Scafell (Place name) mountain in England

Scanlon (Irish) devious
Scan, Scanlin, Scanlun, Scanne

Scant (American) word as name; too little
Scanty

Schae (American) safe; careful
Schay

Schaffer (German) watchful
Schaffur, Shaffer

Schawn (American) form of Shawn/Sean: God is gracious

Schelde (Place name) river in Europe; calm
Shelde

Schelte (German) sheltie

Schmidt (German) hardworking; blacksmith
Schmit

Schneider (German) stylish; tailor
Sneider, Snider

Schubert (German) cobbler
Shubert

Schumann (Last name as first) famous composer; romantic

Schuyler (Dutch) protective
Skylar, Skyler

Scipio (Greek) leader

Scirocco (Italian) warmth of
the wind
Cirocco, Sirocco

Scopus (Biblical) place name

Scorpio (Latin) lethal
Scorp, Scorpioh

Scotland (Place name) from
Scotland

Scott (English) from
Scotland; happy
Scot, Scotty

Scotty (English) happy
Scottee, Scottey, Scotti

Scout (French) hears all;
scouts for information

Scribner (English) the one
who writes

Scully (Irish) vocal
Scullee, Sculley, Scullie

Scupi (Biblical) place name

Seabert (English) shines like
the sea
Seabright, Sebert, Seibert

Seabrook (English)
outdoorsy
Seabrooke

Seabury (English) lives by the
sea
Seaberry, Seabry

Seaby (American) form of
Sebastian: dramatic;
honorable

Seaman (English) seafarer

Seamus (Gaelic)
replacement; bonus
Seemus, Semus

Sean ☉ (Irish) God is gracious
Seann, Shaun, Shaune, Shawn

Searcy (English) fortified
Searcee, Searcey

Searles (English) fortified
Searl, Searle, Serles, Serls

Seaton (Place name) seaton
Seaten, Seeten, Seeton

Seaver (Last name as first
name) safe
Seever

Sebastian ☉ (Latin)
dramatic; honorable
*Bastian, Seb, Sebashun,
Sebastien, Sebastion,
Sebastuan, Sebo*

Sebbie (American) form of
Sebastian: dramatic;
honorable

Sebe (Latin) form of
Sebastian: dramatic;
honorable
*Seb, Sebo, Seborn, Sebron,
Sebrun*

Secondo (Italian) second-
born boy
Segundo

Sedgley (American) classy
Sedg, Sedge, Sedgeley, Sedgely

Sedgwick (English) from the
place of swords; defensive
*Sedgewick, Sedgewyck,
Sedgwyck*

Seely (Last name as first
name) fun-loving
Sealy, Sealey, Seeley

Seerath (Indian) great

Sef (Egyptian) yesterday

Seferino (Spanish) flying in
the wind
*Cefirino, Sebarino, Sephirio,
Zefarin, Zefirino, Zephir,
Zephyr*

Sefre (Welsh) peace

Sefton (English) from the town in the rushes; safe

Seger (Last name as first name) singer
Seager, Seeger, Sega, Segur

Segundo (Spanish) second child

Seidon (Greek) from Greek mythology Poseidon; Earth

Sekani (African) laughing

Sela (Hebrew) from the cliff; dares
Selah

Selby (English) from a village of mansions; rich
Selbey, Shelbey, Shelbie, Shelby

Seldon (English) from the willow valley; swaying
Selden, Sellden, Shelden

Selestino (Spanish) heavenly
Celeste, Celestino, Celey, Sele, Selestyno

Selig (German) blessed boy
Seligman, Seligmann, Zelig

Selim (Turkish) safe haven

Selkirk (Scottish) church home boy; conflicted

Sellers (English) dweller of marshland; sturdy
Sellars

Selmo (Spanish) form of Anselmo: protected by God

Selmy (French) form of Anselme: protective

Selo (Biblical) place name

Selvin (English) from the woods

Selvon (American) gregarious
Sel, Selman, Selv, Selvaughn, Selvawn

Selwyn (English) friend from the mansion; wealthy
Selwin, Selwinn, Selwynn, Selwynne

Semaj (Turkish) named

Semath (American) unites

Semeon (Biblical) form of Simon: good listener; thoughtful

Seminole (Native American) tribe name; unyielding

Semion (Slavic) form of Simon: good listener; thoughtful

Senath (Biblical) belongs

Sender (Hebrew) form of Alexander: great leader; helpful

Seneca (Native American) tribe name; revered

Senen (Irish) wise boy

Senior (French) older
Sennyur, Senyur, Sinior

Sennen (English) aged

Sennett (French) old spirit
Sennet

Sentino (Italian) form of Santino: sacred

Seppel (German) loved

Sepph (Biblical) place name

Septimus (Latin) seventh child; neglected

Sequoia (Native American) tree; sturdy

Serafin (Spanish) form of Seraphim: full of fire

Seraphim (Hebrew) full of fire
Sarafim, Saraphim, Serafim, Serephim

Sereno (Latin) serene
Cereno

Serf (Spanish) serves

Serge (French) gentle man
Serg

Sergeant (French) officer;
leader
Sarge, Sargent

Sergei (Russian) good
looking
Serg, Serge, Sergie, Sergy, Surge

Sergio (Italian) handsome
Serge, Sergeeo, Sergeoh, Sergyo

Serguej (Slavic) serves well

Sero (Italian) sun

Servacio (Spanish) saved

Servando (Spanish) services

Servas (Latin) saved
Servaas, Servacio, Servatus

Sesame (Botanical) seed;
flavors
Sesamey, Sessame, Sessamee

Seth ✪ (Hebrew) chosen
Sethe

Seton (English) from the sea
town; loves the water

Sevastian (American) form
of Sebastian: dramatic;
honorable

Seven (American) dramatic;
seventh child
Sevene, Sevin

Several (American)
multiplies
Sevral, Sevrull

Severence (French) strict
Severince, Severynce

Severin (Latin) severe
Saverino, Sverinus, Seweryn

Severn (English) having
boundaries

Severo (Italian) unbending;
harsh

Sevester (American) form of
Sylvester: forest-dweller;
heavy-duty
Seveste, Sevy

Sevrin (Scandinavian) severe

Seward (English) guarding
the sea
Sew, Sewerd, Sward

Sewell (Last name as first
name) seaward
Seawell, Seawel, Sewel

Sexton (English) church-
loving
Sextan, Sextin, Sextown

Sextus (Latin) sixth child;
mischievous
Sesto, Sixto, Sixtus

Seymour (French) prayerful
Seamore, See, Seye, Seymore

Shaamar (Biblical) name
spelled backward

Shabat (Hebrew) the end
Shabbat

Shachar (Hebrew) the dawn

Shad (African) joyful

Shade (English) secretive
Shadee, Shadey, Shady

Shadman (Hebrew) farm

Shadow (English) mystique
Shade, Shadoe

Shadrach (Biblical) godlike;
brave
*Shad, Shadd, Shadrack,
Shadreck, Shadryack*

Shadrie (Biblical) form of
Shadrach: godlike; brave

Shaff (American) companion

Shafiq (Arabic) forgiving
Shafeek, Shafik

Shafir (Hebrew) handsome
Shafeer, Shafer, Shefer

Shago (American) casual

Shahzad (Persian) royalty;
king

Shai (Hebrew) the gift

Shaikh (French) severe

Shak (Arabic) attracts

Shakil (Arabic) attractive
*Shakeel, Shakill, Shakille,
Shaqueel, Shaquil, Shaquille*

Shakir (Arabic) appreciative
Shakee, Shakeer

Shakunt (Indian) bluebird

Shakur (Arabic) thankful
Shakurr

Shale (Hebrew) form of
Shalev: calm
Shaile, Shayle

Shalev (Hebrew) calm

Shalom (Hebrew) peaceful
Sholem, Sholom

Shalu (American) peace

Sham (Biblical) armed

Shaman (Russian) mystical
Shamain, Shamon, Shayman

Shamar (Indian) proud

Shamir (Hebrew) thorn
Shameer

Shammah (Biblical) devout

Shamus (Irish) seizing
Schaemus, Schamus, Shamuss

Shan (Hindi) bright sun

Shanahan (Irish) giving
Shanihan, Shanyhan

Shance (American) form of
Chance: good fortune; happy
Shan, Shanse

Shand (English) loud
Shandy

Shandee (English) noisy
Shandi, Shandy

Shane (Irish) easygoing
Shain, Shay, Shayne

Shani (African) a wonder;
Hebrew
red

Shanley (Irish) old soul
Shannley

Shannon (Irish) wise
*Shana, Shanan, Shane,
Shanen, Shann, Shannen,
Shanon*

Shantam (Hindi) bright sun

Shantan (Sanskrit) peaceful

Shante (American) poised
Shantae, Shantay

Shap (English) form of Shep:
watchful

Shapleigh (English) form of
Shepley: from the sheep
meadow; tender

Shaq (Arabic) form of
Shaquille: handsome
Shack, Shak

Shaquille (Arabic) handsome
*Shak, Shakeel, Shaq, Shaquil,
Shaquill*

Sharad (Indian) fall season

Sharif (Arabic) truthful
Shareef, Sheref

Sharkie (American) crafty

Sharman (American) magic
man

Sharp (Word as name) bright

Shashee (Indian) moon

Shashhi (Hindi) moon

Shasta (Place name) oregon mountain; high hopes

Shaun (Irish) form of Sean: God is gracious
Seanne, Shaune, Shaunn

Shaw (English) safe; in a tree grove
Shawe

Shawn (Irish) form of Sean: God is gracious
Shawnay, Shawne, Shawnee, Shawney

Shawnell (African American) talkative
Shaunell

Shawner (American) form of Shawn: God is gracious

Shawon (African American) optimistic
Shawan, Shawaughn, Shawaun

Shay (Irish) form of Shamus: seizing
Shai

Shayan (Native American) from Cheyenne; tribe; erratic

Shayde (Irish) confident
Shaedy, Sheade

Shaykeen (African American) successful
Shay, Shaykine

Shea (Irish) vital
Shay

Sheamus (Irish) form of James: he who supplants

Sheban (Biblical) sworn

Shechem (Biblical)

Sheehan (Irish) clever
Shehan, Shihan

Sheen (English) bright and shining; talented
Shean, Sheene

Shehzad (Arabic) prince

Shel (Hebrew) mine

Shelah (Biblical) vivacious

Shelby (English) established
Shel, Shelbee, Shelbey, Shelbie, Shell, Shelly

Sheldon (English) quiet
Shel, Sheld, Shelden, Sheldin, Shell, Shelly

Shell (English) form of Sheldon: quiet

Shelley (English) form of Shelby: established
Shelly

Shelton (English) from the village of ledges

Shem (Hebrew) famous

Shen (Chinese) introspective

Shenandoah (Place name) valley; nostalgic

Sheng (Chinese) winning

Shep (English) watchful
Shepp, Sheppy

Shepal (English) herds sheep

Shepher (English) sheep herder

Shepherd (Last name as first name) vigilant
Shepard, Sheperd, Shephard

Shepherd (English) herds sheep

Shepho (Biblical) herds sheep

Shepley (English) from the sheep meadow; tender
Sheplea, Shepleigh, Shepply, Shipley

Sherag (Jewish) bright

Sherborn (English) from the bright shiny stream; careful
Sherborne, Sherbourn, Sherburn, Sherburne

Sheridan (Irish) wild-spirited
Sharidan, Sheridon, Sherr, Sherrey, Shuridun

Sheridun (Irish) confident

Sherill (English) from the shining hill; special
Sherrill

Sherlock (English) fair-haired; smart
Sherlocke, Shurlock

Sherm (English) worker; shears
Shermy

Sherman (English) tough-willed
Cherman, Shermann, Shermy, Shurman

Sherrerd (English) from open land; rancher
Sherard, Sherrard, Sherrod

Sherrick (Last name as first name) already gone
Sherric, Sherrik, Sherryc, Sherryck, Sherryk

Sherris (English) herds sheep

Sherwin (English) fleet of foot
Sherwind, Sherwinn, Sherwyn, Sherwynne

Sherwood (English) bright options
Sherwoode, Shurwood, Woodie, Woody

Shevon (African American) zany
Shavonne, Shevaughan, Shevaughn

Shiloh (Hebrew) gift from God; charmer
Shile, Shilo, Shy, Shye

Shimron (Biblical) place name

Shin (Korean) faithful

Shine (American) shines

Shiney (American) luminescent

Shing (Chinese) wins

Shingo (Japanese) clutch

Shipley (English) meadow of sheep
Ship

Shipton (English) from the ship village; sailor

Shire (Place name) english county; humorous
Shyre

Shirely (English) of the shire

Shishir (Indian) season

Shiva (Hindi) of great depth and range; life/death
Shiv

Shlomo (Hebrew) form of Solomon: peaceful and wise
Shelomi, Shelomo, Shlomi

Shmuel (Hebrew) form of Samuel: man who heard God; prophet

Shomer (Hebrew) watches

Shon (American) form of Shawn: God is gracious
Sean, Shaun, Shonn

Shontae (African American) hopeful
Shauntae, Shauntay, Shawntae, Shontay, Shontee, Shonti, Shontie, Shonty

Shorty (American) small in stature
Shortey, Shorti

Shoshone (Native American) tribe; wanderer
Shoshoni

Shoval (Hebrew) on the right path

Shreya (Indian) best

Shuan (Mythology) dark place

Shunem (Biblical) place name

Shur (Biblical) place name

Shura (Russian) protective
Schura, Shoura

Shuu (Japanese) responsible

Shyam (Hindi) dark

Si (Hebrew) form of Simon: good listener; thoughtful
Sy

Sichuan (Place name) chinese

Sicily (Place name) traveler
Sicilly

Sid (French) form of Sidney: attractive
Cyd, Sidd, Siddie, Siddy, Syd, Sydd

Side (Biblical) place name

Sidel (English) valley child

Sidney (French) attractive
Ciddie, Cidnie, Cyd, Cydnee, Sidnee, Sidnie, Syd, Sydney

Sidon (Biblical) place name

Sidonio (Spanish) form of Sidney: attractive

Sidor (Russian) gifted
Isidor, Sydor

Sidromio (Spanish) form of Sydney: attractive

Sidus (Latin) star
Sydus

Siegbert (German) wins

Siegfried (German) victor
Siegfred, Sig, Sigfred, Sigfrid, Siggee, Siggie, Siggy

Siello (Indian) superb

Sierra (Spanish) dangerous
See-see, Serra, Siera, Sierrah

Sig (German) form of Sigmund and Siegfried: victor
Siggey, Siggi, Sigi, Syg

Sigga (Scandinavian) form of Siegfried: victor
Sig

Sigge (German) form of Sigmund: victor

Sigmund (German) victor
Siegmund, Sig, Siggi, Siggy, Sigi, Sigmon, Sigmond

Signe (Scandinavian) victor
Signy

Sigoph (Biblical) place name

Sigurd (Scandinavian) winning personality

Sigus (German) winner

Sigwald (German) leader
Siegwald

Sil (Spanish) light

Silar (American Indian) leader

Silas (Latin) saver
Si, Siles, Silus

Sill (English) beam of light
Sills

Silo (Scandinavian) legendary

Siloam (Biblical) place name

Silous (American) form of Silas: saver
Si, Silouz

Silvano (Latin) of the woods;
unique
Silvan, Silvani, Silvio, Sylvan

Silvanus (Mythology)
woodland

Silver (Latin) silver
Sylver

Silverman (German) works
with silver; craftsman

Silverton (English) from the
town of silversmiths
Silvertown

Silvester (Latin) from the
woods
Silvestre, Silvestro, Sylvester

Silvio (Italian) sylvan

Sim (African) form of Simba:
lionlike

Simba (African) lionlike

Simcha (Hebrew) joyful

Siment (Scandinavian) form
of Simon: good listener;
thoughtful

Simeon (French) listener
*Si, Simion, Simone, Simyon,
Sy*

Simington (English) devout

Simmon (Hebrew) devout

Simms (Hebrew) good
listener
Sims

Simon (Hebrew) good
listener; thoughtful
*Si, Siman, Simen, Simeon,
Simmy, Sye, Symon, Syms*

Simpson (Hebrew) simplistic
Simpsen, Simpsun, Simson

Simran (Indian) God loves

Simus (Biblical) form of
Onesimus: profits

Sinc (Native American) leader

Sinclair (French) prayerful
Clair, Sinc, Sinclare, Synclaire

Sinclar (French) prays

Sindbad (Literature) from
The Arabian Nights; daring
Sinbad

Sindry (Mythology) shines

Singer (Last name as first
name) vocalist
Synger

Singh (Hindi) lion's courage

Singo (American) genuine

Sinjin (English) form of St.
John

Sion (Hebrew) heavenly peak
Zion

Sione (African) believer

Sipher (American) treasure

Siraj (Arabic) shines

Sirion (Biblical) place name

Siris (Egyptian) starlike

Sirius (Star) shining

Sissel (Greek) difficult

Sisto (American) cowboy

Sisyphus (Greek) in
mythology

Sivney (Irish) satisfied
Sivneigh, Sivnie

Six (American) number as
name
Syx

Sixto (Greek)
Well-mannered

Sixtus (Latin) sixth child

Skay (Native American) white

Skeeter (English) fast
Skeater, Skeet, Skeets

Skeetz (American) zany
Skeet, Skeeter, Skeets

Skelly (Irish) bard
Scully

Skerry (Scandinavian) from the island of stone; pragmatist

Ski (Scandinavian) sends out

Skilling (English) masterful
Skillings

Skinner (English) skins for a living

Skip (American) form of Skipper: shipmaster
Skipp, Skyp, Skyppe

Skipper (American) shipmaster

Skippy (American) fast
Skippee, Skippie, Skyppey

Skye (Dutch) goal-oriented
Sky

Skylar (Dutch) protective
Skilar, Skye, Skyeler, Skylir

Slade (English) quiet child
Slaid, Slaide, Slayd, Slayde

Sladen (English) valley child

Sladkey (Slavic) glorious
Sladkie

Slam (American) friendly
Slams, Slamz

Slane (Irish) good health

Slap (American) casual

Slater (Last name as first name) precocious
Slaiter, Slayter

Slatter (English) works on roofs

Slav (Russian) glorified

Slava (Russian) form of Stanislav: glory in leading

Slavek (Polish) smart; glorious
Slavec, Slavik

Slavin (Irish) mountain man; hermit
Slawin, Slaven

Slawomir (Slavic) great glory; famed
Slavek, Slavomir

Slim (English) nickname for slim guy

Sloan (Irish) sleek
Sloane, Slonne

Slocum (Last name as first name) happy
Slo, Slocom, Slocumb

Slover (Last name as first name) slove

Sly (Latin) form of Sylvester: forest-dweller; heavy-duty

Smedley (English) of the flat meadow
Smedleigh, Smedly

Smerdyakov (Russian) sinister

Smith (English) crafty; blacksmith
Smid, Smidt, Smit, Smitt, Smitti, Smitty

Smithson (Last name as first name) son of Smith; craftsman

Smitty (English) craftsman
Smittey

Smokey (American) smokin'
Smoke, Smokee, Smoky

Snake (Place name) U.S. river

Snead (English) last name as first name

Snowden (English) from a snowy hill; fresh
Snowdon

Snyder (German) tailor's clothing; stylish
Schneiger, Snider

So (Vietnamese) smart

Socorro (Spanish) helpful
Sokorro

Socrates (Greek) philosophical; brilliant
Socratez, Socratis, Sokrates

Soeren (Scandinavian) sun ray

Sofian (Arabic) devoted

Sofus (Greek) wise
Sophus

Sogane (Biblical) place name

Sohan (Hindi) charmer

Sohan (Indian) handsome

Sohil (Hindi) beautiful

Sol (Hebrew) form of Solomon: peaceful and wise
Solly

Solano (Latin) from the east

Solly (Hebrew) form of Solomon: peaceful and wise
Sollee, Solley, Solli, Sollie

Solomon (Hebrew) peaceful and wise
Salamon, Sol, Sollie, Solly, Soloman

Somerby (English) from the summer village; lighthearted
Somerbie, Somersby, Sommersby

Somerley (Irish) summer sailor
Somerled, Sorley

Somers (English) loving summer
Sommers

Somerset (English) talented
Somer, Somers, Sommerset, Summerset

Somerton (English) from the summer town
Somervile, Somerville

Sommar (English) summer
Somer, Somers, Somm, Sommars, Sommer

Son (English) boy
Sonni, Sonnie, Sonny

Sonny (English) boy
Son, Sonney, Sonni, Sonnie

Sonteeahgo (Invented) form of Santiago: sainted; valuable

Sophocles (Greek) playwright

Sorel (Botanical) form of Sorrel: reddish-brown horse; horse lover

Soren (Scandinavian) good communicator
Soryn

Sorrel (French) reddish-brown horse; horse lover
Sorre, Sorrell, Sorrey

Sorren (Scandinavian) sun ray

Sosimo (Spanish) promise

Sothern (English) from the south; warmhearted
Southern

Sound (American) word as a name; dynamic

Sousan (French) underdog

Southwell (English) living by the southern well

Sovann (Asian) golden

Spanky (American) outspoken; stubborn
Spank, Spankee, Spankie

Sparks (English) happy

Sparky (Latin) ball of fire; joyful
Spark, Sparkee, Sparkey, Sparki, Sparkie

Sparta (Biblical) place name

Spas (Slavic) saved by God

Spaulding (Last name as first name) comic
Spalding, Spaldying, Spauldyng

Specie (American) special child

Speed (English) plucky

Speedy (English) fast

Speers (English) good with spears; swift-moving
Speares, Spears, Spiers

Spence (English) form of Spencer: giver; provides well
Spens, Spense

Spencer (English) giver; provides well
Spence, Spencey, Spenser, Sponsor, Spensy

Sperry (Last name as first name) inventive
Sperrey

Spider (American) scary
Spyder

Spidey (American) zany

Spike (American) word as name
Spiker

Spiker (English) go-getter
Spike, Spikey, Spyk

Spillane (American) funloving

Spiridon (Greek) like a breath of fresh air
Speero, Spero, Spiridon, Spiro, Spiros, Spyridon, Spyros

Spiro (Greek) coil; spiral
Spi, Spiroh, Spiros, Spy, Spyro

Sprague (French) high-energy

Springer (English) fresh
Spring

Sprinter (American) runner

Spud (English) energetic

Spunk (American) spunky; lively
Spunki, Spunky

Spurgeon (Botanical) from the shrub spurge; natural
Spurge

Spurs (American) boot devices used to spur horses; cowboy
Spur

Spyros (Greek) round

Squire (English) land-loving
Squirre, Skwyre

Sravanthi (Indian) old soul

Stace (English) optimist
Stayce

Stacey (English) hopeful
Stace, Stacee, Stacy, Stase, Stasi

Stackler (Last name as first name) aligned

Stadler (Last name as first name) staid
Stadtler

Staffan (Slavic) crowned

Stafford (English) dignified
Staff, Staffard, Stafferd, Staffi, Staffie, Staffor, Staffy

Stagio (Italian) of the stage

Stajonne (Slavic) form of Stoyan: loyal

Stamos (Greek) reasonable
Stammos, Stamohs

Stan (Latin) form of Stanley: traveler

Stanbury (English) fortified
Stanberry, Stanbery, Stanburghe, Stansberry, Stansburghe, Stansbury

Stancliff (English) from the stone cliff; prepared
Stancliffe, Stanclyffe, Stanscliff, Stanscliffe

Standa (Slavic) glory

Standish (English) farsighted
Standysh

Standley (English) travels

Stanfield (English) from the stone field; able
Stansfield

Stanford (English) dignified
Stan, Stanferd, Stann

Stanislaus (Latin) glorious
Staneslaus, Stanis, Stanislus, Stann, Stanus

Stanislav (Russian) glory in leading
Slava, Stasi

Stanley (English) traveler
Stan, Stanlea, Stanlee, Stanli, Stanly

Stanmore (English) lake of stones; ill-fated

Stanton (English) stone-hard
Stan

Stanway (English) came from the stone road
Stanaway, Stannaway, Stannway

Stanwick (English) born in village of stone; hard
Stanwicke, Stanwyck

Stanwood (English) stone woods man; tough

Stark (German) high-energy
Starke, Starkey

Starling (English) singer; bird
Starlling

Starr (English) bright star
Star, Starri, Starrie, Starry

Stash (Russian) form of Stanislav: glory in leading

Stavros (Greek) winner
Stavrohs, Stavrows

Stavrus (Greek) cross

Steadman (English) landowner; wealthy
Steadmann, Sted, Stedmann

Steaven (Scottish) form of Steven: victorious

Steed (English) horse of high spirits

Steele (English) hardworking
Steel, Stille

Stefan (Scandinavian) crowned; German
chosen one, Stefawn, Steff, Steffan, Steffie, Steffon, Steffy, Stefin, Stephan

Stefano (Italian) supreme ruler
Stef, Steffie, Steffy, Stephano, Stephanos

Stehlin (Last name as first name) genius
Staylin, Stealan, Stehlan

Stein (German) stonelike
Steen, Sten, Steno

Steinar (Scandinavian) muse; rock
Steinard, Steinart, Steinhardt

Steinbeck (Last name as first) writer John

Stelios (Greek) community hero

Stellan (Swedish) star

Sten (Scandinavian) star stone
Stene, Stine

Stennis (Scottish) prehistoric standing stones; eternal

Stepan (English) form of Stephen: victorious
Stepen, Stepyn

Steph (English) form of Stephen: victorious
Stef, Steff, Steffy

Stephan (Greek) form of Stephen: victorious

Stephanos (Greek) crowned; martyr
Stef, Stefanos, Steph, Stephanas

Stephen (Greek) victorious
Stephan, Stephon, Stevee, Steven, Stevey, Stevi, Stevie, Stevy

Stephene (French) form of Stephen: victorious
Stef, Steff, Steph

Stephine (French) wins

Sterl (English) valuable

Sterling (English) worthwhile

Stern (German) bright; serious
Stearn, Sterns

Stetson (American) cowboy
Stetsen, Stetsun, Stettson

Steubing (Last name as first name) stepping
Steuben, Stu, Stuben, Stubing

Steve (Greek) form of Steven or Stephen: victorious
Stevie

Steven ✪ (Greek) victorious
Stevan, Steve, Stevey, Stevie

Steveo (American) form of Steve: victorious

Stevie (English) form of Steven: victorious
Stevee, Stevey, Stevi, Stevy

Stevland (English) steve's place

Stewart (English) form of Stuart: careful; watchful
Stewert, Stu, Stuie

Stian (Scandinavian) traveler

Stieran (Scandinavian) wandering
Steeran, Steeren, Steeryn, Stieren, Stieryn

Stig (Scandinavian) upwardly mobile
Stigg, Styg, Stygg

Stiles (English) practical
Stile, Stiley, Styles

Stillman (English) quiet boy

Sting (English) spike of grain

Stoat (English) small mammal also called ermine; white
Stoate, Stote

Stobart (German) harsh
Stobe, Stobey, Stoby

Stock (American) macho
Stok

Stockard (English) dramatic
Stock, Stockerd, Stockord

Stockdale (English) from meadow with trees

Stocker (English) foundation
Stock

Stockett (English) from meadow with trees

Stockley (English) in a field of tree stumps stock; rooted in reality

Stockton (English) strong foundation
Stockten

Stockwell (English) from the well by tree stumps; grounded

Stoddard (English) caretaker of horses
Stoddart

Stokley (English) stokes the fire

Stoli (Russian) celebrant

Stone (English) athletic
Stonee, Stoney, Stonie, Stony

Stonewall (English) fortified
Stone, Stoney, Wall

Stoney (American) form of Stone: athletic
Stonee, Stoni, Stonie

Stonne (English) stone

Storey (English) one story of a house; storyteller
Story

Storm (English) impetuous; volatile
Storme, Stormy

Stowe (English) secretive
Stow, Stowey

Stoy (Slavic) steadfast

Stoyan (Slavic) loyal

Strahan (Irish) sings stories
Strachan

Stratan (Greek) from the army

Stratford (English) river-crossing boy; happy
Strafford

Strato (Invented) strategic
Strat, Stratt

Stratton (Scottish) home-loving
Straton, Strattawn

Straus (German) ostrich; in disbelief
Strauss

Strausser (Last name as first name)

Stretch (American) easygoing
Stretcher

Strickland (English) field of flax; outdoorsy

Strider (Literature) from Tolkien's *Lord of the Rings*; great warrior

Strike (American) word as name; aggressive
Striker

Stroheim (Last name as first name) great director

Strom (German) water-lover
Strome, Stromm

Strong (English) strength of character

Strother (Irish) strict
Strothers, Struther, Struthers

Struther (Last name as first name) flowing
Strother, Strothers, Struthers

Stu (English) form of Stuart: careful; watchful
Stew, Stue, Stuey

Stuart (English) careful; watchful
Stewart, Stu, Stuey

Studs (American) cocky
Studd, Studds

Studs (English) wears studs;
masculine

Sture (Scandinavian) difficult
Sturah

Styles (English) practical
Stile, Stiles, Style

Stylianos (Greek) stylish
Styli

Sudal (Indian) good

Sudarshan (Indian)
handsome

Sudbury (English) southern
town boy; lackadaisical
Sudbery, Sudberry, Sudborough

Sudhakar (Indian) good;
sweet nectar

Suede (Arabic) leader

Suffield (English) man from
the south field

Suffolk (English) from
southern folks

Sugar-Ray (American)
strong; singer
Sugar Ray

Sujay (Hindi) good
Sujit

Sujit (Indian) wins

Sulaiman (Arabic) loves
peace
Suleiman, Suleyman

Sullivan (Irish) dark-eyed;
quiet
*Sullavan, Sullie, Sullivahn,
Sully*

Sully (Irish) melancholy;
hushed
Sull, Sullee, Sulley, Sullie

Sultan (American) bold
Sultane, Sulten, Sultin

Suman (Hindi) ingenious

Sumano (Spanish) smart

Sumarto (Indian) good

Sumit (Indian) measured

Sumner (Last name as first
name) honorable; fortified

Sumney (American) ethereal
*Summ, Summy, Sumnee,
Sumnie*

Sunder (Indian) handsome

Sunil (Hindi) blue; sad

Sunil (Indian) blue

Sunny (American) happy
baby boy
Sunney, Sunnie

Suresh (Indian) sun

Surian (Sanskrit) sun

Surinder (Indian) believes in
Indra

Surya (Indian) sun

Sutcliff (English) from the
south cliff; edgy
Sutcliffe

Sutherland (Scandinavian)
sunny; southerner
Southerland

Sutter (English) southern
Sutt, Suttee, Sutty

Sutter (English) southerner

Sutterly (English) southerner

Sutton (English) sunny;
southerner

Suvomoy (Indian) religious

Suvrat (Indian) devout

Svatomir (Slavic) known for
being spiritual

Svatoslav (Slavic) having the
glory of being devout

Sven (Scandinavian) young boy
Svein, Svend, Swen

Svendin (Scandinavian) young

Svere (Scandinavian) untamed

Swahili (Arabic) language of East Africa; verbal

Swain (English) rigid; leading the herd
Swaine, Swayne

Swanton (English) where swans live; sylvan boy

Swapnil (Indian) fantasy

Sween (Irish) ambitious

Sweeney (Irish) hero
Schwennie, Sweeny

Swen (Scandinavian) form of Sven: young

Swift (English) fast
Swifty

Swinburne (English) seeing pigs in the stream
Swinborn, Swinbourne, Swinburn, Swinbyrn, Swynborne

Swindell (English) polished
Schwindell, Swin, Swindel

Swinford (English) seeing pigs in the ford
Swynford

Swinton (English) from the town of swine

Swithin (English) swift
Swithinn, Swithun

Sy (Latin) form of Silas: saver
Sylas, Si

Sychar (Biblical) place name

Sydney (French) form of Sidney: attractive
Cyd, Syd, Sydie

Sye (Latin) form of Silas: saver

Syfron (American) form of Saffron: spice/plant; orange-haired

Sylvain (Latin) reclusive
Syl

Sylvan (Spanish) nature-loving
Silvan, Syl, Sylvany, Sylvin

Sylvester (Latin) forest dweller; heavy-duty
Sil, Silvester, Sly, Syl

Symms (Last name as first name) landowner

Symotris (African American) fortunate
Sym, Symetris, Symotrice, Syms

Synklair (American) form of Sinclair: prayerful

Syon (Sanskrit) lucky boy

Syrtis (Biblical) place name

T

Taanach (Biblical) place name

Tab (German) intelligent
Tabby, Tabbey, Tabby

Tabbai (Hebrew) good boy

Tabbebo (Native American) boy of the sun

Tabib (Turkish) physician
Tabeeb

Tabor (Aramaic) unfortunate
Taber, Taibor, Tayber, Taybor

Tack (American) popular

Taco (Spanish) thoughtful

Tad (Greek) form of
Thaddeus: courageous
*Tadd, Taddee, Taddey, Taddie,
Taddy*

Tadashi (Japanese) loyal

Taddeo (Italian) form of
Thaddeus: courageous

Taden (Native American)
bountiful

Tadeu (Slavic) praised

Tadeusz (Polish) praiseworthy
Tad, Taduce

Tadeusz (Slavic) worthy

Tadhg (Irish) poetic
Taidghin, Teague, Teige

Tadi (Native American) wind
child

Tadmor (Biblical) place name

Tadros (Slavic) brave

Tadzi (Polish) praised

Tae (Irish) poetic

Tafar (African) impressive

Taff (American) sweet
Taf, Taffee, Taffey, Taffi, Taffy

Taft (English) flowing
Tafte, Taftie, Taffy

Taggart (Last name as first
name) keeps track; singer

Taghee (Native American)
chief
Taighe, Taihee, Tyee, Tyhee

Tague (Scandinavian) star of
the day

Taha (Polynesian) first
Tahatan

Taher (Arabic) cleansed

Taheton (Native American)
like a hawk

Tahi (Polynesian) by the sea

Tahir (African) pure

Tahj (African) crowned

Tahl (Hebrew) rainy

Tahoe (Place name) lake
Tahoe
Taho

Tahoma (Native American)
mountain peak; high hopes
Tohoma

Tahti (Scandinavian) shining
star

Tai (Vietnamese) talented

Taillam (French) works iron

Taima (Native American)
storm baby

Taimah (Native American)
thunder

Tair (Arabic) form of Tahir:
pure

Taisto (Scandinavian) fighter

Tait (Scandinavian) form of
Tate: happy

Taiwo (African) first of twins

Taizo (Japanese) third son

Taj (Sanskrit) royal; crowned

Takao (Asian) strong

Takeshi (Japanese)
unbending

Taklishim (Native American)
gray-haired

Takoda (Native American)
friend

Tal (Hebrew) worrier
Tallee, Talley, Talli, Tally

Talal (Indian) prayerful

Talan (American)
opportunistic

Talat (Arabic) prays

Talbot (French) skillful
*Tal, Talbert, Talbott, Tallbot,
Tallbott, Tally*

Talcot (English) lake-cottage
dweller; laidback

Tale (African) green; open

Talfryn (Welsh) on the high
hill

Talib (African) looking for
enlightenment

Taliesin (Welsh) head that
shines
Taltesin

Talli (Hebrew) dew; fresh

Talm (Aramaic) hurt

Talmadge (English) natural;
living by lakes
Tal, Tally, Tamidge

Talmai (Aramaic) born on a
hill

Talman (Hebrew) from my
hill
Tallie, Tally, Talmon

Talon (French) wily
Tallie, Tallon, Tally, Tawlon

Talor (French) cutter; tailor

Tam (Hebrew) truthful
Tammy

Taman (Hindi) needed

Tamar (Hebrew) grows dates

Tamarius (African American)
stubborn
*Tam, Tamerius, Tammy,
T'Marius*

Tamer (Arabic) tall

Tamir (Arabic) owner

Tammany (Native American)
friendly boy
Tamanend

Tammy (English) form of
Thomas: twin; look-alike;
form of Tamarius: stubborn
Tammee, Tammie, Tammey

Tan (Japanese) high achiever

Tanafa (Polynesian)
drumbeat

Tanaki (Polynesian) boy who
counts

Tanay (Hindi) son

Tandie (African American)
virile

Tandy (English) together

Tane (Polynesian) sky god;
fertile
Tain

Tangaloa (Polynesian) gutsy

Tangie (French) battles

Tanh (Vietnamese) having his
way

Tani (African American) form
of Tanier: tanner of skins

Tank (American) big; bullish

Tankie (American) large
Tank, Tankee, Tanky

Tanmay (Indian)
mesmerizing

Tanner ♂ (English) tanner of
skins
*Tan, Tanier, Tann, Tannar,
Tanne, Tanney, Tannie, Tannor,
Tanny*

Tano (Ghanese) named for
the river

Tanom (American) creative

Tanton (English) town of tanners

Tanveer (Indian) informed

Taos (Place name) town in New Mexico
Tao, Tayo

Tap (American) light touch
Tapp, Tappi, Tappy

Tapan (Indian) sun

Tarek (Indian) star

Tarem (American) the son

Taren (French) God's gift

Tarentum (Biblical) place name

Tarhe (Native American) strength of a tree

Tarick (American) form of Tarek: star

Tarik (Arabic) knocks
Taril, Tarin, Tariq

Tariq (African American) conqueror
Tarik

Tarking (Arabic) summons

Tarlach (Hebrew) wild

Tarleton (English) stormy
Tally, Tarlton

Tarm (Scandinavian) energy

Tarmo (Scandinavian) energy

Taro (Japanese) firstborn son

Tarquin (Roman clan) impulsive

Tarrance (Latin) smooth
Terance, Terrance, Terry

Tarrant (Place name) county in Texas; lawful

Tarri (American) form of Terry: tender
Tari, Tarree, Tarrey, Tarry

Tarso (Italian) dashing

Tarsus (Biblical) place name

Tarum (Indian) young

Tarun (Arabic) knocks

Tarvin (English) on the hill

Tary (American) form of Terry: calm

Taryll (American) form of Terrell: puller
Tarell

Tas (Place name) from Tasmania
Taz

Tashunka (Native American) horse lover
Tasunke

Tasi (Greek) on the makr

Taso (Greek) on the mark

Tassilo (Scandinavian) fearless protector

Tasso (Greek) on the mark

Tassos (Italian) dark

Tatankamimi (Native American) the buffalo walks

Tate (English) happy
Tait, Taitt, Tatey, Tayt, Tayte

Taten (Scandinavian) happy

Tatlock (English) happy

Tatonga (Native American) deer; swift

Tatry (Place name) mountains in Poland
Tate, Tatree, Tatri

Tau (African) lionine

Taufiq (Arabic) wins

Tauney (English) form of Tawny: tan-skinned

Taurean (African American)
reclusive; quiet
Taureen

Taurino (Italian) reserved

Taurus (Astrological sign)
macho
Tar, Taur, Tauras, Taures

Tava (Polynesian) fruit; fertile

Tavares (African American)
hopeful
Tavarus

Tavarius (African American)
fun-loving
Tav, Taverius, Tavurius, Tavvy

Tavas (Hebrew) peacock;
handsome

Taven (Scandinavian) form of
Tavi: good

Tavi (Aramaic) good

Tavi (Scandinavian) form of
David: beloved

Tavish (Scottish) upbeat
Tav, Taven, Tavis, Tevis

Tavium (Biblical) place name

Tavor (Aramaic) unfortunate
Tabor

Taw (African) form of Tau:
lion's roar

Tawa (Native American) sun
boy

Tawagahe (Native American)
builder

Tawanima (Native American)
measures the sun
Tewanima

Tawfiq (Arabic) fortunate
Tawfi

Tawl (Arabic) tall
Taweel

Tawno (American) small

Tay (Scottish) river in
Scotland; jaunty
Tae, Taye

Tayhan (Last name as first
name)

Tayib (Arabic) city in Israel;
spiritual

Taylor (English) tailor
Tailor, Talor, Tayler, Tayley

Tayton (American) form of
Payton: soldier's town
*Tate, Taye, Tayte, Tayten,
Taytin*

Tayve (Scandinavian) form of
David: beloved

Taz (Arabic) cup; vibrant

Teagu (Irish) poetic

Teague (Celtic) poet
Teaguey, Tege

Teal (English) duck

Tearlach (Scottish) adult
man; bold

Techomir (Czech) famed
comfort

Techoslav (Native American)
glorious comfort

Tecumseh (Native American)
shooting star; bright

Ted (English) form of
Theodore: God's gift; a
blessing
Teddee, Teddey, Teddi, Teddy

Teddy-Blue (American)
smiley
*Blu, Blue, Teddie-Blue, Teddy,
Teddyblu, Teddy-Blu, Teddyblue*

Tedmund (American) shy
Tedmond

Tedrick (African American)
form of Cedric: leader
Ted, Tedrik

Tegan (Celtic) doe
Tege, Tegen, Tegun, Teige

Tego (Irish) form of Teague:
poetic

Tehaney (English) reddish-brown

Tejomay (Hindi) glorious
Tej

Tejraj (Indian) sharp

Teklad (Slavic) wonder

Tekoa (Biblical) place name

Tekonsha (Native American)
caribou

Telamon (Greek)
mythological hero

Telek (Polish) ironworker

Telem (Hebrew) their dew;
their shadow

Telemachus (Mythological)
son of Ulysses

Telesforo (Spanish) country
boy

Telesphoros (Greek) leading
to an end; centered

Telford (English) cutting iron;
targeted
Telfer, Telfor, Telfour

Teller (English) relates stories;
storytelling
Tellie, Telly

Tello (German) reformed

Telmo (English) works earth

Telvis (American) form of
Elvis: all-wise
Telly

Tem (African) form of Teman:
spiritual

Tema (Biblical) southerner

Teman (Hebrew) spiritual
(Temani are Jews from
Yemen)

Tempest (French) stormy;
volatile
Tempie, Tempy, Tempyst

Templar (Spanish) temple;
spiritual

Templar (Latin) form of
Temple: spiritual

Temple (Latin) spiritual
Tempie, Templle, Tempy

Temple (Latin) temple

Templeton (English) from a
religious place
Temp, Tempie, Temple, Temps

Temre (American) spices

Ten (American) tenth

Tendoy (Native American) he
who climbs higher
Tendoi

Teneangopte (Native
American) bird; flies high

Tennant (American) capable
Tenn

Tennessee (Native American)
able fighter; U.S. state
Tenns, Tenny

Tennison (English) creates

Tenny (English) creative

Tennyson (English)
storyteller
*Tenie, Tenn, Tenney, Tenneyson,
Tennie, Tenny, Tennysen*

Tensk (Native American)
open

Teo (Greek) gift of God

Teodo (Greek) form of
Theodore: God's gift; a
blessing

Teodoro (Spanish) God's gift
Tedoro, Teo, Teodore, Theo

Teofanes (Spanish) God-loving

Teofilo (Greek) God-loving

Tephon (Biblical) place name

Teppo (Scandinavian) from Stephen: victorious

TeQuarius (African American) secretive
Teq, Tequarius, Tequie

Terach (Hebrew) wild goat; contentious
Tera, Terah

Terak (Biblical) established

Terard (Invented) form of Gerard: brave
Terar, Tererd, Terry

Tercer (Spanish) third baby

Tercero (Spanish) third baby

Terence (Irish) tender
Tarrance, Terencio, Terrance, Terrence, Terrey, Terri, Terry

TeRez (African American) creative

Terhea (American) from the oak tree

Terl (German) ruler

Term (Latin) terminates

Termell (Invented) form of Terrell: puller
Termel

Teron (Greek) hunter; calms

Terrance (Latin) calm
Terance, Terence, Terre, Terree, Terrence, Terrie, Terry

Terrell (French) puller

Terrelle (German) thunderous; outspoken
Terel, Terele, Terell, Teril, Terille, Terral, Terrale, Terre, Terrel, Terril, Terrill, Terrille, Terry, Tirill, Tirrill, Tyrel, Tyril

Terrien (Greek) hunts; calms

Terron (Greek) hunts

Terry (English) form of Terence: tender
Terree, Terrey, Terri, Terrie

Tesher (Hebrew) gift

Teshombe (African American) able

Tet (Vietnamese) vietnamese New Year

Teunis (Dutch) form of Antonio: superb

Teva (Hebrew) natural
Tevah

Tevaughn (African American) tiger
Tev, Tevan, Tevaughan, Tivan, Tivaughan

Tevey (Hebrew) good
Tev, Tevi, Tevie

Tevin (African American) outgoing
Tev, Tevan, Tivan

Tevis (American) flamboyant
Tev, Tevas, Teves, Teviss, Tevy

Tex (American) from Texas; cowboy
Texas, Texx

Texas (Place name) U.S. state; cowboy
Tex

Thabiti (African) real man

Thabo (African) joyful

Thad (Greek) form of
Thaddeus: courageous
Thadd, Thaddy

Thaddeous (Greek) form of
Thaddeus: courageous

Thaddeous (African) brave

Thaddeus (Greek)
courageous
*Taddeo, Tadeo, Tadio, Thad,
Thaddaus, Thaddius, Thaddy,
Thadeus, Thadius*

Thaddus (African) brave

Thady (Irish) thankful
*Thad, Thaddee, Thaddie,
Thaddy, Thads*

Thai (Vietnamese) winner

Thais (Asian) flourishes

Thalan (Irish) charming

Thamar (Biblical) form of
Ithamar: island of the palm
trees

Thamer (American) helpful

Thanatos (Greek) dies

Thandiwe (African) loved

Thane (English) protective
Thain, Thaine, Thayn, Thayne

Thang (Vietnamese)
victorious

Thanh (Vietnamese) tops

Thanos (Greek) praiseworthy
Thanasis

Thanus (American)
landowner; wealthy
Thainas, Thaines

Thao (American) variant on
Theo: godlike

Thatcher (English) practical
*Thacher, Thatch, Thatchar,
Thaxter*

Thavin (Greek) shows love
for God

Thaw (Word as name) cool

Thayer (English) protected;
sheltered
Thay, Thayar

Thayle (Jewish) form of Tal:
worrier

Thebez (Biblical) place name

Thel (Hebrew) upper story

Themba (African) hopeful

Themis (Greek) lawful

Thena (Greek) honoree

Thenan (Greek) honored

Thenard (American) form of
Leonard: courageous

Theo (Greek) godlike

Theobald (German) brave
man
*Thebaud, Thebault, Thibault,
Thibaut, Tibold, Tiebold*

Theodis (English) spirited

Theodore (Greek) God's gift;
a blessing
*Teador, Ted, Tedd, Teddey,
Teddie, Teddy, Tedor, Teodor,
Teodoro, Theeo, Theo, Theodor,
Theos*

Theodoric (African
American) God's gift
Thierry

Theodoros (Greek) God's gift
Theo, Theodor

Theodorus (Greek) form of
Theodore: God's gift; a
blessing

Theophilos (Greek) loved by
God
Teofil, Theo, Theophile

Theopoline (Greek) open

Therman (Scandinavian)
thunderous
Thur, Thurman, Thurmen

Theron (Greek) industrious
Therron, Theryon

Theseus (Mythology) brave

Thessal (Biblical) martyr

Thiago (Spanish) saint

Thiassi (Scandinavian) wily
Thiazi, Thjazi

Thibaud (French) form of
Theobald: brave man

Thibaut (French) form of
Theobald: brave man

Thierno (American) humble
Therno, Their

Tho (Vietnamese) long-living

Tho (American) form of
Thomas: twin; look-alike

Thomas ☉ (Greek) twin;
look-alike
*Thom, Thomes, Thommy,
Thomus, Tom, Tomas, Tommi,
Tomus*

Thompson (English)
prepared
*Thom, Thompsen, Thompsun,
Thomson, Tom, Tommy*

Thor (Scandinavian)
protective; god of thunder
Thorr, Tor, Torr

Thorald (Scandinavian)
thundering
Thorold, Torald

Thoralf (Scandinavian)
thunder

Thorbert (Last name as first
name) warring

Thorburn (Last name as first
name) warlike

Thord (Scandinavian)
thunder

Thorer (Scandinavian)
warrior
Thorvald

Thorin (Scandinavian) form
of Thor: protective; god of
thunder
Thorrin, Thors

Thorley (Last name as first
name) warrior
*Thorlea, Thorlee, Thorleigh,
Thorly, Torley*

Thormond (Last name as
first name) world of thunder
Thurmond, Thurmund

Thorn (English) thorny;
bothersome

Thorndike (Last name as first
name) powerful
Thorndyck, Thorndyke

Thorne (English) complex
*Thorn, Thornee, Thorney,
Thornie, Thorny*

Thornley (Last name as first
name) empowered
Thornlea, Thornleigh, Thornly

Thornston (Scandinavian)
protected
Thornse, Thors

Thornton (English) difficult
Thorn, Thornten

Thorpe (English) homebody
Thor, Thorp

Thrace (Place name) region
in southeast Europe
Thrase

Thu (Vietnamese) born in the
fall

Thuan (Asian) aware

Thuc (Vietnamese) alert

Thuel (Biblical) form of
Bethuel: religious

Thunor (Mythology) thunder

Thuong (Vietnamese) in pursuit

Thurlow (Last name as first name) helping

Thurm (Greek) form of Theron: industrious

Thurman (Last name as first name) popular
Thurmahn, Thurmen, Thurmie, Thurmy

Thurmond (Norse) sheltered
Thurman, Thurmon

Thurso (Scandinavian) thunders

Thurston (Scandinavian) thundering
Thor, Thors, Thorst, Thorstan, Thorstein, Thorsteinn, Thorsten, Thur, Thurs, Thurstain, Thurstan, Thursten, Torstein, Torsten, Torston

Thurstron (Scandinavian) volatile
Thorst, Thorsten, Thorstin, Thurs, Thurstran

Thuy (Vietnamese) kind

Tiago (Hispanic) brave
Ti, Tia

Tiaone (Spanish) form of Tiago: brave

Tiarnach (Irish) Lordlike
Tighearnach

Tiber (Biblical) place name

Tiberius (Biblical) place name

Tibor (Czech) artist
Tybald, Tybalt, Tybault

Ticio (Spanish) heroic

Tien (Vietnamese) first and foremost

Tiernan (Irish) regal
Tierney

Tifton (English) last name as first name

Tige (American) easygoing
Tig, Tigg

Tiger (American) ambitious; strong
Tig, Tige, Tigur, Tyg, Tyge, Tyger, Tygur

Tigny (Irish) poetic

Tigran (Latin) tiger

Tigrano (Biblical) place name

Tiki (Mythology) first man

Tilak (Hindi) leader; troubled

Tilak (Indian) spot on forehead

Tildan (English) man who tills

Tilden (Place name) tilden

Tilene (Slavic) religious

Tilford (Last name as first name) tilling the soil

Till (German) form of Tillman: tiller of soil

Tillery (German) ruler
Till, Tiller

Tillman (German) tiller of soil
Tilman

Tillo (German) devout

Tilon (Hebrew) mound; giver

Tilton (English) prospering
Till, Tillie, Tylton

Tim (Greek) form of Timothy: reveres God
Timmy, Tym

Timber (American) word as name
Timb, Timby, Timmey, Timmi, Timmy

Timenn (Indian) child from the sea

Timin (Irish) honors God

Timmy (Greek) truthful
Timi, Timmee, Timmey, Timmie

Timna (Biblical) place name

Timnah (Biblical) place name

Timo (Finnish) form of Timothy: reveres God; form of Timon: from Shakespeare's *Timon of Athens*; wealthy man

Timon (Literature) from Shakespeare's *Timon of Athens*; wealthy man
Tim

Timothy ○ (Greek) reveres God
Tim, Timathy, Timmie, Timmothy, Timmy, Timo, Timon, Timoteo, Timothe, Timothey, Timothie, Timuthy, Tymmothy, Tymothy

Timur (African) timid

Timur (Slavic) conqueror

Timus (Scandinavian) powerful

Tin (Vietnamese) proud; pondering

Tingo (Italian) grateful

Tinks (American) coy
Tink, Tinkee, Tinki, Tinky, Tynks, Tynky

Tino (Spanish) respected
Tyno

Tinsley (English) personable
Tensley, Tins, Tinslee, Tinslie, Tinsly

Tinus (Slavic) leader

Tiombe (African) faith

Tione (American) form of Tyrone: self-starter; autonomous

Tip (American) small boy
Tipp, Tippee, Tippey, Tippi, Tippy, Typp

Tippen (American) last name as first name

Tippie (Scandinavian) from Stephen: victorious

Tipu (Hindi) tiger

Tiras (Biblical) thoughtful

Tirso (Greek) religious

Tiru (Hindi) pious

Tisa (African) ninth child

Titan (Greek) powerful giant
Titun, Tityn

Tito (Latin) honored
Teto, Titoh

Titon (American) concerned

Titus (Latin) heroic
Titas, Tite, Tites

Titus (Latin) heroic

Tivon (African American) popular

Tizian (Italian) creative

Tjaru (Biblical) place name

Toa (Polynesian) brave-hearted

Toafo (Polynesian) in the wild; spontaneous

Toal (Irish) from strong roots

Toal (Irish) leader; willful

Tob (Biblical) place name

Tobbar (African American) physical

Tobby (African) excellent

Tobert (French) believer

Tobes (Hebrew) form of Tobias: believing the Lord is good
Tobee, Tobi, Tobs

Tobian (Hebrew) form of Tobias: believing the Lord is good

Tobias (Hebrew) believing the Lord is good
Tobe, Tobey, Tobi, Tobiah, Tobie, Tobin, Toby, Tobyas, Tovi

Tobias (Hebrew) believer

Tobikuma (Japanese) cloud; misty

Tobin (Hebrew) form of Tobias: believing the Lord is good
Toban, Toben, Tobun, Tobyn

Tobit (Biblical) form of Tobias: believing the Lord is good

Toblin (American) form of Tobias: believing the Lord is good

Toby (Hebrew) form of Tobias: believing the Lord is good
Tobe, Tobee, Tobey, Tobie, Toto

Todd (English) sly; fox
Tod, Toddy

Todor (Slavic) dignity

Todros (Hebrew) gifted; treasure
Todos

Togar (Biblical) place name

Togo (Place name) country in West Africa; jaunty

Tohon (Native American) loves the water

Tokala (Native American) fox; sly

Tokar (German) lucky

Toks (American) carefree

Tokutaro (Japanese) virtuous son

Tolan (American) studious
Tolen, Toll

Tolbert (English) bright prospects
Talbart, Talbert, Tolbart, Tolburt, Tollee, Tolley, Tollie, Tolly

Toledo (Place name) city in Ohio; casual
Tol, Tolly

Tolerence (American) unbiased

Tolero (Spanish) tolerant

Tolfe (American) outgoing

Tolin (American) form of Colin: young; quiet; peaceful; the people's victor

Toliver (American) combo of T and Oliver

Tolome (Spanish) strong

Tolomey (French) planner

Tom (English) form of Thomas: twin; look-alike
Thom, Tommy

Tomaro (Spanish) form of Thomas: twin; look-alike

Tomas (Spanish) form of Thomas: twin; look-alike

Tomasso (Italian) doubter
Maso, Tom

Tomer (Hebrew) tall

Tomi (Spanish) form of Tomas: twin; look-alike

Tomiko (Japanese) born to riches

Tomio (Italian) twin

Tomioson (Italian) son of twin

Tomlin (Last name as first name) ambitious

Tommie (Hebrew) tomee
Tommee, Tommey, Tommi, Tomy

Tomochichi (Hawaiian) seeking truth and beauty
Tomocheechee

Tomok (Slavic) twin

Tond (Slavic) form of Tony: priceless

Tondeloro (Spanish) loud thunder

Tondy (Slavic) form of Tony: priceless

Tong (Chinese) name of a secret society; keeps a secret

Tongo (Asian) sweet aroma

Toni (Greek) tonee
Toney, Tonie, Tony

Tonin (Italian) form of Antonio: superb

Tonion (American) form of Tony or Anthony: priceless

Tonny (Spanish) form of Antonio: superb

Tony (Greek) priceless

Tooling (American) vibrant

Toopweets (Native American) strong man

Toph (Greek) valued

Topher (Greek) form of Christopher: the bearer of Christ; form of Christian: follower of Christ

Toppin (English) from the hill

Tops (American) best

Topwe (American) jovial

Tor (Scandinavian) thunder; brash
Thor, Torr, Torri, Torrie, Torry

Torao (Japanese) tiger male; wild

Torb (Scandinavian) form of Tor: thunder; brash

Torben (Scandinavian) form of Tor: thunder; brash

Torbie (Scandinavian) form of Tor: thunder; brash

Torcall (Scandinavian) summoned by thunder

Tord (Dutch) peaceful

Tordin (Scandinavian) form of Tor: thunder; brash

Torell (English) form of Tor: thunder; brash

Toreth (Biblical) from Ashtoreth

Torey (English) form of Tor: thunder; brash

Torger (Scandinavian) thor's spear
Terje, Torgeir

Torgne (American) form of Tor: thunder; brash

Torial (Irish) form of Tor: thunder; brash

Torian (Irish) form of Torin: like thunder

Toribio (Spanish) strong; bullish

Toril (Hindi) having attitude

Torin (African American) like thunder

Torio (Spanish) fierce

Torkel (Scandinavian) protective
Thorkel, Torkil, Torkild, Torkjell, Torquil

Torless (Literature) from *The Confusions of Young Torless by Musil*

Torm (Scandinavian) armed

Tormod (Scottish) man of the north

Torn (Last name as first name) whirlwind
Torne, Tornn

Toro (Spanish) bull

Toroh (Spanish) bull

Torolf (Scandinavian) wolf of Thor
Thorolf, Tolv, Torolv, Torulf

Toronto (Place name) jaded
Torontoe

Torq (Scandinavian) form of Thor: protective; god of thunder
Tork

Torquil (Scandinavian) a kettle of thunder; trouble

Torr (English) tower; tall
Torre

Torrence (Latin) smooth
Torrance, Torence, Torey, Tori, Torr, Torrance, Torrie, Tory

Torrent (Irish) form of Torrence: smooth

Torri (English) calming
Toree, Tori, Torre, Torree, Torrey, Torry

Torst (Scandinavian) thunders

Toru (Scandinavian) thundering

Torun (Scottish) manly

Tosan (Spanish) bull

Tosh (American) form of Josh: devout

Toshiro (Japanese) smart

Totan (Scandinavian) beloved

Toth (Egyptian) life in balance

Toussaint (French) saints; valued

Tov (Hebrew) good
Tovi, Toviel, Tovya, Tuvia, Tuviah, Tuviya

Tova (Hebrew) good
Tov

Tovar (Hebrew) form of Tova: good

Tovaris (Spanish) good

Tove (Scandinavian) ruling; leads
Tuve

Townie (American) jovial
Townee, Towney, Towny

Townley (Last name as first name) citified
Townlea, Townlee, Townleigh, Townlie, Townly

Townsend (Last name as first name) went to town

Toyah (Place name) town in Texas; saucy
Toy, Toya, Toye

Trace (French) careful
Trayse

Tracy (French) spunky
Trace, Tracee, Tracey, Traci

Traddesus (Greek) form of Thaddeus: brave

Trae (American) form of Trey: third-born; creatively brilliant

Trahaearn (Welsh) strong man
Trahern, Traherne

Trahan (English) handsome
Trace, Trahahn, Trahain, Trahane, Trahen

Trai (Vietnamese) pearl in the oyster

Trajan (American) form of Trahan: handsome

Trakis (American) vibrant

Tram (Scottish) form of Tramaine: protector

Tramar (Scottish) form of Tramaine: protector

Trampus (American) talkative
Amp, Tramp, Trampy

Tranis (Irish) thunders

Tranquilino (Spanish) calm

Trap (American) word as name; masculine
Trapp, Trappy

Trapezus (Biblical) place name

Trau (German) loyal

Trauti (French) believer

Travers (English) helpful

Traverse (French) form of Travers: helpful

Traves (American) traversing different roads
Trav, Travus, Travys

Travis (English) conflicted
Tavers, Traver, Travers, Traves, Travess, Travey, Travus, Travuss, Travys

Travo (American) form of Travis: conflicted

Travon (African American) brash
Travaughn

Travon (Slavic) happy

Travor (English) form of Trevor: wise

Trawin (English) friend of Trevor

Trayton (English) third
Tray, Trey

Treat (English) pleasing

Treavon (American) form of Trevon/Trevaughan: studious

Treb (Irish) wise

Treebeard (Literature) from Tolkien's *The Lord of the Rings*; noble; strong

Trefor (Welsh) form of Trevor: wise

Treiber (Irish) form of Treber/Trevor: wise

Treil (American) form of Terrell: puller

Treit (American) form of Treat: pleasing

Tremayne (French) protector
Tramaine, Treemayne, Trem, Tremain, Tremaine, Tremane, Tremen

Tremetrice (American) loved

Trent (Latin) quick-minded
Trente, Trenten, Trentin, Trenton, Trenty, Trint, Trynt

Trento (Spanish) form of Trent: quick-minded

Trenton (Latin) fast-moving
Trent, Trentan, Trenten, Trentin

Trer (Irish) form of Trevor: wise

Trest (Welsh) form of Tristan: sad; wistful

Treton (Welsh) form of Tristan: sad; wistful

Trev (Irish) strong

Treva (Irish) wise
Trevan

Trevan (African American) outgoing
Trevahn, Trevann

Trevelyan (English) from Elyan's home; comforted

Trevey (Irish) strong

Trevin (American) form of Trevon: studious

Trevine (American) strong

Trevis (English) form of Travis: conflicted

Trevon (African American) studious
Trevaughan

Trevor (Irish) wise
Trefor, Trev, Trevar, Trever, Trevis, Trevur, Treve

Trevour (American) form of Trevor: wise

Trex (American) combo of T and Rex (as in the dinosaur)

Trey (English) third-born; creatively brilliant
Trae, Tray, Tre, Treye

Trigg (American) from Trigger; quick-witted
Trig, Trygg

Triman (English) form of Truman: honest man

Trinee (Spanish) musical
Triney, Trini

Trinity (Latin) triad
Trinitie

Trint (American) holy trinity

Trinton (American) town of trinity (holy)

Trip (English) wanderer
Tripe, Tripp

Triplett (American) one of the triplets

Tripolis (Biblical) place name

Tripsy (English) dancing
Trippsie, Tryppsi

Tripton (English) town of travelers

Tris (Welsh) form of Tristan: sad; wistful

Tristan (French) form of Triste: sad; wistful
Trestan, Trestyn, Trist, Tristen, Tristie, Triston, Tristy, Tristyn

Tristannel (Welsh) form of Tristan: sad; wistful

Triste (French) sad; wistful
Tristan

Tristian (English) form of Tristan: sad; wistful

Tristram (Welsh) sorrowful

Trivett (Last name as first name) trinity
Trevett, Triv

Trivin (American) form of Devin: poetic; writer
Trevin

Troas (Biblical) place name

Trocky (American) manly
Trockey, Trockie

Troclus (Greek) glorified

Trond (Scandinavian) from Norway

Trotter (American) quick

Trovillion (English) home-loving

Trowbridge (Place name) trowbridge Park

Troy (French) good-looking
Troi, Troye, Troyie

Troyal (Irish) form of Troy: good-looking

Trudell (English) remarkable for honesty
Trude, True

Truitt (English) honest
Tru, True, Truett, Truitte

Truk (Place name) islands in the West Pacific; tough
Truck

Truls (Scandinavian) truth

Truman (English) honest man
Tru, true, Trueman, Trumaine, Trumann

Trumble (Last name as first name) sincere
Trumball, Trumbell, Trumbull

Trusdale (English) truthful
Dale, Tru, true

Truslowe (English) truth

Tryg (Scandinavian) trustworthy

Trygve (Scandinavian) trustworthy

Trym (Scandinavian) new

Trysten (Welsh) form of Tristan: sad; wistful

Trystene (American) laughter

Trystenn (American) laughter

Tsalani (African) says good-bye; leaving

Tsatoke (Native American) hunter on a horse

Tsela (Native American) star

Tsin (Native American) riding a horse

Tsoai (Native American) tree; big

Tu (Vietnamese) fourth

Tuan (Vietnamese) simple

Tuar (Native American) eagle-eyed

Tubal (Biblical) place name

Tucker (English) stylish
Tuck, Tucky, Tuckyr

Tucks (English) form of Tucker: stylish
Tuk

Tuder (Welsh) form of Tudor/Theodore: leader; God's gift

Tudor (Welsh) leader; special

Tue (Danish) form of Thor: protective; god of thunder

Tufe (American) energetic

Tukuli (African) moon child

Tulio (Spanish) energetic

Tullis (Latin) important
Tull, Tullice, Tullise, Tully

Tully (Irish) form of Tullis: important
Tull, Tulley, Tulli, Tullie

Tulsa (Place name) city in Oklahoma; rancher

Tulse (American) from Tulsa (place name)

Tulsi (Hindi) holy

Tumaini (African) optimist

Tune (American) dancer; musical
Toone, Tuney

Tung (Vietnamese) medium

Tunney (Welsh) leader

Tunu (Place name) from Tununak

Tuong (Vietnamese) everything

Tupaar (Welsh) God's child

Tupi (Spanish) a language family with Brazilian roots

Turah (Native American) thyme

Turang (Biblical) wave

Turck (Biblical) place name

Ture (Scandinavian) form of Thor: protective; god of thunder

Turer (Scandinavian) soldier

Turgut (German) believer

Turi (Hindi) growth

Turk (English) tough
Terk, Turke

Turlough (Hebrew) form of Tuvia: good

Turlow (Irish) thunder child

Turn (Latin) turner

Turner (Latin) skilled
Turn

Turone (African American) form of Tyrone: self-starter; autonomous
Ture, Turrey, Turry

Turston (Greek) form of Thurston: thundering

Tushar (Indian) droplets

Tut (Arabic) brave
Tuttie, Tutty

Tuttle (Scottish) strong

Tutts (American) unique

Tuvia (Hebrew) good
Tuvyah, Tuvyeh

Tuwa (Native American) earth-loving

Tuyen (Vietnamese) angelic

Twain (English) dual-faceted
Twaine, Tway, Twayn

Twyford (English) debonair

Twymon (English) double

Ty (English) form of Tyler: industrious
Ti, Tie, Tye

Tybalt (Greek) always right

Tyce (American) lively
Tice

Tycho (Scandinavian) focused
Tyge, Tyko

Tydeus (Mythology) determined

Tyee (African American) goal-oriented

Tyerson (English) son of Tye

Tygie (American) energetic
Tygee, Tygey, Tygi

Tyke (Scandinavian) determined

Tyko (Greek) form of Tycho: focused

Tyler ✪ ✪ (English) industrious
Tile, Tiler, Ty, Tye, Tylar, Tyle, Tylir, Tylor

Tylus (Scandinavian) impact

Tyman (Scandinavian) high integrity

Tymon (Polish) honored by God

Tynan (Place name) a town in Northern Ireland

Tynan (Irish) dark

Tyobaldo (Slavic) form of
Theobald: brave man

Tyones (American) form of
Tyrone: self-starter;
autonomous

Tyonne (African American)
feisty
Tye, Tyon

Tyounes (American) form of
Tyrone: self-starter;
autonomous

Typhoon (English) volatile
Tifoon, Ty, Tyfoon, Tyfoonn

Tyr (Scandinavian) norse god;
daring warrior

Tyran (American) form of
Tyrone: self-starter;
autonomous

Tyre (English) thunders
Tyr

Tyree (African American)
courteous
Ty, Tyrae, Tyrie, Tyry

Tyreece (African American)
combative
Tyreese

Tyrell (African American)
personable
*Trelle, Tyrel, Tyrelle, Tyril,
Tyrrel*

Tyrellon (American) form of
Tyrell: personable

Tyrese (American) form of
Tyrone: self-starter;
autonomous

Tyresen (American) form of
Tyrese: self-starter;
autonomous

Tyron (African American)
self-reliant
Tiron, Tyronn

Tyrone (Greek) self-starter;
autonomous
*Terone, Tiron, Tirone, Tirus, Ty,
Tyronne, Tyron, Tyroon, Tyroun*

Tyroneece (African
American) ball of fire
Tironeese, Tyronnee

Tys (American) fighter
Thysen, Tyes, Tys, Tyse, Tysen

Tyson (French) son of Ty
*Tieson, Tison, Tyse, Tysen,
Tysson, Tysy*

Tzach (Hebrew) unblemished
Tzachai, Tzachar

Tzadik (Hebrew) fair
*Tzadok, Zadik, Zadoc, Zadok,
Zaydak*

Tzadkiel (Hebrew) righteous
Zadkiel

Tzalmon (Hebrew) dark
Zalmon

Tzephaniah (Hebrew) man
protected by God
*Tzefanya, Zefania, Zefaniah,
Zephania, Zephaniah*

Tzevi (Hebrew) graceful; deer
Tzeviel, Zevi, Zeviel

Tzuriel (Hebrew) depends on
God
Zuriel

U

Ualtar (Irish) strong
Ualtarr

Uan (Irish) form of Owen:
well-born; high principled

Uba (African) rich

Ubald (French) brave one
Ubaldo, Ube

Ubanwa (African) wealth in children

Uben (German) practice
Ubin, Ubyn

Ubiwe (African) of the heart

Ubrig (German) big
Ubrigg, Ubryg, Ubrygg

Ubrigens (German) bothered
Ubrigins, Ubrigyns

Uchtred (English) cries
Uchtrid, Uchtryd, Uctred, Uctrid, Uctryd, Uktred, Uktrid

Udall (English) certain; valley of trees
Eudall, Udahl, Udawl, Yudall

Udeep (Indian) flood

Udeh (Hindi) praised

Udel (English) growing

Udell (English) from a tree grove
Del, Dell, Udale, Udall

Udenwa (African) thriving

Udo (German) shows promise

Udolf (German) stodgy

Ufer (German) dark mind

Ugo (Italian) bright mind

Uhr (German) disturbed

Uilleac (Irish) ready
Uilleack, Uilleak, Uilliac, Uilliack, Uilliak, Uillyac, Uillyack, Uillyak

Uilleog (Irish) prepared
Uilliog, Uillyog

Ukel (American) player
Ukal, Uke, Ukil

Ukraine (Place name) republic

Ulan (Place name) city in Russia
Ulane

Uland (African) firstborn twin
Ulande

Ulas (German) noble

Ulbrich (German) aristocratic

Ulfat (Norse) wolf

Ulff (Scandinavian) wolf; wild
Ulf, Ulv

Ulfred (Norse) noble

Ulgar (German) highborn

Ulhas (Indian) mirth

Ulices (Latin) form of Ulysses: forceful
Uly

Ulick (Irish) for William; up-and-coming

Ulise (Latin) form of Ulysses: forceful

Ulissus (Invented) form of Ulysses: forceful

Ulland (English) noble Lord
Uland, Ullund

Ullock (Irish) nobleman

Ulman (German) the wolf's infamy
Ulmann, Ullman, Ullmann

Ulmer (German) wolf; cagy

Ulriah (German) form of Ulrich: ruling; power
Ulria, Ulrya, Ulryah

Ulrich (German) ruling; power
Ric, Rick, Rickie, Ricky, Ulrek, Ulric, Ulriche, Ulrick, Ulrico

Ulrid (German) leader

Ulster (Scandinavian) wolf

Ultan (Irish) noble
Ultann

Ultar (Scandinavian) wolf
Ultarr

Ultman (Hindi) godlike

Ulton (German) highborn

Ulysses (Latin) forceful
Ule, Ulesses, Ulises, Ulisses

Umang (Indian) excited

Umar (Hindi) doing well

Umbard (German) form of
Humbert: famous giant;
renowned warrior
Umbarde

Umber (French) brown; plain

Umberto (Italian) earthy

Umed (Hindi) has an aim

Umek (Japanese) blossoms

Umher (Arabic) controlling

Umi (African) life

Unique (American) word as
name
Uneek, Unik

Unitas (American) united

Univers (American)
universal; man for all

Unser (Last name as first
name) drives hard and fast

Unten (English) not a friend
Untenn

Unus (Latin) one
Unuss

Unwin (Last name as first
name) modest

Updike (Last name as first
name) from up above

Upjohn (English) creative
Upjon

Upton (English) highbrow
writer
*Uppton, Uptawn, Upten,
Uptown*

Upwood (Last name as first
name) upper woods is home

Uranus (Greek) the heavens

Urban (Latin) city dweller
*Urb, Urbain, Urbaine, Urbane,
Urben, Urbin, Urbun, Urby*

Urho (Scandinavian)
courageous

Uri (Hebrew) form of Uriel:
light; God-inspired

Uriah (Hebrew) bright; led by
God
Uri, Urie, Uryah

Urian (Irish) from heaven
Urion

Urias (Hebrew) Lord as my
light; old-fashioned
Uraeus, Uri, Uria, Urius

Uriel (Hebrew) light; God-
inspired

Urielon (American) form of
Uriel: light; God-inspired

Urien (Mythology) lights life

Urs (Scandinavian) bear;
growly
Urso

Ursan (French) form of
Orson: strong as a bear
Ursen, Ursyn

Ursino (Spanish) dark

Urteil (German) judgment
Urteel, Urtiel

Uruk (Slavic) form of Urias:
Lord as my light; old-
fashioned

Urv (Biblical) place name

Urvano (Spanish) city boy
 Urbano

Urvine (Place name) form of
 Irvin: attractive
 Urveen, Urvene, Urvi

Ury (Hispanic) God-loving

Ury (Hebrew) shining

Usaid (Arabic) laughs

Usaku (Japanese) moonlit

Usher (Latin) decisive

Usman (Arabic) friend

Usry (Slavic) cultured

Utah (Place name) U.S. state

Uthman (Arabic) bird
 Uthmann

Utz (American) befriends all

Uwe (Welsh) gentle

Uz (Hebrew) passion

Uzal (Hebrew) strong in God

Uziah (Hebrew) believes

Uziel (Hebrew) soothed by
 God's strength

Uzondu (African) attracts
 others

Uzu (Biblical) strength in God

Uzzi (Biblical) place name

Uzziel (Hebrew) powerful in
 God

Vachel (French) keeps cows
 Vachell

Vadim (French) creative
 Vadeem

Vadin (Hindi) speaks well

Vaduz (Place name) city in
 Germany

Vahan (Slavic) protected

Vail (English) serene
 *Bail, Bale, Vaile, Vaill, Vale,
 Valle*

Vaino (Scandinavian)
 wagonbuilder

Val (Latin) form of Valeri:
 athletic; mighty; form of
 Valentine: robust
 Vall

Vala (Latin) form of Valentine:
 robust

Valare (Latin) water-loving

Valdem (Scandinavian) rules

Valdemar (Scandinavian)
 famous leader
 Waldemar

Valensi (Spanish) valiant

Valente (Italian) form of
 Valentin: valient

Valenti (Italian) mighty;
 romantic
 *Val, Valence, Valentin,
 Valentyn*

Valentin (Russian) valiant
 Val, Valeri

Valentine (Latin) robust
Val, Valentijn, Valentin,
Valentinian, Valentino,
Valentinus, Valentyn,
Valentyne, Valyntine

Valentino (Italian) strong;
healthy
Val

Valeri (Russian) athletic;
mighty
Val, Valerian, Valerio, Valry

Valerian (Russian) strong
leader
Valerien, Valerio, Valerius,
Valery, Valeryan

Vali (Scandinavian) brave man

Vali (Italian) form of Valentin:
valiant

Valin (Latin) form of Valentin:
valiant
Valen, Valyn

Vallance (Last name as first
name) tenacious

Vallie (Romanian) valor

Valmar (Slavic) peaceful

Valu (Polynesian) eight

Van (Dutch) descendant
Vann, Von, Vonn

Vance (English) brash
Vans, Vanse

Vanco (Slavic) form of
Vincent: victorious

Vanda (Russian) form of
Walter: army leader

Vandan (Hindi) saved

Vander (Greek) form of
Evander: manly; champion
Vand

Vandiver (American) quiet
Van, Vand, Vandaver, Vandever

Vandwon (African American)
covert
Vandawon, Vandjuan

Vandyke (Last name as first
name) educated

Vane (Last name as first
name) gifted

Vangle (Greek) brings good
news

Vanhue (Armenian) protected

Vannevar (Scandinavian)
form of Evander: manly;
champion

Vanni (Italian) form of
Giovanni: jovial; happy
believer

Vanny (Slavic) form of Vanya:
right

Vanslow (Scandinavian)
sophisticated
Vansalo, Vanselow, Vanslaw

Vanya (Russian) right
Van, Yard, Yardy

Varady (Slavic) fortified

Vardon (French) green hill is
home
Varden, Verdon, Verdun

Varen (Hindi) rain god Varun

Varesh (Hindu) God is
superior

Varg (American) vigorous

Vargu (Scandinavian) wolflike

Varick (German) defender
Varrick, Warick, Warrick

Varil (French) faithful

Varkey (American) boisterous

Varlan (American) tough
Varland, Varlen, Varlin

Varma (Hindi) fruitful

Varner (Last name as first name) formidable
Varn

Varo (Last name as first name)

Vartan (Russian) gives roses

Vartkes (History) king of all

Varun (Hindi) water Lord; excellent
Varoun

Vas (Slavic) protective
Vaston, Vastun, Vasya

Vasant (Sanskrit) brings spring

Vasch (Slavic) clarity

Vasco (Hindi) excellent

Vash (Spanish) from Velasco, Texas

Vashon (American) delightful
Vashaun, Vashonne

Vasil (Slavic) form of William: staunch protector
Vasile, Vasilek, Vasili, Vasilis, Vasilos, Vasily, Vassily

Vasile (Greek) form of Vasilis: king

Vasilis (Russian) king
Vasileios, Vasilij, Vasily, Vaso, Vasos, Vassilij, Vassily, Vasya, Wassily

Vasin (Hindi) rules all

Vasken (Slavic) quiet

Vassil (Bulgarian) king
Vass

Vassilios (Greek) king

Vasu (Sanskrit) rich boy

Vasu (Indian) rich

Vatche (Armenian) loving

Vaughn (Welsh) compact
Vaughan, Vaunie, Von

Vea (Vietnamese) form of Veasna: fortunate

Veasna (Vietnamese) fortunate

Vedn (Latin) sees

Vee (Hebrew) ash tree

Veejay (American) talkative
V.J., Vee-Jay, Vejay

Veer (English) form of Vere: springlike

Vegas (Place name) from Las Vegas
Vega

Vejis (Invented) form of Regis: kingly
Veejas, Veejaz, Vejas, Vejes

Velamo (Scandinavian) of the sea

Velle (American) tough
Vell, Velley, Velly, Veltree

Veltry (African American) hopeful

Velvet (American) smooth
Vel, Velvat, Velvit

Venancio (Spanish) glorious

Venard (Spanish) starry

Venaventura (Spanish) hurts

Vencel (Hungarian) king

Vendon (Indian) fortified

Venedict (Greek) form of Benedict: blessed man
Venedikt, Venka, Venya

Venezio (Italian) glorious
Venetziano, Veneziano

Venkat (Hindi) godlike

Venkata (Hindi) godlike

Ventura (Spanish) good fortune

Venturo (Italian) lucky
Venturio

Verdun (French) green knoll

Vere (Latin) springlike

Vered (Hebrew) rose-loving

Vergel (Spanish) writer
Vergele, Virgil

Verile (German) macho
Verill, Verille, Verol, Verrill

Verissimo (Spanish) truthful

Verlan (Latin) flourishes

Verle (American) truthful

Verlie (American) form of Verle: truthful
Verley

Verlyn (African American) growing
Verle, Verlin, Verllin, Verlon, Verlyn, Virle, Vyrle

Vermont (Place name) U.S. state

Vern (Latin) form of Vernon: fresh and bright
Verne, Vernie, Verny

Vernados (Greek) hearty

Verner (German) resourceful
Vern, Verne, Vernir, Virner

Verniamin (Greek) form of Benjamin: son of the right hand; son of the south

Vernie (Latin) form of Vernon: fresh and bright

Vernon (Latin) fresh and bright
Lavern, Vern, Vernal, Verne, Vernen, Vernin, Verney

Verona (Italian) man of Venice or Verona
Verone

Verrier (French) faithful

Verrill (German) manly
Verill, Verrall, Verrell, Verroll, Veryl

Verron (Latin) form of Vernon: fresh and bright

Vesa (Scandinavian) young

Vest (English) church child

Vester (Latin) form of Sylvester: forest-dweller; heavy-duty

Vestin (English) church child

Vesuvio (Place name) mount Vesuvius; spontaneous

Vetch (German) comforts

Vetis (Latin) life

Vettorio (Italian) victor

Vezeleo (Spanish) form of Basil: regal

Vic (Latin) form of Victor: victorious
Vick, Vickey, Vik

Vicason (English) son of Victor

Vicente (Spanish) winner
Vic, Vicentay, Visente

Vicken (Latin) victor

Vico (Italian) form of Victor: victorious

Vico (Italian) winning

Victen (American) form of Victor: victorious

Victor (Latin) victorious
Vic, Vick, Vickter, Victer, Victorien, Victorin, Vidor, Vikki, Viktor, Vitorio, Vittorio

Victoriano (Spanish) form of
Victor: victorious

Vid (Spanish) form of Vidal:
full of vitality

Vida (Hebrew) beloved;
vibrant

Vidal (Spanish) full of vitality
Bidal, Videl, Videlio

Vidalo (Spanish) energetic
Vidal

Vidar (Scandinavian) soldier

Viddell (Spanish) vital

Vidkun (Scandinavian) gives

Vidor (Hungarian) delightful

Vidya (Indian) smart

Vidyalakshmi (Indian) bright

Viggo (Scandinavian)
exuberant
Viggoa, Vigo

Vigile (American) vigilant
Vegil, Vigil

Vihs (Hindu) increase

Vijay (Hindi) winning
Bijay, Vijun

Vikas (Indian) growth

Vila (Czech) form of William:
staunch protector
Vili, Ville

Vili (Indian) bright

Viliam (Slavic) form of
William: staunch protector

Viliami (Slavic) form of
William: staunch protector

Villalvazo (Spanish) home of
peace

Villantes (French) valiant

Villard (French) village man

Villen (Russian) form of
Lennon: renowned; caped

Villiers (French) kindhearted

Vilmos (Italian) happy
Villmos

Vilnis (Slavic) form of
Vilmos: happy

Vilok (Hindu) to see

Vimal (Hindi) unblemished

Vin (Italian) form of Vincent:
victorious
Vinn, Vinney, Vinni, Vinnie

Vinay (Hindi) good manners

Vinay (Indian) polite

Vince (English) form of
Vincent: victorious
Vee, Vence, Vins, Vinse

Vincent (Latin) victorious
*Vencent, Vicenzio, Vin, Vince,
Vincens, Vincente, Vincentius,
Vincents, Vincenty, Vincenz,
Vincenzio, Vincenzo, Vincien,
Vinicent, Vinnie, Vinny,
Vinzenze, Wincenty, Vinciente,
Vinn, Vinny*

Vincenzo (Italian) conqueror
Vincenze, Vinnie, Vinny

Vine (Latin) form of Vin:
victorious

Vinicius (Indian) victor

Vinod (Hindi) effervescent

Vinod (Indian) joy

Vinson (English) winning
attitude
Venson, Vince, Vinny, Vins

Vinton (English) town of
wine; reveler

Vinus (Slavic) ready

Vio (Indian) form of Vijay:
winning

Vip (Hindi) bounty

Vir (Indian) large

Viral (Indian) mannered

Virat (Indian) big

Vireo (Latin) brave

Virgil (Latin) holding his own;
writer
*Verge, Vergil, Vergilio, Virge,
Virgie, Virgilio, Virgy*

Virginius (Latin) virginal
Virginio

Virrgilio (Spanish) form of
Virgil: holding his own;
writer

Virtus (Greek) virtuous

Vischer (Last name as first
name) longing
Visscher

Vishal (Indian) grand

Vishnu (Indian) pervasive

Vison (Hindi) persuades

Vitale (Italian) important

Vitaliano (Italian) vital

Vitalis (Latin) bubbly; vital

Vitas (Latin) animated
Vidas, Vite

Viticus (Biblical) from
Leviticus

Vito (Italian) form of Vittorio:
lively; victor
*Veto, Vital, Vitale, Vitalis,
Vitaly, Vitas, Vite, Vitus, Witold*

Vitone (Italian) form of Vitas:
animated

Vitrano (Indian) great

Vittorio (Italian) lively; victor
Vite, Vito, Vitor, Vitorio, Vittore

Vittorios (Italian) victor

Vitus (Latin) winning

Vivaldo (Italian) celebrant

Vivar (Greek) alive
Viv

Vivek (Hindi) wise

Vivek (Indian) knowing

Vivian (Latin) lively
*Viviani, Vivien, Vivyan,
Vyvian, Vyvyan*

Vlad (Russian) form of
Vladimir: glorious leader

Vladimir (Russian) glorious
leader
*Vlada, Vladameer, Vladamir,
Vlademar, Vladimeer,
Vlakimar, Wladimir, Wladimyr*

Vladislav (Czech) glorious
leader

Vladislava (Slavic) glorious
ruler

Vladja (Russian) form of
Vladislav: glorious leader

Vodie (Scandinavian) victor

Volf (Hebrew) form of Will:
staunch protector

Volkan (Slavic) defends

Volker (German) prepared to
defend
Volk

Volney (Greek) hidden

Volun (Latin) flies

Volya (Slavic) hopes

Von (German) bright
Vaughn, Vonn, Vonne

Vong (Scandinavian) tough

Vonko (Slavic) form of Vanco:
victorious

Vontaire (French) noisy

Vonzie (American) form of Fonzie: distinguished
Vons, Vonze, Vonzee, Vonzey, Vonzi

Vorris (Latin) versatile

Voshon (Slavic) generous

Vui (African) saves

Vuk (Slavic) wolf-like; Eloquent

Vuok (Scandinavian) flower

Vurl (American) form of Verle: truthful

Vusen (Dutch) vain

Vyacheslav (Russian) glorious child

Vyom (American) vocal

Waclaw (Polish) glorified

Wacy (Arabic) knowledgeable

Wade (English) mover; crossing a river
Wadie, Waide, Wayde

Wadell (English) southerner
Waddell, Wade

Waden (American) form of Jaden: Jehovah has heard
Wade, Wedan

Wadley (Last name as first name) by the water
Wadleigh, Wadly

Wadsworth (English) homebody
Waddsworth, Wadswurth

Wady (Slavic) water boy

Wael (English) from Wales

Wagner (German) musical; practical
Wagg, Waggner, Waggoner, Wagnar, Wagnur

Wagon (American) conveyance
Wag, Wagg, Waggoner

Wai (Asian) form of Wei: excellent

Wain (English) industrious

Wainwright (Last name as first name) works hard
Wain, Wainright, Wayne, Wayneright, Waynewright, Waynright, Wright

Waisim (Arabic) attractive

Wait (American) word as name; patient
Waite

Wake (Place name) island in the Marshall Islands

Wakefield (English) the field worker
Field, Wake

Wakely (Last name as first name) wet

Wakeman (Last name as first name) wet
Wake

Wal (Arabic) form of Waleed: newborn

Walbert (German) protective; stodgy

Walcott (Last name as first name) steadfast
Wallcot, Wallcott, Wolcott

Waldemar (German) famous leader
Valdemar, Waldermar, Waldo

Walden (English) calming
*Wald, Waldan, Waldi, Waldin,
Waldo, Waldon, Waldy, Welti*

Waldo (German) form of
Oswald: divine power
Wald, Waldoh, Waldy

Waldron (English) leader

Waleed (Arabic) newborn
Waled, Walid

Walenty (Polish) strong

Walerian (Polish) powerful

Wales (English) from Wales
*Wael, Wail, Wails, Wale,
Waley, Wali, Waly*

Walford (English) wealthy;
from Wales

Walfred (English) from
Wales; loyal

Wali (Arabic) newborn

Walker (English) distinctive
Walk, Wally

Wall (English) from Wales

Wallace (English) from
Wales; charming
*Wallas, Walley, Walli, Wallice,
Wallie, Wallis, Wally, Walsh,
Welsh*

Waller (English) from Wales;
confident

Wallis (English) from Wales;
smooth

Walls (American) walled
Walen, Wally, Waltz, Walz

Wally (English) form of
Walter: army leader
Wall, Walley, Walli, Wallie

Walmir (Slavic) ruler

Walmond (Last name as first
name) laidback

Walsh (English) inquisitive
*Walls, Welce, Welch, Wells,
Welsh*

Walt (German) army leader
Waltey, Waltli, Walty

Walter (German) army leader
*Walder, Wallie, Wally, Walt,
Walther, Waltur, Walty, Wat*

Walther (German) army
leader; powerful

Walton (English) shut off;
protected
Walt, Walten, Waltin

Waltrau (German) strong
leader

Walu (American) form of
Wally: army leader

Walworth (English) introvert

Walwyn (English) reticent
*Walwin, Walwinn, Walwynn,
Walwynne, Welwyn*

Waman (American) form of
Wymann: contentious

Wang (Chinese) hope; wish

Waqar (Arabic) talkative

Warburton (Last name as
first name) still

Ward (English) vigilant; alert
Warde, Warden, Worden

Wardell (English) guarded

Warden (English) watchful
*Warde, Wardie, Wardin,
Wardon*

Wardley (English) careful
Wardlea, Wardleigh

Ware (English) aware;
cautious
Warey, Wary

Warfield (Last name as first
name) cautious

Warford (Last name as first name) defensive

Waring (English) dashing
Wareng, Warin, Warring

Wark (American) watchful

Warley (Last name as first name) worthy people

Warlito (Spanish) warring

Warner (German) protective
Warne

Warren (German) safe haven
Ware, Waren, Waring, Warrenson, Warrin, Warriner, Warron, Warry, Worrin

Warton (English) defended town

Warvin (American) form of Marvin: steadfast friend

Warwen (American) defensive
Warn, Warwun, Warwun

Warwick (English) lavish
War, Warick, Warrick, Warweck, Warwyc, Warwyck, Wick

Washburn (English) bountiful
Washbern, Washbie, Washby

Washington (English) leader
Wash, Washe, Washing

Wasim (Arabic) pretty baby

Wason (Arabic) form of Wasim: pretty baby

Wat (English) form of Watkins: able

Watford (Last name as first name) soft-spoken

Watkins (English) able
Watkens, Wattie, Wattkins, Watty

Watson (English) helpful
Watsen, Watsie, Watsun, Watsy, Wattsson

Waulkie (English) form of Wilkie: willful

Wave (American) word as a name
Waive, Wave, Wayve

Waverley (Place name) city in New South Wales
Waverlee, Waverli, Waverly

Way (English) landed; smart
Waye

Wayel (English) the road

Wayland (English) from the path land

Wayling (English) the right way
Waylan, Wayland, Waylen, Waylin

Waylon (English) form of Wayland: from the path land
Wallen, Walon, Way, Waylan, Wayland, Waylen, Waylie, Waylin, Waylond, Waylun, Wayly, Weylin

Wayman (English) traveling man
Way, Waym, Waymon, Waymun

Waymon (American) knowing the way
Waymond

Wayne (English) wheeler and dealer
Wain, Wanye, Way, Wayn, Waynell, Waynne

Wazir (Arabic) minister

Weather (Native American) dark

Webb (English) intricate
mind
Web, Webbe, Weeb

Weber (German) intuitive
Webb, Webber, Webner

Webley (English) weaves;
intuitive
Webbley, Webbly, Webly

Webster (English) creative
Web, Webstar, Webstur

Weddel (Last name as first
name) has an angle

Wedon (Last name as first
name) inspired

Weebie (American) wily
Weebbi

Wegner (American) form of
Wagner: musical; practical

Wehrle (last name as first
name)

Wei (Chinese) excellent

Weido (Italian) bright;
personable
Wedo

Welborne (Last name as first
name) where the well is
*Welborn, Welbourne, Welburn,
Wellborn, Wellborne,
Wellbourn, Wellburn*

Welby (German) astute
Welbey, Welbi, Welbie, Wellby

Welby (German) farmer by
the well

Weld (English) from the well

Weldom (American) form of
Weldon: where the well is

Weldon (Last name as first
name) where the well is

Welford (English) unusual
Walferd, Wallie, Wally

Wellington (English) nobility
Welling

Wellis (American) form of
Willis: youthful

Wells (English) unique
Well, Wellie, Welly

Wel-Quo (Asian) bothered
Wel

Welsh (English) form of
Walsh: inquisitive
Welch, Wellsh

Welton (English) spring town

Wen (American) winter baby

Wenceslaus (Polish)
glorified king
*Wenceslas, Wenzel,
Wiencyslaw, Wenczeslaw*

Wendell (German) full of
wanderlust
*Wandale, Wend, Wendall,
Wendel, Wendey, Wendie,
Wendill, Wendle, Wendull,
Wendy*

Wendolid (Spanish) form of
Wendell: full of wanderlust

Wenford (English) confessing
Wynford

Wenjic (Slavic) wanders

Wenli (American) form of
Wendell: wanderlust

Went (American) ambitious
Wente, Wentt

Wentworth (English) last
name as first name

Wenworth (English)
adventures

Werley (English) last name as
first name

Werner (German) warrior

Werther (German) worthy

Wes (English) form of
Wesley: bland
Wess, Wessie, Wessy

Wesh (German) from the
west

Wesley (English) bland
*Wes, Weslee, Wesleyan, Weslie,
Wesly, Wessley, West, Westleigh,
Westley, Westly, Wezlee, Wezley*

Wessell (English) westerner

Wessey (English) westerner

Wesson (American) from the
west
Wess, Wessie

West (English) westerner
Weste, Westt

Westbrook (Last name as
first name) from the west
brook; nature-loving
Brook, West, Westbrooke

Westby (English) near the
west

Westcott (English) from a
western cottage
Wescot, Wescott, Westcot

Westel (English) westerner

Westie (American) capricious
*West, Westee, Westey, Westt,
Westy*

Westleigh (English) western
Westlea, Westlie, Wezlee

Westley (English) from the
west fields

Westoll (American) open
West, Westall

Weston (English) good
neighbor
*West, Westen, Westey, Westie,
Westy, Westin*

Wesze (English) westerner

Weszel (English) westerner

Wether (English) lighthearted
*Weather, Weth, Wethar,
Wethur*

Wetherby (English)
lighthearted
*Weatherbey, Weatherbie,
Weatherby, Wetherbey,
Wetherbie*

Wetherell (English)
lighthearted

Wetherly (English)
lighthearted

Wex (English) the fjord of the
flats

Whalen (English) from the
woods

Whalley (Last name as first
name) predicts

Wharton (Last name as first
name) provincial
Warton

Wheat (Invented) fair-haired
*Wheatie, Wheats, Wheaty,
Whete*

Wheatley (Last name as first
name) fair-haired; fields of
wheat
*Whatley, Wheatlea,
Wheatleigh, Wheatly*

Wheaton (Last name as first
name) blond; wheat town

Wheel (American) important
player
Wheele

Wheeler (English) likes cars;
wheel maker
Weeler, Wheel, Wheelie, Wheely

Wheeless (English) off track
Whelus

Wheelie (American) big-wig
Wheeley, Wheels, Wheely

Whesk (American) self-serving

Whip (American) friendly

Whistler (English) melodic
Whis, Whistlar, Whistle, Whistlerr

Whit (English) form of Whitman: man with white hair
Whitt, Whyt, Whyte, Wit, Witt

Whit (English) form of Whitman: man with white hair

Whitby (English) white-haired; white-walled town

Whitcomb (English) light in the valley; shining
Whitcombe, Whitcumb

White (English) white

Whitelaw (English) white
Whitlaw

Whitey (English) fair-skinned
White

Whitfield (English) from a white field

Whitford (English) the light source

Whitley (English) white area is home
Whitlea, Whitlee, Whitleigh

Whitman (English) man with white hair
Whit, Whitty, Witman

Whitmore (English) white
Whitmoor, Whittemore, Witmore, Wittemore

Whitney (English) likes white spaces
Whit, Whitnee, Whitnie, Whitt, Whittney, Widney, Widny, Witt

Whitson (English) son of Whit
Whitt, Witt

Whittaker (English) outdoorsy
Whitaker, Whitt, Witaker, Wittaker

Whitter (English) white

Whittson (English) white son

Wick (American) burning
Wic, Wik, Wyck

Wickham (Last name as first name) living in a hamlet
Wick

Wickley (Last name as first name) coming from a small home
Wicley

Wier (German) famous

Wieslaw (Polish) known

Wijnand (Slavic) form of Wymon; soldier

Wilberforce (German) wild and strong

Wilbert (German) smart
Wilberto, Wilburt

Wilbur (English) fortified
Wilbar, Wilber, Willbur, Wilburt, Willbur, Wilver

Wilburn (German) brilliant
Bernie, Wil, Wilbern, Will

Wilder (English) wild man
Wildar, Wilde, Wildey

Wildon (Last name as first name) willing support
Wilden, Willdon

Wilee (English) form of Wylie: charmer

Wilen (English) form of William: staunch protector

Wiles (American) tricky
Wyles

Wiley (English) cowboy
Wile, Willey, Wylie

Wilf (English) form of
Wilford: willowy; peaceful
wishes

Wilford (English) willowy;
peaceful wishes

Wilfre (German) peaceful

Wilfred (German)
peacemaker
*Wilferd, Wilfrid, Wilfride,
Wilford, Wilfried, Wilfryd, Will,
Willfred, Willfried, Willie, Willy*

Wilfredo (Italian) peaceful
Fredo, Wifredo, Willfredo

Wilhelm (German) resolute;
determined
Wilhelmus, Wilhem, Willem

Wilke (German) form of
Wilkins: affectionate

Wilkie (English) willful

Wilkins (English) affectionate
*Welkie, Welkins, Wilk, Wilkens,
Wilkes, Wilkie, Wilkin, Willkes,
Willkins*

Wilkinson (English) son of
Wilkin; capable
Willkinson

Will (English) form of
William: staunch protector
Wil, Wilm, Wim, Wyll

Willard (German) courageous
Wilard, Willerd

Willeo (Spanish) form of
William: staunch protector

Willer (American) form of
Willard: courageous

Willerson (English) son of
Willard

Willialdo (Spanish) form of
William: staunch protector

William ✪ ✝ (English)
staunch protector
*Bill, Will, Willeam, Willie,
Wills, Willy, Willyum, Wilyam*

Williams (German) brave
Williamson

Willie (German) form of
William: staunch protector
*Will, Wille, Willey, Willeye,
Willi, Willy, Wily*

Willis (German) youthful
*Willace, Willece, Willice, Wills,
Willus*

Willits (Scandinavian)
protective

Willoughby (Last name as
first name) lives with grace
Willoughbey, Willoughbie

Wills (English) willful

Wilmer (German) resolute;
ambitious
*Willmar, Willmer, Wilm,
Wilmar, Wilmyr, Wylmar,
Wylmer*

Wilmot (German) tough-
minded

Wilson (English)
extraordinary
*Willson, Wilsen, Wilsun,
Willson*

Wilt (English) talented
Wiltie

Wilton (English) practical and
open
*Will, Wilt, Wiltie, Wylten,
Wylton*

Wiltson (English) son of Will

Wim (Slavic) go-getter

Wimmy (American) form of
William: staunch protector

Win (German) flirtatious
Winn, Winnie, Winny

Wincate (English) form of
Vincent: victorious

Winchell (English)
meandering
Winchie, Winshell

Wind (American) word as
name; breezy
Windy

Windell (German) wanderer
Windelle, Windyll

Windsor (English) royal
*Win, Wincer, Winnie, Winny,
Winsor, Wyndsor, Wynser*

Winfield (English) peace in
the country
*Field, Winifield, Winnfield,
Wynfield, Wynnfield*

Winfried (English) peaceful

Wing (Chinese) in glory
Wing-Chiu, Wing-Kit

Wingate (Last name as first
name) glorified

Wingi (American) spunky

Wings (American) soaring;
free
Wing

Wink (American) vigorous

Winkel (American) bright;
conniving
Wink, Winky

Winkle (American) vigorous

Winlove (Filipino) winning
favor

Winn (English) form of Wyn:
gregarious

Winnell (English) fair-haired

Winslone (English) form of
Winslow: friendly

Winslow (English) friendly
Winslo, Wynslo, Wynslow

Winsome (English)
gorgeous; charming
Wins, Winsom, Winz

Winston (English) dignified
*Win, Winn, Winnie, Winny,
Winstan, Winsten, Winstonn,
Winton, Wynstan, Wynsten,
Wynston*

Winter (English) born in
winter
*Win, Winnie, Winny, Wintar,
Winterford, Wintur, Wynter,
Wyntur*

Winthrop (English) winning;
stuffy
*Win, Winn, Winnie, Winny,
Wintrop*

Winton (English) winning
Wynten, Wynton

Winward (English) friendly

Wiss (American) carefree
Wissie, Wissy

Wit (Polish) life
Witt, Wittie, Witty

Witek (Polish) form of Victor:
victorious

Witha (Arabic) vibrant

Witold (Polish) lively

Witt (Slavic) lively
Witte

Witter (Last name as first
name) alive

Witton (Last name as first
name) lively

Witty (American) humorous
Wit, Witt, Witte, Wittey, Wittie

Wize (American) smart
Wise, Wizey, Wizi, Wizie

Wladymir (Polish) famous
ruler
Vladimir

Wladyslaw (Polish) good
leader
Slaw

Wlodek (Polish) rules

Wohn (African American)
form of John: God is gracious

Wojciech (Polish) comforts

Wojtek (Polish) comforter;
warrior

Wolcott (English) home of
wool

Wolf (German) form of
Wolfgang: talented; a wolf
walks
Wolff, Wolfie, Wolfy

Wolfe (German) wolf;
ominous
Wolf, Wolff, Wulf, Wulfe

Wolfgang (German) talented;
a wolf walks
*Wolf, Wolff, Wolfgans, Wolfy,
Wulfgang*

Wolfram (Jewish) ominous

Wolley (American) form of
Wally: army leader
Wolly

Wolsh (Slavic) form of Walter:
army leader

Wolter (Slavic) form of
Walter: army leader

Wood (English) form of
Woodrow: special
Woode, Woody

Woodery (English)
woodsman
*Wood, Wooderree, Woodree,
Woodri, Woodry, Woods,
Woodsry, Woody*

Woodfield (Last name as first
name) enjoys the woods

Woodfin (English) attractive
*Wood, Woodfen, Woodfien,
Woodfyn, Woodie, Woody*

Woodford (Last name as first
name) forester

Woodrow (English) special
Wood, Woodrowe, Woody

Woodruff (Last name as first
name) smooth; natural

Woodson (Last name as first
name) son of Wood; suave

Woodville (Last name as first
name) from the town of trees

Woodward (English)
watchful
*Wood, Woodie, Woodard,
Woodwerd, Woody*

Woodwer (Native American)
mourning

Woody (American) jaunty
*Wooddy, Woodey, Woodi,
Woodie*

Woolsey (English) leader
Wools, Woolsi, Woolsie, Woolsy

Worcester (English) secure

Word (American) talkative
Words, Wordy, Wurd

Worden (American) careful
Word, Wordan, Wordun

Wordsworth (English) poetic
Words, Worth

Worie (English) cautious

Worsh (American) from
worship; religious
Wor

Worth (English) deserving;
special
*Werth, Worthey, Worthie,
Worthington, Worthy, Wurth*

Wortham (English) worthy

Worthington (English) fun; worthwhile
Worth, Worthey, Worthing, Worthingtun, Wurthington

Wouter (German) power figure

Wrae (English) corner

Wrangle (American) cowboy
Wrang, Wrangler, Wrangy

Wrangle (American) wrangler

Wray (American) cornered

Wren (American) leader of men
Ren, Rin, Rinn, Wrenn

Wright (English) clear-minded; correct
Right, Rite, Wrighte, Write

Wrigley (Place Name) city in Tennessee

Wrisley (American) smart
Wrisee, Wrislie, Wrisly

Wriston (American) good proportions
Wryston

Wulf (Hebrew) wolf
Wolf

Wunig (Native American) believer

Wurei (Native American) windy

Wyam (American) form of Wyoming

Wyanll (Scandinavian) arises

Wyant (American) strong-willed

Wyatt ✪ (French) ready for combat
Wiatt, Wy, Wyat, Wyatte, Wye, Wyeth

Wybert (Last name as first name) good profile

Wyborn (Last name as first name) wellborn

Wyck (English) light

Wyclef (American) trendy
Wycleff

Wycliff (English) edgy
Cliffie, Cliffy, Wicliff, Wyclif, Wycliffe

Wydee (American) form of Wyatt: ready for combat
Wy, Wydey, Wydie

Wykeum (American) different

Wyland (English) charismatic

Wyler (German) creative

Wylie (English) charmer
Wiley, Wye, Wylee

Wylon (English) charismatic

Wymann (English) contentious
Wimann, Wye, Wyman

Wymel (English) famous

Wymen (English) soldier

Wymer (English) rambunctious; fighter

Wymon (English) soldier

Wyn (Welsh) gregarious

Wyndham (English) from a hamlet
Windham, Wynndham

Wynell (English) companion

Wynne (English) dear friend
Winn, Wyn, Wynn

Wynter (English) born in winter

Wynton (English) winter town child

Wyshawn (African American) friendly
Shawn, Shawny, Why, Whysean, Wieshawn, Wye, Wyshawne, Wyshie, Wyshy

Wystan (English) struggles

Wythe (English) fair

Wythel (English) of willows

Wyton (English) fair-haired; crowd-pleaser
Wye, Wytan, Wyten, Wytin

Wyze (American) sizzle; capable
Wise, Wye, Wyse

Xan (Greek) form of Alexander: great leader; helpful

Xander (Greek) form of Alexander: great leader; helpful
Xan, Xande, Xandere, Xandre

Xanthin (Greek) gold hair

Xanthos (Greek) attractive

Xanthus (Greek) golden-haired child

Xaque (American) unique

Xat (American) saved
Xatt

Xaver (Spanish) form of Xavier: home; shining

Xaverius (Spanish) form of Xavier: home; shining
Xaverious, Xaveryus

Xavier Ⓐ (Arabic) home; shining
Saverio, Xaver, Zavey, Zavier

Xavion (Spanish) form of Xavier: home; shining

Xaxon (American) happy
Zaxon

Xayvion (African American) dwells in new house
Savion, Sayveon, Sayvion, Xavion, Xayveon, Zayvion

Xebec (French) from Quebec; cold
Xebeck, Xebek

Xen (African American) original
Zen

Xenik (Russian) sly
Xenic, Xenick, Xenyc, Xenyck, Xenyk

Xeno (Greek) gracious
Xenoes, Zene, Zenno, Zenny, Zeno, Zenos

Xenon (Greek) gracious

Xenophon (Greek) gracious

Xenos (Greek) with grace
Xeno, Zenos

Xerarch (Greek) dancing
Xerarche

Xeres (Persian) form of Xerxes: leader
Xeries

Xerxes (Persian) leader
Xerk, Xerky, Zerk, Zerkes, Zerkez

Xhosas (African) south African tribe
Xhoses, Xhosys

Xiaoping (Chinese) brightest star

Ximen (Spanish) obeys
Ximenes, Ximon, Ximun

Ximena (Spanish) good
listener

Xing-Fu (Chinese) happy

Xi-Wang (Chinese) optimistic

Xochitl (Spanish) flowers

Xuthus (Last name as first
name) long-suffering

Xyle (American) helpful
Zye, Zyle

Xylo (Greek) form of Xylon:
forester

Xylon (Greek) forester

Xyshaun (African American)
zany
Xye, Zye, Zyshaun, Zyshawn

Xyst (English) a portico;
systematic
Xist

Xystum (Greek) promenade
Xistoum, Xistum, Xysoum

Xystus (Greek) promenade
Xistus

Yaameen (Hebrew) right
hand

Yachna (Hebrew) gracious

Yadid (Hebrew) friend

Yadon (Last name as first
name) different
Yado, Yadun

Yadua (Hindi) judged

Yael (Hebrew) teacher
Yail, Yaley, Yalie

Yagil (Hebrew) celebrant

Yagna (Indian) devout

Yahir (Hebrew) enlightened

Yahne (Hebrew) adored

Yahya (Arabic) vital
Yahiya

Yair (Hebrew) strong

Yakar (Hebrew) adored

Yakez (Scandinavian) celestial

Yale (German) producer

Yalen (English) old soul

Yall (English) form of Yalman:
old man

Yalman (English) old man

Yalon (English) form of Jalen:
vivacious

Yamato (Japanese) mountain;
scaling heights

Yamen (Indian) death god

Yan (Slavic) form of John:
God is gracious

Yana (Native American)
bearlike

Yance (American) from
England

Yancy (American) vivacious
Yanci, Yancie, Yancy, Yanzie

Yanis (Hebrew) God's gift
Yannis, Yantsha

Yank (American) yankee
Yanke

Yankel (Hebrew) supportive
Yaki, Yakov, Yekel

Yannis (Greek) believer in
God
Yannie

Yannis (Greek) form of John: God is gracious

Yanny (Hebrew) learns

Yanto (French) confident

Yanton (Hebrew) form of Jonathan: gift of God

Yao (Chinese) athletic; Thursday's child

Yao (African) Thursday's child

Yaphet (Hebrew) form of Japheth: grows
Yapheth, Yefat, Yephat

Yar (English) forest

Yarb (Gypsy) spicy

Yarbon (English) surname

Yarbrough (English) surname

Yarden (Hebrew) flowing
Yard, Yardan, Yarde, Yardene, Yardun

Yardley (English) adorned; separate
Yard, Yarde, Yardie, Yardlea, Yardlee, Yardly, Yardy

Yared (Hebrew) form of Jared: descendant; giving

Yaren (Hebrew) form of Jaren: vocal

Yarkon (Hebrew) green

Yarom (Hebrew) sings
Yaron

Yash (Hindi) famous

Yashy (Indian) wealthy

Yasin (Arabic) seer

Yasir (Arabic) rich

Yasmuji (Asian) flowering

Yassah (Indian) famed

Yasuo (Japanese) calm

Yasutaro (Japanese) peaceful

Yates (English) smart; closed
Yate, Yattes, Yeats

Yati (Indian) beloved

Yave (Hindi) giving

Yavin (Hebrew) believes

Yaw (Akan) Thursday's child

Yawo (African) Thursday's child

Yay (African) Thursday's child

Yazeed (Arabic) growing in spirit

Yeardley (Indian) victor

Yeats (English) gates
Yates

Yeb (English) form of Jeb/Jacob: jolly; one who supplants

Yediel (Hebrew) loved by Jehovah

Yehem (Biblical) place name

Yehoshua (Hebrew) alive by God's salvation

Yehuda (Hebrew) praised
Yehudi

Yemin (Hebrew) guarded

Yemyo (Asian) serene

Yen (Chinese) calming; capable

Yenny (Biblical) place name

Yens (Vietnamese) yen; calm

Yeoman (English) helping
Yeomann, Yo, Yoeman, Yoman, Yoyo

Yered (Jewish) form of Jared: descendant; giving

Yerel (Indian) careful

Yero (African) studious

Yesel (Hebrew) won by God

Yeshaya (Hebrew) treasured

Yesher (Hebrew) God's salvation

Yeshurun (Hebrew) focuses on God

Yeshya (Hebrew) gifted

Yevgeny (Russian) life-giving

Yianni (Greek) creative

Yigal (Turkish) lively

Yimer (Scandinavian) giant

Yiron (Czech) form of George: land-loving; farmer

Yishai (Hebrew) form of Jesse: wealthy

Yisrael (Hebrew) struggles with God

Yitro (Hebrew) form of Jethro: fertile

Yitzhak (Hebrew) laughing
Yitz, Yitzchak

Yngvar (Scandinavian) god of fertility
Ingvar;

Yo (Vietnamese) truthful

Yoav (Hebrew) form of Joab: praising God; hovering

Yobachi (African) prayerful

Yochanan (Hebrew) form of John: God is gracious
Yohanan

Yoel (Hebrew) form of Joel: Jehovah is the Lord

Yogesh (Hindi) another name for Hindu god Shiva

Yogi (Japanese) yoga practicer

Yoginee (Indian) yoga enthusiast

Yohance (Hebrew) form of John: God is gracious

Yohane (Hebrew) form of Johane: God is gracious

Yohann (German) form of Johann: God is gracious
Yohan, Yohn

Yohanys (German) form of Johane: God is gracious

Yoi (Hebrew) bounty

Yojiro (Japanese) hopes

Yolan (French) generous

Yolander (French) violet

Yonah (Hebrew) form of Jonah: peacemaker

Yonatan (Hebrew) form of Jonathan: gift of God
Yonathan, Yonathon

Yong (Chinese) brave

Yoosef (Hebrew) favorite
Yosef

Yoran (Hebrew) to sing

Yorick (Literature) Hamlet's jester

Yorik (English) farms

York (English) affluent
Yorke, Yorkee, Yorkey, Yorki, Yorky

Yorker (English) rich
York, Yorke, Yorkur

Yosef (Hebrew) form of Joseph: He will add
Yose, Yoseff, Yosif

Yosefu (Hebrew) form of Joseph: He will add

Yosemite (Place name)
natural wonder

Yosh (Japanese) son

Yoshe (Hebrew) wise

Yoshiaki (Japanese) attractive

Yoshikatsu (Japanese) good

Yoshinobu (Japanese)
goodness

Yoshio (Japanese) giving

Yossel (Hebrew) favored
Yoska, Yossi

Yosuke (Japanese) helps

Yosvani (Slavic) form of
Johanne: God is gracious

Younes (Hebrew) form of
Jonah: peacemaker

Young (English) fledgling
Jung, Younge

Younger (Scandinavian)
young

Yoursie (American) form of
Juri: farms

Yov (Russian) reliable

Yovan (Slavic) form of Jovan:
gifted

Yri (Hebrew) form of Joseph:
He will add

Yu (Chinese) shiny; smart

Yuan (Chinese) circle

Yudel (Hebrew) jubilant
Yudi

Yui (Chinese) moon;
universal

Yuji (Japanese) snow

Yuke (American) form of
Yukon: individualist

Yuki (Japanese) loves snow

Yukichi (Japanese) lucky
snow

Yukien (Japanese) of the
snows

Yukio (Japanese) man of
snow

Yukon (Place name)
individualist

Yul (Chinese) infinity

Yule (English) christmas-born
Yuel, Yul, Yuley, Yulie

Yuli (Basque) childlike

Yuma (Place name) city in
Arizona; cowboy
Yumah

Yunuen (Spanish) seer

Yunus (Turkish) young

Yurcel (Turkish) the best

Yuri (Russian) dashing
*Yurah, Yure, Yurey, Yurie,
Yurri, Yury*

Yurik (Japanese) yuri's child

Yurik (Slavic) form of Yorick:
Hamlet's jester

Yuris (Latin) farmer
Yures, Yurus

Yuritzi (Slavic) form of Yuri:
dashing

Yursa (Japanese) lily; delicate

Yurza (Slavic) form of George:
land-loving; farmer

Yusuf (Arabic) form of
Joseph: He will add

Yuta (Native American) hunts

Yutu (African) hunter

Yuval (Hebrew) celebrant

Yuvaraj (Indian) prince

Yux (Spanish) form of Joshua: devout

Yuz (Scandinavian) form of John: God is gracious

Yuzhi (Slavic) form of Joseph: He will add

Yves (French) honest; handsome
Eve, Ives

Yvonn (French) attractive
Von, Vonn, Yvon

Zaavan (Biblical) God hides him

Zab (American) slick
Zabbey, Zabbi, Zabbie, Zabby

Zabel (Biblical) place name

Zac (Hebrew) form of Zachariah: Lord remembers
Zacary, Zach, Zachary, Zachry

Zaca (Hebrew) water movement

Zacary (Hebrew) form of Zachary: spiritual
Zac, Zacc, Zaccary, Zaccry, Zaccury

Zaccheus (Hebrew) unblemished
Zac, Zacceus, Zack

Zace (American) pleasure-seeking
Zacey, Zacie, Zase

Zach (Hebrew) form of Zachary: spiritual
Zac, Zachy

Zachariah (Hebrew) Lord remembers
Zac, Zacaria, Zacarias, Zacary, Zacaryah, Zaccaria, Zaccariah, Zaccheus, Zach, Zachaios, Zacharia, Zacharias, Zacharie, Zachary, Zacheriah, Zachery, Zacheus, Zachey, Zachi, Zachie, Zachy, Zack, Zackariah, Zackerias, Zackery, Zak, Zakarias, Zakarie, Zakariyyah, Zakery, Zechariah, Zekariah, Zekeriah, Zeke, Zhack

Zacharias (Hebrew) devout
Zacharyas

Zachary ♂ ♀ (Hebrew) spiritual
Zacary, Zacchary, Zach, Zackar, Zackarie, Zak, Zakari, Zakri, Zakrie, Zakry

Zack (Hebrew) form of Zachary: spiritual
Zacky, Zak

Zade (Arabic) flourishing; trendy
Zaid

Zadok (Hebrew) unyielding
Zadek, Zaydie, Zadik, Zayd, Zaydok

Zafar (Hindi) victor
Zaphar

Zafir (Arabic) wins
Zafeer, Zafyr

Zahavi (Hebrew) golden child

Zaher (American) exceeds

Zahir (Hebrew) bright
Zaheer, Zahur

Zahur (Arabic) flourishes

Zain (American) zany
Zane, Zayne

Zaire (Place name) country in Africa; brash

Zakary (Hebrew) form of Zachary: spiritual

Zakhar (Hebrew) pure of heart

Zakhary (Hebrew) form of Zachary: spiritual

Zaki (Arabic) virtuous
Zak

Zale (Greek) strong
Zail, Zaley, Zalie, Zayle

Zalman (Hebrew) peaceful
Salman, Zaloman

Zalmon (Jewish) form of Solomon: peaceful and wise

Zamar (Hebrew) sings

Zamen (Hebrew) form of Zalman: peaceful

Zamil (German) form of Samuel: man who heard God; prophet
Zameel, Zamyl

Zamir (Hebrew) lyrical
Zameer, Zamyr

Zammet (Slavic) head of household

Zamuel (Hebrew) variant on Samuel: man who heard God; prophet

Zan (Hebrew) well-nourished
Xan, Zander, Zandro, Zandros, Zann

Zanchet (French) homebody

Zand (Greek) form of Zander: great leader; helpful

Zander (Greek) form of Alexander: great leader; helpful
Zande, Zandee, Zandey, Zandie, Zandy

Zandy (American) high-energy
Zandee, Zandi

Zane (English) debonair
Zain, Zay, Zayne, Zaynne

Zano (American) unique
Zan

Zanoni (Unknown) from god Zeus

Zaphon (Biblical) God hides him

Zappa (American) zany
Zapah, Zapp

Zappe (Persian) happy

Zappy (Persian) jovial

Zar (African) watchful

Zared (Arabic) gold

Zarek (Aramaic) light

Zarel (Slavic) watchful

Zarethan (Biblical) helped by God

Zario (Biblical) place name

Zartavious (African American) unusual
Zar, Zarta

Zashawn (African American) fiery
Zasean, Zash, Zashaun, Zashe, Zashon, Zashone

Zasu (Slavic) form of Jose: asset; favored

Zauk (Slavic) form of Zac: Lord remembers

Zaul (American) form of Saul: gift

Zavel (American) youthful

Zavier (Arabic) form of Xavier: home; shining

Zavion (American) smiling
Zavien

Zayn (English) form of Zane:
debonair

Zazel (Arabic) handsome

Zbigniew (Polish) free of
malice; calming

Zbigniew (Polish)
relinquishes anger

Zeb (Hebrew) form of
Zebediah: gift from God
Zebe

Zebby (Hebrew) believer;
rambunctious
Zabbie, Zeb, Zebb, Zebbie

Zebediah (Hebrew) gift from
God
*Zeb, Zebadia, Zebb, Zebbie,
Zebby, Zebedee, Zebediah, Zebi,
Zebidiah*

Zebul (Hebrew) respected

Zebulon (Hebrew) uplifted
*Zebulen, Zebulun, Zevulon,
Zevulun*

Zebulun (Hebrew) revered

Zechariah (Hebrew) form of
Zachariah: Lord remembers
Zeke

Zed (Hebrew) energetic
Zedd, Zede

Zedediah (Hebrew) form of
Zebediah: gift from God
Zededia, Zedidia, Zedidiah

Zedekiah (Hebrew) believing
in a just God
*Zed, Zeddy, Zedechia,
Zedechiah, Zedekias*

Zeeman (Dutch) seafaring
Zeaman

Zeevy (American) sly
Zeeve, Zeevi, Zeevie

Zef (Hebrew) wolf

Zeffy (American) explosive
Zeff, Zeffe, Zeffi, Zeffie

Zekarias (Dutch) impulsive

Zeke (Hebrew) friendly;
outgoing
Zeek, Zekey, Zeki

Zekel (Hebrew) form of
Ezekial: God's strength

Zeker (Hebrew) form of
Ezekial: God's strength

Zekie (Turkish) bright mind

Zel (American) hearty

Zelalem (Biblical) form of
Zel: hearty

Zelbie (Hebrew) delicate

Zelig (Hebrew) holy; happy
Selig, Zel, Zeligman, Zelik

Zelmon (English) man of
peace

Zemaraim (Biblical) lion-like

Zen (Japanese) spiritual

Zenas (Greek) form of Zeus:
powerful
Zenios, Zenon

Zenen (Biblical) place name

Zenib (Greek) life of Zeus

Zenith (Word as name)
famous

Zeno (Greek) philosophical;
stoic
Zeney, Zenie, Zenno, Zeny

Zenobios (Greek) living
Zeus; lively
Zenobius, Zinov, Zinovi

Zenon (Greek) form of
Xenon: gracious

Zenotis (Greek) form of
Zeus: powerful

Zenovial (Greek) form of
Zeus: powerful

Zent (American) zany
Zynt

Zeph (Greek) form of Zephyr:
breezy

Zephaniah (Hebrew)
protected by God
Zeph, Zephan

Zephariah (Hebrew)
Jehovah's light

Zephen (Greek) form of
Zephyr: breezy

Zepho (Greek) form of
Zephyr: breezy

Zephyr (Greek) breezy
*Zayfeer, Zayfir, Zayphir, Zefar,
Zefer, Zefir, Zeffer, Zefur,
Zephir, Zephiros, Zephirus,
Zephyrus*

Zerah (Biblical) light

Zero (Arabic) nothing
Zeroh

Zerond (American) helpful
Zerre, Zerrie, Zerry, Zerund

Zes (Biblical) place name

Zeshon (African American)
zany
Zeshaune, Zeshawn

Zeson (Spanish) fair

Zestler (Last name as first
name)

Zete (Hebrew) shiny

Zeth (American) form of
Seth: chosen
Zethe

Zeus (Greek) powerful
Zues

Zev (Hebrew) form of
Zebulon: uplifted
Zevv

Zevediah (Hebrew) form of
Zebediah; broken dreams
Zevedia, Zevidia, Zevidiah

Zevi (Hebrew) brisk
Zevie

Zevry (Biblical) place name

Zevulon (Hebrew) form of
Zebulon: uplifted
Zevulonn

Zexi (Asian) hopeful

Zhen (Chinese) pure

Zhivago (Russian) dashing;
romantic
Vago

Zhobin (Slavic) form of
George: land-loving; farmer

Zhong (Chinese) middle
brother; loyal

Zia (Hebrew) in motion
Zeah, Ziah

Ziad (Arabic) of the light

Zibeon (Arabic) vibrant
growth

Zichri (American) form of
Zachary: spiritual

Zie (American) compelling
Zye, Zyey

Ziggy (American) zany

Zigmand (American) form of
Sigmund: victor
Zig, Ziggy

Ziklag (Biblical) place name

Zikomo (African) grateful

Zilph (Biblical) place name

Zimran (Hebrew) sacred

Zimri (Hebrew) valued

Zin (Biblical) praised

Zinc (Biblical) place name

Zindel (Yiddish) form of
Alexander: great leader;
helpful
Zindil

Zingo (American) zany

Zino (Greek) philosopher
Zeno

Zion (Hebrew) sign
Sion, Zeione, Zi, Zione, Zye

Zion (Hebrew) omen

Zional (Biblical) place name

Zior (African) sky

Ziph (Biblical) place name

Zipkiyah (Native American)
archer

Zirkle (Biblical) place name

Zito (Italian) growth

Ziv (Hebrew) energetic
Zeven, Zevy, Ziven, Zivon

Ziven (Polish) lively
Ziv, Zivan, Zyvan

Ziya (Turkish) light

Ziz (Hebrew) sign

Zlatko (Slavic) gold

Zoan (Biblical) place name

Zoar (Biblical) place name

Zobah (Biblical) place name

Zobel (Biblical) place name

Zober (African) strong

Zocco (American) form of
Zach: spiritual

Zochi (Turkish) form of
Zekie: bright mind

Zohar (Hebrew) light

Zohreh (Indian) blooms

Zoilo (Greek) life

Zoilo (Spanish) lively

Zol (American) jaunty
Zoll

Zoltan (Hungarian) lively

Zolten-Penn (Hungarian)
lively

Zoma (American) loquacious
Zome

Zook (American) form of
Zach: spiritual

Zoran (Slavic) dawn

Zorba (Greek) pleasure
seeker
Zorbah, Zorbe

Zorby (Greek) tireless
Sorby, Zorb, Zorbie

Zorshawn (African
American) jaded
*Zahrshy, Zorsh, Zorshie,
Zorshon, Zorshy*

Zowie (Greek) life
Zowey, Zowy

Zoy (English) life-giving

Zuad (American) devout

Zuadan (American) invented
from Sudan

Zub (Russian) toothy

Zuba (Iranian) attractive

Zuberi (African) powerful
Zooberi, Zubery

Zubren (African) strength

Zucker (English) penitent

Zuhair (Arabic) shines

Zuhayr (Arabic) flowers
Zuhair

Zuhier (American) shines

Zulfer (American) leads

Zumrud (American) unique

Zuni (Native American)
creative

Zuriel (Hebrew) believer

Zurlo (American) zany

Zury (Spanish) believer

Zuzel (Spanish) sweet

Zvon (Croatian) form of
Zvonimir: sound of peace
Zevon, Zevonn

Zvonimir (Croatian) sound of
peace

Zwie (Spanish) from Jose

Zygmunt (Slavic) form of
Sigmund: victor

Zyke (American) high-energy
Zykee, Zyki, Zykie, Zyky

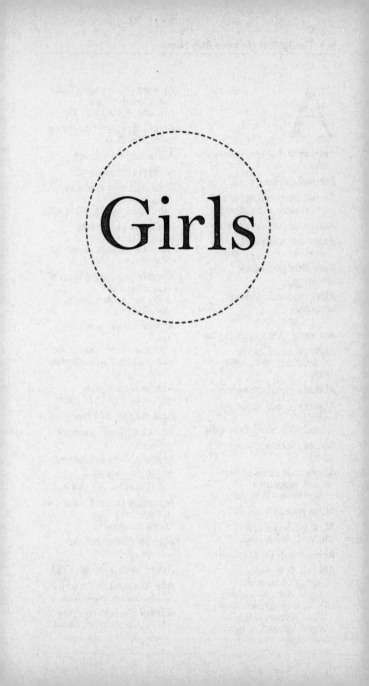

Girls

Aaliyah ✪ (Hebrew) moving up
Aliya

Aamori (African) good

Aarika (Welsh) form of Erika: honorable; leading others

Aarionne (Welsh) knowing

Aaronita (American) knowing

Aaronitia (American) knowing

Abay (Native American) growing
Abai, Abbay, Abey, Abeye

Abayomi (African) giving joy

Abby (English) happy
Abbee, Abbey, Abbi, Abbie, Abbye

Abdulia (Spanish) certain

Abella (French) vulnerable; capable
Abela, Abele, Abell, Bela, Bella

Abena (African) Tuesday's child

Abery (Last name as first name) supportive
Abby, Aberee, Abrie, Abry

Abha (Hindi) lustrous

Abia (Arabic) excellent
Ab, Aba, Abiah, Abbie

Abida (Arabian) worships

Abigail ✪ ⚀ (Hebrew, English, Irish) joyful
Abagail, Abbegayle, Abbey, Abbie, Abby, Abegail, Abey, Abigal, Abigale, Abigayle, Abygail, Abygale, Abygayle, Gail, Gayle

Abilene (Place name) Texas town; southern girl
Abalene, Abi, Abiline, Aby

Abiola (Spanish) God-loving
Abby, Abi, Biola

Abira (Hebrew) strong

Abisael (Biblical) joyful

Abra (Hebrew) example; lesson
Aba, Abbee, Abbey, Abbie, Abby

Abrianna (American) insightful
Abriana, Abryana, Abryanna, Abryannah

Abrielle (American) form of Abigail: joyful
Abby, Abree, Abrey, Abrie, Abriella, Abryelle

Acacia (Greek) everlasting; tree
Akaysha, Cacia, Cacie, Case, Casey, Casha, Casia, Caysha, Kassy, Kaykay

Acadia (Algonquian-Wakashian) place of plenty

Acalena (English) ready

Acantha (Greek) thorny; difficult

Acatia (Greek) forever tree

Accalia (Latin) stand-in
Accal, Accalya, Ace, Ackie

Achantay (African American) reliable
Achantae, Achanté

Ackalin (Greek) beloved nymph

Ackee (American) fall child

Ada (German) noble; joyful
Adah, Addah, Adeia, Aida

Adaani (French) pretty; noble
Adan, Adane, Adani, Daani, Dani

Adaeze (African) prepared
Adaese

Adah (Biblical) decorated
Ada, Adie, Adina, Dina

Adair (Scottish) innovative
*Ada, Adare, Adayr, Adayre,
Adda*

Adalia (Spanish) spunky
*Adahlia, Adailya, Adallyuh,
Adaylia*

Adalind (American) form of
Adeline: sweet

Adalinda (French) form of
Adelle: giving

Adamina (Hebrew) earth
child

Adamita (Spanish) first on
earth

Adanna (Spanish) beautiful
baby
Adana

Adar (Hebrew) respected

Adara (Greek) lovely
Adarah, Adrah

Addison (English) awesome
*Addeson, Addie, Addisen,
Addison, Addy, Addyson,
Adeson, Adisen, Adison*

Addy (English) nickname for
Addison: distinctive; smiling
*Addee, Addie, Addy, Addye,
Adie, Ady*

Adea (English) decorative

Adeen (American) decorated
*Addy, Adeene, Aden, Adene,
Adin*

Adekunle (African) crowned
at sea

Adela (Polish) peacemaker

Adelaida (Spanish) noble

Adelaide (German) calming;
distinguished
*Ada, Adalaid, Adalaide,
Adelade, Adelaid, Laidey*

Adelbola (Spanish) brave

Adeline (English) sweet
*Adaline, Adealline, Adelenne,
Adelina, Adelind, Adlin, Adline*

Adelita (Spanish) form of
Adela: peacemaker
*Adalina, Adalita, Adelaina,
Adelaine, Adeleta, Adey,
Audilita, Lita, Lite*

Adelka (German) form of
Adelaide: calming;
distinguished
*Addie, Addy, Adel, Adelkah,
Adie*

Adelle (German) giving
Adel, Adell, Addy

Adelpha (Greek) beloved
sister
Adelfa, Adelphe

Adena (Hebrew) precious
*Ada, Adenna, Adina, Adynna,
Deena, Dena*

Adeniji (Biblical) believer

Adern (Welsh) birdlike
Adyrn

Aderyn (Hebrew) form of
Adira: strong

Adesina (African) threshold
child

Adess (Hebrew) decorated

Adhelia (Spanish) of the stars

Adia (African) God's gift

Adiel (African) goat; tough-
willed
Adie, Adiell, Adiella

Adil (English) noble born

Adina (Hebrew) high hopes
Addy, Adeen, Adeena, Adine, Deena, Dena, Dina

Adira (Hebrew) strong

Adisa (Hispanic) friendly
Adesa, Adissa

Aditi (Hindi) free

Adiva (Arabic) gracious

Adjanys (Hispanic) lively
Adjanice, Adjanis

Adline (German) reliable
Addee, Addie, Addy, Adleen, Adlene, Adlyne

Adolpha (German) noble wolf; strong girl
Adolpham

Adonia (Greek) beauty
Adona, Adonea, Adoniah, Adonis

Adora (Latin) adored child
Adorae, Adoray, Dora, Dore, Dorey, Dori, Dorree, Dorrie, Dorry

Adoracion (Spanish) adores

Adoraia (Spanish) adoration

Adoral (Spanish) adored baby

Adoria (Spanish) adored

Adorna (Latin) adorned

Adra (Greek) beauty

Adria (Latin) place name
Adrea

Adrian (English) rich
Adrien, Adryan, Adryen

Adriana (Latin) rich; exotic
Addy, Adree, Adrianna, Adrie, Adrin, Anna

Adrienne (Latin) wealthy
Adreah, Adreanne, Adrenne, Adriah, Adrian, Adrien, Adrienn, Adrin, Adrina

Aegle (Greek) radiant

Aereale (Hebrew) form of Ariel: God's lion
Aereal, Aeriel, Areale

Aerena (Welsh) feminine form of Aaron: revered; sharer

Aeronwenn (Welsh) white; aggressor
Awynn

Affrica (Irish) nice

Afiniti (American) affinity

Afiny (Hebrew) doe

Afra (Arabic) deer; lithe
Aphra, Aphrah, Ayfara

Afra (Arabic) reddish

Africa (Place name) continent
Afrika

Afton (English) confident
Aft, Aftan, Aften, Aftie

Afua (African) baby born on Friday
Afuah

Agafi (Greek) form of Agnes: pure
Ag, Aga, Agafee, Agaffi, Aggie

Agapi (Greek) love
Agapay, Agappe, Agape

Agasha (Greek) form of Agatha: kindhearted
Agashah, Agashe

Agata (Italian) good girl

Agate (English) gemstone; precious girl
Agatte, Aget, Aggey, Aggie

Agatha (Greek) kindhearted
Agath, Agathah, Agathe, Aggey, Aggie, Aggy

Agatta (Greek) form of
Agatha: kindhearted
Ag, Agata, Agathi, Aggie, Agi,
Agoti, Agotti

Agave (Botanical) strong-
spined; genus of plants
Ag, Agavay, Aggie, Agovay

Agentina (Spanish) form of
Argentina: confident; land of
silver
Agen, Agente, Tina

Aggie (Greek) kindhearted
Aggee, Aggy

Aggieth (English) form of
Agnes: pure

Aglae (French) splendid

Aglaia (Greek) goddess of
beauty; splendid

Agnes (Greek) pure
Ag, Aggie, Aggnes, Aggy, Agnas,
Agnes, Agness, Agnie, Agnus,
Nessie

Agnesa (Spanish) pure

Aharona (Hebrew) beloved
Arni, Arnina, Arona

Ahimsa (Hindu) virtuous

Ahisa (Spanish) pure

Ahtena (Hebrew) aware

Ahulani (Hawaiian) heavenly
place

Ahvanti (African) focused
Avanti

Aida (Arabic) gift
Aeeda, Ayda, Ayeeda, Ieeda

Aidan (Irish) form of the
masculine name Aidan: bold
spirit
Aden, Aiden, Aidyn

Aileen (Gaelic) fair-haired
beauty
Aleen, Alene, Alenee, Aline,
Allee, Alleen, Allene, Allie, Ally

Ailey (Irish) form of Aileen:
fair-haired beauty
Aila, Ailee, Ailie, Ailli, Allie

Ailsa (Irish) noble

Aimee (French) beloved
Aime, Aimey, Aimi, Aimme,
Amee, Amy

Aimer (German) leader; loved
Aimery, Ame, Amie

Ainda (American) sure

Aine (Irish) blissful
Ayne

Ainsley (Scottish) meadow;
outdoorsy
Ainslea, Ainslee, Ainsleigh,
Ainslie, Anes, Anslie, Aynslee,
Aynsley

Aintre (Irish) joyous estate
Aintree, Aintrey, Antre, Antry

Aisha (Arabic) life; lively
Aaisha, Aaysha, Aeesha,
Aiesha, Aieshah, Ayeesha,
Ayisha, Aysha, Ieashia,
Ieeshah, Iesha

Aisha (Arabic) living

Aisling (Irish) dreamy
Aislinn, Ashling, Isleen

Aislinn (Irish) dreamy
Aisling, Aislyn, Aislynn

Aislinning (Irish) dreamy

Aithne (Irish) fiery
Aine, Eithne, Ena, Ethne

Aja (English) leads

Ajalae (Egyptian) leader

Aka (Hawaiian) regal

Akako (Japanese) red; blushes

Akala (Hawaiian) respected

Akiva (African) morning's baby

Aky (American) lively

Ala (Arabic) excellent
Alla

Alabama (Place name) western
Bama

Alaine (Gaelic) lovely
Alaina, Alaiyne, Alenne, Aleyna, Aleyne, Allaine, Allayne

Alala (Roman mythology) sister of Mars; protected
Alalah

Alalia (German) joyful

Alama (American) lovely

Alameda (Spanish) poplar tree; growth

Alana (Scottish) pretty girl
Alahna, Alahnah, Alaina, Alainah, Alanah, Alanna, Alannah, Allana, Allie, Ally

Alanie (Hawaiian) peace

Alanis (French) shining star
Alaniss, Alannis, Alannys, Alanys

Alaoha (American) dear child

Alason (German) form of Allison: kindhearted
Ala, Alas

Alathea (English) heals and helps
Aleta, Letitia, Letty

Alaula (English) heals and helps

Alaygrah (Invented) form of Allegra: snappy
Alay, Allay

Alaytheea (Invented) form of Alethea: truthful
Alay, Thea, Theea

Alba (Italian) white

Alberta (French) bright-eyed
Alb, Albertah, Albie, Albirta, Alburta, Bertie, Berty

Albertina (Portuguese) bright

Albertine (English) feminine form of Albert: distinguished
Albertyne, Albie, Albyrtine, Teeny

Albie (American)
Albee, Albey, Alby, Albye

Albina (Italian) white
Albyna

Alcina (Greek) magical; strong-willed
Alcee, Alcie, Als, Alsena, Alsie. Cina, Seena, Sina

Alda (German) the older child

Aldine (Place name) elder

Aldona (American) sweet
Aldone

Alea (Arabic) excellent
Alaya, Aleah, Aleeah, Alia, Ally

Alechia (Greek) everlasting

Aleeza (Hebrew) joy
Aliza

Alegria (Spanish) beautiful movement
Allegria

Alejandra (Spanish) defender
Alijandra, Alyjandra

Alejandrina (Spanish) defender of friends

Aleksandra (Russian) form of Alexandra: defender of mankind

Alencia (German) cleansed

Aleshia (Greek) honest
Aleeshia, Aleeshya, Aleshya,
Alyshia, Alyshya

Alessa (Italian) helper
Alesa

Alessandra (Italian) form of
Alexandra: defender of
mankind
Aless, Alessa

Alessia (Italian) nice
Alesha, Alyshia, Allyshia

Alethea (Greek) truthful
Alathea, Aleethia, Aletha,
Aletie, Altheia, Lathea, Lathey

Aletta (Greek) carefree
Aleta, Aletta, Eletta, Letti,
Lettie, Letty

Aleviyah (Arabic) helpful

Alex (English) protector

Alexa ○ (Greek) form of
Alexandra: defender of
mankind
Alecksa, Aleksah, Alex, Alexia,
Alixa, Alyxa

Alexandra ○ (Greek)
defender of mankind
Alejandra, Alejaundro, Alex,
Alexandrah, Alexandria,
Alexis, Alezandra, Allesandro,
Ally, Lex, Lexi, Lexie

Alexandrine (French) helpful
Alexandrie, Alex, Ally, Lexi,
Lexie

Alexcia (English) gracious

Alexi (Greek) form of Alexis:
defender of mankind
Alexie, Alexy, Alixi, Alixie,
Alixy, Alyxi, Alyxie

Alexia (Greek) helpful; bright
Alexea, Alexiah, Alixea, Lex,
Lexey, Lexie, Lexy

Alexina (Scottish) helper

Alexis ○ ⊙ (Greek) form of
Alexandra: defender of
mankind
Aleksus, Alexius, Alexus,
Alexys, Lex, Lexey, Lexi, Lexie,
Lexis, Lexus

Alfonsith (German)
aggressive
Alf, Alfee, Alfey, Alfey, Alfie,
Alfonsine, Allfrie, Alphonsine,
Alphonsith

Alfre (English) form of
Alfreda: wise advisor
Alfree, Alfrey, Alfri, Alfrie, Alfry

Alfreda (English) wise advisor
Alfi, Alfie, Alfred, Alfredah,
Alfrede, Alfredeh, Freda, Freddy

Alfreida (English) wisdom

Algorita (Spanish) eager

Ali (Greek) form of Alexandra:
defender of mankind
Aley, Allee, Alley, Ally, Aly

Alia (Arabic) sky girl

Alianet (Spanish) honest;
noble
Alia, Aliane

Alice (Greek) honest
Alece, Alicea, Alise, Alliss, Ally,
Allys, Alyse, Alysse, Lisie, Lisy,
Lysse

Alicea (Spanish) noble

Alicha (Slavic) joy

Alicia (Greek) delicate; lovely
Alisha

Alida (Greek) stylish
Aleda, Aleta, Aletta, Alidah,
Alita, Lee, Lida, Lita, Lyda

Alima (Hebrew) strong

Alin (Scottish) lovely

Alina (Slavic) form of Helen:
beautiful; light
*Aleena, Alene, Aline, Allene,
Allie, Ally, Allyne, Alyna, Lena,
Lina*

Alinalette (Spanish) noble

Aline (Polish) form of Alina:
beautiful; light

Alisa (Hebrew) happy
Alissa, Allisa, Allissah, Alyssa

Alisha (Greek) happy;
truthful
*Aleesha, Alesha, Alicia, Ally,
Allyshah, Alysha, Lesha, Lisha*

Alison (Scottish) noble
Alisen

Alissa (Greek) pretty
*Alesa, Alessa, Alise, Alissah,
Allee, Allie, Ally, Allyssa,
Alyssea*

Alita (Native American)
sparkling

Alix (Greek) form of
Alexandra: defender of
mankind

Aliya (Hebrew) rises;
sweetheart
Aleeya, Alya

Aliza (Jewish) joy child

Alka (Polish) distinctive
Alk, Alkae

Alke (English) form of Elke:
distinguished

Allaire (Scottish) open-
minded

Allegra (Italian) snappy
*Aligra, All, Allagrah, Allie,
Alligra, Ally*

Allena (Greek) outstanding
*Alena, Alenah, Allana, Allie,
Ally*

Allene (Greek) wonderful
Alene, Alyne

Allesia (English) alyssum
flower girl

Allessandra (Italian)
kindhearted
Allesandra

Allicent (English) form of
Alice: honest

Allie (Greek) smiling
Ali, Allee, Alli, Ally, Allye

Allison ○ ✿ (English)
kindhearted
*Alisen, Alison, Allicen, Allie,
Allisan, Allisen, Allisun, Ally,
Allysen, Allyson, Alysen,
Alyson, Sonny*

Allura (Hispanic) alluring
Alura

Ally (Greek) pure heart
Allee, Alleigh, Alley, Alli, Allie

Allyson (English) another
form of Allison: sweet
*Alisaune, Allysen, Allysun,
Alyson*

Allysse (Greek) smooth
Allice, Allyce, Allyss

Alma (Latin) good; soulful
Almah, Almie, Almy

Almaree (Spanish) smart

Almeida (Spanish) shines;
goal-oriented

Almeria (Arabic) princess
*Alma, Almara, Almaria,
Almer, Almurea, Als*

Almira (Arabic) princess
*Allmeerah, Almirah, Elmira,
Mira*

Alodia (Spanish) thrives; free

Alodie (Origin unknown)
thriving
Alodee

Aloha (Hawaiian) love

Aloma (Jewish) form of
Alona: defends fellow man

Alona (Jewish) sturdy oak
Allona

Alonda (Spanish) form of
Alexandra: defender of
mankind
Alona

Alondra (Spanish) bright
Alond, Alondre, Alonn

Alouette (French) birdlike
*Allie, Allo, Allou, Allouetta,
Alou, Alowette*

Aloyse (German) renowned
Aloice, Aloise, Aloyce

Alpha (Greek) first; superior
*Alf, Alfa, Alfie, Alph, Alphah,
Alphia, Alphie*

Alphareen (Spanish) first
chosen

Alston (English) a place for a
noble
*Allie, Ally, Alstan, Alsten,
Alstun*

Alta (Latin) high place; fresh

Altagracia (Spanish) in God's
grace

Altea (Polish) healer

Althaea (Greek) pure

Althea (Greek) wholesome
*Althe, Althey, Althia, Althie,
Althy, Thea, They*

Altisha (English) other girl

Alula (Arabic) little maiden
girl

Alundey (American) jaunty

Alva (Spanish) fair; bright
Alvah

Alvada (American) evasive
Alvadah, Alvayda

Alverna (English) elf friend
Alver, Alverne, Alvernette

Alvernise (English) form of
Alverna: elf friend
Alvenice

Alvina (English) beloved;
friendly
*Alvee, Alveena, Alvie, Alvine,
Alvy*

Alvinetta (English) popular
friend

Alvita (Latin) charismatic

Alyasha (Arabic) heaven's
child

Alyda (French) soaring
Aleda, Alida, Alita, Lida, Lyda

Alynn (Dutch) intelligent

Alys (English) noble

Alysea (English) high-born

Alysia (Greek) compelling
*Aleecia, Alesha, Alicia, Alish,
Alycia*

Alyssa ✪ (Greek) flourishing
*Alissa, Allissa, Allissae, Ilyssah,
Lissa, Lyssa, Lyssy*

Alysse (English) form of
Alice: honest

Alyx (English) form of Alex:
protector

Amaba (African) amiable

Amabe (Latin) loved
Ama

Amabelle (American) loved
Amabel, Amahbel

Amada (Spanish) form of
Amanda: fit to be loved
Ama, Amadah

Amal (Arabic) optimistic
Amahl

Amalia (Hungarian/Spanish)
industrious

Amalina (German) worker
*Am, Ama, Amaleen, Amaline,
Amalyne*

Amalita (Spanish) hopeful

Amalthea (Greek) perseveres

Amanda ✪ (Latin) fit to be
loved
*Amand, Amandah, Amandy,
Manda, Mandee, Mandi,
Mandy*

Amandra (American) form of
Amanda: fit to be loved
*Amand, Mandee, Mandi,
Mandra, Mandree, Mandry,
Mandy*

Amara (Latin) everlasting
*Am, Amarah, Amareh, Amera,
Amura, Mara*

Amarillo (Spanish) yellow
*Ama, Amari, Amarilla, Amy,
Rillo*

Amaris (Hebrew) beloved;
dedicated
Amares

Amaryllis (Greek) fresh
flower
Ama, Amarillis

Amber (French) gorgeous
and golden; semiprecious
stone
*Ambar, Amberre, Ambur,
Amburr*

Ambike (Hindi) fertile

Amboree (Last name as first
name) precocious
Ambor, Ambree

Ambre (French) kinetic
energy

Ambree (French) amber color

Ambrin (Greek) long life

Ambrosette (Greek) eternal
*Amber, Ambie, Ambro,
Ambrosa, Ambrose*

Ambrosia (Greek) eternal
*Ambroze, Ambrozeah,
Ambrozia*

Ambrosina (Greek)
everlasting
Ambrosine

Amelia ✪ (German)
industrious
*Amalee, Amaylyuh, Amele,
Ameleah, Ameli, Amelie,
Amelya, Amilia*

Amelina (Spanish) diligent

Ameline (French) diligent

Amelita (Spanish) diligent

Amera (Arabic) of regal birth
Ameera, Amira

America (American) patriotic
*Amer, Amerca, Americah,
Amerika, Amur*

Ameth (Greek) precious gem;
Amethyst

Amethyst (Greek) precious
gem
Amathist, Ameth

Amia (German) loved

Amica (Latin) good friend
Ameca, Ami, Amika

Amici (Italian) friend
Amicie, Amie, Amisie

Amie (French) loved one

Amig (Slavic) loved

Amiga (Spanish) friend
Amigah

Amilla (Slavic) form of
Camilla: wonderful

Amina (Arabic) trustworthy
Amena, Amine

Aminta (Latin) protects

Amira (Arabic) nurturer

Amirreza (Spanish) eloquent

Amity (Latin) a good friend
Amitee, Amitey, Amiti

Amiya (Slavic) defense

Amna (Indian) gracious

Amnette (American) haven

Amone (American) harmony

Amor (Spanish) love
Amora, Amore

Amora (Spanish) love

Amorelle (French) lover
*Amoray, Amore, Amorel,
Amorell*

Amoretta (French) little love
Amoreta, Amorreta, Amorretta

Amorette (French) tiny love
Amorrette

Amorita (Spanish) loved

Ampar (Spanish) protected

Amrita (Indian) nectar of
immortality

Amvi (Hindi) goddess

Amy ✪ (Latin) loved one
*Aimee, Amee, Amey, Ameyye,
Ami, Amie, Amye, Amye*

Amyrka (Spanish) lively
*Amerka, Amurka, Amyrk,
Amyrrka*

Anabelia (Slavic) well-loved

Anabril (Spanish) merciful;
pretty
Anabrelle, Anna, Annabril

Anadare (Hawaiian) graceful

Anahi (Biblical) responsive

Anahita (Hindi) graceful

Anaid (Slavic) kind

Anais (French) form of **Anne:**
loving; hospitable

Anala (Hindi) fiery

Analae (Hindi) excellent

Analeese (Scandinavian)
gracious
Analece, Analeece, Annaleese

Analia (Hebrew) gracious;
hopeful
*Ana, Analea, Analeah,
Analiah, Analya*

Analisa (American) lovely

Analy (American) graceful;
gracious
Analee, Anali

Anamita (Spanish) enamored

Anand (Hindi) joyful;
profound
Anan, Ananda

Anandy (Indian) joy girl

Anapua (Hawaiian)
flourishes

Anareli (Spanish) happy

Anastace (Spanish) form of
Anastasia: resurrection
*Anastayce, Anestace, Anestayce,
Anystace, Anystayce*

Anastasia (Greek)
resurrection
Anastasiya, Anastasya

Anastay (Greek) born again;
renewed
Ana, Anastae, Anastie

Anastice (Latin) form of
Anastasia: resurrection
*Anasteece, Anesteece, Anestice,
Anysteece, Anystice*

Anatola (Greek) from the
east
Anatol, Anatole

Anaysis (Latin) form of
Anastasia: resurrection
Anaysys

Anca (Scandinavian) alone

Ancheene (American)
creative

Anchoret (Welsh) beloved
girl

Ancita (Spanish) favorite

Ancret (Welsh) form of
Anchoret: beloved girl

Ander (Greek) feminine

Anders (Scandinavian)
stunning
Andars, Andie, Andurs, Andy

Andes (Greek) feminine
Andee

Andi (English) casual
Andee, Andey, Andie, Andy

Andraa (Greek) feminine
Andrah

Andrea ✪ (Greek) feminine
*Andee, Andi, Andie, Andra,
Andrae, Andre, Andreah,
Andreena*

Andreana (Greek) bold heart
*Andreanna, Andriana,
Andrianna, Andryana,
Andryanna*

Andree (Greek) strong
woman
Andrey, Andrie, Andry

Andrenna (Scottish) pretty;
gracious
Andreene, Adrena

Andrianna (Greek) feminine
Andree, Andy

Andromeda (Greek)
beautiful star
Andromedah

Aneechia (Slavic) pure

Anees (Indian) grace

Aneeta (Indian) grace

Aneith (Slavic) pure

Aneka (Polish) forgiving

Anela (Hawaiian) angelic

Anelica (Spanish) pleasant

Anelka (Slavic) forgives

Anemone (Greek) breath of
fresh air

Anetra (Slavic) gracious

Anewk (Invented) form of
Anouk: loving; hospitable

Anganetta (Slavic) angelic

Ange (Greek) form of Angela:
angelic; divine

Angeele (English) lithe angel

Angel (Latin) sweet; angelic
Angelle, Angie, Anjel, Annjell

Angela (Greek) divine;
angelic
*Angelena, Angelica, Angelina,
Angelle, Angie, Gela, Nini*

Angelia (American) angelic
messenger
Angelea, Angeliah

Angelica (Latin) angelic
messenger
*Angie, Anjeleka, Anjelica,
Anjelika, Anjie*

Angelika (Greek) angel
*Angelyka, Angilika, Angilyka,
Angylika*

Angelina ✪ (Latin) angelic
*Ange, Angelyna, Angie, Anje,
Anjelina, Anjie*

Angeline (American) angelic
Angelene, Angelline

Angelique (French) form of
Angelica: angelic messenger
*Angel, Angeleek, Angelik,
Angie, Anjee, Anjel, Anjelique*

Angelle (Latin) angelic
*Ange, Angell, Anje, Anjell,
Anjelle*

Angerona (Mythology)
angelic

Angha (Hindi) beauty

Angharad (Welsh) graceful
Angahard

Angie (Latin) angelic
Angey, Angi, Angye, Anjie

Aniani (Hawaiian) lovely
reflection

Anice (Slavic) form of Anne:
gracious

Anick (Hebrew) gracious

Aniece (Hebrew) gracious
*Ana, Anesse, Ani, Anice,
Annis, Annissa*

Aniela (Polish) sent by God
Ahneela

Anika (Hebrew) hospitable
*Anec, Anecca, Aneek, Aneeka,
Anic, Anica, Anik, Annika*

Anila (Hindi) wind girl

Anina (Aramaic) answer my
prayer

Aninda (German) form of
Anina: answer my prayer

Anisha (English) purest one
Aneesha, Anysha

Anissa (Greek) a completed
spirit
*Anisa, Anise, Anysa, Anyssa,
Anysse*

Anita (Spanish) gracious
Aneda, Aneeta, Anitta, Anyta

Anitia (Spanish) favored

Anitria (Spanish) favored

Aniyalla (Scandinavian)
beloved

Anjali (Hindi) pretty; honored
Anjaly

Anjana (Hindi) merciful;
pretty
Anjann

Anjelica (Latin) angelic
Anjelika

Anjeliett (Spanish) little
angel
*Anjel, Anjeli, Jelette, Jeliett,
Jeliette, Jell, Jelly*

Anjul (French) jovial
*Angie, Anjewel, Anji, Anjie,
Anjool*

Anka (Polish) favorite

Anmol (Hindi) valued

Ann (Hebrew) loving;
hospitable
*Aine, An, Ana, Anna, Anne,
Annie, Ayn*

Anna ✪ ✿ (Hebrew) gracious
*Ana, Anae, Anah, Annah,
Anne, Anuh*

Annabella (Italian) lovely girl
Anabela, Anabella, Annabela

Annabelle (English) lovely
girl
Anabell, Anabelle, Annabell

Annal (Slavic) form of Anna:
gracious

Annalee (English) form of
Anne: gracious

Annalie (Scandinavian) form
of Annalee: gracious

Annaliea (English) form of Annalee: gracious

Anna-Margarita (Spanish) devout

Ann-Dee (American) courage
Andee, Andey, Andi, Andy, Ann Dee, Anndi

Anne (English) gracious

Anneka (Scandinavian) form of Anne: gracious
Anneke

Annelie (German) girl of grace

Anneliese (Scandinavian/German) form of Anna: gracious, and Liesa: God is bountiful
Aneliece, Aneliese

Annella (Scottish) graceful
Anell, Anella, Anelle

Annemarie (German) bitter grace
Anmarie, Ann Marie, Anne-Marie, Annmarie

Annena (Slavic) chosen

Annes (Hebrew) hospitable

Annette (American) vivacious; giving
Anette, Ann, Anne, Annett, Annetta, Annie, Anny

Anngelite (Slavic) angel

Annice (English) pure of heart

Annie (English) form of Anne: gracious
Ann, Annee, Anney, Anni, Anny

Annika (Scandinavian) gracious
Anika

Anninka (Russian) gracious; graceful

Annis (English) pure
Annys

Annissa (Greek) gracious; complete
Anissa, Anni, Annie, Annisa

Annjanette (Mythology) quiet goddess

Annletta (English) little Ann

Annunciata (Italian) noticed

Anona (Botanical) pineapple; fresh

Anora (Latin) honored

Anouk (French) form of Ann: loving; hospitable

Anoush (Armenian) sweetness

Anselma (German) helmet of God

Ansley (English) happy in the meadow
Annesleigh, Ans, Anslea, Anslee, Ansleigh, Ansli, Anslie

Ansonia (Scandinavian) pure

Anstass (Greek) resurrected; eternal
Ans, Anstase, Stace, Stacey, Stass, Stassee

Anstice (Greek) everlasting
Anst, Steece, Steese, Stice

Answer (Word as name) the answer

Ansylene (English) God protects

Antenise (English) flowering

Anthea (Greek) flowering
Anthia

Antigone (Greek) impulsive; defiant

Antique (Word as name) old
soul
Anteek, Antik

Antoinette (French) priceless
Antoine, Antoinet, Antwanett,
Antwonette, Antwonette,
Toinette, Tonette

Antonella (French) form of
Antoinette: priceless

Antonetta (Greek) praised
Antoneta

Antonia (Latin) perfect
Antone, Antonea, Antoneah

Antonian (Latin) valuable
Antoinette, Antonetta, Toni,
Tonia, Tonya

Antonine (Greek) praised
Antonyne

Antronette (English) form of
Antoinette: priceless

Antwanette (African
American) prized
Antwan, Antwanett

Anupama (Indian) unusual

Anusha (Armenian) sweet

Anya (Russian) grace

Aoife (Irish) beauty

Apalonia (Greek) girl with
strength and light

Aphra (Hebrew) earthy;
sentimental
Af, Affee, Affey, Affy, Afra,
Aphree, Aphrie

Aphrodite (Greek) goddess of
love and beauty
Afrodite, Aphrodytee

Api (Latin) rejoice

Apolinaria (Spanish) form of
Apollonia: sun goddess
Apolinara

Apollonia (Greek) sun
goddess
Apolinia, Apolyne, Appollonia

Apple (Botanical) fruit; quirky
Apel, Appell

April (Latin) month;
springlike
Aprel, Aprile, Aprille, Apryl

Aptha (Biblical) growing

Aqua (Spanish) colorful
Akwa

Aquanetla (Invented)
spontaneous

Aqueelah (Arabic) vigilant

Aquen (Native American)
calm

Aquilline (American) eagle
eye

Arabella (Latin) answer to a
prayer; beauty
Arabel, Arabela, Arabelle,
Arbel, Arbella, Bella, Belle,
Orabele, Orabella

Arabelle (Latin) divine
Arabell

Araceli (Latin) heavenly
Ara, Aracelli, Ari

Aracelle (Spanish)
flamboyant; heavenly
Ara, Aracel, Aracell, Araseli,
Celi

Arachne (Greek) weaver;
spider

Araiza (Spanish) innovator

Araminta (English) unique;
precious dawn
Ara, Arama, Aramynta, Minta

Araxie (Spanish) creative

Arayalle (English) form of
Arielle: God's lion

Araylia (Latin) golden
Araelea, Aray, Rae, Ray

Arbela (Biblical) place name

Arbra (American) form of
Abra: example; lesson
Arbrae

Arce (Spanish) gift

Arcelia (Spanish) treasured
Arcey, Arci, Arcilia, Arla, Arlia

Arcelious (African American)
treasured
*Arce, Arcel, Arcelus, Arcy,
Arselious*

Archana (Indian) loyal
worshipper

Archon (American) capable
Arch, Archee, Archi, Arshon

Ardana (English) ardent

Ardath (Hebrew) ardent
Ardee, Ardie, Ardith, Ardon

Ardele (Latin) enthusiastic;
dedicated
Ardell, Ardella, Ardelle, Ardine

Ardelphia (Place name)
flourishes

Arden (Latin) ardent; sincere
*Ardan, Ardena, Ardin, Ardon,
Ardyn*

Ardery (English) form of
Arden: ardent; sincere

Ardiana (Spanish) ardent
Ardi, Ardie, Diana

Ardie (American)
enthusiastic; special
Ardee, Ardi

Ardienne (American) ardent

Ardina (English) ardent

Ardithan (American) sincere

Ardyss (American) ardent

Areika (Spanish) pure
Areka, Areke, Arika, Arike

Arekah (Greek) virtuous;
loving

Arelie (Latin) golden girl
Arelee, Arely, Arlea

Aretha (Greek) virtuous;
vocalist
Areetha

Aretta (Greek) virtuous
Arette, Arie

Argelia (Spanish) treasured

Argenta (Latin) silver

Argentina (Place name)
confident; land of silver
*Arge, Argen, Argent, Argenta,
Argie, Tina, Tinee*

Argosy (French) bright
Argosee, Argosie

Argus (Greek) bright
Arguss

Ari (Hebrew) form of Ariel:
God's lion
Aree, Arey, Arie, Ary

Aria (Hebrew) form of Ariel:
God's lion
Arya

Aria (English) song

Ariadna (Slavic) holiest

Ariadne (Greek) holiness
Aryadne

Ariana ✪ (Greek) righteous
Arianna

Arianda (Greek) helper
Ariand

Ariane (Greek) very gracious
Arianne, Aryahn

Arianne (French) kind
Ana, Ari, Ariann

Arianwen (Welsh) form of
Aeronwenn: white; aggressor

Arica (Scandinavian) form of
Erica: honorable; leading
others

Aridatha (Hebrew)
flourishing
Ar, Arid, Datha

Aridna (English) form of
Ariadne: holiness

Aridne (English) form of
Ariadne: holiness

Ariedsol (Spanish) blessed

Ariel (Hebrew) God's lion
Aeriel, Airey, Arielle

Ariella (French) lioness
Ariela, Aryela, Aryella

Aries (Latin) zodiac sign of
the ram; contentious
Arees

Arin (Arabic) spreads truth
Aryn

Arina (Russian) peaceful

Aris (Greek) best

Arisca (Greek) form of Arista:
wonderful
Ariska, Ariske, Arista

Arista (Greek) wonderful

Aristelle (Greek) wonder
Aristela, Aristella

Arith (Hebrew) believes

Aritha (Greek) virtuous
Arete, Aretha

Arizona (Place name) U.S.
state; grand
Zona

Arketta (Invented) outspoken
Arkett, Arkette, Arky

Arlais (Welsh) magical

Arlanda (Slavic) dedicated

Arlea (Greek) heavenly
*Airlea, Arlee, Arleigh, Arlie,
Arly*

Arleana (American) form of
Arlene: dedicated
Arlena, Arlina

Arlen (Irish) devoted
Arlin, Arlyn

Arlena (Irish) dedicated
*Arlana, Arlen, Arlenna, Arlie,
Arlina, Arlyna, Arrlina, Lena,
Lina, Linney*

Arlene (Irish) dedicated
*Arlee, Arleen, Arlie, Arline,
Arlyne, Arlynn, Lena, Lina*

Arlette (French) loyal
Arlet

Arli (English) proactive; girl
from rabbit field

Arlind (American) strong;
loyal

Arlitra (American) strength of
character

Arlyn (Irish) dedicated

Armanda (French)
disciplined

Armani (Italian) fashionable
*Armanee, Armanie, Armond,
Armonee, Armoni, Armonie*

Armanth (English)
goal-oriented

Armelle (French) armed

Armetrice (Spanish) armed

Armida (Latin) armed;
prepared
Armi, Armid, Army

Arminda (Spanish) armed

Armineh (Slavic) defends

Arminell (Latin) nobility
Arminel

Arminta (Slavic) armed

Arna (Slavic) eagle watch
Arnetta

Arnette (English) little eagle; observant
Arn, Arnee, Arnet, Arnett, Ornette

Arnica (American) eagle; intense

Arnite (American) eagle; intense

Arnyx (American) eagle-eyed

Arosa (Spanish) rose

Arosell (Last name as first name) loyal
Arosel

Arpine (Romanian) dedicated
Arpyne

Array (Word as name) colorful

Arrissie (American) the sea

Artemis (Greek) moon goddess

Artemisia (Greek) belonging to artemis
Arta, Arte, Artema

Arthel (Greek) rich

Arthlese (Irish) rich
Arth, Arthlice, Artis

Arthurena (American) feminine form of Arthur: bear; stone
Arthurene

Artranese (American) hunts

Artriece (Irish) stable
Artee, Artreese, Arty

Artulia (Spanish) high position

Aruna (Hindi) baby of dawn

Arunice (English) silver girl

Arvilla (English) climber

Arvis (American) special
Arvee, Arvess, Arvie, Arviss, Arvy

Arya (Jewish) lioness

Aryana (English) form of Ariana: righteous

Asabi (African) outstanding

Asalia (Spanish) morning child

Asenath (Biblical) possessed of God's spirit

Ash (Hebrew) form of Asha: lucky
Ashe

Asha (Hebrew) lucky
Aasha, Ashah, Ashra

Ashandra (African American) dreamer
Ashan, Ashandre

Ashanti (African) graceful
Ashantay, Anshante

Ashantia (American) outgoing
Ashantea, Ashantiah

Asharaf (Hindi) wishful
Asha, Ashara

Ashby (English) farm of ash trees
Ashbee

Asher (Hebrew) blessed
Ash

Ashla (English) form of Ashley: woodland sprite

Ashland (Irish) dreamlike
Ashelyn, Ashlan, Ashleen, Ashlin, Ashlind, Ashline, Ashlinn

Ashlei (English) form of Ashley: woodland sprite
Ashee, Ashie, Ashly, Ashy

Ashleigh (English) from the ash tree meadow
Ashlynn, Ashton

Ashley ✿ ☯ (English) woodland sprite
Ash, Ashie, Ashlay, Ashlea, Ashlee, Ashleigh, Ashli, Ashlie, Ashly

Ashlyn (English) natural
Ashlin, Ashlinn, Ashlynn

Ashna (Indian) hopeful

Ashonika (African American) pretty
Ashon, Ashoneka, Shon

Ashton (English) from an eastern town; sassy
Ashe, Ashten, Ashtun, Ashtyn

Asia (Greek) sunrise
Ashah, Asiah, Asya, Aysia, Azhuh

Asli (Turkish) authentic

Asma (Arabic) exalted; loyal

Asmay (Origin unknown) special
Asmae, Asmaye

Asmillinda (Spanish) loyal

Asminda (Arabic) loyal

Asoka (Japanese) morning baby

Asp (Greek) form of Aspasia: witty

Aspasia (Greek) witty
Aspashia, Aspasya

Aspen (Place name) city in Colorado; earth mother
Aspin, Aspyn, Azpen

Asphodel (Greek) lily beauty

Asra (Hindi) pure
Azra

Asrika (Slavic) striking

Asta (Greek) star

Astar (Greek) starry-eyed

Astera (Greek) starlike
Asteria, Astra, Astree, Astrie

Astra (Greek) starlike
Astrah, Astrey

Astraea (Greek) starlike

Astrid (Scandinavian/German) fair; beautiful goddess
Aster, Asti, Astred, Astri, Astridd, Astryd, Astrydd, Atty, Estrid

Asusena (Slavic) lovely fragrance

Asysa (Arabic) lively
Aesha, Asha, Aysah

Atalanta (Greek) athletic; fleet-footed
Addi, Atlante, Attie

Atanasia (Spanish) form of the name Anatasia: devout
Reborn

Atara (Hebrew) crowned

Athalet (American) believes

Athalia (Hebrew) ambitious

Athamadia (Greek) believer

Athelean (Greek) eternal; precocious
Athey, Athi

Athena (Greek) wise woman; goddess of wisdom in mythology
Athene, Athenea, Athina, Xena, Zena

Athene (Chinese) wise

Atherine (Spanish) form of Katherine: pure

Athie (Hebrew) wise
Athee, Athey, Athy

Athinoulla (American)
praiseworthy

Atianna (American) believer

Atifa (Arabic) compassionate
Ateefah

Atornett (American)
off-center

Atropos (Mythology) one of
the Greek Fates; cutter

Atu (American) treasured

Aube (French) form of
Aubrey: ruler

Auber (French) bright

Aubrey (French/German)
ruler
*Aubery, Aubey, Aubrea, Aubree,
Aubreye, Aubri, Aubrie, Aubry*

Auburne (American) tough-
minded
*Aubee, Aubern, Auberne,
Aubey, Aubi, Aubie, Auburn,
Auby*

Auden (English) oldest friend

Audia (French) noble

Audie (English) noble
strength
*Audee, Audey, Audi, Audy,
Audye*

Audra (English) exciting
Audrah, Audray

Audrea (English) highborn

Audrette (French) highborn

Audrey ✪ (Old English)
strong and regal
*Audi, Audie, Audra, Audree,
Audreen, Audreye, Audri,
Audrianna, Audrianne, Audrie,
Audrina, Audry*

Augusta (Latin) revered
*Augustah, Auguste, Augustia,
Augustyna, Austina*

Augustene (English) serious

Augustina (Latin) great
*Agustico, Agustin, Augusine,
Augustine, Gusty, Tina, Tino*

Augustine (Latin) dignified;
worthwhile
*Augestinn, Augusta, Augustina,
Augustyna, Augustyne, Austie,
Austina, Austine, Tina*

Aundra (Scandinavian)
highborn

Aunjanue (French) sparkling

Aunshaunte (African
American) believer
*Anshauntay, Aunshauntay,
Aunshawntay, Aunshawnte,
Shauntae, Shauntay, Shaunte*

Aunzell (American) magical

Aupra (Slavic) form of Audra:
exciting

Aura (Greek) breeze
Arra

Aurelia (Latin) dawn goddess
*Arelia, Aura, Auralea, Aurel,
Aurelie, Auria, Auriel, Aurielle*

Aurelien (Slavic) golden
ornament

Aurian (English) form of
Arianne: kind

Auriel (Latin) gold
Auriol

Auristela (Latin) star

Aurora (Latin) morning glow
Aurorah, Aurore, Rory

Aury (American) golden dawn

Aurysia (Latin) gold
Arys, Arysia, Aurys

Austeena (American)
statuesque
Austeenah, Austie, Austina

Austen (Literature) for author
Jane Austen; charming
Austyn

Austine (Latin) respected
Austen, Austene, Austine,
Austin

Authorea (American)
dawning

Autminia (Spanish) child of
autumn

Autra (Latin) gold

Autumn ✪ (Latin) joy of
changing seasons
Autum, Autumm

Ava ✪ ✱ (Latin) pretty;
delicate bird
Avah, Eva

Avalon (Celtic) paradise

Avedis (Spanish) welcomes

Avena (Latin) basic; oat field

Avengelica (Spanish)
avenging
Angelica, Avenga, Avengele,
Gelica

Averil (French) flighty
Ava, Averile, Averill, Averyl,
Averyll, Aviril

Avery ✪ (French) flirtatious
Avary, Averee, Averi, Averie

Aves (Greek) breath of fresh
air

Aviana (Latin) fresh

Avianca (Latin) fresh

Avino (Hebrew) believes in
God

Avis (Latin) little bird

Avisae (American) springlike
Ava, Avas, Aves, Avi

Aviva (Hebrew) springlike
Avivah

Avivi (Jewish) spring child

Avolonne (African American)
happy
Avalonn, Ave, Avelon, Avlon,
Avo, Avolon, Avolunne

Avon (English) graceful
Avaughn, Avaugn, Avonn,
Avonne

Avonnia (English) graceful;
of Avon

Avril (French) april; springlike

Avrit (Hebrew) fresh
Avie, Avree, Avret, Avrie

Awen (Welsh) wise and gentle

Axelle (French) serene
Axel, Axell

Aya (Hebrew) bird in flight

Ayan (Hindi) pure
Ayun

Ayanna (Hindi) innocent
Ayunna

Ayda (Arabic) comes back

Ayeisha (Arabic) feminine
Aeesha, Aieshah, Asha,
Ayeeshea, Ayisa, Iasha, Yeisha,
Yeishee, Yisha, Yishie

Ayena (Native American)
joyful; pure

Ayesha (Arabic) living

Ayla (Hebrew) strong as an
oak

Aylee (Hebrew) light

Ayleen (Hebrew) lighthearted
Aylene

Aylin (Spanish) strong
Aylen

Aylun (Hebrew) strong

Aylwin (Welsh) beloved
Ayle, Aylwie

Aynet (Spanish) grace

Aynona (Hebrew) form of
Anne: gracious
*Ayn, Aynon, Aynonna,
Aynonne*

Ayo (African) joyful

Ayva (American) form on
Ava: pretty; delicate

Azadeth (Biblical) form of
Asenath: possessed of God's
spirit

Azalea (Latin) earthy;
flowering
Azalee, Azelea

Azalia (Spanish) flower girl

Azami (Japanese) flower

Azenet (Spanish) sun God's
gift
Aza, Azey

Azenett (Spanish) God's child

Azimah (Japanese) azami:
flower

Aziza (African) beloved;
vibrant
Asisa

Azriella (Hebrew) form of
Ariella: lioness
Azriela, Azryela, Azryella

Azsure (American) form of
Azure: blue-eyed

Azucena (Spanish) lily pure
Azu, Azuce, Azucina

Azura (French) blue-eyed
*Azuhre, Azur, Azure, Azurre,
Azzura*

B

Baako (Japanese) promising;
happy

Baba (American) fun-loving

Babe (Latin) little darling;
baby

Babette (French) little
Barbara

Babs (American) form of
Barbara: traveler from a
foreign land

Baca (Biblical) place name;
happy

Bachi (Japanese) happy
Bachee, Bachey, Bachie, Bochee

Bachiko (Japanese) happy

Baden (German) friendly
Boden, Bodey

Baderinwa (African) worthy

Badger (Irish) badger
Badge

Badri (African) moon baby

Badriyyah (Arabic) surprise

Baek (Origin unknown)
mysterious

Baffin (Place name)

Bagent (Last name as first
name) baggage
Bage

Bagula (German) enthused

Bahaar (Hindi) spring

Bahama (Place name)
islands; sun-loving
Baham

Bahati (African) lucky girl
Baha, Bahah

Bahija (Arabic) excelling
Bahiga

Bahir (Arabic) striking
Bah, Baheer, Bahi

Bahira (Arabic) bright mind

Bai (Chinese) outgoing

Baiben (Irish) sweet; exotic
*Babe, Babe, Bai, Baib, Baibe,
Baibie, Baibin*

Bailey (English) bailiff
Bailee, Baylee, Bayley, Baylie

Bailon (American) form of
Bailey: bailiff
Bai, Baye, Baylon

Bain (American) thorn; pale
Baine, Bane, Bayne

Baird (Irish) ballad singer
Bayrde

Bairn (Scottish) child
Bairne

Baka (Hindi) crane; long-
legged
Baca

Bakara (African) noble

Bakul (Hindi) flowering
Bakula

Bakura (Hebrew) ripe; prime
Bikura

Balala (Hindi) hopes

Balaniki (Hawaiian) angelic

Balbina (Latin) stammers
Balbine

Baldree (German) brave;
loquacious
Baldry

Bali (Place name) island near
Indonesia; exotic

Balinda (Slavic) form of
Belinda: beautiful

Ballou (American) outspoken
Bailou, Balou

Balvino (Spanish) powerful
Balvene, Balveno

Bambi (Italian) childlike;
baby girl
*Bambee, Bambie, Bambina,
Bamby*

Banan (Punjabi) held close

Banht (Hindi) fire

Banita (Hindi) girl;
thoughtful

Banjoko (Asian) joy

Banner (Word as name)
flamboyant

Bano (Persian) bride
*Bannie, Banny, Banoah,
Banoh*

Bao (Chinese) adorable;
creative

Bao-Jin (Chinese) precious
gold

Bao-Yo (Chinese) jade; pretty

Baptista (Latin) one who
baptizes
*Baptiste, Batista, Battista,
Bautista*

Bara (Hebrew) chosen
Bari, Barra

Barb (Latin) form of Barbara:
traveler from a foreign land

Barbara (Greek) traveler from
a foreign land
*Babb, Babbett, Babbette, Babe,
Babett, Babette, Babina,
Babita, Babs, Barb, Barbary,
Barbe, Barbette, Barbey, Barbi,
Barbie, Barbra, Barby, Basha,
Basia, Bobbie, Bobi*

Barbarette (English) form of
Barbara: traveler from a
foreign land

Barbrette (English) ill-fated

Barbro (Swedish) extraordinary
Bar, Barb, Barbar

Barcelona (Place name) city in Spain; exotic
Barce, Lona

Barcie (American) sassy
Barsey, Barsi

Bariah (Arabic) does well

Barika (Hebrew) chosen one

Barkait (Arabic) shines
Barkat

Baronetta (English) feminine form of Baron: noble leader

Barran (Arabic) song

Barrent (Last name as first name) hill child

Barrett (Last name as first name) happy girl
Bari, Barret, Barrette, Barry, Berrett

Barrie (Irish) markswoman; *form of masculine name Barry*

Barron (Last name as first name) bright
Bare, Baron, Barrie, Beren, Beron

Barrow (Last name as first name) sharp; sly
Barow

Basey (Last name as first name) beauty
Bacie, Basi

Bashiyra (Arabic) joyful

Basia (Greek) regal
Basha, Basya

Basilia (Greek) regal
Basila, Basilea, Basilie

Basimah (Arabic) smiling
Basima, Basma

Baskama (Biblical) place name; fragrant

Bassen (American) queen

Bastienna (French) form of masculine name Bastien: respected
Bastee, Bastienne

Bat (German) female warrior
Bet

Bathia (German) warrior woman
Basha, Baspa, Batia, Batya, Bitya

Bathilda (German) woman in war
Bathild, Bathilde, Berthilda, Berthilde

Bathsheba (Hebrew) beautiful; daughter of Sheba
Bathseva, Batsheba, Batsheva, Batshua, Sheba

Bathshira (Arabic) happy; seventh

Batia (Hebrew) daughter of God
Batea, Batya

Batice (American) warrior; attractive
Bateese, Batese, Batiece, Batty

Batini (African) ponders much

Batzra (Hebrew) daughter of God

Bay (Vietnamese) saturday's child; patient; unique
Bae, Baye

Bayani (Indian) joy

Bayla (Indian) young girl
Bala

Baylor (French) of the bay; water-loving
Bayler

Baynes (American) feminine form of Baines: pale
Bain, Baines, Bayne

Bayo (African) bringing joy

Bayonne (Greek) joyful victor
Bay, Baye, Bayonn, Bayonna, Bayunn

Bea (American) form of Beatrice: blessed woman

Beama (English) blessed

Beata (German) blessed
Bayahta, Beate

Beatha (Latin) blessed
Betha

Beatrice (Latin) blessed woman
Beat, Beatrisa, Beatrise, Reattie, Bebe, Bee, Beitris, Beitriss, Bibi, Treece, Trice

Beatrix (Latin) happy

Beatriz (Spanish) form of Beatrice: blessed woman

Bebe (French) baby
Babee, Baby, Bebee

Bebhinn (Irish) sweet girl

Becca (Hebrew) form of Rebecca: loyal
Bekka

Becerra (Spanish) safe haven

Bechira (Hebrew) chosen child

Becky (English) form of Rebecca: loyal
Becki, Beki

Bedelia (Irish) form of Bridget: powerful

Bedriska (Irish) form of Bedelia: powerful

Bee (American) form of Beatrice: blessed woman

Beegee (American) laidback; calm
B.G., Begee, Be-Gee

Beeja (Hindi) the beginning; happy
Beej

Bee-Sun (Filipino) nature-loving; glad
Bee Sun

Bego (Hispanic) spunky
Beago

Begonia (Botanical) flower

Behira (Hebrew) shines

Behorah (Invented) friend
Be, Behi, Behie, Behora

Beige (American) tawny; calm
Bayge

Beige-Dawn (American) clear morning
Bayge-Dawn, Beige Dawn

Beila (Spanish) beautiful

Bejoy (American) filled with joy

Bel (Latin) beauty

Bela (Czech) white
Belah

Belann (Spanish) pretty
Bela, Belan, Belana, Belane, Belanna

Belay (English) white

Belem (Spanish) pretty
Bel, Beleme, Bella

Belems (American) relinquishes

Belen (Latin) beauty

Belgica (American) white
Belgika, Belgike, Belgyke, Bellgica

Belia (Spanish) beauty
Belea, Beliano, Belica, Belicia, Belya, Belyah

Belicia (Spanish) believer
Belia

Belinda (Spanish) beautiful
Belynda

Belita (Spanish) little beauty

Bella (Italian) beautiful

Bellace (Invented) pretty
Bellase, Bellece, Bellice

Belle (French) beautiful
Bela, Bele, Bell, Bella

Bellina (French) beautiful

Bellona (Mythology) strong and lovely

Belva (Latin) beautiful view

Belvia (Invented) practical
Bell, Belva, Belve, Belveah

Bemedikta (Scandinavian) form of Benedicta: blessed
Benedikte

Bena (Native American) pheasant; highbrow

Bendite (Latin) well blessed
Ben, Bendee, Bendi, Bennie, Benny, Binni

Bene (Latin) blessed

Benecia (Latin) form of Benedicta: blessed

Benedeto (Italian) form of Benedicta: blessed
Benedetto

Benedetta (Latin) form of Benedicta: blessed
Benedicta, Benedicte, Benedikta, Benetta, Benita, Benni, Benoite

Benedicta (Latin) feminine form of Benedict: blessed
Benna, Benni

Benigna (Spanish) kind

Benilda (German) struggles

Bening (Filipino) blessing

Benita (Latin) feminine form of Benedict: blessed
Bena, Benetta, Benitri, Bennie, Binnie

Benneta (Spanish) pretty

Bennetteta (Spanish) blessing

Benni (Latin) form of Benedicta: blessed
Bennie, Binny

Benson (Last name as first name) ben's child

Benta (Latin) much blessed

Bente (Latin) blessed

Bentley (English) meadow; luxury life
Bentlea, Bentlee, Bentleigh, Bently

Beon (Biblical) place name

Beonn (American) good girl

Bera (German) bearish

Berachan (Hebrew) blessing
Beracha, Berucha, Beruchiya, Beruchya

Berdina (German) bright; robust
Berd, Berdie, Berdine, Berdyne, Burdine, Burdynne, Dina, Dine

Berdine (German) glows

Berecyntia (Mythology) earth goddess

Berenjena (Spanish) eggplant

Bergen (American) pretty
Berg, Bergin

Berget (Irish) form of
Bridget: powerful
Bergette

Berit (Scandinavian) glorious
Beret, Berette

Berkley (American) smart
Berkeley, Berkie, Berklie, Berkly

Bermuda (Place name)
island; personable
Bermudoh

Bernadette (French) form of
Bernadine: brave
*Berna, Bernadene, Bernadett,
Bernadina, Bernadine,
Bernarda, Bernardina,
Bernardine, Berneta, Bernetta,
Bernette, Berni, Bernie,
Bernita, Berny*

Bernadine (German) brave
Bernadene, Berni, Bernie

Bernardita (Spanish) brave
little bear

Berneen (Irish) hearty

Berney (English) brave bear

Bernice (Greek) victorious
*Beranice, Berenice, Bernelle,
Berneta, Bernetta, Bernette,
Berni, Bernicia, Bernie,
Bernyce*

Bernie (American) winning
Bernee, Berney, Berni, Berny

Bernita (Greek) form of
Bernice: victorious

Berry (Botanical) tiny;
succulent
Berree, Berri, Berrie

Bersaida (American)
sensitive
*Bersaid, Bersaide, Bersey, Bersy,
Sada, Saida*

Berta (German) bright

Bertel (Slavic) smart

Bertha (German) bright
*Barta, Berta, Berte, Berthe,
Berti, Bertie, Bertilda, Bertilde,
Bertina, Bertine, Bertita,
Bertuska, Berty, Bird, Birdie,
Birdy, Birtha*

Bertie (German) bright
Bert, Bertee, Bertey, Berty

Bertille (German) form of
Bertha: bright

Bertina (German) feminine
form of Bert: shining bright

Bertrice (French) form of
Beatrice: blessed woman

Berule (Greek) bright; pure
Berue, Berulle

Berura (Hebrew) chaste
Beruria

Beryl (Greek) bright and
shining gem
*Beril, Berlie, Berri, Berrill,
Berry, Beryla, Beryle, Beryn*

Bess (Hebrew) form of
Elizabeth: God's promise
Bessie

Bet (Hebrew) daughter

Beta (Greek) from Greek
alphabet; beginning
Betka, Betuska

Beth (Hebrew) form of
Elizabeth: God's promise

Betha (Welsh) devoted to God
Bethah, Bethanne

Bethamie (English) form of
Bethany: God's disciple

Bethann (English) combo of
Beth and Ann; devout
*B-Anne, Bethan, Beth-ann,
Bethanne*

Bethany (Hebrew) God's
disciple
*Beth, Bethanee, Bethani,
Bethania, Bethanie, Bethann,
Bethanne, Bethannie,
Bethanny, Betheny, Bethina*

Bethel (Hebrew) in God's
house; holy child

Bethesda (Hebrew) child of a
merry home

Bethia (Hebrew) Jehovah's
daughter
Betia, Bithia

Beti (English) small woman

Betricia (American) form of
Patricia: woman of nobility;
unbending

Betriss (Welsh) blessed
Betrys

Bets (Jewish) God's child

Betsayra (Spanish)
abundance

Betsy (Hebrew) form of
Elizabeth: God's promise
Bet, Betsey, Betsi, Betsie, Betts

Betta (Italian) form of
Bettina: God's promise
Blessed

Bette (French) lively; God-
loving

Betty (Hebrew) form of
Elizabeth: God's promise
Bett, Betti, Bettye

Betuel (Hebrew) in God's
house
Bethuel

Betula (Hebrew) dedicated;
religious
*Bee, Bet, Bethula, Bethulah,
Bett, Betulah*

Beulah (Hebrew) married
Bealah, Beula, Bew, Bewla

Beulahma (Biblical) marries

Bev (English) form of Beverly:
beavers by the stream; friendly

Beverly (English) beavers by
the stream; friendly
*Bev, Beverelle, Beverle, Beverlee,
Beverley, Beverlie, Beverlye,
Bevvy, Verly*

Bevina (Irish) vocalist
*Beavena, Bev, Beve, Beven,
Bevena, Bevin, Bevy, Bovana*

Bevinn (Irish) royal
Bevan

Bezetha (Bibllical) place name

Bhamini (Hindi) beautiful
girl

Bhanumati (Hindi) bright

Bharaati (Hindi) careful

Bhavika (Hindi) devoted girl

Bhuma (Hindi) of the earth

Bian (Vietnamese) hides from
life

Bianca (Italian) white
*Beanka, Beonca, Beyonca,
Biancha, Biancia, Biankah,
Bionca, Bionka, Blanca,
Blancha*

Bibi (Arabic) lady
*Bebe, Bibiana, Bibianna,
Bibianne, Bibyana*

Bibiane (Latin) vibrant

Bice (Last name as first
name) axe; sharp talent

Bidelia (Irish) form of
Bridget: powerful
Bedilia, Biddy, Bidina

Bienvenida (Spanish)
welcomed baby

Bijou (French) jewel
*Bejeaux, Bejou, Bejue, Bidge,
Bija, Bijie, Bijy*

Bik (Chinese) jade

Bikini (Place name) island
girl; fun-loving
Bikinee

Bilhah (Biblical) summer's
child

Billie (German) feminine
form of Bill: staunch
protector
*Billa, Billee, Billey, Billi, Billy,
Billye*

Billina (English) feminine
form of Bill: staunch
protector
Belli, Bill, Billee, Billie, Billy

Billings (American) bright
*Billey, Billie, Billing, Billy,
Billye, Billyngs, Byllings*

Bina (Indian) instrument of
music

Bina (Hebrew) perceptive
woman
Bena, Binah, Byna

Binali (Hindi) music girl

Binase (Hebrew) bright
*Beanase, Benace, Bina, Binah,
Binahse*

Binti (African) dancer

Binyamina (Hebrew) right
hand

Bionda (Italian) black
Beonda, Biondah

Bira (Hebrew) fortified;
strong
Biria, Biriya

Bircit (Scandinavian) form of
Bridget: powerful

Bird (English) birdlike
Birdy

Birdie (English) bird
Birdee, Birdey, Birdi, Byrdie

Birdron (German) of birds

Birgit (Scandinavian)
spectacular
*Bergette, Berit, Birgetta, Birgite,
Britta, Byrget, Byrgitt*

Birgitta (Scandinavian) form
of Bridget: powerful
*Birgette, Brita, Byrgetta,
Byrgitta*

Birgitte (Scandinavian)
strong

Birte (Scandinavian) form of
Bridget: powerful
Berty, Birt, Birtey, Byrt, Byrtee

Birthenne (American) born
lucky

Bishop (Last name as first
name) loyal
Byshop

Bita (Hebrew) form of Bithia:
Jehovah's daughter

Bitha (Biblical) blessed
daughter

Bithia (Hebrew) Jehovah's
daughter

Bithron (Biblical) resounding

Bitina (Mythology) darkness
Libitina

Bitki (Spanish) form of
Beatrix: happy

Bitsie (American) small
Bitsee, Bitzee, Bitzi, Bytsey

Bitta (Scandinavian) form of
Bridget: powerful
Bit, Bitt, Bittey

Bittan (Origin unknown)
gives joy

Bivona (African American)
feisty
BeBe, Biv, Bivon, Bivonne

Bjork (Icelandic) unique
Byork

Blade (English) glorified
Blaide, Blayde

Blaine (Irish) thin
Blane, Blayne

Blair (Scottish)
plains-dweller
Blaire, Blayre

Blaise (Latin/French) lisp;
stutter
Blaize, Blasé, Blaze

Blake (English) dark

Blakely (English) dark
Blakelee, Blakeley, Blakeli

Blanca (Spanish) white
Blancah, Blonka, Blonkah

Blanche (French) white
*Blanca, Blanch, Blancha,
Blanchette, Blanka, Blanshe,
Blenda*

Blanchefleur (French) white
flower; pretty

Blanchine (French) white

Blanda (Latin) seductive
Blandina, Blandine

Blanka (Spanish) form of
Blanca: white

Blasia (Spanish) form of
Blaise: stutters; lisp

Blasie (French) blaze;
stammering

Blath (Irish) flower

Blaze (Englush) fiery
Blaize, Blayze

Bleinda (American) form of
Belinda: beautiful

Blesida (Spanish) blessed

Bless (American) blessed
Blessie

Blessing (English) dedicated

Blessy (American) blessed

Bleu (French) blue
Blue

Blima (Hebrew) blossoming
girl
Blimah, Blime

Bliss (English) blissful girl

Blodwen (Welsh) white
flower
Blodwyn, Blodyn

Blom (Hebrew) form of
Blum: flower

Blonda (English) blonde

Blondelle (French) blonde
girl
Blondell, Blondie, Blondy

Blondie (American) blonde
Blondee

Blossom (English) flower

Bluebell (Botanical) pretty
*Belle, Blu, Blubel, Blubell, Blue,
Bluebelle*

Blum (Hebrew) flower
Bluma

Blumelle (English) flowers

Blush (American) pink-
cheeked
Blushe

Bly (American) soft; sensual
Blye

Blyde (English) obliging

Blydece (English) obliging

Blythe (English) carefree
Blithe, Blyth

Bo (Chinese) precious girl

Boanah (American) good
Boana, Bonaa, Bonah, Bonita

Bobbi (American) form of
Roberta: brilliant mind
Bobbee, Bobbette, Bobbie,
Bobby, Bobbye, Bobi, Bobina

Bobett (American) form of
Roberta: brilliant mind
Brilliant

Bodil (Polish) heroic
Bothild, Botilda

Bogdana (Polish) gift from
God
Boana, Bocdana, Bogda,
Bogna, Bohdana, Bohdana,
Bohna

Bogdanka (Slavic) God's gift

Bogumila (Polish) loved by
God

Boguslawa (Polish) in God's
glory

Boinaiv (Native American)
girl in the grass

Bola (Origin unknown) clever
Bolo

Bolade (African) honored girl

Bolanile (African) rich in
spirit

Bolda (Slavic) embolden

Boleslawa (Polish) strong

Bona (Italian) good
Bonah, Bonna

Bonbon (American)
goodness

Boncela (Spanish) good

Boncie (Spanish) good

Bonda (Spanish) good
Bona

Bondeau (American) pretty

Bonett (Spanish) pretty

Bonfilia (Italian) good
daughter

Bong-Cha (Korean) excellent
daughter

Bonille (Italian) goodness

Bonita (Spanish) good; pretty
Bo, Bona, Boni, Bonie,
Bonitah, Nita

Bonn (French) satisfied; good
Bon, Bonne

Bonnefin (Spanish) good end

Bonnevie (Scandinavian)
good life

Bonnie (Scottish) fine;
attractive; pretty
Boni, Bonie, Bonne, Bonnebell,
Bonnee, Bonni, Bonnibel,
Bonnibell, Bonnibelle, Bonny

Bonosse (American)
generous

Booth (German) from the
dwelling; home-loving
Boothe

Bootsey (American) cowgirl
Boots, Bootsie

Bopelo (African) confident

Borghild (Scandinavian)
prepared

Borgny (Scandinavian)
fortified; strong

Bors (Latin) foreign
Borse

Boske (Hungarian) strays

Boston (Place name) city in
Massachussets; courteous
Boste, Bosten, Bostin

Boswell (Last name as first
name) intellectual
Boz, Bozwell

Boupha (Vietnamese) flower
girl

Boussaina (Arabic) smiles

Bowdy (American) outgoing
Bow, Bowdee, Bowdey, Bowdie

Boxidara (Slavic) divine
Boza, Bozena, Bozka

Bozena (Polish) treasured

Bracha (Hebrew) blessed;
sways in wind
Brocha

Bradley (English) girl of the
broad meadow; carefree
*Bradlee, Bradleigh, Bradlie,
Bradly*

Brady (Irish) spirited child
Bradee, Bradey, Bradi, Bradie

Braisly (American) cautious
Braise, Braislee, Braize, Braze

Branca (American) form of
Blanca: white

Branda (Spanish) brandy

Brandisa (English) brandy

Brandise (English) brandy

Brandy (Dutch) sweet as
wine; fun-loving
*Bran, Brandais, Brande,
Brandea, Brandee, Brandeli,
Brandi, Brandye, Brandyn,
Brani, Branndea*

Branka (Czech) glory
Bran, Branca, Bronca, Bronka

Braxton (English) from town
of Brock: safe
Braxten

Brayden (American)
humorous
*Braden, Brae, Braeden, Bray,
Brayd, Braydan, Braydon*

Breana (Irish) form of
Briana: virtuous; strong
*Bre-Anna, Breanne, Breeana,
Briana, Briane, Briann,
Brianna, Brianne, Briona,
Bryanna, Bryanne*

Breann (Irish) form of
Briana: virtuous; strong
*Bre-Ann, Bree, Breean,
Breeann*

Breathine (English) breath of
fresh air

Breck (Irish) freckled

Breckina (Irish) little freckled
girl

Bree (Irish) upbeat
Brea, Bria, Brie, Brielle

Breela (Irish) esteemed

Breelya (Irish) popular

Breena (Irish) glowing
Brena

Breene (English) palace child

Breeshonna (African
American) happy-go-lucky
Bree, Brie, Brieshonna

Breezy (American) easygoing
Breezee, Breezie

Brehea (American) self-
sufficient
Breahay, Brehae, Brehay

Breken (English) freckled

Bren (American) form of
Brenda: royal; glowing
Breyn

Brena (Irish) strong-willed
Brenna

Brenda (Irish) royal; glowing
*Bren, Brendalynn, Brenn,
Brenna, Brennda, Brenndah,
Brinda, Brindah, Brinna*

Brendelle (American)
distinctive

Brendette (French) small and
royal

Brendie (American) form of
Brenda: royal; glowing
Brendee, Brendi

Brenita (Spanish) form of
Brenda: royal; glowing

Brenna (Irish) form of
Brenda: royal; glowing
Bren, Brenn, Brenie

Brenth (Welsh) hill child

Brenyatta (Welsh) hill child

Brenza (Spanish) quiet

Bresan (American) nice

Brescia (American) nice

Bretislava (Polish) glorious
Breeka, Breticka

Brett (Latin) jolly
Bret, Bretta, Brette

Breyawna (African
American) form of Brianna:
virtuous; strong
Bryawn, Bryawna, Bryawne

Bria (Irish) form of Briana:
virtuous; strong

Briandi (Irish) honorable

Brianna ♀ ♂ (Irish)
virtuous; strong
*Breana, Breann, Bria, Briana,
Briannah, Brie-Ann, Bryanna*

Brianne (Irish) strong
Briane, Brienne, Bryn

Briar (French) heather
Brear, Brier

Briar-Rose (Literature) from
Sleeping Beauty: princess

Briazine (English) honored

Brice (English) quick

Briceidy (English) precocious
*Brice, Bricedi, Briceidee,
Briceidey*

Bricene (American) aware

Bride (Scottish) form of
Bridget: powerful

Bridey (Irish) wise
Bredee, Breedee, Bride, Bryde

Bridged (Scottish) has the
strength of fire
Bridgid, Briged, Brigid

Bridget (Irish) powerful
*Birgit, Birgitt, Birgitte, Breeda,
Brid, Bride, Bridge, Bridgett,
Bridgette, Bridgitte, Bridgey,
Brigantia, Briget, Brigette,
Brighid, Brigid, Brigida, Brigit,
Brigitt, Brigitta, Brigitte,
Brijette, Brygett, Brygida,
Brygitka*

Brie (French) from the French
town Rozay-en-Brie
Bree, Brielle

Brienne (French) honored

Brier (French) heather
Briar

Briesha (African American)
giving
Bri, Brieshe

Brigida (Italian) strong
Brigeeda

Brigitta (Romanian) strong
Brigeeta, Brigeetta, Brigita

Bril (American) strong
Brill

Briley (Last name as first
name) popular
BeBe, Bri, Brile

Brina (Latin) form of Sabrina:
passionate
*Breena, Brena, Brinna, Bryn,
Bryna, Brynn, Brynna, Brynne*

Brindha (Indian) tulasi
Sorrowful

Brindie (American) form of Brenda: royal; glowing

Brindle (Irish) versatile
Bryndle

Brine (Irish) strong
Bryne

Brinkelle (American) independent nature
Binkee, Binky, Brinkee, Brinkel, Brinkell, Brinkie

Brinlee (American) sweetheart
Brendlie, Brenlee, Brenly

Brionna (Irish) happy
Breona, Briona

Brisa (Spanish) beloved
Breezy, Breza, Brisha, Brisia, Brissa, Briza, Bryssa

Brisalle (Spanish) loved

Brisco (American) high-energy woman
Briscoe, Briss, Brissie, Brissy

Briseis (Mythology) prized; loved

Briseyda (Spanish) happy

Brissellies (Spanish) happy
Briselle, Briss, Brisse, Brissel, Brissell, Brissey, Brissi, Brissies

Brit (Latin) British

Britaney (English) girl from Britain
Britanee, Britani, Briteny, Brittaney, Brittenie, Britnee, Britney, Britni

Brites (Spanish) strong

Britt (Latin) girl from Britain
Brit

Britta (Swedish) strong woman
Brita

Brittany (English) girl from Britain
Brinnee, Britany, Briteney, Britney, Britni, Brittan, Brittaney, Brittani, Brittania, Brittanie, Brittannia, Britteny, Brittni, Brittnie, Brittny

Brittenne (English) girl from Britain

Britty (Irish) form of Brittney: girl from Britain
Britee, Britey, Briti, Britie, Brittee, Brittey, Britti, Brittie, Brity

Brizalette (English) beloved

Brody (Irish) girl from the canal
Brodee, Brodey, Brodi, Brodie

Brona (Italian) brown-haired girl

Bronislava (Polish) protective
Brana, Branislava, Branka, Brona, Bronicka, Bronka

Bronislawa (Polish) protective
Bronya

Bronte (Literature) for authors Charlotte and Emily Bronte; romantic
Brontae, Brontay

Bronty (American) form of author surname Bronte: for authors Emily and Charlotte Bronte; romantic

Bronwyn (Welsh) white-breasted
Bron, Bronwen, Bronwhen, Bronwynn

Brooke ✿ (English) sophisticated
Brook, Brooky

Brookette (American) girl from the brook

Brooklyn ☻ (Place name) neighborhood in New York
Brookelyn, Brookelynn, Brooklynn, Brooklynne

Broolyn (American) form of Brooklyn: neighborhood in New York

Browning (Literature) for poet Elizabeth Barrett Browning; pensive

Brucie (French) feminine form of Bruce: complicated; from a thicket of brushwood
Brucina, Brucine

Bruenetta (French) brown-haired
Bru, Brunetta

Bruna (Italian) brown-haired girl

Bruneita (German) brown-haired
Broon, Brune, Bruneite, Brunny

Brunella (German) intelligent
Brun, Brunela, Brunella, Brunelle, Brunetta, Brunette, Brunilla, Brunne

Brunetta (Slavic) brunette

Brunhilda (German) warrior
Brunhild, Brunhilde, Brunnhilda, Brunnhilde, Brynhild, Brynhilda, Hilda

Bruni (Spanish) brown hair

Bruno (Italian) brown

Bryanna (Gaelic) powerful female
Breanna, Brianna, Bryana

Bryanta (American) feminine form of Bryan: ethical; strong
Brianta, Bryan, Bryianta

Bryce (Welsh) aware

Bryce (American) happy
Brice

Bryleigh (English) form of Brittany: jovial
Brilee, Briley, Brily, Brilye, Brylee, Brylie

Bryn (Welsh) hopeful; climbing a hill
Brenne, Brinn, Brynn, Brynne, Brynnie

Brynn (Welsh) hopeful
Brenn, Brinn, Brynne

Brynna (Welsh) optimistic
Brinn, Brinna

Bryonie (Latin) clinging vine
Breeonee, Brioni, Bryony

Bryony (Latin) vine; clingy
Briony, Bronie, Bryonie

Bua (Vietnamese) fortunate
Boo, Bu

Bubbles (American) perky
Bubb

Buena (Spanish) goodness

Buffy (American) plains-dweller
Buffee, Buffey, Buffie

Bukola (African) wealthy
Bucola

Bule (Biblical) wed
Beul, Beulah

Bunard (American) good
Bunerd, Bunn, Bunny

Bunita (Spanish) wins

Bunmi (Hindi) earth

Bunmi (Slavic) lady

Bunny (English) little rabbit; bouncy
Bunnee, Bunni, Bunnie

Burcetta (Slavic) sweet

Burgundy (French) red wine; unique
Burgandi, Burgandy

Burke (American) loud
Berk, Burk, Burkie

Burkeley (English) birches; outdoorsy
Burkelee, Burkeleigh, Burkeli, Burkelie, Berkeley, Burkely, Burklee, Burkleigh, Burkley, Burkli, Burklie, Burkly

Burma (Place name)

Burns (Last name as first name) presumptuous
Bernes, Berns, Burn, Burnee, Burnes, Burney, Burni, Burny

Buseje (African) interesting

Buthaayna (Arabic) lovely body
Busayna, Buthaynah

Butte (Place name) landscape

Butter (American) smooth

Button (American) sensitive

Buz (Biblical) angry

Buzzie (American) spirited
Buzz, Buzzi

Bwyana (African American) smart
Bwya, Bwyanne

Byhalia (Native American) strong oak

Byria (Place name)

Byronae (American) feminine form of Byron: reclusive; small cottage
Byrona, Byronay

Bythia (American) virtuous

Cabot (French) fresh-faced

Cabriole (French) adorable
Cabb, Cabby, Cabriolle, Kabriole

Cacalia (Botanical) accommodating

Cachay (African American) distinctive

Cachet (French) fetching
Cache, Cachee

Cadasa (Biblical) place name

Caddy (American) elusive; alluring

Cade (American) precocious
Kade, Kaid

Cadena (Latin) rhythmic

Cadence (American) musical
Kadence

Cadencia (Spanish) in cadence

Cadenie (American) in cadence

Cadou (French) rhythmic

Cady (English) fun-loving
Cadee, Cadey, Cadye, Caidee, Caidy, Kadee, Kady

Caesaria (Greek) feminine form of Caesar: focused leader

Cahara (American) coherent

Cai (Chinese) wealthy; girlish

Cailida (Spanish) passionate

Cailidora (Greek) gifted with a beautiful face

Cailin (American) happy
*Cailyn, Cailynn, Calyn,
Cayleen, Caylin, Caylyn,
Caylynne*

Caimile (Spanish) helps

Cainwen (Welsh) lovely
treasure
Ceinwen, Kayne, Keyne

Cairo (Place name) Egypt's
capital; confident
Kairo, Kayro

Caissa (American) form of
Cassandra: insightful

Cait (Greek) purest
Cate, Kate

Caitlin (Irish) virginal
*Cailin, Caitleen, Caitlen,
Caitlinn, Caitlyn, Catlin,
Catlyn, Catlynne*

Caitrin (Irish) pure of heart

Caitronia (Irish) pure

Cakusola (African)
lionhearted

Cala (Arabic) strong
Calla, Callah

Calandra (Greek) lark
Calendra, Calondra, Kalandra

Calanrea (Greek) form of
Calantha: gorgeous flower
Calendrea

Calantha (Greek) gorgeous
flower
*Calanth, Calanthe, Callantha,
Calli, Calanthia*

Calatea (Greek) flowering
Calatee

Cale (Latin) respected
Kale

Caledonia (Latin) from
Scotland
Kaledonia

Caleigh (American) beauty
Calleigh

Calenda (Irish) form of
Cailin: happy
Calendun

Calent (Irish) form of Cailin:
happy

Caley (American) warm
Caleigh, Kaylee

Calhoun (Last name as first
name) surprising

Calia (American) beauty

Calida (Spanish) sincere

Calida (Spanish) warmth

California (Place name) U.S.
state; cool
Callie, Kalifornia, Kallie

Caliopa (Greek) singing
beautifully
Kaliopa

Calise (Greek) gorgeous

Calista (Greek) most
beautiful
*Calysta, Kali, Kalista, Kalli,
Kallista, Callista*

Call (American) summoned

Calla (Greek) beautiful
Cala, Callie, Cally

Callen (Irish) loquacious

Callian (Irish) beauty

Callidora (Greek) gift of
beauty

Callie (Greek) beautiful
*Caleigh, Callee, Calley, Calli,
Cally, Kali, Kallee, Kallie*

Calligenia (Italian) beauty's
child

Calliope (Greek) poetry muse
Kalliope, Kallyope

Callista (Greek) most
beautiful
*Calesta, Calista, Callista,
Calysta, Kallista*

Callistua (Greek) most
beautiful

Callula (Latin) beautiful

Caltha (Latin) gold flower

Calumina (Scottish) calm

Calvina (Latin) has no hair
Calvine

Calypso (Greek) sea nymph

Cam (American) form of
Cameron: popular; crooked
nose
Cami, Camie, Cammie

Camaren (American) form of
Cameron: popular; crooked
nose

Cambay (American) saucy
Cambaye, Kambay

Cambee (English) of the
people

Camber (American) form of
Amber: gorgeous and golden;
semiprecious stone
*Cambie, Cambre, Cammy,
Kamber*

Cambree (Welsh) form of
Cambria: the people
*Cambre, Cambrie, Cambry,
Cambry, Kambree, Kambrie*

Cambria (English) the people

Camden (American) glorious
face
*Cam, Camdon, Cammi,
Cammie, Cammy*

Cameka (African American)
form of Tamkia: lively
*Cammey, Cammi, Cammy,
Kameka, Kammy*

Camelina (American) form
of Camilla: wonderful

Camellia (Italian) flower
Camelia, Kamelia

Camelot (English) elegant
Cam, Cami, Camie, Camy

Cameo (French) piece of
jewelry; singular
Cameoh, Cammie, Kameo

Camera (Word as name)
stunning
Kamera

Camerino (Spanish)
unblemished
Cam, Cammy

Cameron (Scottish) popular;
crooked nose
*Cameran, Camren, Camryn,
Kameron, Kamryn*

Cameshia (American) pretty

Cametria (American) pretty

Cami (French) form of
Camellia: flower
*Camey, Camie, Cammie,
Cammy*

Camilla (Latin/Italian)
wonderful
*Cam, Camelia, Camellia,
Camila, Camile, Camille,
Camillia*

Camille (French) swift
runner; great innocence
*Camila, Cammille, Cammy,
Camylle, Kamille*

Cammy (American) form of
Camilla: wonderful

Camp (American) outsider
Cam, Campy

Campbell (Last name as first
name) amazing
*Cam, Cambell, Camey, Cami,
Camie, Camy*

Camrin (American) form of
Cameron: popular; crooked
nose
Camren, Camryn

Canace (American) form of
Candace: glowing girl

Canada (Place name) country
in North American; decisive
Cann, Kanada

Canain (Biblical) patient

Candace (Greek) glowing girl
*Caddy, Candice, Candis,
Candys, Kandace*

Candelara (Spanish) spiritual
*Cande, Candee, Candelaria,
Candi, Candy, Lara*

Candene (English) glows

Candenza (Italian) form of
Candace: glowing girl

Candice-Rae (American)
glows

Candida (Latin) white

Candis (American) form of
Candace: glowing girl

Candlia (American)
candlelight

Candra (Latin) she who glows
Candria, Kandra

Candy (American) form of
Candace: glowing girl
Candee, Candi, Candie

Caneadea (Native American)
the horizon; far-reaching
goals

Caneeka (American) clever

Canei (Greek) pure

Canela (Spanish) pure

Cannes (Place name) town in
France; selective
Can, Kan

Cannon (American) vital

Cantara (Arabic) bridge
Canta, Kanta, Kantara

Capelta (American) fanciful
Capeltah, Capp, Cappy

Caper (American) mischief

Caplice (American)
spontaneous
Capleece, Capleese, Kapleese

Capote (Spanish) cloak;
protected

Capri (Place name) island off
coast of Italy
Caprie, Kapri

Caprice (Italian) playful;
capricious
*Caprece, Capreese, Capricia,
Caprise*

Caprik (Spanish) capricious

Capucine (French) cloak
Cappy

Car (American) driven
Carr, Kar, Karr

Cara (Latin/Gaelic) beloved
friend
Carah, Kara

Caramea (Italian) dear girl

Caramenia (Spanish) dear
girl

Caramia (Italian) my dear
Cara Mia, Cara-Mia

Cardea (Mythology) pivotal

Cardia (Spanish) giving
Cardi, Kardia

Careletta (Spanish) smart

Caren (American) dear
Carine, Caryn, Karen, Karyn

Caresse (Greek) well-loved

Carey (Welsh) by a castle;
fond
Caree, Cari, Carrie, Cary

Cari (Latin) giving

Caria (Biblical) place name

Caribe (Place name)

Caridad (Spanish) giving
Cari

Caridad (Spanish) loving

Carie (Latin) generous

Carina (French/Italian) pure;
darling
*Careena, Carena, Carin,
Carine, Kareena, Karina*

Carinthia (Place name) city
in Austria; dear girl

Carissa (Greek) loving
*Carisa, Caryssa, Karessa,
Karissa*

Carita (Latin) giving; loved
*Caritta, Carrita, Carritta,
Karita*

Carla (German) feminine
form of Charles: well-loved
*Carlah, Carlee, Carli, Carlia,
Carlie, Carly, Karla, Karlah*

Carlanda (American) darling
*Carlan, Carland, Carlande,
Carlee, Carlie, Carly, Karlanda*

Carle (English) winner

Carleas (American) form of
Carlissa: pleasant

Carlee (German) darling
*Carleigh, Carley, Carli, Carly,
Karlee, Karley*

Carlen (English) winner

Carlene (American) sweet
*Carleen, Carlina, Carline,
Carlyn*

Carlett (Spanish) affectionate
*Carle, Carlet, Carletta, Carlette,
Carley, Carli*

Carlice (Spanish) pleases

Carlin (Gaelic) little
champion
Caline, Carlan, Carlen

Carlisle (Place name) city on
the border of England and
Scotland; sharp
Carlile, Carrie, Karlisle

Carlissa (American) pleasant
Carleeza, Carlisse

Carlita (Italian) outstanding

Carlone (Italian) winning

Carlotta (Italian) sensual
Karlotta

Carly (German) darling
*Carlee, Carley, Carli, Carlie,
Karlee*

Carlysle (English) island of
Carla

Carm (Italian) garden
paradise

Carma (Hebrew) form of
Carmel: garden
*Car, Carmee, Carmi, Carmie,
Karma*

Carmel (Hebrew) garden
Carmela, Carmella, Karmel

Carmela (Hebrew) form of
Carmel: garden
*Carmalla, Carmel, Carmella,
Carmie, Carmilla*

Carmen (Hebrew) crimson
*Carma, Carman, Carmela,
Carmelinda, Carmita,
Carmynne, Chita, Mela, Melita*

Carmensita (Spanish) dear
girl
*Carma, Carmens, Carmense,
Karmence*

Carmi (English) garden

Carmiela (Hebrew) form of Carmel: garden

Carmina (Italian) garden paradise

Carmine (Italian) attractive
Carmyne, Karmine

Carminia (Italian) dearest
Carma, Carmine, Carmynea, Karm, Karminia, Karmynea

Carmiya (Hebrew) form of Carmel: garden

Carmona (Italian) garden paradise

Carmone (Spanish) garden

Carmyle (American) garden

Carna (Latin) horn; sound of joy

Carnation (Botanical) abundant flower
Carn, Carna, Carnee, Carney, Carny

Carnelian (American) gemstone

Carnelle (American) gem

Carnethia (Invented) fragrant
Carnee, Carney, Carnithia, Karnethia

Carni (Latin) horn; vocal
Carna, Carney, Carnia, Carnie, Carniela, Carniella, Carniya, Carny, Karni, Karnia, Karniela, Karniella, Karniya

Carnie (American) happy
Carni, Karni, Karnie

Carody (American) humorous
Caridee, Caridey, Carodee, Carodey, Carrie, Karodee, Karody

Carol (English) feminine; joyful song
Carole, Carroll, Caryl, Karol, Karrole

Carole (French) joyous song
Karol, Karole

Carolena (Italian) happy

Caroli (Last name used as first name) joyous

Carolina (Italian) form of Carla: well-loved
Carrolena, Karolina

Caroline ✪ (German) little; womanly
Caraline, Carilene, Cariline, Caroleen, Carolin, Carrie, Karalyn, Karolina, Karoline, Karolyn, Karolynne

Carolleen (American) form of Carol: feminine; joyful song

Carolye (English) form of Carolina: well-loved

Carolyn (English) womanly
Carilyn, Carilynn, Carolyne, Carolynn, Karolyn

Caron (Welsh) giving heart
Carron, Karon

Caronsy (American) form of Caron: giving heart
Caronnsie, Caronsi, Karonsy

Caroun (Slavic) springtime

Carran (American) generous

Carrell (American) form of Carol: feminine; joyful song

Carrelle (American) lively
Carrele

Carrie (English) form of Caroline: little; womanly
Carey, Cari, Carri, Carry, Kari

Carron (English) form of Karen: purehearted

Carson (Nordic) dramatic
*Carse, Carsen, Carsun,
Karrson, Karsen, Karson*

Carsyn (American) form of
Carson: dramatic

Caryn (Danish) form of
Karen: purehearted
Caren, Carrin, Caryne, Carynn

Carys (Welsh) love

Casey (Gaelic) alert; watchful
*Casie, Cassee, Cassey, Casy,
Caysee, Caysie, Caysy, Kasey*

Casha (American) radiant

Cashandra (American) form
of Cassandra: insightful

Cashonya (African
American) monied; lively
Kashonya

Casilda (Latin) from the
dwelling

Casilde (Spanish) combative
*Casilda, Casill, Cass, Cassey,
Cassie*

Cason (Greek) seer; spirited
Case, Casey, Kason

Cassandra (Greek) insightful
*Casandra, Casandria, Cass,
Cassie, Cassondra, Kassandra*

Cassia (Greek) spicy;
cinnamon

Cassidy (Irish) clever girl
*Casadee, Cass, Cassidee,
Cassidi, Kassidy*

Cassie (Greek) form of
Cassandra: insightful
Cassey, Cassi

Cassiopeia (Greek) starry-
eyed
Cass, Cassi, Kass, Kassiopia

Cassis (American) form of
Carson: dramatic

Cassundra (American) form
of Cassandra: insightful

Casta (Spanish) form of
Castalina: pure

Castalia (Mythology) ill-fated

Castalina (Spanish) form of
Catalina: chaste

Castara (Greek) form of
Catherine: pure
Castera, Castora

Castille (Spanish) traditional

Cata (Spanish) pure

Catalina (Spanish) pure
Catalena, Katalena, Katalina

Catalynn (American) form of
Catalina: pure

Catarina (Greek) pure
Caterina, Catrina, Katarina

Catava (Greek) uncorrupted

Catesa (American) form of
Contessa: pretty

Catharina (Greek) form of
Catherine: pure

Cather (Literature) for author
Willa Cather; earthy
Kather

Catherine (Greek) pure
*Cartharine, Cathrine, Cathryn,
Katherine*

Catherique (French) pure

Cathleen (Irish) pure;
immaculate
*Cathelin, Cathleyn, Cathlinne,
Cathlyn, Cathy*

Cathresha (African
American) pure; outspoken
*Cathrisha, Cathy, Kathresha,
Resha*

Cathryn (Greek) form of
Catherine: pure

Cathy (Greek) pure; innocent
Cathee, Cathey, Cathie, Kathy

Catima (Greek) pure
Cattima

Catina (Italian) pure
Catin, Catine, Catinean

Catline (Irish) form of
Caitlin: virginial
*Cataleen, Catalena, Catleen,
Catlen, Katline*

Catresia (Italian) form of
Catima: pure

Catrice (Greek) form of
Catherine: pure
*Catrece, Catreece, Catreese,
Katreece, Katrice*

Catrina (Greek) pure
*Catreena, Catreene, Catrene,
Katrina*

Catriona (Greek) form of
Catherine: pure
Katriona

Cauda (Biblical) place name

Cavaray (American) celestial

Cavender (American)
emotional
Cav, Cavey, Kav, Kavender

Cavinessa (American) form
of Kavinli: pretty; gentle

Cawleen (American) vocal

Cayen (American) form of
Kay: happy; rejoicing

Cayenne (Word as name)
peppery; spice

Cayla (American) form of
Kayla: pure

Cayla (Hebrew) unblemished
*Cailie, Calee, Cayley, Caylie,
Kayla*

Cayley (American) joyful
*Caelee, Caeley, Cailey, Cailie,
Caylea, Caylee, Cayleigh,
Caylie*

Cayman (Place name) the
islands; free spirit
Caman, Caymanne, Kayman

Cayne (American) generous
Cain, Kaine

Ceanatha (American) form
of Ciana: old soul

Ceara (Irish) form of Ciara:
brunette

Ceaskarshenna (African
American) ostentatious
Ceaskar, Karshenna, Shenna

Cece (Latin) form of Cecilia:
blind

Ceci (Latin) form of Cecilia:
blind

Cecile (Latin) form of Cecilia:
blind
Cecily

Cecilia (Latin) blind
*Cacelia, Cece, Cecelia, Ceil,
Celia, Cice, Cicilia, Cilley,
Secilia, Sissy*

Cedrica (English) chief;
leader

Cedrice (American) feminine
form of Cedric: leader
Ced, Cedrise

Ceil (Latin) blythe
Ceel, Ciel

Ceinwen (Welsh) blessed
baby

Ceirra (Irish) clear-eyed
CeAirra, Cierra

Ceiteag (Scottish) purest

Celand (Latin) heavenward
Cel, Cela, Celanda, Celle

Celandine (Greek)
wildflower; natural beauty

Celandine (Color) yellow

Celaya (Spanish) serene

Celebration (American) word
as name; celebrant
Cela, Sela

Celena (Greek) form of
Selena: like the moon
Celeena, Celene

Celerina (Spanish) moves fast

Celery (Botanical) refreshing
*Cel, Celeree, Celree, Celry, Sel,
Selery, Selry*

Celes (Latin) heavens

Celeslie (Latin) celestial

Celesta (English) celestial

Celeste (Latin) gentle and
heavenly
*Celest, Celestial, Celestine,
Seleste*

Celestia (Latin) heavenly
*Celeste, Celestea, Celestiah,
Seleste, Selestia*

Celestina (Spanish) celestial

Celestral (American) celestial

Celestyna (Polish) heavenly
*Cela, Celeste, Celesteenah,
Celestinah, Celestyne*

CeLetha (Spanish) heavenly

Celina (Greek) form of
Celena: like the moon
Selina, Celena

Celinda (American) lovely

Celine (Greek) lovely
Celeen, Celene

Celisha (Greek) flaming;
passionate

Celka (Latin) celestial
Celk, Celkee, Celkie, Selk, Selka

Celkee (Latin) form of
Celeste: gentle and heavenly
Celkea, Celkie, Cell, Selkee

Cellene (French) celestial
leader

Celnie (French) heavenly

Celosia (Greek) flaming

Celta (American) form of
Delta: fourth letter of Greek
alphabet

Cena (English) special
Cenna, Sena

Cene' (French) knowing

Cennetta (American)
knowing

Cenobia (Spanish) power of
Zeus; strong girl
Cenobie, Zenobia, Zenobie

Censey (American) knowing

Ceola (American) clarity

Ceoline (American) clarity

Ceporah (Hebrew) form of
Zipporah: bird in flight

Cera (French) colorful

Cera (Spanish) growth

Cerbrenda (American) young
raven

Cerea (Greek) thriving
Serea

Cerelia (Latin) spring
Cerallua, Cerellia, Cerelly

Cerelia (Latin) spring baby

Cerella (Latin) springlike

Ceres (Latin) joyful

Ceressa (Spanish) growth

Cerestina (Spanish) growth

Ceridwen (Welsh) poetic;
blessed
Ceri, Ceridwyn

Cerina (Latin) form of
Serena: calm

Cerise (French) cherry red
Cerese, Cerice, Cerrice, Ceryce

Cerlan (Spanish) growing

Cerrisa (French) cherry red

Cerys (Mythology) harvest
goddess
Ceri, Ceries, Cerri, Cerrie

Cesaria (Latin) feminine
form of Caesar: focused
leader

Cesarina (Latin) strong spirit
Cesarea, Cesarie, Cesarin

Cesary (Polish) outspoken
Cesarie, Cezary, Ceze

Cesia (Spanish) celestial
Cesea, Sesia

Ceylon (Place name)

Chablay (American) wine

Chablis (French) white wine
Chabli

Chabulon (Biblical) place name

Chacita (Spanish) lively girl
*Chaca, Chacie, Chaseeta,
Chaseta*

Chadawndra (African)
excitable

Chadee (French) goddess
Shadee

Chadra (Indian) peacock

Chaemarique (Invented)
pretty
*Chae, Chaemareek, Marique,
Shaymarique*

Chafin (Last name as first
name) sure-footed
Chaffin, Shafin

Chahna (Hindi) she lights
the world

Chai (Hebrew) life-giving
Chae, Chaeli

Chaitali (Hindi) light

Chakena (African) energy

Chakra (Sanskrit) energy
*Chak, Chaka, Chakara,
Chakyra*

Chala (African American)
exuberant
Chalah, Chalee, Chaley, Chalie

Chalese (French) goblet;
toasts life

Chalette (American) good
taste
*Chalett, Challe, Challie,
Shalette*

Chalica (American) drinks
life fully

Chalice (French) a goblet;
toasting
*Chalace, Chalece, Chalyse,
Chalyssie*

Chalina (Spanish) rose;
fragrant

Chaline (American) smiling
Chacha, Chaleen, Chalene

Chalis (African American)
sunny disposition
Chal, Chaleese, Chalise

Chalissa (African American)
optimistic
Chalisa, Chalysa, Chalyssa

Challie (American)
charismatic
Challee, Challi, Chally

Chalondra (African
American) pretty
*Chacha, Chalon, Chalondrah,
Cheilonndra, Chelondra*

Chalsey (American) variation of Chelsea: safe harbor
Chalsea, Chalsee, Chalsi, Chalsie, Chalsie

Chamania (Hebrew) sunflower; bright
Chamaniya, Hamania, Hamaniya

Chamaran (Hebrew) form of Chamania: sunflower; bright

Chamayne (American) form of Sharmaine; form of Charles: bountiful orchard

Chambray (French) fabric; hardy
Chambree

Chameli (Hindi) jasmine; fragrant

Chamion (American) changes

Champagne (French) sparkling; luxurious

Chan (Vietnamese) fragrant

Chana (Hindi) moonlike

Chanah (Hebrew) graceful
Chanach, Channah

Chanal (American) moonlike

Chanchall (Hindi) energetic

Chanda (Hindi) moon goddess
Chandi, Chandie, Shanda

Chandani (Hindi) moonbeams
Chandni, Chandree, Chandrika

Chandelle (French) candle-lighter
Chandal, Shandalle, Shandel

Chandi (Sanskrit) goddess

Chandler (English) romantic; candle-maker
Chandlee, Shandler

Chandra (Hindi) of the moon
Chandre, Shandra, Shandre

Chandrika (Indian) moon

Chanel (French) fashionable; designer name
Chan, Chanell, Chanelle, Channel, Shanel, Shanell, Shanelle

Chanelle (American) stylish
Shanell, Shanelle

Chaney (English) form of Chandler: romantic; candlemaker
Chanie, Chaynee, Chayney

Chania (Hebrew) blessed by Lord's grace
Chaniya, Hania, Haniya

Chanicka (African American) loved
Chaneeka, Chani, Chanika, Nicka, Nika, Shanicka

Chanina (Hebrew) knows a gracious Lord

Chanise (American) adored
Chanese, Shanise

Chanit (Hebrew) spear; ready for combat
Chanita, Hanit, Hanita

Channa (Hindi) chickpea; little thing

Channary (Vietnamese) moon girl

Channing (Last name as first name) clever

Chanon (American) shining
Chanen, Chann, Channon, Chanun

Chansanique (African American) girl singing
Chansan, Chansaneek, Chansani, Chansanike, Shansanique

Chantal (French) singer of songs
Chandal, Chantale, Chantalle, Chante, Chantee, Chantel, Chantell, Chantelle, Chantile, Chantille, Chawntelle, Shanta, Shantel, Shawntel, Shontelle

Chantee (American) singer
Chante, Chantey, Chanti, Chantie, Shantee, Shantey

Chanterelle (French) singer; prized

Chanthoeun (American) chantress

Chanti (American) melodious
Chantee, Chantie

Chantill (French) singer

Chantilly (French) beautiful lace
Chantille, Shantilly

Chantou (French) singer

Chantre (French) singer

Chantrea (Vietnamese) moonlight

Chantrice (French) singer of songs
Shantreece, Treece

Chanya (Hebrew) blessed by Jehovah's love

Chanyce (American) risk-taker
Chance, Chancie, Chaneese, Chaniece, Chanycey

Chapa (Native American) beaver

Chapawee (Native American) active

Chapin (Last name used as first name) factual

Chaquanne (African American) sassy
Chaq, Chaquann, Shakwan

Chara (Greek) form of Charis: graceful
Charo

Charbonnet (French) loving and giving
Charbonay, Charbonet, Charbonnay, Sharbonet, Sharbonnet

Charde (French) wine
Charday, Chardea, Shardae

Chardonnay (French) white wine
Char, Chardonee, Chardonnae, Shardonnay

Charelle (French) feminine

Chari (American) cherish

Chariah (Hebrew) God's child

Charian (French) womanly

Charie (Greek) form of Charis: graceful
Chari

Charille (French) form of Charlotte: little woman
Char, Chari, Charill, Shar, Sharille

Charis (Greek) graceful
Charice, Charisse

Charish (American) cherished
Chareesh

Charisma (American) charming
Char, Karismah

Chariss (English) cherish

Charissa (Greek) giving
*Char, Charesa, Charisse,
Charissey*

Charissma (American)
magnetic

Charita (Spanish) sweet
Cherita

Charity (Latin) loving;
affectionate
*Carisa, Charis, Charita,
Chariti, Charry, Cherry,
Chirity, Sharity*

Charla (French) form of
Charlotte: little woman
Char

Charlaine (English) form of
Charlene: petite and beautiful
Charlane

Charlana (American) form of
Charlene: petite and beautiful
Chalanna

Charle (English) feminine
form of Charles: well-loved

Charlene (French) petite and
beautiful
*Charla, Charlaine, Charleen,
Charline, Sharlene*

Charlesetta (German)
feminine form of Charles:
well-loved
Charlesette, Charlsetta

Charlesey (American)
expansive; generous
*Charlesee, Charlie, Charlsie,
Charlsy*

Charlesia (American)
feminine form of Charles:
well-loved
*Charlese, Charlisce, Charlise,
Charlsie, Charlsy, Sharlesia*

Charlezet (American)
feminine form of Charles:
well-loved

Charli (English) feminine

Charlie (American) easygoing
Charl, Charlee, Charley, Charli

Charlize (American) pretty

Charlotee (French) small

Charlotta (French) womanly

Charlotte (French) little
woman
*Carly, Charla, Charle, Charlett,
Charletta, Charlette, Charlott,
Charolot, Char*

Charlottie (French) small
Charlotty

Charlsheah (American)
happy

Charlsie (French) womanly

Charlton (English) feminine
form of Charles: well-loved

Charluce (American)
feminine form of Charles:
well-loved
Charl, Charla, Charluse

Charlyn (Spanish) feminine

Charm (Greek) form of
Charmian: charming; joy-
baby
Charma, Charmay, Sharm

Charmaine (Latin) bountiful
orchard
*Charma, Charmagne,
Charmain, Charmane,
Charmayne, Charmian,
Charmine, Charmyn,
Sharmaine, Sharmane,
Sharmayne, Sharmyne*

Charmian (Greek) joy baby;
charming

Charmine (French) charming
Charmen, Charmin

Charminique (African
American) dashing
Charmineek

Charmonique (African American) charming
Charm, Charmi, Charmon, Charmoneek, Charmoni, Charmonik, Sharmonique

Charna (Slavic) darkness

Charnee (American) effervescent
Charney, Charnie, Charny

Charneeka (African American) obsessive
Charn, Charnika, Charny

Charneli (Slavic) dark

Charnelle (American) sparkling
Charn, Charnel, Charnell, Charney, Sharnell, Sharnelle

Charnesa (African American) noticed
Charnessa, Charnessah

Charnesie (American) dark hair

Charnette (American) little Charna; dark

Charney (American) dark

Charnise (American) dark

Charo (Spanish) flower
Charro

Charon (Dutch) dreamer

Charra (French) womanly

Charron (African American) form of Sharon: open heart; desert plain
Charryn, Cheiron

Charry (Spanish) rosary

Charsetta (American) form of Charlene: petite and beautiful
Charsee, Charsette, Charsey, Charsy

Chartra (American) classy
Chartrah

Chartres (French) planner
Chartrys

Charu (Indian) beauty

Charu (Hindi) gorgeous

Charudetta (Combo of Charu and Detta)

Charumat (Hindi) lovely and smart

Charvi (Hindi) lovely

Charvonneia (Combo of Charvon and Vonneia)

Charysse (Greek) graceful girl
Charece, Charese, Charisse

Chashmona (Hebrew) princess

Chasia (Hebrew) sheltered
Chasya, Hasia, Hasya

Chasida (Hebrew) religious
Chasidah, Hasida

Chasina (Aramaic) strength of character

Chasity (Latin) pure
Chassity

Chasmum (Hindi) lovely eyes

Chassie (Latin) form of Chastity: pure woman
Chass, Chassey, Chassi

Chastaine (English) chaste

Chastity (Latin) pure woman
Chasta, Chastitie

Chateria (Vietnamese) moonlight

Chatie (Spanish) lively

Chatree (Indian) daring

Chau (Aramaic) strength of character

Chaucer (English) demure
Chauser, Chawcer, Chawser

Chava (Hebrew) life-giving
Chavah, Chave, Hava

Chavi (Gypsy) girlish

Chaviva (Hebrew) beloved

Chavon (Hebrew) life
Chavonne

Chaya (Jewish) living

Chayan (Native American) form of Cheyenne: Native American tribe
Chay, Chayanne, Chi, Shayan, Shy

Chazmin (American) form of Jasmine: fragrant; sweet
Jasmine

Chazona (Hebrew) seer

Chea (American) witty
Chea, Cheeah

Chedra (Hebrew) happy

Cheer (American) joyful

Cheesa (American) forgiving

Cheifa (Hebrew) enjoys a safe harbor

Chekia (Invented) cheeky
Chekie, Shekia

Chela (Spanish) exuberant
Chelan, Chelena

Cheletha (African American) smiling
Chelethe, Cheley

Chelle (American) form of Chelsea or Michelle: safe harbor; like the Lord
Shell

Chelsea (Old English) safe harbor
Chelcy, Cheli, Chellsie, Chelse, Chelsee, Chelsei, Chelsey, Chelsie, Kelsey, Shelsee

Chemarin (French) fertile; dark

Chemash (Hebrew) servant of God
Chema, Chemesh, Chemosh

Chemda (Hebrew) charismatic

Chemdiah (Hebrew) loves God
Chemdia, Chemdiya, Hemdia, Hemdiah

Chemelle (American) form of Chanel: fashionable; designer name

Chemikaln (American) hip

Chenchayya (American) responsible

Chenecua (Native American) peace

Chenia (Hebrew) lives by the grace of God
Chen, Chenya, Hen, Henia, Henya

Chenicha (Native American) at odds

Chenille (American) soft
Chenelle, Chenile, Chinille

Chenlei (Asian) wise

Chenoa (American) form of Genoa: playful
Cheney, Cheno

Chenzia (American) peace

Cheops (Egyptian) pyramid builder

Cher (French) dear
Chere, Sher

Cherelle (French) dear
Charell, Cherrelle, Sharelle

Cherian (English) darling

Cherie (French) dear
*Cherey, Cheri, Cherice, Cherree,
Cherrie, Cherry, Cherye*

Cheriel (American) darling

Cherika (French) form of
Cherry: cherry red
Chereka, Cherikah

Cherinne (American) happy
Charinn, Cherin, Cherry

Cheris (American) cherished

Cherise (French) cherry
*Cherece, Cherice, Cherish,
Cherrise*

Cherish (French) precious
girl
Charish, Cherishe, Sherishe

Cherisha (American)
endearing
Cherishah, Cherishuh

Cherita (Spanish) dearest
Cheritt, Cheritta, Cherrita

Cherith (Biblical) place name;
charitable

Cheritt (American) charitable

Cheritte (American) held
dear
Cher, Cherette, Cheritta

Cherly (American) form of
Shirley: bright meadow;
cheerful girl
Cherlee, Sherly

Chermelia (American) charm

Chermelle (American) charm

Chermey (American) charm

Chermona (Hebrew) goes to
the sacred mountain

Chero (American) dearest

Cherokee (Native American)
indian tribe member

Cherone (Italian) dear

Cherria (American) dear

Cherrill (American) form of
Cheryl: beloved

Cherron (American) graceful
dancer
Cher, Cheron, Cherronne

Cherry (English/French)
cherry red
Cheree, Cherey, Cherrye, Chery

Cheryce (American) cherish

Cheryl (French) beloved
*Charyl, Cherel, Cherelle,
Cheryll*

Chesley (English) pretty;
meadow
*Ches, Cheslay, Cheslea,
Chesleigh*

Chesma (Slavic) peace-loving

Chesna (Slavic) peace
Ches, Chesnah

Chesney (English)
peacemaker
*Chesnee, Chesni, Chesnie,
Chessnea*

Chessa (Slavic) peace

Chesskwana (African
American) evoker
*Chesskwan, Chessquana,
Chessy*

Chessteen (American)
needed
*Ches, Chessy, Chesteen,
Chestene*

Chestnut (Botanical) unique

Chet (American) vivacious
Chett

Chevona (Irish) loves a
gracious God

Chevy (American) funny
Chev, Chevee

Cheyann (Native American)
form of Cheyenne: Native
American tribe

Cheye (American) form of
Cheyenne: Native American
tribe

Cheyenne (Native American)
native American tribe
*Chayanne, Cheyan, Cheyanna,
Cheyene, Chynne, Shayan,
Shayann, Sheyenne*

Chezuka (Asian) quiet
Shizuka

Chhaya (Hebrew) life; vibrant

Chhaya (Indian) shadow

Chi (African) ibo God; light

Chiante (Italian) wine
Chianti

Chiara (Italian) bright and
clear
Cheara, Chiarra, Kiara, Kiarra

Chiarina (Italian) clear

Chiba (Hebrew) love

Chic (Spanish) little; strong

Chica (Spanish) girl
Chika

Chick (American) fun-loving
Chicki, Chickie

Chickadee (American) cute
little girl
*Chicka, Chickady, Chickee,
Chickey, Chicky*

Chidi (Spanish) cheerful

Chidori (Japanese) shorebird

Chika (Japanese) dear girl;
wise

Chikira (Spanish) dancer
Shakira

Chiku (African) loquacious

Chilali (Native American)
snowbird

Childe (American) offspring
Child

Childers (Last name as first
name) dignified
*Chelders, Childie, Chilldres,
Chylders*

Chillon (American) polished

Chimalis (Native American)
snowbird

Chimene (French) self-
starter; eager

China (Place name) unique
Chinnah, Chyna, Chynna

Chinadoll (Word as name)
delicate
*China Doll, China-Doll,
Chynadoll*

Chinasia (Place name) China
and Asia; different

Chinenye (Place name) form
of China

Chinesia (Chinese) delicate

Chinnamma (Asian) wonder;
summer

Chinnereth (Biblical) place
name; God's child

Chinue (African) blessed by
Chi

Chionne (Egyptian) kind and
obedient

Chipo (African) gift

Chiquida (Spanish) form of
Chiquita: small girl
Chiquide

Chiquita (Spanish) small girl
*Chica, Chick, Chickie, Chikita,
Chiquitia, Chiquitta, Shiquita*

Chiriga (African) triumphant; capable

Chirline (American) form of Charline: petite and beautiful
Chirl, Chirlene, Shirl, Shirline

Chislaine (French) loyal

Chita (Spanish) girlish; form of Chica

Chitsa (Spanish) form of Carmen: crimson

Chivonne (American) happy
Chevonne, Chivaughan, Chivaughn, Chivon, Chivonn

Chiyena (Hebrew) in the Lord's grace

Chiyoko (Japanese) forever

Chizoba (African) well-protected; strong

Chizu (Japanese) a thousand storks; bountiful

Chizuko (Japanese) abundant

Chloe ✿ (Greek) flowering
Chloee, Clo, Cloe, Cloee, Cloey, Khloe, Kloe

Chloris (Greek) pale-skinned
Chloras, Cloris, Kloris

Cho (Japanese) dawn of day
Choko, Choyo

Chofa (Polish) able

Cholena (Native American) birdlike; sings

Chonzette (English) risk-taker

Chotsani (Asian) adoring

Choye (Asian) pretty

Chris (Greek) form of Christina: follower of Christ
Chrissie, Chrissy, Kris

Chrisana (American) boisterous
Chris, Chrisanah, Crisane

Chriselda (German) form of Griselda: patient

Chrissa (Greek) form of Christina: follower of Christ
Crissa, Cryssa, Krissa

Chrissy (English) form of Christina
Chrissie, Chrysie, Krissy

Christa (Latin) anointed one; Christian
Crista, Krista

Christal (Latin) form of Crystal: clear; open-minded
Christall, Christalle, Christel

Christanda (American) smart
Christandah, Christawnda

Christauna (American) spiritual
Christaun, Christawna, Christown, Christwan

Christen (Greek) form of Christiana: follower of Christ
Christan, Christin, Cristen, Kristen

Christiana (Greek) follower of Christ
Christa, Christianna, Christianne, Christie, Chystyana, Crystianne, Crysty-Ann, Kristiana

Christie (Greek) form of Christina: follower of Christ
Christi, Kristi, Kristie

Christina (Greek) form of Christiana: follower of Christ
Chris, Chrissie, Christi, Christiana, Chrystina, Crista, Kristina

Christine (French/English) form of Christina: follower of Christ
Christene, Christin, Cristine, Kristine

Christle (German) form of Christina: follower of Christ
Christian

Christmas (English) Christmas baby

Christopher (Greek) devout Christian
Kris, Krissie, Krissy, Krista, Kristofer, Kristopher

Christy (Scottish) Christian
Christee, Christi, Christie

Chrysanthemum (American) flower
Chrys, Chrysanthe, Chrysie, Mum

Chrysanthum (Invented) from flower chrysanthemum; flowering
Chrys, Chrysan, Chrysanth

Chrysolite (American) gemstone

Chuke (African) hopes

Chuki (African) born in a sour time

Chula (Native American) flower; colorful

Chulda (Hebrew) fortune-teller
Hulda, Huldah

Chulisa (Invented) clever
Chully, Ulisa

Chuma (Hebrew) warm
Chumi, Huma, Humi

Chumana (Native American) dew; morning fresh

Chumani (Native American) dewdrop

Chumba (African) darling

Chumina (Hebrew) warmth

Chun (Chinese) springlike

Chyan (American) form of Cheyenne: Native American tribe

Chylene (American) form of Cheyenne: Native American tribe

Chyler (American) feminine form of Kyler: peaceful

Chynna (Chinese) china; wise; musical
Chyna

Ciana (Irish) old soul

Ciandra (Italian) light

Ciani (Irish) old soul

Cianna (Italian) old soul

Ciannait (Irish) an old soul

Ciannata (Latin) old spirit

Ciannedra (Irish) old soul

Ciara (Irish) brunette
Cearra, Ciarah, Ciarra, Ciera, Keera, Keerah

Cicely (Latin) form of Cecilia: blind
Cicelie, Cici, Sicely

Cicylia (English) form of Cicely: clever

Cid (American) fun
Cyd, Syd

Cida (American) form of Cindy: moon goddess

Cidni (American) jovial
Cidnee, Cidney, Cidnie

Cidrah (American) unusual
Cid, Ciddie, Ciddy, Cidra

Cieara (Spanish) dark
CiCi, Ciear, Sieara

Ciemone (American) form of
Simone: wise and thoughtful

Ciera (Irish) dark
Clera, Cia, Cieera, Cierra,
Cierre

Cilicia (Biblical) place name

Cilla (Greek) vivacious
Cika, Sica, Sika

Cille (American) form of
Lucille: bright-eyed
Ceele

Cilvia (Spanish) form of
Sylvia: girl of the forest
Sylvan

Cima (Place name) form of
Cimarron: western

Cimarra (Last name used as
first name) aware

Cimm (Place name) form of
Cimarron: western

Cinderella (Literature) cinder
chld

Cinderella (French) girl in
the ashes
Cinda, Cindi, Cindie, Cindy

Cindy (Greek) form of
Cynthia: moon goddess
Cindee, Cindi, Cyndee, Cyndi,
Cyndie, Sindee, Syndi, Syndie,
Syndy

Cinnamon (English) savory
spice
Cenamon, Cinna,
Cinnammon, Cinnamond,
Cinamen, Cynamon

Cinta (Spanish) mountain of
good

Cinthya (American) form of
Cynthia: moon goddess

Cinzia (Italian) mountain;
reasonable

Ciona (American) steadfast
Cinonah, Cionna, Cyona

Cipriana (Italian) form of
Cyprus: island south of
Turkey; outgoing
Cipri, Cipriannah, Cypriana,
Cyprianna, Cyprianne,
Sipriana, Siprianna, Ciprianna

Circe (Greek) sorceress deity;
mysterious
Circee, Cirsey, Cirsie

Ciri (Latin) regal
Ceree, Ceri, Seree, Siri

Cirila (Latin) heavenly
Ceri, Cerila, Cerilla, Cerille,
Cerine, Ciria, Cirine

Cissy (American) sweet
Ciss, Cissey, Cissi, Sissi

Cita (American) from the
musical instrument sitar

Citalin (American) starlike

Citare (Greek) musical; form
of the Indian lute sitar
Citara, Sitare

Citlali (Native American)
starry
Citlee

Claire ✿ (Latin/French) form
of Clara: clear; bright
Clair, Clairee, Claireen,
Claireta, Clairy, Clare, Clarette,
Clarry, Klair

Clancey (American)
a devil-may-care attitude
Clance, Clancee, Clancie,
Clancy

Clara (Latin) clear; bright
Clarie, Clarine, Clareta,
Clarette, Clare, Claire, Clary

Claresta (Greek) form of
Clarissa: smart; clear-minded

Clareta (Latin) clarity;
distinguished
Clarita

Clarice (Latin) form of Clara:
clear; bright
*Clairece, Claireece, Clairice,
Clarece, Clareece, Clariece,
Clarise*

Clarie (French) clear

Clarieca (Latin) bright
*Claire, Clare, Clari, Clarieka,
Clary, Klarieca, Klarieka*

Clarimond (Latin) shining
defender; bright

Clarinda (Latin) form of
Claire: clear; bright

Clarion (American) clear

Claris (Italian) insightful

Clarisha (Invented) clarissa

Clarissa (Latin/Greek) smart;
clear-minded
*Claressa, Clarice, Clarisa,
Clarise, Clerissa*

Clarissima (Italian) clear

Clarity (Word as name) clear-
minded
Clare, Claritee, Claritie

Claronne (French) clear

Clasina (Latin) bright

Classie (American) class act

Claudette (French) persistant
*Claude, Claudee, Claudet,
Claudi, Claudie, Claudy*

Claudia (German) crippled

Claudia (Latin) lame
*Claudelle, Claudie, Claudina,
Clodia, Klaudia*

Clava (Spanish) earnest;
sincere

Clavenna (American)
aggressive

Clea (Invented) form of
Cleanthe: famed
Clia, Klea, Klee

Cleandrea (American) form
of Cleanthe: famed

Cleanthe (English) famed
*Clea, Cleantha, Cliantha, Klea,
Kleanth*

Cleatris (American) form of
Cleanthe: famed

Clelia (Latin) glorious girl

Clem (Latin) gentle; vine

Clematia (Greek) winding
vine

Clematis (Greek) vine; clings

Clemence (Latin) easygoing;
merciful
*Clem, Clemense, Clements,
Clemmie, Clemmy*

Clementina (Spanish) kind;
forgiving
*Clementas, Clementi,
Clementis, Clementyna,
Clymentyna, Klementina*

Clementine (French/Latin)
merciful
*Clemencie, Klementine,
Klementynne*

Cleo (Greek) form of
Cleopatra: Egyptian queen

Cleodal (Latin) glory
Cleodel, Cleodell

Cleofe (Greek) glorified

Cleopatra (Greek) egyptian
queen
Cleo, Clee, Kleeo, Kleo

Cleopatrea (American) form
of Cleopatra: Egyptian queen

Cleora (American) famed

Cleotilda (French) form of Clotilda: famed fighter

Clerafina (Spanish) clear finish

Cleta (Greek) busy

Cletalline (Greek) busy

Cletenne (Greek) busy

Cleva (English) from the hill

Cliantha (Greek) flower of glory
Cleantha, Cleanthe, Clianthe

Clio (Greek) history muse
Kleeo, Klio

Cliodhna (Irish) dark
Clidna, Cliona

Cliona (Greek) form of Clio: history muse

Clipper (American) topnotch

Cloe (Greek) flourishing
Cloee, Cloey

Cloi (Greek) spins life

Clois (Greek) thrives

Cloise (English) cloissone

Cloreen (American) happy
Clo, Cloreane, Cloree, Cloreene, Corean, Klo, Klorean, Kloreen

Cloressa (American) consoling
Cloresse, Kloressa

Clorinda (Latin) happy
Cloee, Cloey, Clorinde, Clorynda, Klorinda

Cloris (Latin) pale
Chloris

Clory (Spanish) smiling
Clori, Clorie, Kloree, Klory

Closetta (Spanish) secretive
Close, Closette, Klosetta, Klosette

Clotho (Mythology) one of the Greek Fates; spins web of fate

Clotilda (German) famed fighter
Clotilde, Clothilde, Tilda, Tillie, Tilly

Clotilde (French) combative

Cloud (Word as name) airy
Cloudee, Cloudie, Cloudy

Clove (Botanical) distinctive spice
Klove

Clover (Botanical) lucky
Clovah, Clove, Kloverr

Cluette (American) savvy

Clydette (American) feminine form of Clyde: adventurer
Clidette, Clidett, Clydie, Klyde, Klydette

Clymene (Greek) famous

Clytie (Greek) excellent; in love with love
Cly, Clytee, Clytey, Clyty, Klytee, Klytie

Co (American) jovial
Coco, Ko, Koko

Coahoma (Native American) panther; stealthy

Coby (American) glad
Cobe, Cobey, Cobie

Cochava (Hebrew) star girl

Cocheta (Italian) Concetta: pure female

Coco (Spanish) coconut
Koko

Cocoa (Spanish) chocolate; spunky girl

Cody (English) softhearted; pillow
Codi, Codie, Kodie

Coffey (American) lovely
Cofee, Caufey

Cofta (Last name used as first name) audacious

Coiya (American) coquettish
Coyuh, Koya

Cokey (American) intelligent
Cokie

Colanda (African American) form of Yolanda: pretty as a violet flower

Colby (English) enduring
Cobie, Colbi, Kolbee

Cole (Last name as first name) laughing
Coe, Colie, Kohl

Colemand (American) adventurer
Colmyand

Colene (American) girl

Coleteen (Invented) created; trusted

Coletta (French) wins

Colette (French) spiritual; victorious
Coey, Collette, Kolette

Colina (English) girl

Colina (American) righteous
Colena, Colin, Colinn

Coline (Greek) victory
Colinette

Colisa (English) delightful
Colissa, Collisa, Collissa

Colleen (Irish) young girl
Coleen, Colene, Coley, Colleene, Collen, Colli, Kolene, Kolleen

Collena (English) girl

Colletta (English) girl

Colley (English) fearful; worrier
Col, Collie, Kolley

Collie (English) female child

Colmbyne (Latin) form of Columbine: dove; flower

Coloma (Spanish) calm
Colo, Colom, Colome

Colossae (Biblical) place name; colossal

Columbia (Latin) form of Columbine: dove; flower
Colombe, Columba, Columbine

Columbine (Latin) dove; flower

Colure (French) color

Colynne (American) form of Colleen: young girl

Comfort (American) comforting; easygoing
Komfort

Comfortyne (French) comforting
Comfort, Comfortine, Comfurtine, Comfy

Comora (African) moon
Komoria

Comsa (Greek) form of Cosma: of the universe

Concepcion (Spanish) conceived; begins
Conception

Concetta (Italian) pure female

Conchetta (Spanish) wholesome
Concheta, Conchette

Conchie (Latin) conception
Conchee, Conchi, Konchie

Conchita (Spanish) girl of the conception
Chita, Concha, Conchi

Conchiteen (Spanish) pure
Conchita, Conchitee, Connie

Conchobarre (Irish) willful

Concordia (Latin) goddess of peace

Condoleezza (American) smart; with sweetness
Condeleesa, Condilesa, Condolissa

Coneisha (African American) giving
Coneisha, Conisha, Conishah, Conniesha

Conene (American) smart

Conerly (Last name used as first name) worthy

Conesa (American) free-flowing nature
Conisa, Connesa, Konesa

Conita (Dutch) consistent

Conlee (American) form of Connelly: radiant
Con, Conlee, Conley, Conlie, Conly, Conly, Connie, Konlee, Konlee, Konlie

Conner (American) brave
Con, Coner, Coni, Connie, Connor, Conny, Conor

Connie (English) form of Constance: loyal
Con, Conni, Conny, Konnie

Connie-Kim (Vietnamese) golden girl
Conni-Kim

Conradina (German) feminine form of Conrad: optimist
Connie, Conradine, Conradyna, Konnie, Konradina

Conroe (Place name) small town in Texas
Conn, Connie, Konroe

Conroy (Last name as first name) stately; literary
Conroi, Konroi, Konroy

Conseja (Spanish) advises

Consilletta (Italian) counsels

Consolata (Spanish) consoles others

Constance (Latin) loyal
Con, Connie, Conny, Constantia, Constantina, Constantine, Constanza

Constantina (Italian) loyal; constant
Conn, Connee, Conni, Connie, Conny, Constance, Constanteena, Constantinah

Constanza (Hebrew) constant
Constanz, Connstanzah

Constanze (German) unchanging
Con, Connie, Stanzi

Consuelo (Spanish) comfort-giver
Chelo, Consolata, Consuela

Contessa (Italian) pretty
Contesa, Contessah, Contesse

Contina (American) countess

Cookie (American) cute
Cooki

Copeland (Last name as first name) adaptable
Copelan, Copelyn, Copelynn

Copper (American) redhead
Coppyr

Coppola (Italian) theatrical
Copla, Coppi, Coppo, Coppy, Kopla, Kopola, Koppola

Coprice (American) form of
Caprice: playful; capricious

Cora (Greek) maid; giving girl
*Corah, Corra, Correna, Corene,
Coretta, Corette, Corrie,
Corinna, Kora*

Coral (Latin) natural; small
stone
*Corall, Coralle, Coraly, Core,
Corel, Koral, Koraly*

Coraline (American) country
girl

Coraz (Spanish) form of
Corazon: heart

Corazon (Spanish) heart
Cora, Corrie, Zon, Zonn

Corazonna (Spanish) form of
Corazon: heart

Corby (Latin) raven; dark

Corday (English) prepared;
heart
*Cord, Cordae, Cordie, Cordy,
Korday*

Cordelia (Latin) warmhearted
woman
*Cordeelia, Cordalia, Cordelie,
Cordi, Cordie, Cordilia,
Kordelia, Kordey, Kordi*

Cordelita (Latin/Spanish)
heartfelt
Cordelia, Cordelite, Cordella

Cordillera (Latin) form of
Cordelia: warmhearted
woman

Cordula (Latin/German)
heart; jewel
*Cord, Cordie, Cordoola,
Cordoolah, Cordy*

Corenda (American)
derivative of Dorenda; adored

Corette (Greek) form of Cora:
maid; giving girl

Corey (Irish) perky
*Cori, Corree, Corrie, Korey,
Korri, Korrie*

Corgie (American) funny
Corgi, Korgee, Korgie

Cori (Greek/Irish) caring
Corey, Corri, Corrie, Cory

Coriander (Botanical)
seasoning; simplistic

Corinna (Greek) young girl
*Corina, Corrinna, Corryna,
Corynna*

Corinne (Greek/French)
maiden; protective
*Coreen, Corina, Corine,
Corinna, Corrina, Coryn,
Corynn, Koreene, Korinne*

Corintha (German) maiden

Corinthian (Place name) a
town in Greece; religious

Coris (Greek) singer
Corris, Koris, Korris

Corissa (Greek) kindhearted
Korissa

Corissah (American)
mysterious

Corita (Spanish) kind

Corky (American) energetic
*Corkee, Corkey, Corki, Corkie,
Korkee, Korky*

Corliss (English) open-
hearted
*Corless, Corlise, Corly, Korlis,
Korliss*

Corlisse (American) cheerful

Corlissen (American)
cheerful

Corly (American) active
*Corlee, Corli, Corlie, Korli,
Korly*

Corlyn (American) innovative
Corlin, Corlinn, Corlynn,
Corlynne, Korlin, Korlyn

Cormella (Italian) fiery
Cormee, Cormela, Cormelah,
Cormellia, Cormey, Cormie

Cornae (Origin unknown) all
seeing
Coma, Korna, Kornae

Cornecia (Latin) yellow hair;
horn

Corneitha (Latin) horn child

Cornelia (Latin) practical
Carnelia, Corney, Corni

Cornelie (Latin) horn child

Cornelius (Latin) realistic
Corneal, Corneelyus, Corney,
Corny

Cornesha (African
American) talkative
Cornee, Corneshah, Cornesia

Cornish (English) cornish

Corona (Spanish) crowned
Corone, Coronna, Korona

Correne (American) musical
Coree, Coreen, Correen,
Correna, Korrene, Korene

Corri (English) naive
Corry

Corrianna (American) joyful
Coreanne, Corey, Corianna,
Corri, Corriana

Corrie (English) form of
Coral: natural; small stone

Corrinda (French) girlish
Corri, Corrin, Korin, Korinda

Corseta (English)
unsophisticated

Cortanie (American) form of
Courtney: domain of Curtis
Cortanny, Cortany

Cortland (American)
distinctive
Cortlan, Courte, Courtland,
Courtlin

Cortlinn (American) happy
Cortlenn, Cortlin, Cortlyn,
Cortlynn

Corvette (Word as name)
speedy
Corv, Corva, Corve, Korvette

Corvina (Latin) raven;
brunette

Cosetta (French) pretty thing

Cosette (French) warm
Cossette

Cosima (Greek) universe;
harmony
Coseema, Koseema, Kosima

Cosma (Greek) of the
universe

Cosmee (Greek) organized
Cos, Cosmi, Cosmie

Cosmiss (American)
harmony with the cosmos

Cossette (French) winning
Coss, Cossie, Cossy, Kossee,
Kossette

Costanza (Last name as first
name) strong-willed; funny

Costner (American)
embraced
Cosner, Cost, Costnar, Costnor,
Costnur

Cota (Spanish) lively

Cotcha (African American)
stylish
Kasha, Katcha, Katshay,
Kotsha

Cotia (Spanish) full of vitality

Cotilia (Spanish) vital

Cotrena (American) form of Katrina: melodious
Catreena, Catrina, Catrine, Cotrene, Katrine, Kotrene

Cotton (American) comforting
Cottie

Countess (English) blueblood
Contessa

Courday (French) courteous

Couria (French) courteous

Cournette (American) form of Coronet: regal
Courney, Kournette

Courney (English) form of Courtney: domain of Curtis

Courtney (English) domain of Curtis
Cortney, Courtenay, Courteney, Courtnay, Courtnee, Courtny, Kortnee, Kortney

Covelina (Spanish) cave child

Covin (American) unpredictable
Covan, Cove, Coven, Covyn

Coy (American) sly
Coye, Koi, Koy

Coyah (American) singular
Coya, Coyia

Coyote (American) wild
Coyo, Kaiote, Kaiotee

Cozeth (English) rainbow

Cozetta (English) rainbow

Cozette (French) darling

Cramer (American) jolly
Cramar, Cramir, Kramer

Cramisa (Invented) nice
Cramissa, Kramisa

Creda (English) giving credence

Cree (American) wild spirit
Crea, Creeah

Creed (American) boisterous
Crede, Cree, Kreed

Creesha (English) flower

Creirwy (Welsh) lucky amulet

Cremone (French) wanted

Creola (American) desires

Cresa (English) fickle

Crescena (German) grows

Crescente (American) impressive
Crescent, Cresent, Cress, Cressie

Crescentia (Spanish) crescent-faced; smiling
Creseantia, Crescent, Cressentt

Cresenda (American) explosive

Cressa (Greek) form of Cressida: infidel
Cresa, Cressah, Cresse, Cress, Kressa

Cressell (American) growth

Cressida (Greek) infidel
Cresida, Cresiduh, Cresside

Cressie (American) growing; good
Cress, Cressy, Kress, Kressie

Creston (American) worthy
Crest, Crestan, Creste, Cresten, Crestey, Cresti, Crestie

Cresusa (English) fickle

Cricket (American) energetic
Kricket

Crimson (American) deep
Cremsen, Crims, Crimsen, Crimsonn, Crimsun

Crisanta (American) form of Chrysanthemum: flower

Crisel (English) form of Crystal: clear; open-minded

Criselda (Spanish) wild
Crisselda

Criselle (English) crystal

Crishonna (American) beautiful
Crishona, Crisshone, Crissie, Crissy, Krishona, Krishonna

Crisiant (Welsh) crystal; clear
Cris, Crissie

Crispa (Latin) curly hair

Crispina (Latin) curly-haired girl

Crispy (Invented) fun-loving; zany
Crispee, Krispy

Crista (Italian) form of Christina: follower of Christ
Krista

Cristella (English) crystal

Cristin (Irish) dedicated
Cristen, Crystyn, Kristin, Krystyn

Cristina (Greek) form of Christina: follower of Christ
Christina, Kristina

Cristos (Greek) dedicated
Criss, Crissie, Christos

Cristy (English) spiritual
Cristi, Crysti, Krystie, Kristi

Crusitee (Spanish) of the cross

Cruzita (Spanish) of the cross

Cruzitte (Spanish) of the cross

Cryange (Place name)

Crystal (Latin) clear; open-minded
Christal, Chrystal, Cristal, Cristalle, Crys, Crystelle, Krystal

Crystilis (Spanish) focused
Chrysilis, Crys, Cryssi, Cryssie, Crystylis

Csaba (Hungarian) shepherd; wanderer

Csilla (Hungarian) defensive

Cuasha (American) goodness

Cuba (Place name) island; fun-loving girl

Cullen (Irish) attractive
Cullan, Cullie, Cullun, Cully

Cumale (American) open-hearted
Cue, Cuemalie, Cue-maly, Cumahli

Cumthia (American) open-minded
Cumthea, Cumthee, Cumthi, Cumthie, Cumthy

Cupertina (Spanish) covert

Cupid (American) romantic
Cupide

Curine (American) attractive
Curina, Curinne, Curri, Currin

Curisten (Invented) form of Kirsten: follower of Christ

Curry (American) languid
Curree, Currey, Curri, Currie

Cursten (American) form of Kirsten: follower of Christ
Curst, Curstee, Curstie, Curstin

Cushaun (American) elegant
Cooshaun, Cooshawn, Cue, Cushawn, Cushonn, Cushun

Cximara (Spanish) greatness

Cyan (American) colorful
Cyanne, Cyenna, Cyun

Cyanea (Greek) blue-eyed baby

Cyanetta (Greek) little blue
Cyan, Cyanette, Syan, Syanette

Cybele (Greek) conflicted

Cybill (Latin) prophetess
Cybell, Cybelle, Cybil, Sibyl, Sibyle

Cydell (American) country girl
Cydee, Cydel, Cydie, Cydile, Cydy

Cydney (American) perky
Cyd, Cydni, Cydnie

Cylee (American) darling
Cye, Cyle, Cylea, Cyli, Cylie, Cyly

Cylene (American) melodious
Cylena, Cyline

Cyllene (American) sweet

Cyma (Greek) does well

Cymantha (English) form of Simone: wise and thoughtful

Cymbeline (Greek) benevolent ruler
Beline, Cymba, Cymbe, Cymbie, Cyme, Cymmie, Symbe

Cyn (Greek) form of Cynthia: moon goddess
Cynnae, Cynnie, Syn

Cynara (Greek) prickly; particular
Cynarra

Cynder (English) having wanderlust
Cindee, Cinder, Cindy, Cyn, Cyndee, Cyndie, Cyndy

Cynista (English) leader

Cyntanah (American) singer
Cintanna, Cyntanna

Cynthia (Greek) moon goddess
Cindy, Cyn, Cyndee, Cyndy, Cynthea, Cynthee, Cynthie

Cynthiah (American) form of Cynthia: moon goddess

Cyntia (Greek) form of Cynthia: moon goddess
Cyn, Cyntea, Cynthie, Cyntie, Syntia

Cyntrille (African American) gossipy
Cynn, Cyntrell, Cyntrelle, Cyntrie

Cypress (Botanical) swaying
Cypres, Cyprice, Cypris, Cypriss, Cyprus

Cyra (American) willing
Cye, Cyrah, Syra

Cyreen (American) sensual
Cyree, Cyrene, Cyrie

Cyrena (American) form of Serena: calm

Cyrene (Greek) mythological nymph

Cyrenian (American) bewitching
Cyree, Cyren, Cyrenean, Cyrey, Siren, Syrenian

Cyrenna (American) straightforward
Cyrena, Cyrennah, Cyrinna, Cyryna, Cyrynna

Cyriece (American) artistic
Cyreece, Cyree, Cyreese, Cyrie

Cyrilla (Latin) royal; little minx
Cirila

Cyrise (English) serene

Cytherea (Greek) from the island of Cythera; celestial

Cyvie (American) clean

Czara (Slavic) leads

Czaree (American) czar-like

Czarina (Russian) royal

D'Anna (Hebrew) special

Daba (Hebrew) kindhearted

Dabaloth (Biblical) angelic

Dabaritta (Biblical) angelic

Daberath (Biblical) angelic

Dabire (Biblical) angelic

Dacey (Irish) a southerner
Dace, Dacee, Daci, Dacia,
Dacie, Dacy, Daicie, Daycee

Dacia (Latin) old soul
Dacie, Dachia, Dachi

Dae (English) day
Day, Daye

Daelan (English) aware
Dael, Daelan, Daeleen,
Daelena, Daelin, Daely,
Daelyn, Daelynne, Dale, Daley,
Daylan, Daylin, Daylind, Dee

Daevrissa (American) girl of
the day

Daeze (African) day

Daffodil (Botanical) flower
Daffy

Dafna (Slavic) form of
Daphne: pretty nymph

Dafnee (Greek) form of
Daphne: pretty nymph
Dafney, Dafnie

Dafo (American) form of
Daffodil: flower

Dagmar
(Scandinavian/German)
glorious day
Dag, Dagmara, Dagmarr

Dagny (Scandinavian) day
Dagna, Dagnanna, Dagne,
Dagney

Dahlia (Scandinavian) flower
Dahl, Dollie

Dahri (American) form of
Dahlia: flower

Dai (Welsh/Japanese) beloved
one of great importance

Dailah (American) form of
Dahlia: flower

Dainikya (Slavic) form of
Danica: star of the morning

Daira (American) outgoing
D'Aira, Daire, Dairrah,
Darrah, Derrah

Daisha (American) sparkling
D'Aisha, Daish, Daishe,
Dasha, Dashah

Daisy (English) flower; day's
eye
Daisee, Daisey, Daisi, Daisia,
Daisie, Daissy, Daizee, Daizi,
Daizy, Dasey, Dasi, Dasie,
Dasy, Daysee, Daysie, Daysy

Daisy-Boo (American)
frivolous; flower

Daiton (American) wondrous
Day, Dayten, Dayton

Daja (American) intuitive
Dajah

Dajanae (African American)
persuasive
Daije, Daja, Dajainay,
Dayjanah

Dajon (American) gifted
D'Jon, Dajo, Dajohn, Dajonn,
Dajonnay, Dajonne

Dakara (American) firebrand
Dacara, Dakarah, Dakarea, Dakarra

Daking (Asian) friendly

Dakota (Native American) tribal name; solid friend
Dacota, Dakohta, Dakotah, Dakotha, Dakotta, Dekoda, Dekota, Dekotah, Dekotha

Dalacie (American) brilliant
Dalaci, Dalacy, Dalasie, Dalce, Dalci, Dalse

Dalaina (American) spirited
Dalana, Dalayna, Delaina, Delaine, Delayna

Dalaney (American) hopeful
Dalanee, Dalaynee, Dalayni

Dalaya (English) form of Dahlia: flower

Dale (English) valley-life
Daile, Daleleana, Dalena, Dalina, Dayle

Daleah (American) pretty
Dalea

Daley (Irish) leader
Dailey, Dalea, Daleigh, Dali, Dalie, Daly

Dali (Spanish) of the day

Dalia (Spanish) flower
Daliah, Daliyah, Dayliah, Doliah, Dolliah, Dolya

Dalia (Arabic) flower

Dalian (American) joy
Dalean

Daliana (American) joyful spirit
Daliane, Dalianna, Dilial, Dollianna

Dalice (American) able
Daleese, Dalleece

Dalila (African) gentle
Dahlila, Dahlilla, Dalia, Dalilah, Dalilia

Dalimda (American) form of Dalinda: beautiful; honey; sweetheart

Dalin (American) calm
Dalen, Dalenn, Dalun

Dalinda (American) form of Belinda: beautiful; form of Melinda: honey; sweetheart

Dalita (American) smooth
Daleta, Daletta, Dalite, Dalitee, Dalitta

Dallas (Place name) city in Texas; confident
Dalis, Dalisse, Daliz, Dallice, Dallis, Dallsyon, Dallus, Dallys, Dalyce, Dalys

Dallen (American) outspoken
Dal, Dalin, Dallin, Dalen

Dallise (American) gentle
Dalise, Dallece, Dalleece, Dalleese

Dalmar (German) perseveres

Dalmatia (Biblical) place name

Dalondra (Invented) generous
Dalandra, Dalon, Dalondrah, Delondra

Dalonna (Invented) generous
Dalohn, Dalona, Dalonne

Dalphine (French) form of Delphine: calmness
Dal, Dalf, Dalfeen, Dalfene, Dalphene

Dalton (American) smart
Dallee, Dalli, Dallie, Dallton, Dally, Daltawyn

Daltrey (American) quiet
Daltree, Daltri, Daltrie

Dalva (American) strong

Dalyn (American) smart
*Dalin, Dalinne, Dalynn,
Dalynne*

Dama (Hindi) temptress

Damalla (Greek) fledgling;
young
*Damala, Damalas, Damalis,
Damall*

Damara (Greek) gentle
Damaris, Damarra

Damaris (Greek) calm
*Damalis, Damar, Damara,
Damares, Damaret, Damarius,
Damary, Damarys, Dameress,
Dameris, Damiris, Dammaris,
Dammeris, Damrez, Damris,
Demaras, Demaris, Demarays*

Damecia (Invented) sweet
*Dameisha, Damesha, Demecia,
Demisha, Demeshe*

Dami (Greek) form of Damia:
spirited
Damee, Damey, Damie, Damy

Damia (Greek) spirited
*Damiah, Damya, Damyah,
Damyen, Damyenne, Damyuh*

Damianne (Greek) one who
soothes
Damiana

Damica (French) open-
spirited
*Dameeka, Dameka, Damekah,
Damicah, Damie, Damika,
Damikah, Demeeka, Demeka,
Demekah, Demica, Demicah*

Damita (Spanish) small
woman of nobility
*Dama, Damah, Damee,
Damesha, Dameshia, Damesia,
Dametia, Dametra, Dametrah*

Damitte (Irish) small

Damon (American) sprightly
Damoane, Damone

Damone (American) mighty
Dame

D'Amore (Invented) love

Dana (English) bright gift of
God
*Daina, Dainna, Danae,
Danah, Danai, Danaia,
Danalee, Danan, Danarra,
Danayla, Dane, Danean,
Danee, Daniah, Danie,
Danna, Dayna, Daynah*

Danae (Greek) bright and
pure
*Danay, Danayla, Danays,
Danea, Danee, Dannae,
Danays, Danee, Denae, Denee*

Danala (English) happy;
golden
*Dan, Danalla, Danee, Danela,
Danney, Danny*

Danay (American) happy
D'Nay, D·nay, Danaye

Dancel (French) energetic
*Dance, Dancell, Dancelle,
Dancey, Dancie, Danse,
Dansel, Danselle*

Dancie (American) from the
word dancer
Dancy

Dandelion (Botanical) flower

Daneaa (Welsh) bright day

Daneen (Greek) blessed

Daneil (Hebrew) judged by
God; spiritual
*Daneal, Daneala, Daneale,
Daneel, Daneela, Daneila*

Danelle (Hebrew)
kindhearted
*Danael, Danalle, Danel,
Danele, Danell, Danella, Dani,
Dannele, Danny*

Danelly (Spanish) form of Danielle: judged by God; spiritual
Daneli, Danellie, Dannelley, Dannelly

Danena (Greek) blessed

Danessa (American) dainty
Danesa, Danese, Danesha, Danesse, Daniesa, Daniesha, Danisa, Danisha, Danissa

Danessia (American) delicate child
Danesia, Danieshia, Danisla, Danissia

Danette (American) form of Danielle: judged by God; spiritual
Danetra, Danett, Danetta

Dangela (Latin) form of Angela: divine; angelic
Angee, Angelle, Angie, Dangelah, Dangelia, Dangey, Dangi, Dangie

Dani (Hebrew) form of Danielle: judged by God; spiritual
Danee, Danie, Danne, Dannee, Danni, Dannie, Danny, Dany

Dania (Hebrew) form of Danielle: judged by God; and feminine form of Daniel: spiritual
Daniah, Danya, Danyah

Daniah (Hebrew) judged
Dan, Dania, Danny, Danya

Danica (Latin/Polish) star of the morning
Daneeka, Danika, Danneeka, Dannica, Dannika

Daniella (Italian) form of Danielle: judged by God; spiritual
Danilla

Danielle (Hebrew/French) feminine form of Daniel: judged by God; spiritual
Danelle, Daniell, Daniele, Danniella, Danyel

Danir (American) fresh
Daner

Danit (Hebrew) judged by God
Danett, Danis, Danisha, Daniss, Danita, Danitra, Danitza, Daniz, Danni

Danita (English) form of Danielle: judged by God; spiritual
Danni, Danny, Denita, Denny

Danla (Slavic) form of Danielle: judged by God; spiritual

Danna (American) cheerful
D'Ana, D'Anna, Dannae, Danni, Danny

Danner (American) morning star

Danube (Place name) river; flowing spirit

Danuta (Polish) God's gift

Danyella (Slavic) form of Danielle: judged by God; spiritual

Danyiel (Slavic) form of Danielle: judged by God; spiritual

Danz (Last name used as first name) trendsetter

Daphiney (Greek) form of Daphne: pretty nymph
Daff, Daph

Daphne (Greek) pretty
nymph
*Daphane, Daphaney,
Daphanie, Daphany, Daphiney,
Daphnee, Daphney, Daphnie,
Daphny, Daphonie, Daphy*

Daphoneel (Greek) form of
Daphne: pretty nymph

Daphyne (Greek) form of
Daphne: pretty nymph

Daquisha (African
American) talkative

Dara (Hebrew)
compassionate
*Dahra, Dahrah, Darah, Darra,
Darrah*

Daralice (Greek) beloved
Dara, Daraleese, Daraliece

Daravia (Hebrew) loving

Darby (Irish) a free woman
*Darb, Darbee, Darbi, Darbie,
Darbye*

Darceece (Irish) form of
Darci: dark

Darcelle (American) secretive
Darce, Darcel, Darcell, Darcey

Darci (Irish) dark
*Darce, Darcee, Darcie, Darcy,
Dars, Darsey*

Darda (Hebrew) wise

Dare (Hebrew) compassion

Daretha (Slavic) loved

Dari (Czech) rich

Daria (Persian) queenly
*Dare, Darea, Dareah, Dari,
Darian, Darianne, Darria,
Darya*

Darian (Anglo-Saxon)
precious
*Dare, Darien, Darry, Derian,
Derian*

Darice (English)
contemporary
*Dareese, Darese, Dari, Dariece,
Darri, Darrie, Darry*

Darielle (French) rich
*Darell, Darelle, Dariel, Darriel,
Darrielle*

Darienne (Greek) great

Darika (Indian) young
maiden

Darilyn (American) darling
*Darilin, Darilinn, Darilynn,
Derilyn*

Darina (Greek) rich

Darine (English) feminine
form of Darren: great

Darionne (American)
adventuresome
*Dareon, Darion, Darionn,
Darionna*

Dariya (Russian) sweet
Dara, Darya

Darla (English) form of
Darlene: darling girl
*Darl, Darlee, Darley, Darli,
Darlie, Darly*

Darlee (English) darling
Darl, Darley, Darli, Darlie

Darlene (French) darling girl
*Darlean, Darleen, Darlena,
Darlenia, Darlin, Darling*

Darlenn (French) form of
Darlene: darling girl

Darless (French) form of
Darlene: darling girl

Darlette (French) form of
Darlene: darling girl

Darlina (French) form of
Darlene: darling girl

Darling (American) precious
Darline, Darly, Darlyng

Darlonna (African American) darling
Darlona

Darlusz (Slavic) loved

Darlye (French) darling

Darmetra (American) able

Darnelle (Irish) seamstress
Darnel, Darnell, Darnella, Darnyell

Darnette (American) hides

Daroma (American) treasured

Daron (Irish) great woman
Daren, Darun, Daryn

Darquea (American) different

Darr (Slavic) form of Daria: queenly

Darras (Slavic) rules

Darrelle (English) loved

Darrien (Irish) great

Darrow (Last name as first name) cautious
Darro, Darroh

Darryl (French/English) form of Darlene: darling girl
Darel, Darelle, Daril, Darrell, Darrill, Daryl, Daryll, Derel, Derrell

Darsa (American) bright spirit

Darshelle (African American) confident
Darshel, Darshell

Dart (English) tenacious
Darte, Dartee, Dartt

Darva (Invented) sensible
Darv, Darvah, Darvee, Darvey, Darvi, Darvie

Daryn (Greek/Irish) gift-giver
Daryan, Darynn, Darynne

Daryna (Slavic) form of Daria: queenly

Dash (American) fast-moving
Dashee, Dasher, Dashy

Dasha (Russian) darling
Dashah

Dashanda (African American) loving
Dashan, Dushande

Dashawn (African American) brash
Dashawna, Dashay

Dashawntay (African American) careful
Dash, Dashauntay

Dashea (Hebrew) patient

Dasheena (African American) flashy
Dashea, Dasheana

Dashelle (African American) striking
Dachelle, Dashel, Dashell, Dashy

Dashika (African American) runner
Dash, Dasheka

Dashiki (African) loose shirt; casual
Dashi, Dashika, Dashka, Desheka, Deshiki

Dashilan (American) solemn
Dashelin, Dashelin, Dashlinne, Dashlyn, Dashlynn, Dasialyn

Dasmine (Invented) sleek
Dasmeen, Dasmin, Dazmeen, Dazmine

Dassa (Jewish) form of Hadassah: myrtle tree
Dassah, Dasa

Dassia (American) pretty
Dasie, Dassea, Dasseah, Dassee, Dassi, Dassie, Deassiah

Dathema (Biblical) feminine form of David: beloved

Dati (Hebrew) believer

Dativa (Hebrew) believer

Daufenne (French) of the dolphin

Daulette (American) invented

Dauphinais (French) of the dolphin

Daureen (American) darling
Dareen, Daurean, Daurie, Daury, Dawreen

Dauria (American) form of Daria: queenly

Daveena (Scottish) feminine form of David: beloved
Daveen, Davena, Davey, Davina, Davinna

Davianna (English) beloved

Davida (Hebrew) beloved one
Daveeda, Daveisha, Davesia, Daveta, Davetta, Davette, Davika, Davisha, Davita

Davina (Hebrew) believer; beloved
Dava, Daveena, Davene, Davida, Davita, Devina, Devinia, Devinya

Davincia (Spanish) God-loving; winner
Davince, Davinse, Vincia

Davinique (African American) believer; unique
Davin, Davineek, Vineek

Davis (American) boyish
Daves

Davisnell (Invented) vivacious
Daviesnell, DavisNell

Davonna (Scottish) well-loved
Davon, Davona, Davonda

Davonne (African American) splashy
Davaughan, Davaughn, Davion, Daviona, Davon, Davone, Davonn

Davrush (Yiddish) loves others

Daw (Asian) starlike

Dawa (Tibetan) girl born on Monday

Dawanda (African American) righteous
Dawana, Dawand, Dawanna, Dawauna, Dawonda, Dawonna, Dwanda

Dawn (English) daybreak
Daun, Dawna, Dawne

Dawna (English) eloquence of dawn
Dauna, Daunda, Dawn, Dawnah, Dawnna, Dawny, Dawnya

Dawnesha (American) dawn's child

Dawnika (African American) dawn
Dawneka, Dawneeka, Dawnica, Donika

Dawnisha (African American) breath of dawn
Daunisha, Dawnish, Dawny, Nisa, Nisha

Dawntelle (African American) morning bright
Dawntel, Dawntell, Dontelle

Dawona (African American) smart
Dawonna, Dawonne

Day (English) day; bright

Dayana (American) form of Diana: divine woman; goddess of the hunt and fertility
Dayannah, Dyana

Dayanara (Spanish) form of Deyanira: aggressor
Day, Daya, Dayan, Dianara, Diannare, Nara

Dayita (Indian) loved

Dayla (American) day's joy

Dayle (American) joyful

Daylee (American) calm; reserved
Dailee, Day, Dayley, Dayly

Dayna (English) form of Dana: bright gift of God
Daynah

Daysha (Russian) serene
Dasha, Dayeisha

Dayshanay (African American) saucy
Daysh, Dayshanae, Dayshannay, Dayshie

Dayshawna (American) laughing
Dayshauna, Dayshona, Dashonah

Dayshay (African American) lovable
Dashae, Dashay, Dashea

Dayton (Place name) town in Ohio; fast

Daytona (American) speedy
Dayto, Daytonna

Dayvonne (African American) careful
Dave, Davey, Davonne, Dayvaughn

De (Chinese) virtuous

Deabora (Spanish) form of Debora: prophetess

Deacon (Greek) joyful messenger
Deak, Deakon, Deecon, Deke

Dealba (Irish) Irish girl

Dean (English) practical
Deanie, Deanni

Deana (Latin) divine girl
Deane, Danielle, Deanna

Deandea (English) form of Deanne: mood goddess

Deandria (American) sweetheart
Deandreah, Deandriah

Deanie (English) feminine form of Dean: leader
Deanee, Deaney, Deani

Deanna (Latin/English) divine girl
Deana, Deanne, Dee

Deanne (Latin) form of Diana:
Deann, Dee, Deeann

Dearbhail (Welsh) held close

De-Armone (French) girl of the army

Dearon (American) dear one
Dear, Dearan, Dearen, Deary

Dearoven (American) form of Dearon: dear one
Derovan, Deroven

Deasa (Spanish) delightful

Deatra (English) form of Deitra: goddesslike

DeAyn (Dutch) form of Deann: moon goddess

Debara (Spanish) form of Deborah: prophetess

Debarath (Hebrew) bee; busy
Deborath, Daberath

Debbie (Hebrew) form of
Deborah: prophetess
*Deb, Debbee, Debbey, Debbi,
Debby, Debbye, Debee, Debi,
Debie*

Deborah (Hebrew)
prophetess
*Debbie, Debbora, Debborah,
Debor, Deboreh, Deborrah,
Debra*

Deboria (English) form of
Debora: prophetess

Debra (Hebrew) prophetess
Debbra, Debbrah, Debrah

Debran (American) form of
Deborah: prophetess

Debrani (American) grace

Debray (American) form of
Deborah: prophetess
Dabrae, Deb, Debrae, Debraye

Debrean (Slavic) form of
Deborah: prophetess

Debreka (Slavic) form of
Deborah: prophetess

Dece (Spanish) tenth child

Decena (Latin) form of
Decima: tenth girl
Decia

Deceshia (American) tenth
child

D'Echon (French) echo

Decima (Latin) tenth girl

Decole (French) form of
Nicole: winning

Decolia (American) form of
Nicole: winning

Decuma (Mythology) one of
the Roman Fates; measures

Dedra (American) spirited
*Dee, DeeDee, Deeddra, Deedra,
Deedrea, Deedrie, Deidra,
Deirdre*

Dedranay (American) form
of Deidra: sparkling

Dee (English/Irish) lucky one
*Dedee, Dea, Deah, DeeDee,
Dee-Dee, Didee*

Deedee (American) form of
D names: vivacious
*D.D., Dee Dee, DeeDee, Dee-
Dee*

Deen (English) form of Dean:
practical

Deena (American) soothes

Deepa (Hindi) light

DeErica (African American)
audacious
Dee-Erica

Deesha (American) dancing
*Dedee, Dee, Deesh, Deeshah,
Deisha*

Deianna (English) form of
Deanna: divine girl

Deidra (Irish) sparkling
Deedra, Deidre, Dierdra

Deighan (American) exciting
Daygan, Deigan

Deina (Spanish) soothes

Deiondra (Greek) feminine
form of Dionysis: joyous
celebrant
*Deandrah, Deann, Deanndra,
Dee, Deean, Deeann, DeeDee,
Deondra*

Deirdre (Irish) passionate
*Dedra, Dee, Deedee, Deedrah,
Deerdra, Deerdre, Didi*

Deissy (Greek) form of
Desma: oath
*Deisi, Deissey, Deissie, Desma,
Desmee, Desmer, Dessi*

Deitra (Greek) goddess-like
Deetra, Detria

Deittra (English) form of
Demetria: harvest goddess

Deja (French) already seen
D'Ja, Dejah

Dejan (Slavic) siren

Dejeane (French) born before

Dejoie (French) joy

Dejon (French) she came
before
Daijon, Dajan, Dajona

Deka (African) a pleasure
Dekah, Dekka

Dekeidra (American)
pleasant

Dela (English) dramatic

Delakate (American) delicate

Delana (German) protective
*Dalana, Dalanna, Dalayna,
Daleena, Dalena, Dalenna,
Dalina, Dalinna, Deedee,
Delaina, Delainah, Delena*

Delanah (American) wise
Delana, Dellana, Delano

Delandra (American)
outgoing
Delan, Delande

Delaney (Irish) bouncy;
enthusiastic
*Dalanie, Delaine, Delainey,
Delane, DeLayney, Dellie,
Dulaney*

Delaune (English) form of
Delaney: bouncy; enthusiastic

Delaura (American) prefix De
and Laura

Delcia (Latin) delightful

Delcine (Latin) a delight

Delcy (American) friendly
Del, Delcee, Delci

Dele (American) rash; noble
Del, Dell

Delene (French) dearest girl

Delfin (Spanish) of the
dolphin

Delfina (Latin/Italian)
flowering
Dellfina, Delphina

Delia (Greek) lovely; moon
goddess
*Dehlia, Deilyuh, Del, Delea,
Deli, Dellia, Dellya, Delya,
Delyah*

Delicia (English) delights
*Delesha, Delice, Delisa, Delise,
Delisha, Delisiah, Delya, Delys,
Delyse, Delysia*

Delieca (Spanish) delight

Delight (French) wonderful

Delilah (Hebrew) beautiful
temptress
Dalia, Dalila, Delila, Lilah

Delina (French) dearest

Delinah (American) form of
Adeline: sweet

Delinda (American) form of
Melinda: honey; sweetheart
Delin, Delinde, Delynda

Delinde (French) dearest

Delise (Latin) delicious
*Del, Delice, Delicia, Delisa,
Delissa*

Delite (American) a pleasure
Delight

Delja (Slavic) form of Deja:
already seen

Dell (Greek) kind
Del

Della (Greek) kind
*Dee, Del, Dela, Dell, Delle,
Delli, Dells*

Dellana (Irish) form of
Delaney: bouncy; enthusiastic
*Delaine, Delana, Dell,
Dellaina, Dellane, Dellann*

Dellia (American) pretty

Delmee (American) star
Del, Delmey, Delmi, Delmy

Delmys (American)
incredible
Del, Delmas, Delmis

Delo (Slavic) form of Delos:
beautiful brunette; a small
Aegean isle; stunning

Deloise (Italian) combative

Delon (American) musical
Delonn, Delonne

Delora (Spanish) form of
Delores: woman of sorrowful
leaning
Dellora, Delorita

Delores (Spanish) woman of
sorrowful leaning
*Del, Delora, Delore, Dolores,
Deloria, Delories, Deloris,
Delorise*

Delos (Greek) beautiful
brunette; a small Aegean isle;
stunning
Delas

Delpha (Greek) form of
Delphine: calmness
Delfa

Delphina (Greek) dolphin;
smart

Delphine (Latin) calmness
*Delfina, Delfine, Delpha,
Delphe, Delphene, Delphi,
Delphia, Delphina, Delphinia,
Delvina*

Delphy (Biblical) place name
Delphia, Delphi

Delta (Greek) fourth letter of
the Greek alphabet
Del, Dell, Dellta, Delte, Deltra

Deltrese (African American)
jubilant
*Del, Delltrese, Delt, Delta,
Deltreese, Deltrice*

Delwyn (English/Welsh)
friend from the valley; neat
and fair
Delwen, Delwenne, Delwin

Demareas (Biblical) calf

Demetia (Greek) harvest
goddess

Demetress (Greek) form of
Demetria: harvest goddess
*Deme, Demetra, Demetres,
Demetri, Demetria, Dimi,
Tress, Tressie, Tressy*

Demetria (Greek) harvest
goddess
*Deitra, Demeta, Demeteria,
Demetra, Demetrice, Demetris,
Demetrish, Demetrius, Demi,
Demita, Demitra*

Demetriase (Greek) harvest
goddess

Demi (French) half
Demiah, Demie

Demtrialle (American) regal

Dena (English) laid back;
valley
*Deane, Deena, Deeyn, Denae,
Denah, Dene, Denea, Deney,
Denna*

Denada (American) calm

Denae (Hebrew) form of
Dena: shows the truth
Danay, Denee

Dencie (English) form of
Denise: wine-lover

Denda (American) form of
Dena: laid back; valley

Deneane (English) form of
Denise: wine-lover

Denedra (American) lively;
natural
Den, Dene, Denney

Denee (French) robust

Deneen (American) absolved
Denean, Denene

Deneka (Slavic) star

Denes (English) nature-lover
Denis, Denne, Denny

Denesha (American) rowdy

Denetria (Greek) from God
Denitria, Denny, Dentria

Denetrice (African
American) optimistic
Denetrise, Denitrise, Denny

Denezia (Turkish) of the sea
Denizia, Deniz

Denise (French) wine-lover
*Danice, Daniece, Danise,
Denese, Deni, Denica, Deniece,
Denni, Denny*

Denisha (American) jubilant
*Danisha, Deneesha, Deneesha,
Denesha, Deneshea, Deniesha,
Denishia*

Denna (American) lively

Dennice (American) festive

Denovia (American) reveler

Den'tessa (American) form
of Contessa: pretty

Denton (Place name) town in
Texas; from a holy town
Dent, Dentun, Denty, Dentyn

Denver (English) born in a
green valley
Denv, Denvie

Denyse (American) form of
Denise: wine-lover

Denz (Invented) lively
Dens

Denza (American) fun-loving

Deo (Scottish) God's grace

Deoniece (African American)
feminine
*Dee, DeeDee, Deo, Deone,
Deoneece, Deoneese*

Deonsha (American) form of
Deoniece: feminine

Deonta (American) calm
valley

Deora (English) adored

Deoran (American) adored

Dephoine (American) form
of Delphine: calmness

Dera (Slavic) ocean's child

Derbe (Biblical) place name

Dericka (American) dancer
*D'ericka, Derica, Dericca,
Derika, Derrica, Derricka,
Derrika*

Derie (Hebrew) form of
Derorah: free
Derey, Drora, Drorah

Derline (American) from
land of deer
Derlini

Derneeka (Slavic) of the
ocean

Dernise (American) form of
Denise: wine-lover

Deronique (African
American) unique girl
Deron, Deroneek

Derorah (Hebrew) free
Derora

Derrinda (Spanish) form of
Dorinda: loved

Derrisa (American) form of Merissa: ocean-loving

Derrona (American) natural
Derona, Derone, Derry

Derry (Irish) red-haired woman
Deri, Derrie

Deryn (Welsh) birdlike; small
Derren, Derrin, Derrine, Deryne

Desai (African) desired

Desba (African) desired

Desbiene (American) desired

Desdemona (Greek) tragic figure; destined
Des, Desde, Dez

Desena (American) desired

Deshawna (African American) vivacious
Dashawna, Deshan, Deshanda, Deshandra, Deshane, Deshaun, Deshauna, Deshaundra, Deshaune, Deshawnna, Deshawn, Deshawndra, Desheania, Deshona, Deshonda, Deshonna

Deshette (African American) dishy
Deshett

Deshondra (African American) vivacious
Deshaundra, Deshondrah, Deshondria

Desi (French) form of Desiree: desired
Dezi, Dezzie

Desiah (French) form of Desiree: desired

Desire (English) desired
Dezire

Desiree (French) desired
Des'ree, Desairee, Desarae, Desaray, Desaraye, Desaree, Desarhea, Desary, Deseri, Desree, Des-Ree, Dezaray, Deziree, Dezray

Desireenah (American) desirable

Desirette (American) desires

Desislav (Slavic) glory girl

Deslin (American) tenth

Desma (Greek) oath

Desna (Hindi) giving

Despina (Greek) ladylike

Desreta (Spanish) desires

Dess (Slavic) tenth

Desta (Slavic) joyful

Destin (American) destiny
Destinn, Destyn

Destina (Spanish) destiny
Desteena, Desteenah

Destiny ○ (French) fated
Destanee, Destanie, Desteney, Destinay, Destinee, Destinei, Destini, Destinyi, Destnay, Destney, Destonie, Destony, Destyni

Destry (American) well-fated; western feel
Destrey, Destri, Destrie

Deterrion (Latin) form of Detra: blessed
Deterr, Deterreyon, Detra, Detrae

Detra (Latin) blessed
Detraye

Deva (Hindi) moon goddess; wielder of power
Devi

Devahuti (Hindi) in mythology, daughter of Manu

Devaki (Indian) revered mother of Krishna

Devalca (Spanish) generous
Deval

Devan (Irish) poetic
Devana, Devn

Devashka (Hebrew) honey

Deven (English) dark

Devendra (Indian) dark skin

Devera (Jewish) form of Devorah: heroine

Devette (American) form of Devera: heroine

Devi (Hindi) beloved goddess
Devia, Deviann, Devian, Devie, Devri

Devin (Irish) poetic
Devan, Devane, Devanie, Devany, Deven, Devena, Deveny, Deveyn, Devine, Devinne, Devn, Devyn, Devynne

Devina (Irish) divine; creative
Davena, Devie, Devine, Devy, Divine

Devon (English) poetic
Dev, Devaughan, Devaughn, Devie, Devonne, Devy

Devonna (English) girl from Devonshire; happy
Davonna, Devon, Devona, Devonda, Devondra

Devorah (American) heroine
Devora, Devore, Devra, Devrah

Devy (American) poetic

Devyn (English) poetic

Dew (Word as name) misty; fresh
Dewi, Dewie

Dewanna (African American) clingy
D'Wana, Dewana, Dewanne

Dexhiana (Origin Unknown) nimble

Dexter (English) spunky; dexterous
Dex, Dexee, Dexey, Dexie, Dext, Dextar, Dextur, Dexy

Dextra (Latin) skilled

Deyanira (Spanish) aggressor
Deyan, Deyann, Dianira, Nira

Dezelia (American) desired

Dezena (American) desired

Dezra (American) desirable

Dezral (American) desirable

Dharcia (American) sparkler
Darch, Darsha, Dharsha

Dharika (American) sad
Darica, Darika

Dharini (Indian) earth

Dharma (Hindi) morality; beliefs
Darma, Darmah

Dhazalai (African) sweet
Dhaze, Dhazie

Dhelal (Arabic) coy

Dhessie (American) glowing
Dhessee, Dhessey, Dhessi, Dhessy

Dhira (Indian) flow

Dhivia (Indian) heavenly

Dhumma (Hebrew) form of Dumia: quiet

Di (Latin) form of Diane: goddess-like; divine; or form of Diana: divine woman; goddess of hunt and fertility
Didi, Dy

Di Anna (American) form of Diana: goddesslike; divine

Dia (Greek) shining
Deah

Diaelza (Spanish) divine; pretty
Diael, Dialza, Elza

Diah (American) pretty
Dia

Diamantina (Spanish) sparkling
Diama, Diamante, Mantina

Diamond (Latin) precious gemstone
Diamin, Diamon, Diamonda, Diamonds, Diamonte, Diamun, Diamyn, Diamynd, Dyamond

Diamondah (African American) glowing
Diamonda, Diamonde

Diamondique (African American) sparkling
Diamondik

Diamony (American) gem
Diamonee, Diamoney, Diamoni, Diamonie

Diamrose (Spanish) diamond rose

Diana ✪ (Latin) goddess-like; divine
Dee, Di, Diahana, Diahna, Dianah, Diannah, Didi, Dihanna, Dyanna, Dyannah, Dyhana

Diandro (American) special
Diandra, Diandrea, Diandroh

Diane (Latin) goddess-like; divine
Deane, Deanne, Deeann, Deeanne, Deedee, Di, Diahann, Dian, Diann, Dianne, Didi

Dianelle (American) divine

Diange (American) form of Diane: divine woman; goddess of the hunt and fertility

Dianita (Spanish) divine

Diannie (American) divine girl

Diantha (Greek) flower; heavenly
Dianth

Diarah (American) pretty
Dearah, Di, Diara, Diarra, Dierra

Diathe (Biblical) place name

Diathema (Greek) divine

Diavonne (African American) jovial
Diavone, Diavonna, Diavonni

Dica (Slavic) cautious

Dicey (American) impulsive
Di, Dice, Dicee, Dicy, Dycee, Dycey

Dicia (American) wild
Desha, Dicy

Didah (Biblical) of love

Diedre (Irish) form of Deidre: sparkling
Diedra, DiedrÈ

Diella (Latin) worships
Dielle

Diesha (African American) zany
Diecia, Dieshah, Dieshie, Dieshay

Diethild (German) believer

Difanee (American) form of Daphne: pretty nymph

Diggs (American) tomboyish
Digs, Dyggs

Dihana (American) natural
Dihanna

Dijan (Slavic) divine goddess

Dijana (Slavic) form of
Diana: goddesslike; divine

Dijonnay (American) fun-
loving
*Dijon, Dijonae, Dijonay,
Dijonnae, Dijonnaie*

Dilan (American) form of
Dylan: creative; from the sea
Dillan, Dilon

Dilcia (Spanish) loved

Dileone (Spanish) worships

Dilia (Spanish) worships

Dilly (Welsh) loyal

Dillyana (English) worshipful
Diliann, Dilli, Dillianna, Dilly

Dilsey (American)
dependable; one who endures

Dilva (Slavic) loyal

Dilynn (American) form of
Dylan: creative; from the sea
*Di, Dilenn, Dilinn, Dilyn,
Lynn*

Dilys (Welsh) of the truth

Dima (American) high-
spirited
Deemah, Dema

Dimond (American) form of
Diamond: precious gemstone

Dina (Hebrew/Scottish) right;
royal

Dinah (Hebrew) fair judge
*Dina, Dinah, Dinna, Dyna,
Dynah*

Dinavia (American) form of
Dinah: fair judge

Dinesha (American) happy
Dineisha, Dineshe, Diniesha

Dini (American) joyful
Dinee, Diney, Dinie

Dinora (American) form of
Dinah: fair judge

Dinora (Spanish) judged by
God
Dina, Dino, Nora

Dinorah (Spanish) light

Dinorot (American) form of
Dinah: fair judge

Dioma (Greek) form of
Diona: divine woman

Diona (Greek) divine woman
*Dee, Di, Dion, Dionah,
Dionuh*

Dioneece (American) daring
*Dee, DeeDee, Deon, Deone,
Deonece, Deoneece, Dioniece,
Neece, Neecey*

Dionicia (Spanish) vixen
*Di, Dione, Dionice, Dionise,
Nicia, Nise, Nisee*

Dionis (English) feminine
form of Dion: joyous
celebrant

Dionise (English) feminine
form of Dion: joyous
celebrant

Dionish (American)
feminine form of Dion:
joyous celebrant

Dionndra (American) loving
Diondra, Diondrah, Diondruh

Dionne (Greek) love goddess
*Deona, Deondra, Deonia,
Deonna, Deonne, Dion, Dione,
Dionna*

Dionnesha (American)
feminine form of Dion:
joyous celebrant

Dior (French) stylish
Diora, Diorah, Diore, Diorra, Diorre

Diotima (Latin) in the time of God

Dira (Arabic) soft-spoken

Direll (American) svelte
Di, Direl, Direlle

Dirisha (African American) outgoing
Di, Diresha, Direshe

Dirkae (Scandinavian) feminine form of Dirk: leader

Disa (Scandinavian) goddess

Disano (Italian) wise

Disha (American) fine
Dishae, Dishuh

Dishawna (African American) special
Dishana, Dishauna, Dishawnah, Dishona, Dishonna

Dishi (Indian) the right way

Divina (American) divine being

Divine (Italian) divine soul
Divin, Divina

Divinity (American) sweet; devout
Divinitee, Diviniti, Divinitie

Divora (Indian) divine

Divya (Indian) celestial

Divyanah (Hindi) divine

Dix (French) live wire

Dixie (English/French) from the South in the United States
Dixee, Dixi, Dixy

Diya (Indian) divine

Diyanne (Slavic) form of Diane: divine woman; goddess of the hunt and fertility

Dizian (American) joyful

Dnisha (African American) rejoicing
D'Nisha, Dnisa, Dnish, Dnishay, Dnishe

Dobie (American) cowgirl
Dobee, Dobey, Dobi

Dobra (Polish) kindness

Docia (Latin) form of Docilla: docile
Docie

Docilla (Latin) docile
Docila, Docile

Dodie (Greek/Hebrew) gift of God
Doda, Dodee, Dodi, Dody

Dodona (Greek) ancient city in Greece

Doe (Polish) kind

Doherty (American) ambitious
Dhoertey, Dohertee, Dohertie

Doina (Slavic) lady

Doka (Slavic) dependable

Dolah (Hindi) loved

Dolas (American) sorrows

Dolchil (American) docile

Dolcy (American) a vision
Dolcee, Dolcie, Dolsee

Dollis (American) doleful

Dolly (American) toylike
Dol, Doll, Dollee, Dolli, Dollie

Doloarea (Spanish) sorrows

Dolores (Spanish) woman of sorrowful leaning
Delores

Dolory (Slavic) form of Dolores: woman of sorrowful leaning

Domel (American) steadfast; faithful
Domela, Domella

Dometria (American) form of Demetria: harvest goddess
Dome, Dometrea, Domi, Domini, Domitra

Domina (Latin) ladylike

Dominga (Spanish) her dominion

Domini (Latin) feminine form of Dominic: child of the Lord; saint
Dom, Dominee, Domineke, Dominey, Dominie, Dominika, Domino, Dominy

Dominica (Latin) follower of God
Domenica, Domenika, Domineca, Domineka, Domini, Dominika, Domenika, Domineca, Dom, Domonica, Domonika

Dominique (French) bright; masterful
Dom, Domanique, Domeneque, Domenique, Domino, Domonik

Domitila (Spanish) home-loving

Dona (Latin) always giving
Donail, Donalea, Donalisa, Donay, Donelle, Donetta, Doni, Donia, Donice, Donie, Donise, Donisha, Donishia, Donita, Donitrae

Donalda (Scottish) loves all
Donalda, Donaldina, Donaleen, Donelda, Donella, Donellia, Donette, Doni, Donita, Donnella, Donnelle

Donalie (American) lady

Donata (Italian) celebrating
Donada, Donatah, Donatha, Donatta, Donni, Donnie, Donny

Donatella (Latin/Italian) gift
Don, Donnie, Donny

Donatilde (Spanish) gift

Donava (African) jubilant
Donavah

Dondra (American) ladylike

Dondranea (Invented) ladylike

Donela (Italian) leader
Donella

Donelda (Spanish) giving

Donia (American) form of Donna: ladylike and genteel

Donicia (Spanish) feminine

Donika (African American) form of Donna: ladylike and genteel
Donica

Donisha (African American) laughing; cozy
Daneesha, Danisha, Doneesha

Donna (Italian) ladylike and genteel
Dom, Don, Dona, Dondi, Donnie, Donya

Donnata (Latin) giving
Dona, Donata, Donni

Donnelly (Italian) lush
Donally, Donelly, Donnell, Donnelli, Donnellie, Donni, Donnie, Donny

Donnettella (Italian) giving

Donnis (American) pleasant; giving
Donnice

Donserena (American)
dancer; giving
*Donce, Doncie, Dons, Donse,
Donsee, Donser, Donsey*

Dontilan (American) donates

Donya (Italian) feminine

Donyale (African American)
form of Danielle: judged by
God; spiritual
Donyelle

Donyan (English) feminine

Donyellan (African) upbeat

Dora (Greek) gift from God
*Dorah, Dori, Dorie, Dorra,
Dorrah*

Dorant (American) gifted

Dorat (French) a gift
Doratt, Dorey, Dorie

Dorby (Spanish) devout

Dorcea (Greek) sea girl
Dorcia

Dorcelline (English) fast

Dordea (English) heritage

Dore (Irish) form of Dora:
gift from God

Doree (Hebrew) heritage

Doreen (Greek/Irish)
capricious
Dorene, Dorine, Dory

Dorei (American) form of
Doris: sea-loving; sea nymph

Dorekka (Slavic) form of
Dorika: God's gift

Dorel (Spanish) adored

Dorenda (American) adored

Dorende (American) adored

Doreneah (American) adored

Dorenee (American) form of
Doreen: capricious

Dorentia (American) adored

Doreth (American) form of
Dorit: God's gift; shy

Doretha (American) form of
Dorit: God's gift; shy

Dori (French) adorned
*Dore, Dorey, Dorie, Dory,
Dorree, Dorri, Dorrie, Dorry*

Doria (Greek) form of
Dorian: happy
*Dori, Doriana, Doriann,
Dorianna, Dorianne*

Dorial (American) form of
Dorit: God's gift; shy

Dorian (Greek) happy
*Dorean, Doreane, Doree,
Doriane, Dorri, Dorry*

Dorianna (Greek) of the sea
Dorianne

Dorie (American) faithful

Dorika (Greek) God's gift
Doreek, Dorike, Dory

Dorin (Greek) form of
Dorian: happy

Dorina (Hawaiian) loved

Dorind (American) form of
Doreen: capricious

Dorinda (Spanish) loved

Dorinta (American) gift

Doris (Greek) sea-loving; sea
nymph
*Dor, Dori, Dorice, Dorise,
Doriss, Dorris, Dorrise, Dorrys,
Dory*

Doriscus (Biblical) place name

Dorisette (American) form
of Doris: sea-loving; sea
nymph

Dorit (Greek) God's gift; shy
Dooritt

Dorita (Greek) empress

Dorle (Greek) empress

Dorly (Greek) empress

Dor-Lyn (Combo of Dor and Lyn) empress

Dornay (American) involved
Dorn, Dornae, Dornee, Dorny

Dorothea (Greek) gift from God
Dorethea, Dorotha, Dorothia, Dorotthea, Dorthea, Dorthia

Dorothy (Greek) gift of God
Dorathy, Dorthy

Dorren (Irish) sad-faced
Doren

Dorte (Scandinavian) God's gift

Dortha (Greek) God's gift; studious
Dorth, Dorthee, Dorthey, Dorthy

Dorthe (Scandinavian) God's gift

Dorum (American) God's gift

Dory (French) gilded; gold hair
Dora, Dore, Dorie

Doshene (American) shares

Dosia (Russian) happy

Dossey (Last name as first name) rambunctious
Dosse, Dossi, Dossie, Dossy, Dozze

Dot (Greek) spunky
Dottee, Dottie, Dotty

Dottie (Greek) form of Dorothy: gift of God

Dottye (English) gift

Dottylene (English) gift

Doubta (Slavic) doubtful

Douce (French) sweet
Doucia, Dulce, Dulci, Dulcie

Douet (French) dew

Dove (Greek) dreamy

Dovie (English) dove of peace

Doxey (American) vaiant of Moxie and Dottie

Doxie (Greek) fine
Doxy

Dragana (Slavic) dragon lady

Drahomira (Czech) dearest

Drake (English) dragon

Draleen (American) dragon

Drancine (French) dragon lady

Draven (American) loyal
Dravan, Dravin, Dravine

Draxy (American) faithful
Drax, Draxee, Draxey, Draxi

Draya (Slavic) form of Drake: dragon

Drea (American) adorable

Dream (American) dream girl; misty
Dreama, Dreamee, Dreamey, Dreami, Dreamie, Dreamy

Dreana (Spanish) spiritual

Dreda (Anglo-Saxon) thoughtful
Drida

Dree (American) soft-spoken

Dreena (American) cautious
Dreenah, Drina

Drelan (Origin Unknown) watches

Drena (Spanish) form of Adriana: rich; exotic
Spiritual

Drenda (American) form of
Dorinda: loved

Drenea (American) spiritual

Drestell (American) new

Drew (Greek) woman of valor
Dru, Drue

Driana (American) form of
Adriana: rich; exotic

Dricea (American) form of
Adriana: rich; exotic

Drina (American) form of
Adriana: rich; exotic

Drinda (Spanish) form of
Dorinda: loved

Drisena (Spanish) strong

Dristi (Indian) insightful

Drover (American)
surprising
Drovah, Drovar

Dru (American) bright
Drew, Drue

Druanna (American) bold
*Drewann, Drewanne,
Druanah, Druannah*

Drucelle (American) smart
*Druce, Drucee, Drucel, Drucell,
Drucey, Druci, Drucy*

Druella (Latin) form of
Drusilla: strong

Drummond (Last name used
as first name) drummer's
mountain

Druna (English) leader

Drusa (Latin) form of
Drusilla: strong
Drusie, Drucie

Drusi (Latin) strong girl
*Drucey, Drucie, Drucy, Drusey,
Drusie, Drusy*

Drusilla (Latin) strong
Dru, Drucilla

Dryden (Last name as first
name) special
Dydie

Duana (Irish) dark
Dwana

Dubethza (Invented) sad
Dubeth

Duchess (American) fancy
*Duc, Duchesse, Ducy, Dutch,
Dutchey, Dutchie, Dutchy*

Ducy (Slavic) purest

Duena (Spanish) chaperones;
guards

Duffy (Irish) spunky

Dufvenius (Swedish) lovely
Duf, Duff

Duhnell (Hebrew)
kindhearted
Danee, Danny, Nell

Duiene (Spanish)
accompanies

Dulce-Maria (Spanish) sweet
Mary
Dulce, Dulcey

Dulceria (Spanish) sweet

Dulcibella (Italian) sweet
beauty

Dulcie (Latin/Spanish) sweet
one
Dulce, Dulcey, Dulcy

Dulcinea (Latin) sweet
nature

Dulvio (Italian) helpful

Duma (African) quiet help
Dumah

Dumia (Hebrew) quiet
Dumi

Duna (Spanish) protects

Dune (American) summery
Doone, Dunah, Dunie

Dunesha (African American)
warm
Dunisha

Dunning (Last name used as
first name) alive

Dupre (American) soft-
spoken
Dupray, Duprey

Dura (Biblical) place name

Dureene (Latin) endures

Durice (American) out of
reach

Durrah (Hindi) heroine

Dusanka (Slavic) soulful
*Dusan, Dusana, Dusank,
Sanka*

Duscha (Russian) happy
*Dusa, Duschah, Dusha,
Dushenka*

Duse (Slavic) happy

Dusky (Invented) dreamy

Dusky-Dream (Invented)
dreamy
Duskee-Dream

Dustine (German) go-getter
*Dustee, Dusteen, Dustene,
Dusti, Dustie, Dustina, Dusty*

Dusty (American) southern
Dustee, Dusti, Dustie, Dustey

Dwanda (American) athletic
Dwana, Dwayna, Dwunda

Dwayna (American)
feminine form of Dwayne:
swarthy

Dwyn (Welsh) fairhaired

Dyan (Latin) form of Diane:
goddesslike; divine
*Dian, Dyana, Dyane, Dyani,
Dyann, Dyanna, Dyanne*

Dyandra (Latin) sleek
*Diandra, Dianndrah, Dyan,
Dyandruh*

Dylan (Welsh) creative; from
the sea
*Dilann, Dyl, Dylane, Dylann,
Dylanne, Dylen, Dylin, Dyllan,
Dylynn*

Dylana (Welsh) sea-loving

Dymea (American) crazed

Dymond (American) form of
Diamond: precious gemstone
*Dymahn, Dymon, Dymonn,
Dymund*

Dymphia (Irish) poetic
Dimphia

Dynasty (Word as name)
substantial; rich

Dynet (American) curious

Dyney (American) consoling
others
Diney, DiNey, Dy

Dyonne (American)
marvelous
Dyonn, Dyonna, Dyonnae

Dyronisha (African
American) fine
Dyron

Dyshaunna (African
American) dedicated
*Dyshaune, Dyshawn,
Dyshawna*

Dyshay (American) healthy

Dywon (American) bubbly
*Diwon, Dywan, Dywann,
Dywaughn, Dywonne*

Dzidzo (African) universal
child

E

Eadrianne (American)
standout
*Eddey, Eddi, Eddy, Edreiann,
Edrian, Edrie*

Eamina (American) curious

E'ann (Irish) sunny

Eanna (Irish) sunny

Earla (English) leader
*Earlah, Erla, Erlene, Erletta,
Erlette*

Earlean (Irish) dedicated
*Earla, Earlecia, Earleen,
Earlena, Earlene, Earlina,
Earlinda, Earline, Erla, Erlana,
Erlene, Erlenne, Erlina,
Erlinda, Erline, Erlisha*

Earlette (American) dedicated

Earlinetta (American)
dedicated

Early (American) bright
Earlee, Earlie, Earlye, Erly

Earlyne (American) dedicated

Earnesia (Spanish) sincere

Earth (English) earth child

Eartha (English) earth
mother

Earthelen (American) earthy

Earthine (American) of the
earth

Easter (American) born on
Easter; springlike

Easton (American)
wholesome
*Eastan, Easten, Eeston, Eastun,
Estynn*

Eavan (Irish) beautiful
Evaughn, Eevonne

Ebba (English/Scandinavian)
strong
Eb, Eba, Ebbah

Ebban (American) pretty;
affluent
Ebann, Ebbayn

Ebbie (English) blessed child

Ebony (Greek) hard and dark
*Eb, Ebanie, Ebbeny, Ebbie,
Ebonea, Ebonee, Eboney, Eboni,
Ebonie, Ebonni*

Ebonyishia (American) black

Eboyn (English) form of
Ebony: hard and dark

Ebrel (Cornish) from the
month April
Ebby, Ebrelle, Ebrie, Ebrielle

Echo (Greek) echo

Echo (Greek) smitten
Eko

Ecia (Slavic) royal

Ecstasy (American) joyful
Ecstasey, Ecstasie, Stase

Eda (Irish) form of Edith: a
blessed girl who is a gift to
mankind

Edaena (Irish) fiery;
energetic
*Ed, Eda, Edae, Edana, Edanah,
Edaneah, Eddi*

Edalene (German) refined
*Eda, Edalyne, Edeline, Ediline,
Lena, Lene*

Edana (Irish) flaming energy
Eda, Edan, Edanna

Eddi (English) form of
Edwina: prospering female
Eddie, Eddy, Edy

Edel (German) clever; noble
Edell, Eddi

Eden (Hebrew) paradise of delights
Ede, Edena, Edene, Edin, Edyn

Edessa (Biblical) place name; flourishes

Edia (Hebrew) special

Edie (English) form of Edith: a blessed girl who is a gift to mankind
Eadie, Edee, Edi, Edy, Edye, Eydie

Edieh (American) gifted

Edina (Slavic) affluent

Edith (English) a blessed girl who is a gift to mankind
Eadith, Ede, Edetta, Edette, Edie, Edithe, Editta, Ediva, Edy, Edyth, Edythe, Eydie

Editha (Spanish) blessed

Edithanette (American) blessed

Edju (Origin unknown) giving
Eddju

Edlin (German) noble; sophisticated
Eddi, Eddy, Edlan, Edland, Edlen

Edmea (Scottish) form of Edme: beloved
Beloved

Edmee (American) spontaneous
Edmey, Edmi, Edmy, Edmye

Edmonda (English) feminine form of Edmond: protective
Edmon, Edmond, Edmund, Edmunda, Monda

Edna (Hebrew) youthful
Eddie, Ednah, Edneisha, Ednita, Eydie

Edreanna (American) merry
Edrean, Edreana, Edreanne, Edrianna

Edrika (Scandinavian) forever

Edrina (American) old-fashioned
Ed, Eddi, Eddrina, Edrena, Edrinah

Edsel (American) plain
Eds, Edsell, Edzel

Edshone (American) wealthy
Ed, Eds, Edshun

Edwina (English) prospering female
Eddi, Eddy, Edina, Edweena, Edwena, Edwenna, Edwine, Edwyna, Edwynna

Efanye (African) respected

Effemy (Greek/German) form of Euphemia: well-spoken
Efemie, Efemy, Effee, Effemie, Effey, Effie, Effy

Effen (English) eloquent

Effie (Greek) form of Euphemia: well-spoken
Effi, Effia, Effy, Ephie

Efigenia (Spanish) form of Eugenia: high-born

Efrat (Hebrew) bountiful
Efrata

Egan (American) wholesome
Egen, Egun

Eglantyne (French) flower

Egypt (Place name) country; exotic
Egyppt

Egzanth (Invented) form of Xanthe: beautiful blonde; yellow

Ehrone (Slavic) peaceful

Eileen (Irish) bright and spirited
Eilean, Eilee, Eileena, Eileene, Eilena, Eilene, Eiley, Eilleen, Eillen, Eilyn, Elene, Ellie

Eireen (Scandinavian) peacemaker
Eirena, Erene, Ireen, Irene

Eires (Greek) peaceful
Eiress, Eres, Heris

Eirianne (English) peaceful
Eirian, Eriann

Ekaja (Hindi) only child

Ekanta (Hindi) loyalty

Ekaterina (Slavic) respected

Ekaterini (Slavic) form of Katherine: pure

Eko (American) form of Echo: echo

Eks (Slavic) gleans

Ekta (Indian) together

Elaine (French) dependable girl
Elain, Elaina, Elainia, Elainna, Elan, Elana, Elane, Elania, Elanie, Elanna, Elayn, Elayna, Elayne, Ellaine

Elana (Greek) pretty
Ela, Elan, Elani, Elanie, Lainie

Elanja (Slavic) gleeful girl

Elasa (Biblical) place name

Elata (Latin) bright; well-positioned
Ela, Elate, Elatt, Elle, Elota

Elcida (Spanish) elucidate

Elda (Italian) protective

Eldee (American) light
El, Eldah, Elde

Eldora (Spanish) golden girl
Eldoree, Eldorey, Eldori, Eldoria, Eldorie, Eldory

Eldora (Spanish) golden spirit

Eldulita (Spanish) protective

Eleacie (American) forthright
Acey, Elea, Eleasie

Eleanor (Greek) light-hearted
Elana, Elanor, Elanore, Eleanora, Elenor, Elenorah, Eleonor, Eleonore, Elinor, Elinore, Ellie, Ellinor, Ellinore, Elynor, Elynore, Lenore

Eleanora (Greek) light

Eleanora (Greek) light
Elenora, Eleonora, Eleora, Ella nora, Ellora, Ellenora, Ellenorah, Elnora, Elora, Elynora

Eleatrice (Greek) free girl

Electra (Greek) shining; brilliant
Elec, Elek, Elektra

Elegy (American) lasting
Elegee, Eleggee, Elegie, Eligey

Elek (American) star-like
Elec, Ellie, Elly

Elelvina (Spanish) resilient

Elena (Greek/Russian/Spanish) form of Helen: beautiful; light
Elana, Eleana, Eleen, Eleena, Elen, Elene, Eleni, Ilena, Ilene, Lena, Leni, Lennie, Lina, Nina

Eleni (Greek) sweet
Elenee

Eleonore (French) form of Helen: beautiful; light
Elenore, Elle, Elnore

Eleovina (Spanish) bright
way

Eleri (Welsh) smooth
Elere, Eleree

Elettra (Latin/Italian) form of
Electra: shining; brilliant

Elfin (American) small girl
*El, Elf, Elfan, Elfee, Elfey, Elfie,
Elfun, Els*

Elfreda (English) elf strength;
good counselor

Elfrida (German) peaceful
spirit
*Elfie, Elfrea, Elfredda, Elfreeda,
Elfreyda, Elfryda*

Elgie (Spanish) chosen elegy

Eliana (Hebrew) the Lord
answers
*Eliane, Elianna, Elianne,
Elliana, Ellianne, Ellie, Liana,
Liane*

Eliane (French) cheerful;
sunny

Elicabeth (American) form of
Elizabeth: God's promise

Elicia (Hebrew) dedicated
Ellicia

Eliki (Hawaiian) abundant

Elisa (Spanish) dedicated to
God
*Elecea, Eleesa, Elesa, Elesia,
Elisia, Elissa, Elisse, Elisya,
Ellisa, Ellisia, Ellissa, Ellissia,
Ellissya, Ellisya, Elysa, Elysia,
Elyssia, Elyssya, Elysya, Leese,
Leesie, Lisa*

Elisabet
(Hebrew/Scandinavian) form
of Elizabeth: God's promise
Bet, Elsa, Else, Elisa

Elisabeth
(Hebrew/French/German)
form of Elizabeth: God's
promise
*Bett, Bettina, Elisa, Elise, Els,
Elsa, Elsie, Ilsa, Ilyse, Liesa,
Liese, Lisbeth, Lise*

Elise (French) consecrated to
God
Elice, Elisse, Elle, Ellyse, Lisie

Eliseu (Biblical) abundance in
God

Elisha (Greek) God-loving
*Eleacia, Eleasha, Elecia,
Eleesha, Eleisha, Elesha,
Eleshia, Elicia, Eliesha, Ellie,
Lisha*

Elishama (American) loves
God

Elishca (American) form of
Elizabeth: God's promise

Elisheba (Biblical) form of
Elizabeth: God's promise

Elissa (Greek) from the
blessed isles
*Ellissa, Ellyssa, Elyssa, Ilissa,
Ilyssa*

Elita (French) selected one
*Elida, Elitia, Elitie, Ellita,
Ellitia, Ellitie, Ilida, Ilita, Litia*

Elite (Latin) best
Elita

Eliza (Irish) sworn to God
Aliza, Elieza, Elize, Elyza

Elizabeth ○ ❶ (Hebrew)
God's promise
*Beth, Betsy, Elisabeth,
Elizebeth, Lissie, Liza*

Elizeth (American) form of
Elizabeth: God's promise

Elke (Dutch) distinguished
Elki, Ilki

Elken (American) believer

Elkie (Dutch) form of Elke:
distinguished
Elk, Elka

Ella ✪ ✿ (Greek) beautiful
and fanciful
Ellamae, Elle, Ellia, Ellie, Elly

Ellaina (American) sincere
Elaina, Ellana, Ellanuh

Ellan (American) coy
Elan, Ellane, Ellyn

Elle (Scandinavian) woman
Ele

Ellen (English) open-minded
*El, Elen, Elenee, Eleny, Elin,
Ellene, Ellie, Ellyn, Ellynn, Elyn*

Ellender (American) decisive
Elender, Ellander, Elle, Ellie

Elli (Scandinavian) aged
Ell, Elle, Ellie

Ellice (English) loves God
Ellecia, Ellyce, Elyce

Ellie (English) candid
Ele, Elie, Elly

Ellina (Scandinavian) valuable

Ells (Scandinavian) patient
Els

Ellyce (French) abundance in
God

Elm (Botanical) tree

Elma (Turkish) sweet
El

Elmas (Armenian)
diamondlike
Elmaz, Elmes, Elmis

Elna (American) light

Elnora (American) sturdy
Ellie, Elnor, Elnorah

Elocile (Spanish) easy child

Elodia (Spanish) flowering
Elodi

Elodie (French) melody

Eloina (Spanish) fulfills
destiny

Eloisa (Italian) sun girl

Eloise (German) high-spirited
Eluise, Luise

Elora (American) fresh-faced
Elorah, Flory, Floree

Eloyse (English) form of
Eloise: high-spirited

Eloysee (American) form of
Eloise: high-spirited

Elpidia (Spanish) shining
El, Elpey, Elpi, Elpie

Elrica (German) leader
*Elrick, Elrika, Elrike, Rica,
Rika*

Elsa (German) form of
Elizabeth: God's promise
*Ellsa, Ellse, Ellsey, Els, Elsah,
Elseh, Elsie, Ellsee*

Elsie (German) hard-working
Elsee, Elsi, Elsy

Elsiy (Spanish) God-loving
El, Els, Elsa, Elsee, Elsi, Elsy

Elspeth (Scottish) loved by
God
El, Elle, Els

Elspie (Scottish) regal

Elsy (Spanish) form of
Elizabeth: God's promise

Elton (American)
spontaneous
Elt, Elten, Eltone, Eltun

Eluvia (Spanish) happy

Elva (English) tiny
*Elvenea, Elvia, Elvie, Elvina,
Elvinea, Elvineah, Elvah*

Elverna (American) form of
Elvire: truest of all

Elvetta (American) form of
Elva: tiny

Elvia (Latin) sunny
Elvea, Elviah, Elvie

Elvira (Latin/German) truth
Elva, Elvie, Elvina, Elwire, Vira

Elvire (French) truest of all

Elyana (Spanish) friend

Elyanna (American) good
friend
Elyana, Elyannah, Elyunna

Elyse (English) soft-mannered
*Elice, Elle, Elysee, Elysia,
Ilysia, Ilysia*

Elysia (Latin) joyful
Elyse, Elysee, Elysha, Elyshia

Elyssa (Greek) form of Elissa:
from the blessed isles
Elisa, Elissa, Elysa, Illysa, Lyssa

Elysse (French) God's
abundance

Elzada (Polish) form of
Elizabeth: God's promise

Emalee (German) thoughtful
*Emalea, Emaleigh, Emaley,
Emaline, Emally, Emaly,
Emmalynn, Emmeline,
Emmelyne*

Emann (American) soft-
spoken
Eman

Emaunuela (Spanish)
believes in God

Ember (American)
temperamental
Embere, Embre

Emberatriz (Spanish)
respected
*Emb, Ember, Embera,
Emberatrice, Emberatryce,
Embertrice, Embertrise*

Emberli (American) pretty
*Em, Emb, Ember, Emberlee,
Emberley, Emberly*

Embray (American) form of
Emily: industrious; eager

Eme (Hawaiian) loved
*Em, Emee, Emm, Emmee,
Emmie, Emmy*

Eme (German) form of
Emma: universal; all-
embracing
Emee, Emme, Emmee

Emea (Dutch) competes

Emelle (American) kind
Emell

Emelsa (Spanish) emulates

Emely (German) go-getter
Emel, Emelee, Emelie

Emena (Latin) of fortunate
birth
*Em, Emen, Emene, Emina,
Emine*

Emera (Irish) talented

Emerald (French) bright as a
gemstone
Em, Emmie

Emerenciana (Spanish)
experienced

Emerene (Spanish)
experienced

Emerita (Spanish)
experienced

Emesa (Biblical) place name;
reserved

Emestina (American) form of Ernestine: sincere spirit
Emee, Emes, Emest, Tina

Emigdea (Spanish) enigmatic

Emika (Slavic) charming

Emilee (American) form of Emily: industrious; eager

Emilia (Italian) soft-spirited
Emalia, Emelia, Emila

Emilie (French) charmer

Emily ✪ ✿ (Latin) industrious; eager
Em, Emalie, Emilee, Emili, Emilie, Emmi, Emmie

Emma ✪ ✿ (German) universal; all-embracing
Em, Emmah, Emme, Emmie, Emmi, Emmot, Emmy, Emmye, Emott

Emmaline (French/German) form of Emily: industrious; eager
Em, Emaline, Emalyne, Emiline, Emmie

Emmanuelle (Hebrew/French) believer
Em, Emmi, Emmie, Emmy

Emmatha (Biblical) place name; dedicated

Emme (German) feminine
Em

Emmi (German) pretty
Emmee, Emmey, Emmy

Emoke (Asian) charms

Emperatriz (Spanish) empress

Emroy (American) elegant royal

Emsky (American) fun

Ena (Hawaiian) intense
Eana, En, Enna, Ina

Encetta (Spanish) starts

Enchantay (American) enchanting
Enchantee

Endah (Irish) flighty
Ena, End, Enda

Endia (American) form of India: woman of India
Endee, Endey, Endie, Endy, India, Ndia

Endriss (Slavic) endears

Enedelia (Spanish) praiseworthy

Enedina (Spanish) praised; spirited
Dina, Ened

Enesha (American) warmth

Enette (American) warmth

Engracia (Spanish) ingratiates

Enid (Welsh) lively
Eneid

Enideen (American) vibrant

Enka (Scandinavian) gem

Enna (Greek) ninth child

Ennis (Irish) dignity

Enore (English) careful
Enoor, Enora

Enrichetta (French) enriches the home

Enslie (American) emotional
Ens, Enslee, Ensley, Ensly, Enz

Enya (Irish) fiery; musician
Enyah, Nya

Epatha (African) empathy

Epifania (Spanish) proof
Epi, Epifaina, Epifanea, Eppie, Pifanie, Piffy

Epiphania (Biblical) place name; religious epiphany

Eppy (Greek) lively
Ep, Eppee, Eppey, Eppi, Eps

Equoia (African American) great equalizer
Ekowya

Era (Slavic) from the windy place

Eranth (Greek) spring bloomer
Erantha, Eranthae, Eranthe

Erasema (Spanish) happy
Eraseme

Erathine (American) earth child

Erato (Mythology) pretty poet

Erba (Spanish) feminine

Ercella (Spanish) earnest

Ercie (Spanish) sincere

Ercilia (American) frank
Erci, Ercilya

Erdell (American) of the earth

Erendia (Spanish) calm

Erendira (Spanish) peaceful

Erene (Irish) irish child

Eres (Greek) goddess of chaos
Era, Ere, Eris

Eridania (Spanish) rules

Erika (Scandinavian) honorable; leading others
Erica, Ericah, Ericca, Ericha, Ericka, Erikka, Errica, Errika, Eryka, Erykka, Eryka

Erin (Irish) peace-making
Eran, Eren, Erena, Erene, Ereni, Eri, Erian, Erine, Erinn, Erinne, Eryn, Erynn, Erynne

Erina (American) peaceful
Era, Erinna, Erinne, Eryna, Erynne

Eriqueta (Spanish) ruling

Erla (Spanish) loyal

Erla (Irish) playful

Erlen (Spanish) loyal

Erlina (Spanish) loyal

Erlind (Hebrew) form of Erlinda: loyal
Erlinda, Erlinde

Erlinda (Spanish) loyal

Erma (Latin) wealthy
Erm, Irma

Ermelinda (Spanish) fresh-faced
Ermalinda, Ermelind, Ermelynda

Ermine (Latin) rich
Erma, Ermeen, Ermie, Ermin, Ermina, Erminda, Erminia, Erminie

Erminette (Italian) noble

Erna (English) form of Ernestine: sincere spirit
Emae, Ernea, Ernie

Ernelle (German) earnest

Ernestine (English) sincere spirit
Erna, Ernaline, Ernesia, Ernesta, Ernestina, Ernestyne

Ernme (Scandinavian) sincere

Erona (Welsh) form of Erin: peacemaking

Ersemi (Scandinavian) gem

Ertha (English) form of Eartha; also form of Bertha: earth mother

Erwen (Welsh) blessing

Eryn (Irish) calm

Erynea (English) earnest

Erzsebet (French) form of Elizabeth: God's promise

Es (American) form of Estella: radiant star
Esa, Essie

Esbelda (Spanish) black-haired beauty
Es, Esbilda, Ezbelda

Esdey (American) warmhearted
Esdee, Esdy, Essdey

Esenzia (Spanish) essence

Esha (Slavic) vibrant

Eshah (African) exuberant
Esha

Eshe (African) life
Eshay

Eshey (American) life
Es, Esh, Eshae, Eshay

Esiquio (Spanish) child of Sunday

Esmee (French) much loved
Esma, Esme, Esmie

Esmeralda (Spanish) emerald; shiny and bright
Emelda, Es, Esmerelda, Esmerilda, Esmie, Esmiralda, Esmirilda, Ezmerelda, Ezmirilda

Esmirna (Spanish) noble

Esne (English) happy
Es, Esnee, Esney, Esny, Essie

Esperanza (Spanish) hopeful
Es, Espe, Esperance, Esperans, Esperanta, Esperanz, Esperanza

Essence (American) ingenious
Esence, Essens, Essense

Essene (Slavic) girl of the wind
Essen

Essica (American) form of Jessica: rich

Essie (English) queenly

Essie (English) shining
Es, Essa, Essey, Essie, Essy

Esta (Hebrew) bright star
Es, Estah

Estalyn (English) noble girl

Estana (Slavic) form of Esther: myrtle leaf

Estee (English) brightest
Esti

Estefani (Spanish) crowned

Estefania (Spanish) crowned

Estelita (Spanish) little queen

Estella (French) radiant star
Es, Estel, Estell, Estelle, Estie, Stell, Stella

Estelle (French) glowing star
Es, Essie, Estee, Estel, Estele, Estell, Estie

Esterlea (Scandinavian) star queen

Estevina (Spanish) adorned; wreathed
Estafania, Este, Estebana, Estefania, Estevan, Estevana

Esth (French) star

Esthelia (Spanish) shining
Esthe, Esthel, Esthele, Esthelya

Esther (Persian) myrtle leaf
Es, Essie, Estee, Ester, Esthur

Estherelda (Spanish) form of Esther: myrtle leaf

Estherita (Spanish) bright
Estereta

Estime (French) esteemed
Es

Estine (German) sweet child

Estrella (Latin) shining star
Estrell, Estrelle, Estrilla

Eta (German) form of
Henrietta: home-ruler
Etah

Etaney (Hebrew) focused
Eta, Etana, Etanah, Etanee

Ethel (English) noble
*Ethelda, Ethelin, Etheline,
Ethelle, Ethelyn, Ethelynn,
Ethelynne, Ethyl*

Ethelen (English) strong

Ethelene (American) form of
Ethel: noble
Ethe, Etheline

Ethne (Irish) blueblood
Eth, Ethnee, Ethnie, Ethny

Ethnea (Irish) kernel; piece
of the puzzle
Ethna, Ethnia

Etosha (African) energetic

Etta (German/English) form
of Henrietta: home-ruler
Etti, Ettie, Etty

Eudlina (Slavic) generous;
affluent
Eudie, Eudlyna, Udie, Udlina

Eudocia (Greek) fine
Eude, Eudocea, Eudosia

Eudora (Greek) cherished

Eudore (Greek) treasured

Eudoxia (Spanish) fine

Eufrocina (Spanish)
happiness

Eugenia (Greek) regal and
polished

*Eugeneia, Eugenie, Eugenina,
Eugina, Gee, Gina*

Eula (Greek) specific
Eulia

Eulala (Greek) spoken sweetly
Eulalah

Eulalia (Greek/Italian) well-
spoken
Eula, Eulia, Eulie

Eulanda (American) fair
Eudlande, Eulee, Eulie

Eunice (Greek) joyful;
winning
*Euna, Euniece, Eunique,
Eunise, Euniss*

Eunja (Asian) silver

Eupheme (Greek) form of
Euphemia: well-spoken
*Eu, Euphemee, Euphemi,
Euphemie*

Euphemia (Greek) well-
spoken
*Effam, Eufemia, Euphan,
Euphie, Uphie*

Euphrosyne (Greek) one of
the three Graces; joy

Eureka (Word as name)
surpise

Eurydice (Greek)
adventurous
Euridice, Euridyce, Eurydyce

Eustacia (Greek) industrious
Eustace, Stacey, Stacy

Eustolia (Spanish) tenacious;
moves well

Euvenia (American)
hardworking
Euvene, Euvenea

Eva (Hebrew/Scandinavian)
life
Evah, Evalea, Evalee

Evadne (Greek) pleasing; lucky
Eva, Evad, Evadnee, Evadny

Evaline (French) form of Evelyn: optimistic
Evalyn, Eveleen

Evan (American) bright; precocious
Evann, Evin

Evana (Greek) lovely woman
Eve, Ivana, Ivanna, Evania

Evangelina (Greek) bringing joy
Eva, Evangelia, Evangelica, Evangeline, Evania, Eve, Lina

Evania (Irish) spirited
Ev, Evana, Evanea, Evann, Evanna, Evanne, Evany, Eve, Eveania, Evvanne, Evyan

Evanka (Slavic) form of Ivanka: gracious gift from God

Evanthie (Greek) flowering well
Evanthe, Evanthee, Evanthi

Eve (Hebrew) life
Eva, Evie, Evvy

Evegelina (Spanish) lively

Evelina (Russian) lively
Evalina, Evalinna

Evelyn ☻ (English) optimistic
Aveline, Ev, Evaleen, Evalene, Evaline, Evalenne, Evalyn, Evalynn, Evalynne, Eveleen, Eveline, Evelyne, Evelynn, Evelynne, Evline

Evelyna (Scandinavian) form of Evelyn: optimistic

Ever (Word as name) eternal
Ev

Everilda (Spanish) forever

Everilde (Origin unknown) hunter

Everla (English) ever

Everleen (American) evergreen

Everlin (American) forever

Evette (French) dainty
Evett, Ivette

Evgeniia (Slavic) form of Eugenia: regal and polished

Evie (English) vibrant life

Evine (English) alive

Evlesin (American) lives large

Evline (French) nature girl
Evleen, Evlene, Evlin, Evlina, Evlyn, Evlynn, Evlynne

Evolia (Slavic) form of Evelyn: optimistic

Evonne (French) form of Yvonne: athletic
Evanne, Eve, Evie, Yvonne

Evonnette (American) form of Evelyn: optimistic

Ewelina (Polish) life
Eva, Lina

Exee (American) form of Lexie: helpful; sparkling

Exelda (Spanish) excels

Eydie (American) endearing
Eidey, Eydee

Eyote (Native American) great
Eyotee

Ezra (Hebrew) happy; helpful
Ezrah, Ezruh

Ezza (American) healthy
Eza

F

Faba (Latin) bean; thin
Fabah, Fava

Fabette (Italian) fabulous
little girl

Fabi (Italian) generous

Fabia (Latin) fabulous; special
Fabiann, Fabianna, Fabianne

Fabienne (French) fabulous

Fabienne (French) farming
beans

Fabio (Latin) fabulous
Fabeeo, Fabeo, Fabeoh

Fabiola (Spanish) royalty

Fabrizia (Italian) manual
worker
*Fabrice, Fabricia, Fabrienne,
Fabriqua, Fabritzia*

Fadia (Arabic) saved

Fae (English) form of Faye:
light-spirited

Fael (English) of the fairies

Faffa (American) frivolity

Fahimah (Arabic) form of
Fatima: wise woman

Faida (Arabic) bountiful
Fayda

Faillace (French) delicate
beauty
Faill, Faillaise, Faillase, Falace

Faine (English) happy
Fai, Fainne, Fay, Fayne

Fairlee (English) lovely
Fair, Fairlea, Fairley, Fairly

Faith ○ ● (English) loyal
woman
Fay, Fayth

Faithette (American)
trustworthy

Falesyia (Hispanic) exotic
Falesyiah, Falisyia

Faline (Latin/French) lively
Faleen, Falene

Fall (Word as name)
changeable
Falle

Fallon (Irish) fetching; from
the ruling class
Falan, Fallen, Fallyn, Falyn

Falsette (American) fanciful
Falcette

Famke (Polish) little girl

Fanchon (French) form of
France
*Fan, Fanchee, Fanchie, Fanny,
Fran, Frannie, Franny*

Fancine (French) fancy

Fancy (English) fanciful
Fanci, Fancie

Fandila (Spanish) dancer

Fane (American) strict
Fain, Faine

Fanfara (Last name as first
name) fanfare; excitement
Fann, Fanny

Fang (Chinese) pleasantly
scented

Fanny (Latin) from France
Fan, Fani, Fannie

Fantasia (American)
inventive
*Fantasha, Fantasiah, Fantasya,
Fantazia*

Fantazee (American) fantasy

Fantazie (American) fantasy

Fanteen (English) clever
*Fan, Fannee, Fanney, Fanny,
Fantene, Fantine*

Farah (English) lovely
Farrah

Faray (Arabic) form of Farrah:
good-looking; happy

Faredah (Arabic) special
Farida

Farhanah (Arabic) lovely

Farica (German) leader
Faricka, Fericka, Flicka

Farida (Arabic) wanders far

Farina (Latin) flour
Fareena

Faris (American) forgiving
Fair, Farris, Pharis, Pharris

Farrah (English/Arabic) good-
looking; happy
Fara, Farah

Farren (American) fair
Faren, Farin

Farrow (American) narrow-
minded
Farow, Farro

Faryl (American) inspiring
Farel, Farelle

Farzana (American) wanders

Fashion (American) stylish
Fashon, Fashy, Fashyun

Fatie (Arabic) winning

Fatima (Arabic) wise woman
Fatema, Fatimah, Fatime

Faulk (American) respected
Falk

Fauna (Roman mythology)
goddess of nature
Faunah, Fawna, Fawnah

Faunee (Latin) nature-loving
*Fauney, Fauneye, Fawnae,
Fawni, Fawny*

Fausta (French) desired

Fausta (Italian) lucky

Faustene (French/American)
envied
*Fausteen, Faustine, Fausty,
Fawsteen*

Faustiana (Spanish) good
fortune
Faust, Fausti, Faustia, Faustina

Faustina (Italian) lucky
*Fausta, Faustine, Fawsteena,
Fostina, Fostynna*

Favela (Spanish) favored

Favianna (Italian) confident
Faviana

Faviolia (Indian) lucky

Fawn (French) gentle
Faun, Fawne

Fawna (French) soft-spoken
Fawnna, Fawnah, Fawnuh

Fawntae (English) fawn girl

Fawntay (American) fawn
girl

Faye (English/French) light-
spirited
Fae, Fay, Fey

Fayette (American) southern
Fayet, Fayett, Fayetta, Fayitte

Fayleen (American) quiet
*Faylene, Fayline, Falyn, Falynn,
Faye, Fayla*

Fayrale (American) wins

Fayth (American) form of
Faith: loyal woman
Faithe, Faythe

Fe (Latin) believer

Feather (Native American)
svelte
Feathyr

Febe (Polish/Greek) bright
Febee

February (Latin) icy
Feb

Fedora (Greek) God's gift

Fedyle (American) loyal

Felda (German) field girl

Felder (Last name as first name) bright
Felde, Feldy

Felice (Latin) form of Felicia: happy
Felece, Felise

Felicia (Latin) happy
Faleshia, Falesia, Felecia, Felisha

Felicie (Latin) form of Felicia: happy
Feliccie, Felicee, Felicy, Felisie

Felicita (Spanish) gracious
Felice, Felicitas, Felicitee, Felisita

Felicity (Latin) form of Felicia: happy
Felice, Felicite, Felicitee, Felisitee

Felisa (Spanish) form of Felicia: happy

Felise (German) joyful
Felis

Felixae (Slavic) good fortune

Feliza (Spanish) good fortune

Felyn (Spanish) lucky

Femay (American) classy
Femae

Femi (African) love-seeking
Femmi

Femise (African American) asking for love
Femeese, Femmis

Fena (Scottish) pale

Fenella (Irish) white
Fionola, Fionnuala

Fenia (Scandinavian) gold worker
Fenja, Fenya

Fenn (American) bright
Fen, Fynn

Fennell (Scottish) pale

Feo (Greek) given by God
Fee, Feeo

Feodora (Greek) God-given girl
Fedora

Feodossia (Slavic) influences

Fereda (Spanish) vigorous

Feride (Hawaiian) calm

Ferilen (American) dares

Fern (German/English) fern
Ferne

Fernanda (German) bold
Ferdie, Fernnande

Fernandaline (French) dares

Fernilia (American) successful
Fern, Fernelia, Ferny, Fyrnilia

Fernley (English) from the fern meadow; nature girl

Feven (American) shy
Fevan, Fevun

Ffion (Irish) pale face
Fi

Fia (Scandinavian) perky

Fiamma (Italian) fiery spirit
Feamma, Fee, Fia, Fiama, Fiammette, Fifi

Fiammetta (Italian) fiery

Fiby (Spanish) bright

Fidela (Spanish) loyal
Fidele, Fidella, Fidelle

Fidelia (Italian) faithful
Fidele

Fidelity (Latin) loyal
Fidele, Fidelia

Fidelma (Irish) loyal

Fife (American) dancing eyes; musical
Fifer, Fifey, Fyfe

Fifer (Last name used as first name) fife-player

Fifi (French) jazzy
Fifee

Fifia (African) friday's child
FeeFee, Fifeea

Filia (Greek) devoted
Filea, Feleah, Filiah

Filipa (Italian) loves horses

Fillis (Greek) form of Phyllis: beautiful; leafy bough; articulate; smitten
Filis, Fill, Fillees, Filly, Fillys, Fylis

Filma (Greek) loved

Filomena (Polish) beloved

Fimy (English) form of Femy: regal and polished

Fina (Spanish) blessed by God

Finch (English) bird; sings

Finelle (Irish) fair-faced
Fee, Finell, Finn, Finny, Fynelle

Finesse (American) smooth
Fin, Finese, Finess

Finette (Scottish) pale

Finley (English) fair

Finn (Irish) cool

Finnian (English) fiery

Finny (Irish) blonde

Finola (Italian) white

Fion (Irish) blonde

Fiona (Irish) fair-haired
Fi, Fionna

Fionnuala (Irish) white
Nuala

Fiorella (Irish) spirited
Fee, Feorella, Rella

Fire (American) feisty
Firey, Fyre

Flair (English) stylish
Flaire, Flairey, Flare

Flame (Word as name) fiery

Flaminia (Latin) flaming spirit

Flana (Irish) red-haired
Flanagh, Flanna, Flannerey, Flannery

Flanders (Place name) region of Belgium; creative
Fland, Flann

Flannery (Irish) warm; red-haired
Flann

Flavey (French) fun-filled

Flavia (Latin) light-haired
Flavie

Flaviana (Spanish) pale

Flavine (French) fun

Flax (Botanical) plant with blue flowers
Flacks, Flaxx

Fleming (Last name as first name) adorable
Flemma, Flemmie, Flemming, Flyming

Flemmi (Italian) pretty
Flemmy

Fleur (French) flower
Fleura, Fleuretta, Fleurette, Fleuronne

Flicky (American) vivacious

Flirt (Word as name) flirtatious
Flyrtt

Flis (Polish) form of Felicity: happy

Flo (American) form of Florence: flowering

Flor (Spanish) blooming
Flo, Flora, Floralia, Florencia, Florencita, Florens, Florensia, Flores, Floria, Floriole, Florita, Florite

Flora (Latin/Spanish) flowering
Floria, Florie

Floraba (Spanish) flowering

Florangel (Spanish) angel flower

Florcina (Spanish) flowering

Flordeperla (Spanish) pearly blooms

Florella (Latin) girl from Florence; blooming

Florence (Latin) flowering
Flo, Flora, Florencia, Florense, Florenze, Florie, Florina, Florrie, Flos, Flossie, Floy

Florenina (Spanish) flowering

Florens (Polish) blooming
Floren

Florens (Latin) thrives

Florent (French) flowering
Flor, Floren, Florentine, Florin

Florette (French) flowering

Florian (Dutch) flower-like

Florica (Spanish) flowers

Florida (Place name) U.S. state; flowered
Flora, Flory

Florienna (Italian) flowering

Florin (English) floral

Florinda (English) flower of spring

Florine (American) blooming
Flo, Flora, Floren, Floryne, Florynne

Floris (Latin) flowers

Florizel (Literature) Shakespearean name; in bloom
Flora, Flori, Florisel

Florrie (English) blooms

Flossie (English) grows beautifully

Flower (American) blossoming beauty
Flo

Floy (English) blooms

Floya (Slavic) quick

Fluffy (American) fun-loving
Fluff, Fluffi, Fluffie

Flynn (Irish) red-haired
Flenn, Flinn, Flyn

Fog (American) dreamy
Fogg, Foggee, Foggy

Fola (African) honored
Folah

Folfeen (American) direct

Fonda (American) risk-taker
Fond

Fondee (American) fond

Fondice (American) fond of friends
Fondeese, Fondie

Fontaine (French) fountaining bounty
Fontane, Fontanna, Fontanne

Fontella (American) small fountain

Fontenot (French) special girl; fountain of beauty
Fonny, Fontay, Fonte, Fonteno

Ford (Last name as first name) confident
Forde

Forsythia (Botanical) flower girl

Fortney (Latin) strength
Fortnea, Fortnee, Fortneigh, Fortnie, Fortny

Fortuna (Latin) good fortune
Fortunata

Fortune (Latin) excellent fate; prized

Fotine (Greek) light-hearted
Foty, Fotyne

Fowler (Last name as first name) stylish
Fowla, Fowlar, Fowlir

Foxyn (American) perceptive

Foynt (English) fount

Fozyne (American) fortunate

Fracesca (American) form of Francesca: open-hearted

Frachette (French) fresh

Fran (Latin) form of France: country; French girl
Frann, Franni, Frannie

Franca (Italian) free spirit

France (Place name) country; French girl
Frans, Franse

Francena (English) form of France: country; French girl

Francene (French) free
Francine

Frances (Latin) form of France: country; French girl
Fanny, Fran, Francey, Franci, Francie, Franse

Francesca (Italian) form of France: country; French girl
Fran, Francessca, Franchesca, Francie, Frankie, Frannie

Franchelle (French) form of France: country; French girl
Franshell, Franchelle, Franchey

Franchesca (Italian) form of Francesca: free spirit; form of France
Cheka, Chekkie, Francheska, Francheska, Franchessca

Francina (Italian) form of France: country; French girl

Francine (French) form of France: country; French girl
Fran, Franceen, Francene, Francie

Françoise (French) free

Franicine (American) form of Francine: beautiful

Franisbel (Spanish) beautiful French girl
Franisbella, Franisbelle

Frankie (American) a form of France: country; French girl
Franki, Franky

Frannie (English) friendly
Franni, Franny

Fransabelle (Latin) form of France: country; French girl
Fransabella, Franzabelle

Fraya (Scandinavian) highborn
Freya

Frayda (Scandinavian) fertile woman
Frayde, Fraydel, Freyda, Freyde, Freydel

Frea (Scandinavian) noble; hearty
Fray, Freas, Freya

Fred (English) form of Elfreda: elf strength; good counselor

Freda (German) serene

Freddie (English) form of Frederica: peacemaking
Fredi, Freddy

Frederica (German) peacemaking
Federica, Fred, Freda, Freddie, Freida, Frida, Fritze, Rica

Frederique (German) serene

Fredesminda (English) girl of peaceful mind

Fredna (American) strength of character

Fredy (American) strong

Free (Word as name) liberated spirit

Freesia (Botanical) fragrant flower

Freida (German) form of Frederica: peacemaking and form of Alfreda: wise advisor
Freda, Frida, Frieda

Frelecia (Slavic) form of Felicia: happy

Frenchie (American) saucy
French, Frenchee, Frenchi, Frenchy

Frenda (Asian) fern

Fresnay (American) place name

Fressia (American) form of the flower fresia

Freya (Scandinavian) goddess; beautiful
Freja, Freyja

Frida (Scandinavian) lovely

Frieda (German) happy
Freda

Friedelinde (German) gentle girl
Friedalinda

Frigg (Scandinavian) loved one

Frigga (Scandinavian) beloved
Fri, Friga, Frigg

Fristell (Last name used as first name) stiff

Fritzi (German) leads in peace

Frona (English) practical

Frond (Botanical) growing

Frosty (Word as name) crisp and cool
Frostie

Fructuose (Latin) bountiful
Fru, Fructuosa, Fruta

Frula (German) hardworking

Fruma (Hebrew) devout

Frythe (English) calm
Frith, Fryth

Fuchsia (Botanical) blossoming pink
Fuesha

Fudge (American) stubborn
Fudgey

Fuensanta (Spanish) holy fountain
Fuenta

Fulgencia (Latin) glowing

Fulki (Hindi) sparks

Fullan (Hindi) flourishing

Fuller (English) clotheir

Fulmala (Hindi) wreath

Fulvia (Latin) blonde

Fulvy (Latin) blonde
Full, Fulvee, Fulvie

Fury (Latin) raging anger
Furee, Furey, Furie

Fushy (American) animated;
vivid
Fooshy, Fueshy, Fushee

Gable (German) farming
woman
*Gabbie, Gabby, Gabe, Gabel,
Gabell, Gabl*

Gabor (French) conflicted
Gaber, Gabi

Gabriella ✪ ✿ (Italian/
Spanish) God is her strength
*Caby, Gabela, Gabi, Gabrela,
Gabriela, Gabryela, Gabryella*

Gabrielle ✪
(French/Hebrew) strong
*Gabi, Gabraelle, Gabreelle,
Gabreille, Gabriele, Gabriella,
Gabrilla, Gabrille, Gabryele,
Gabryelle, Gaby, Gaebriell,
Gaebrielle, Garbreal*

Gaby (French) form of
Gabrielle: strong
Gabey, Gabi, Gabie

Gada (Hebrew) fortune

Gadar (Armenian) perfect
girl
Gad, Gadahr, Gaddie, Gaddy

Gadara (Biblical) place name

Gae (Greek) form of Gaea:
earth goddess
Gay, Gaye

Gaea (Greek) earth goddess
Gaia

Gaegae (Greek) form of
Gaea: earth goddess
Gae, Gaege, Gaegie

Gaelle (American) of the
earth

Gaenor (Welsh) beautiful

Gaetane (Italian) form of
Gaeta, Italy

Gagane (American) sky

Gage (American) happy

Gaia (Greek) goddess of earth
Gaea, Gaya

Gail (Hebrew) form of
Abigail: joyful
Gaelle, Gale, Gayle

Gaillen (American) joyful

Gaily (American) fun-loving
Gailai, Galhy

Gailya (Russian) serene
Galya

Gailyn (English) form of
Galen: decisive

Gaines (Last name used as
first name) gainful

Gaitlynn (American) hopeful
*Gaitlin, Gaitline, Gaitlinn,
Gaitlyn, Gaytlyn*

Gala (French) merrymaking;
festivity
*Gaila, Gailah, Galaa, Galuh,
Gayla*

Galatea (Greek) sea nymph
in mythology
Gal, Gala

Galatia (Biblical) place name;
dramatic

Galaxy (American) universal
Gal, Galaxee, Galaxi

Galen (American) decisive
*Galin, Galine, Galyn, Gaye,
Gaylen, Gaylin, Gaylyn*

Galena (Latin) metal; tough
Galyna, Galynna

Galenza (American) calming girl

Galia (Jewish) flows

Galiana (German) vaulted
Galiyana, Galli, Galliana

Galienna (Russian) steady
Galiena, Galyena, Galyenna

Galina (Russian) deserving
Gailina, Gailinna, Galyna, Galynna

Galise (American) joyful
Galeece, Galeese, Galice, Galyce

Gallaine (Last name used as first name) attractive

Galya (Hebrew) redeemed; merry
Galia

Galyan (Hebrew) saved

Gamala (Biblical) place name; lithe; Lovely

Gamin (American) gamine

Ganisia (American) gains

Garcelle (French) flowered
Garcel, Garsell, Garselle

Gardenia (Botanical) sweet flower baby

Gardner (Last name used as first name) gardens

Garetta (American) form of the name Garrett: bashful

Garim (Hindi) warm

Garima (Hindi) sincere

Garland (American) fancy
Garlan, Garlande, Garlinn, Garlynn

Garlanda (French) flowered wreath; pretty girl
Gar, Garl, Garlynd, Garlynda

Garlin (French) form of Garland: fancy
Garlinn, Garlyn, Garlynn

Garner (American) style-setter
Garnar, Garnir

Garnet (English) pretty; semi-precious stone

Garnett (English) red gemstone; valued

Garnetta (French) gemstone; precious
Garna, Garnet, Garnie, Garny

Garrett (Last name as first name) bashful
Garret, Gerrett

Garri (American) energetic
Garree, Garrey, Garry, Garrye

Garrielle (American) competent
Gariele, Garielle, Garriella

Garrison (American) sturdy
Garisen, Garisun, Garrisen, Garrisun

Garrity (American) smiling
Garety, Garrety, Garity, Garritee, Garritie

Gartha (American) feminine form of Garth: sunny; gardener

Garvin (Last name used as first name) craftsperson

Garyn (American) svelte
Garen, Garin, Garinne, Garun, Garynn, Garynne

Gates (Last name as first name) careful
Gate

Gauri (Hindi) golden goddess

Gavin (American) smart
Gave, Gaven, Gavey, Gavun

Gavion (American) daring
Gaveon, Gavionne

Gaviotte (French) graceful
Gaveott, Gaviot, Gaviott

Gavit (French) form of
Gabrielle: strong
Gavitt, Gavyt, Gavytt

Gavotte (French) dancer
Gav, Gavott

Gavrielle (French) form of
Gabrielle: strong
Gavriele, Gavryele, Gavryelle

Gay (French) jolly
Gae, Gaye

Gayathri (Indian) happy

Gayla (American) planner
*Gaila, Gailah, Gala, Gaye,
Gaylah, Gayluh*

Gayle (Hebrew) rejoicing

Gaylene (English) delighted

Gaynor (American)
precocious
Ganor, Gayner, Gaynorre

Gayor (Hebrew) sunny

Gazee (Hebrew) sturdy

Geanna (American)
ostentatious
Geannah, Gianna

Geary (Hebrew) form of
Jerry: hopeful
*Gearee, Gearey, Geari, Gearie,
Geeree, Geerey, Geeri, Geery*

Gebra (Greek) graceful

Gederah (Biblical) place name

Geena (Italian) form of Gena:
wellborn
Gina, Ginah

Geeta (Italian) pearl

Gelacia (Spanish) treasure
Gela, Gelasha, Gelasia

Gelda (American) gloomy
Geilda, Geldah, Gelduh

Gelil (American) smiling

Gem (American) shining
Gemmy, Gim, Jim

Gemesha (African
American) dramatic
*Gemeisha, Gemiesha, Gemme,
Gemmy, Gimesha*

Gemilie (American) gem

Gemini (Greek) twin
Gem, Gemelle, Gemmy

Gemma (Latin) gem; jewel
Gem, Gema, Gemmie, Gemmy

Gemmalis (American) gem

Gemmy (Italian) gem
Gemmee, Gemmi, Gimmy

Gems (American) shining
gem
Gem, Gemmie, Gemmy

Gemze (American) gem

Gena (French) form of Gina:
wellborn
*Geena, Gen, Genah, Geni,
Genia*

Genay (American) form of
Gena: wellborn

Genell (American) form of
Janelle: exuberant
Genill

Genera (Greek) highborn
Gen, Genere

Generosa (Spanish)
generous
Generosah, Generossa

Genesis (Latin) fast starter;
beginning
*Gen, Gena, Genesys, Geney,
Genisis, Genisys, Genysis,
Genysys, Jenesis*

Geneva (French) city in
Switzerland; flourishing; like
juniper
*Gena, Geneeva, Genyva,
Janeva, Jeneva*

Genevera (Spanish)
highborn

Genevieve (German/French)
high-minded
*Gen, Gena, Genna, Genavieve,
Geneveeve,
Genivieve, Genovieve,
Genyveeve, Genyvieve*

Genica (American)
intelligent
*Gen, Genicah, Genicuh,
Genika, Gennica, Jen, Jenika,
Jennika*

Genie (Greek) of high birth;
tricky
*Geenee, Geeney, Geeni, Geenie,
Geeny, Genee, Geney, Geni,
Geny*

Genna (English) womanly
Gen, Genny, Jenna

Gennesaret (Biblical) place
name

Gennese (American) helpful
*Gen, Geneece, Geniece, Genny,
Ginece, Gineese*

Gennette (American) form
of Jeannette: lively

Gennifer (American) form of
Jennifer: white wave
Genefer, Genephur, Genifer

Genny (Greek) of high birth;
loving
Genney, Genni, Gennie

Genoa (Italian) playful
Geenoa, Genoah, Jenoa

Genova (Place name)

Genovesia (Place name)

Genoveva (American) form
of Genevieve: high-minded
Genny, Geno

Gentle (American) kind
Gen, Gentil, Gentille, Gentlle

Gentry (American) sweet
*Gen, Gentree, Gentrie, Jentrie,
Jentry*

Geoma (American)
outstanding
*Gee, GeeGee, Geo, Geomah,
Geome, Gigi, Jeoma, Oma,
Omah*

Geonna (American)
sparkling
*Gee, Geionna, Geone, Geonne,
Geonnuh*

Georgann (English) bright-
eyed
Georganne, Jorgann, Joryann

Georganna (English) form of
Georgia: farmer
*Georgana, Georgeana,
Georgeanna*

Georgene (English)
wandering
*Georgeene, Georgena, Georgene,
Georgyne, Jorgeen, Jorjene*

Georgenia (Dutch) farm girl

Georgette (French) lively and
little
*Georgett, Georgitt, Georgitte,
Jorgette*

Georgia (Greek) farmer
*Georgi, Georgie, Georgina,
Georgya, Giorgi, Jorga, Jorgia,
Jorja*

Georgianna (English)
gracious farmer
*Georganna, Georgeanna,
Jorjeana, Jorgianna,
Georgianne*

Georgie (English) form of
Georgia: farmer
*Georgee, Georgey, Georgi,
Georgy*

Georgina (Latin) feminine
form of George: land-loving;
farmer

Geowanna (African) earthy

Geraldine (German) strong
Geraldyne, Geri, Gerri, Gerry

Geralena (French) leader
*Gera, Geraleen, Geralen,
Geralene, Gerre, Gerrilyn,
Gerry, Jerrileena, Lena*

Gerarda (Spanish) feminine
form of Gerard: brave

Gerardette (American)
feminine form of Gerard:
brave

Gerasa (Biblical) place name

Gerda (Scandinavian) fertility
goddess

Gerdelle (American) fertile

Gerdellyne (American) form
of Geraldine: strong

Gerdi (Scandinavian) guards

Gerdina (Scandinavian)
guarded

Gerdnan (German) guards

Gerisa (English) form of
Geraldine: strong
Gerry

Gerldine (American) form of
Geraldine: strong

Gerly (English) form of
Geraldine: strong

Gerlynne (German)
tenderness
Gerlind

Germaine (French/German)
important
*Germain, Germane, Germayne,
Jermaine*

Gerol (English) rules

Geroldine (American)
geraldine form; Strong

Gerritta (American) strong

Gerry (German) form of
Geraldine: strong

Gertrude (German) beloved
Gerdie, Gerti, Gertie

Gertudis (Slavic) form of
Gertrude: beloved

Gervaise (French) strong
Gerva, Gervaisa

Gessalin (American) loving
*Gessilin, Gessalyn, Gessalynn,
Jessalin, Jessalyn*

Gessica (American) form of
Jessica: rich
Gesica, Gesika, Gessika

Gethsemane (Biblical)
peaceful
*Geth, Gethse, Gethsemanee,
Gethsemaney, Gethsemanie,
Gethy*

Geynille (American)
womanly
Geynel

Gezelle (American) lithe
Gezzelle, Gizele, Gizelle

Gezzi (Asian) believer

Ggana (African) place name

Ghada (Arabic) graceful
Ghad, Ghadah

Ghadeah (Arabic) graceful
Gadea, Gadeah

Ghaeda (Arabic) graceful

Ghandia (African) able
Gandia, Ghanda, Ghandee, Ghandy, Gondia, Gondiah

Ghea (American) confident
Ghia, Jeah, Jeeah

Gherlan (American) forgiving; joyful
Gerlan, Gherli

Ghislaine (French) loyal

Ghita (Italian) pearl
Gita, Gite

Gia (Italian) lovely

Giacinte (Italian) hyacinth; flowering
Gia, Giacin, Giacinta

Giada (Italian) precious jade

Giani (Italian) feminine form of John: God is gracious

Gianina (Italian) believer
Gia, Giane, Giannina, Gianyna, Janeena, Janina, Jeanina

Gianine (American) feminine form of John: God is gracious

Gianna (Italian) forgiving
Geonna, Giana, Gianne, Gianne, Gianni, Giannie, Gianny, Ginny, Gyana, Gyanna

Giannelle (American) hearty
Geanelle, Gianella, Gianelle, Gianne

Giannesha (African American) friendly
Geannesha, Gianesha, Giannesh, Gianneshah, Gianneshuh

Giara (Italian) sensual
Gee, Geara, Gia, Giarah

Gidget (American) cute
Gidge, Gidgett, Gidgette, Gydget

Gift (American) blessed
Gifte, Gyft

Gigi (French) small; spunky
Geegee, Giggi

Gila (Hebrew) joyful
Gilla, Gyla, Gylla

Gilala (Jewish) happy
Gila, Gilah

Gilberta (German) smart
Bertie, Gill

Gilberte (German) shining

Gilda (English) gold-encrusted
Gildi, Gildie, Gill

Gilead (Biblical) place name

Gill (American) intelligent

Gillaine (Latin) young

Gilleese (American) funny
Gill, Gillee, Gilleece, Gillie, Gilly

Gillen (American) humorous
Gill, Gilly, Gillyn, Gyllen

Gilli (American) joyful
Gill, Gillee, Gilly

Gillian (Latin) youthful
Gila, Gili, Gilian, Giliana, Gilien, Gilliana, Gilliane, Gillie, Gillien, Gilly, Gillyan, Gillyen, Gilyan, Gilyen, Jillian

Gillis (Last name as first name) conservative
Gillice, Gillis, Gilise, Gylis, Gyllis

Gillyle (American) smart

Gilma (American) form of Wilma: sturdy
Gee, Gilly

Gilmore (Last name as first name) striking
Gilmoor, Gill, Gillmore, Gylmore

Gina (Italian) wellborn
*Geena, Gena, Gin, Ginah,
Ginny, Gyna, Gynah, Jenah*

Ginae (Biblical) place name

Ginane (French) wellborn
*Gigi, Gina, Gine, Jeanan,
Jeanine*

Ginate (Italian) precious

Giner (English) ginger

Ginet (French) of the earth

Ginette (Italian) flower

Ginevieve (Irish) form of
Genevieve: high-minded
*Gineveeve, Giniveeve, Ginivieve,
Ginyveeve, Ginyvieve*

Ginge (English) feminine
form of George: land-loving;
farmer

Ginger (Botanical) ginger
plant
Gin, Ginny, Jinger

Gingerly (American) careful

Ginnifer (American) form of
Jennifer: white wave
*Gini, Ginifer, Giniferr, Ginifir,
Ginn*

Ginny (English) form of
Virginia: pure female
Ginnee, Ginney, Ginni, Ginnie

Gioconda (Italian) pleasing
Gio, Giocona

Giolla (Italian) helper

Giono (Last name as first
name) delight; friendly
Gio, Gionna, Gionno

Giorgio (Italian) feminine
form of George: land-loving;
farmer
Giorgi, Giorgie, Jorgio

Giovanna (Italian) gracious
believer; great entertainer
*Geo, Geovanna, Gio,
Giovahna, Giovana*

Giovanne (Italian) form of
Giovanna: gracious believer;
great entertainer

Giovannina (Italian) little
Giovanna; believes in God

Giritha (Sri Lankan) melodic
Giri, Girith

Girty (English) form of
Gertie: graceful; gracious

Gisbelle (American) lovely
girl
Gisbel

Gisella (German) pledged for
service
Gisela

Giselle (French) a promise
*Gis, Gisel, Gisela, Gisele, Gisell,
Gissel, Gissell, Gissella, Gisselle,
Gissie, Jizele*

Gita (Sanskrit) song
Geta, Gete, Git, Gitah

Gitaleen (German) held in
high esteem

Gitana (Spanish) gypsy

Gitele (Hebrew) good
Gitel

Githa (Slavic) form of Gita:
song
Gytha

Gitika (Sanskrit) little singer
Getika, Gita, Giti, Gitikah

Gitka (Indian) singing

Gitta (German) highly
regarded

Giuletta (Italian) tiny girl

Giulia (Italian) little girl

Giva (Sanskrit) form of Gita: song
Givah, Gyva, Gyvah

Givonnah (Italian) loyal; believer
Gevonna, Gevonnuh, Givonn, Givonna, Givonne, Jevonah, Jevonna, Jivonnah, Juvona

Gizela (Polish) dedicated
Giz, Gizele, Gizella, Gizzy

Gizelle (German) pledged to serve
Giselle, Gizel, Gizele, Gizell

Gizmo (American) tricky
Gis, Gismo, Giz

Glad (Welsh) form of Gladys: flower; princess

Gladdies (American) form of Gladys: flower; princess

Gladiola (Botanical) blooming; flower
Glad, Gladdee, Gladdy

Gladyce (Spanish) princess

Gladys (Welsh) flower; princess
Glad, Gladice, Gladis, Gladise, Gladiss, Gladdie

Glafira (Spanish) giving
Glafee, Glafera, Glafi

Glasira (Spanish) uncanny

Gleam (American) bright girl
Glee, Gleem

Glease (American) gleeful

Glee (American) gleeful

Glenda (Welsh) bright; good
Glinda, Glynda, Glynn, Glynnie

Glendora (English) form of Glenda: good; bright

Glenn (Irish) glen; from a sylvan setting
Glen

Glenna (Irish) valley-living
Glena, Glenah, Glenuh, Glyn, Glynna

Glennesha (African American) special
Glenesha, Gleneshuh, Gleniesha, Glenn, Glenneshah, Glenny, Glinnesha

Glennice (American) top notch
Glenis, Glennis, Glenys, Glenysse, Glynnece, Glynnice

Glennish (American) unique

Glensheen (French) from the home by the glen

Glenys (Welsh) holy
Glenice, Glenis

Glenys (Welsh) holy
Glenis, Gleniss, Glenyss

Glikeria (Slavic) cheerful

Gliselda (American) loyal

Glorene (American) form of Gloria: glorious

Gloria (Latin) glorious
Glorea, Glorey, Glori, Gloriah, Glorrie, Glory

Glorielle (American) generous
Gloriel, Gloriele, Glory, Gloree, Glori

Gloris (American) glorious
Gloeeca, Glores, Gloresa, Glorisa, Glorus, Gloryssa

Glory (Latin) shining
Gloree, Glorey, Glori, Glorie

Gloss (American) showy
Glosse, Glossee, Glossie, Glossy

Glow (American) glowing

Glyde (American) smooth

Glynis (Welsh) from the glen
Glyniss, Glynys, Glynyss

Glynisha (African American) vibrant
Glynesh, Glynn, Glynnecia, Glynnesha, Glynnie, Glynnisha

Glynn (Welsh) from the glen
Glin, Glinn, Glyn

Glynnis (Welsh) vivacious; glen
Glenice, Glenis, Glennis, Glinice, Glinnis, Glynn, Glynnie, Glynny

Goala (American) goal-oriented
Go, GoGo, Gola

Gobnat (Irish) cuddly

Goddess (American) gorgeous
Godess, Goddesse

Godiva (English) God's gift; brazen
Godeva, Godivah

Golda (English) golden
Goldi, Goldie

Golden (American) shining
Goldene, Goldon, Goldun, Goldy

Goldie (English) bright and golden girl
Goldee, Goldey, Goldi, Goldy

Goliad (Spanish) goal-oriented
Goleade, Goliade

Gomery (Biblical) all there

Gomti (Hindi) river

Goneril (Literature) Shakespearean name; ruthless
Gonarell, Gonarille, Gonereal

Gordie (American) girl who is watchful

Gordyene (Biblical) place name

Gormie (Scottish) lady

Govindi (Sanskrit) devout; faithful

Grable (American) handsome woman
Gray, Graybell

Grace ✪ ✝ (Latin) graceful
Graci, Gracie, Gracy, Graice, Gray, Grayce

Graceann (American) girl of grace
Gracean, Grace-Ann, Graceanna, Graceanne, Gracee, Gracy

Gracell (American) graceful girl

Gracia (Spanish) gracious

Gracie ✪ (Latin) graceful
Gracee, Gracey, Graci, Gracy, Graecie, Gray

Graciela (Spanish) pleasant; full of grace
Chita, Gracee, Gracella, Gracey, Gracie, Graciella, Gracilla, Grasiela, Graziela

Gracilia (Latin) graceful girl
Gracillia, Gracillya, Gracilya

Grady (Irish) hardworking; diligent

Graham (American) sweet
Graehm, Grayhm

Graichen (American) pearl-like

Grainne (Irish) loving girl
Graine, Grayne, Graynne

Grana (Irish) form of Grania: love

Grania (Irish) love
Grainee, Graini

Grant (Last name used as first name) good values

Grantyne (American) generous

Granya (Russian) breech baby

Gratia (Scandinavian) graceful; gracious
Gart, Gert, Gertie, Grasha, Gratea, Grateah, Gratie

Gray (Last name as first name) quiet
Graye, Grey

Graysha (American) gray hair

Grayson (Last name as first) child of quiet one
Graison, Grasen, Greyson

Grazie (Italian) graceful; pleasant
Grasie, Grazee, Grazy

Grazyna (Polish) graceful; pleasant

Grecian (Place name) form of Greece

Greer (Scottish) aware
Greere, Grear, Greare, Grier

Gregory (American) scholarly
Gregoree, Gregge, Greggy, Gregoria, Gregorie

Greshawn (African American) lively
Greeshawn, Greshaun, Greshawna, Greshonn, Greshun

Gresia (American) compelling
Grecia, Grasea, Graysea, Grayshea

Greta (German) pearl
Gretah, Grete, Gretie, Grette, Grytta

Gretchen (German) pearl
Grechen, Grechin, Grechyn, Gretch, Gretchin, Gretchun, Gretchyn, Grethyn

Grete (Dutch) pearl girl

Gretel (Dutch) manipulative

Gretel (German) pearl; fanciful
Gretal, Grettel, Gretell, Gretelle

Grethel (Dutch) form on Gretel: manipulative or pearl; fanciful

Grewn (American) supporter

Greyland (American) focused
Grey, Greylin, Greylyn, Greylynne

Gricie (Spanish) form of Griselda: patient

Griffie (Welsh) royal
Griff, Griffee, Griffey, Griffi, Gryffie

Griffin (Welsh) royal
Griff

Griffith (Last name used as first name) confident

Grindelle (American) live wire
Dell, Delle, Grenn, Grin, Grindee, Grindell, Grindy, Renny

Griselda (German) patient
Grezelda, Grisel, Grissy, Grizel, Grizelda, Grizzie

Griselia (Spanish) gray; patient
Grise, Grisele, Grissy, Seley, Selia

Grisham (Last name as first name) ambitious
Grish

Gritta (German) pearl

Grittith (American) form of
Griffith: confident

Grizel (Spanish)
long-suffering
Griz, Grizelda, Grizelle, Grizzy

Grove (Botanical) child of the
outdoors

Grushenka (Russian)
desirable

Guadalupe (Spanish) patron
saint; easygoing
Guadelupe, Guadrylupe, Lupe,
Lupeta, Lupita

Guadarrama (Spanish) river
of saints

Gubby (Irish) cuddly
Gub, Gubee, Gubbie

Gudrun (Scandinavian) wise
Gudren, Gudrenne, Gudrin,
Gudrinne

Guendolen (Welsh) fair born

Guenevere (Welsh) soft;
white

Guenna (Welsh) soft
Guena

Guessa (American) kind

Guinevere (Welsh) queen;
white
Guenevere, Guenyveere, Guin,
Gwen

Gulab (Hindi) darken

Gulanara (Spanish) needy

Gulenia (Spanish) wanted

Gullermina (Spanish) willful
protector

Gumercindo (Spanish)
famed

Gunda (German) combative

Gunilla (Scandinavian)
warlike
Gun, Gunn

Gunta (German) form of
Gunda: combative

Gunun (German) lively
Gunan, Gunen

Gurlene (American) smart
Gurl, Gurleen, Gurleene,
Gurline

Gurshawn (American)
talkative
Gurdie, Gurshauna,
Gurshaune, Gurshawna, Gurty

Gussie (Latin) form of
Augusta: revered
Gus, Gussy, Gustie

Gusta (German) form of
Gustava: royal
Gussy, Gustu, Gustana, Gusty

Gustava (Scandinavian) royal

Guy (French) guiding;
assertive
Guye

Guyette (French) ambitious

Guyla (French) asserts

Guyna (American) aggressor

Gwen (Welsh) form of
Gwendolyn: mystery goddess;
bright
Gwyn, Gweni, Gwenn, Gwenna

Gwenda (Welsh) beautiful
Guenda

Gwendolyn (Welsh) mystery
goddess; bright
Gwenda, Gwendalinne,
Gwendalyn, Gwendelynn,
Gwendolen, Gwendolin,
Gwendoline, Gwendolynn,
Gwennie, Gywnne

Gwenless (Invented) fair
Gwen, Gwenles, Gwenny

Gwenllian (Welsh) lovely

Gwenna (Welsh) beautiful
Gwena

Gwitira (American) fair

Gwladys (Welsh) form of
Gladys: flower; princess

Gwyn (Welsh) form of
Gwyneth: blessed
*Gwenn, Gwinn, Gwynn,
Gwynne*

Gwynedd (Welsh) blessed

Gwyneth (Welsh) blessed
*Gwennie, Gwinith, Gwynethe,
Gwynith, Gwynithe, Gwynne,
Gwynneth, Win, Winnie*

Gyanll (African) genuine

Gyda (Scandinavian) celestine

Gygi (French) form of GiGi:
small; spunky

Gylla (Spanish) feminine
form of Guillermo: attentive
Guilla, Gye, Gyla, Jilla

Gynette (American) form of
Jeanette: lively
Gyn, Gynett, Gynnee, Gynnie

Gypsy (English) adventurer
Gippie, Gipsie, Gypsie

Gyselle (German) form of
Giselle: a promise
Gysel, Gysele

Gyta (American) young

Gythae (English) feisty
Gith, Gyth, Gythay

H

Ha (Vietnamese) happy

Haafizah (Arabic) librarian
Hafeezah

Haalah (Arabic) librarian

Haarisah (Hindi) sun girl

Haarithah (Arabic) angel

Habbai (Arabic) well-loved

Habiba (Arabic) well-loved
Habeebah, Habibah

Habika (Arabic) loved and
cherished

Hadassah (Hebrew) myrtle
tree
*Hadasa, Hadasah, Hadaseh,
Hadassa, Haddasah, Haddee,
Haddi, Haddy*

Hadil (Arabic) cooing

Hadlee (English) girl in
heather
Hadlea, Hadley, Hadli, Hadly

Hady (Greek) soulful
*Haddie, Hadee, Hadie, Haidee,
Haidie*

Hadyn (American) smart
Haden

Haelee (English) form of
Hailey: natural; hay meadow

Hagai (Hebrew) abandoned;
alone
Haggai, Haggi, Hagi

Hagar (Hebrew) stranger
Haggar, Hager, Hagur

Hagen (Last name used as
first name) defender

Hagir (Arabic) wanderer
Hajar

Haidee (Greek) humble
Haydee

Hailey ✪ ✿ (English)
natural; hay meadow
*Haile, Hailea, Hailee, Hailie,
Haily, Halee, Haley, Halie,
Hallie*

Haiti (Place name)

Halalah (Slavic) serenity

Halcyone (Greek) calm
Halceonne, Halcyon

Halda (Scandinavian) half-
Danish
*Haldaine, Haldana, Haldane,
Haldayne*

Halden (Scandinavian) half-
Danish girl
Haldin, Haldyn

Haldi (Scandinavian) form of
Halda: half-Danish
Haldie, Haldis

Halea (Hawaiian) halo

Haleemah (Arabic) speaks
quietly

Halena (Russian) form of
Helen: beautiful; light
Haleena, Halyna

Halene (Russian) staunch
Haleen, Haleen, Halyne

Haletta (Greek) little country
girl from the meadow
*Hale, Halette, Hallee, Halletta,
Halley, Hallie, Hally, Letta,
Lettie, Letty*

Halfrida (German) peaceful

Hali (English) heroic

Halia (Hawaiian)
remembering

Halima (Arabic) gentle

Halimeda (Greek) sea-loving
Hallie, Hally, Meda

Halina (Russian) faithful
Haleena, Halyna

Hall (Last name as first name)
distinguished
Haul

Halle (German) home ruler

Hallela (Hebrew)
praiseworthy

Hallie (German) high-spirited
*Halle, Hallee, Haleigh, Hali,
Halie, Hally, Hallye*

Halona (Native American)
lucky baby
Halonna

Halsey (American) playful
Halcie, Halsea, Halsee, Halsie

Halston (American) stylish
Hall, Halls, Halsten

Halzey (American) leader
*Hals, Halsee, Halsi, Halsy,
Halze, Halzee*

Hameedah (Arabic) grateful

Hamilton (American)
wishful
*Hamil, Hamilten, Hamiltun,
Hamma, Hamme*

Hamony (Latin) form of
Harmony: synchrony

Hana (Arabic) delight

Haneefah (Arabic) true
believer

Hanh (Vietnamese) moral

Hani (Hawaiian) sways

Hanifa (Arabic) righteous

Hanna (Polish) grace

Hannabelle (German)
feminine form Hannibal:
happy; beauty
*Hannabell, Hannahbell,
Hannahbelle*

Hannah ✪ ✿ (Hebrew)
merciful; God-blessed
*Hanae, Hanah, Hanan,
Hannaa, Hanne, Hanni*

Hanne (Scandinavian) girl of
grace

Hannelore (American) form
of Hannah: merciful; God-
blessed

Hannette (American) form
of Jannette: lovely
Hann, Hanett, Hannett

Hannia (Polish) graceful

Hannie (German) believer

Hansa (Indian) swanlike
Hans, Hansah, Hansey, Hanz

Happy (English) joyful
Hap, Happee, Happi

Haralda (Scandinavian) rules
the army
Harelda, Hallie, Hally, Harilda

Hardin (Last name used as
first name) keeps rabbits

Harla (English) country girl
from the fields
*Harlah, Harlea, Harlee,
Harlen, Harlie, Harlun*

Harlan (English) athletic
Harlen, Harlon, Harlun

Harlene (French) energetic

Harlequine (Invented)
romantic
Harlequinne, Harley

Harley (English) wild thing
*Harlea, Harlee, Harleey, Harli,
Harlie, Harly*

Harlie (English) in the field;
dreamy

Harlinne (American)
vivacious
*Harleen, Harleene, Harline,
Harly*

Harlow (American) brash
Harlo, Harly

Harmon (Last name as first
name) attuned
*Harmen, Harmone, Harmun,
Harmyn*

Harmonita (Greek) in
harmony

Harmony (Latin) in
synchrony
*Harmonee, Harmoni,
Harmonia, Harmonie*

Harolyn (American) form of
Carolyn: womanly

Harper (English) musician;
writer
Harp

Harrah (English) rejoicing;
merriment
Hara, Harah, Harra

Harrell (American) leader
Harell, Harill, Haryl, Harryl

Harriet (French) homebody
*Harri, Harrie, Harriett,
Harriette, Harrott, Hat, Hattie,
Hatty, Hatti, Hattie*

Harrisah (Indian) happy

Harsha (Indian) joyful

Harshita (English) form of
Harriet: homebody

Hart (American) romantic
*Harte, Hartee, Hartie, Harty,
Heart*

Hartley (Last name as first
name) having heart
*Hartlee, Hartleigh, Hartli,
Hartlie, Hartly*

Hasina (African) beauty

Hassaanah (African) first
girl born

Hattie (English) home-loving
Hatti, Hatty, Hettie, Hetty

Hattina (Biblical) place name; homebody

Haute (French) high
Hautie

Hava (Hebrew) life; lively
Chaba, Chaya, Haya

Havana (Cuban) loyal
Havanah, Havane, Havanna, Havvanah, Havanuh

Haven (American) safe place; open
Havin, Havun

Havilah (Hebrew) beloved

Haviland (American) lively; talented
Havilan, Havilynd

Hawkins (American) wily
Hawk, Hawkens, Hawkey, Hawkuns

Hawlee (American) negotiator
Hawlea, Hawleigh, Hawlie, Hawley, Hawly

Haydee (American) capable
Hady, Hadye, Haydie

Haydeeline (English) sweet

Haydell (Last name used as first name) hill child

Hayden (Last name used as first name) hill child

Haydon (American) knowing
Hayden, Hadyn

Hayfa (Arabic) slim

Hayla (Arabic) moon's halo

Hayley (English) natural; hay meadow
Hailey, Haley, Haylee, Hayleigh, Hayli, Haylie

Haze (American) word as a name; spontaneous
Haise, Hay, Hays, Hazee, Hazey, Hazy

Hazel (English) powerful
Hazell, Hazelle, Hazie, Hazyl, Hazzell

Hazen (Hindi) joyful

Healy (Last name used as first name) healthy

Heart (American) romantic
Hart, Hearte

Heath (English) open; healthy
Heathe

Heather (Scottish) flowering
Heath, Heathar, Heathor, Heathur

Heaven (English) happy and beautiful
Heavyn, Hevin

Heavenly (American) spiritual
Heaven, Heavenlee, Heavenley, Heavynlie, Hevin

Heba (Greek) child; goddess of youth
Hebe

Hecate (Greek) goddess of witchcraft

Hedda (German) capricious; warring
Heda, Heddi, Heddie, Hedi, Hedy, Hetta

Heddalin (Scandinavian) contender

Hedley (German) excites

Hedley (Greek) sweet
Hedlee, Hedleigh, Hedli, Hedlie, Hedly

Hedviga (Scandinavian) excites

Hedy (German) mercurial
Hedi

Hedya (Hebrew) joy girl
Hedia, Hedva

Hedy-Marie (German)
capricious

Heidi (German) noble;
watchful; perky
*Heide, Heidee, Heidie, Heidy,
Hidi*

Heidrun (German) form of
Heidi: noble; watchful; perky

Heija (Korean) bright
Hia, Hya

Heilala (Asian) sun child

Heirnine (Greek) form of
Helen: beautiful; light

Heirrierte (English) form of
Harriet: homebody

Hela (Biblical) olden

Helaine (French) ray of light;
gorgeous
*Helainne, Helle, Helyna,
Hellyn*

Helanna (Greek) lovely
*Helahna, Helana, Helani,
Heley, Hella*

Helayne (American) pretty
girl

Helbon (Greek) form of
Helen: beautiful; light
*Helbona, Helbonia, Helbonna,
Helbonnah*

Held (Welsh) light

Helen (Greek) beautiful; light
*Hela, Hele, Helena, Helyn,
Lena, Lenore*

Helena (Greek) beautiful;
ingenious
*Helana, Helayna, Heleana,
Helene, Hellena, Helyena, Lena*

Helene (French) form of
Helen: beautiful; light
Helaine, Heleen, Heline

Helenore (Greek) form of
Helen: beautiful; light
*Hele, Helen, Helenoor, Helenor,
Helia, Helie, Hellena, Lena,
Lennore, Lenora, Lenore,
Lenory, Lina, Nora, Norey,
Norie*

Helfine (Scandinavian)
blessed

Helga (Anglo-Saxon) pious
Helg

Helia (Greek) sun
Heleah, Helya, Helyah

Helice (Greek) form of
Helen: beautiful; light

Helie (Greek) sunny
Heley, Heli

Helina (Greek) delightful
Helinah, Helinna, Helinnuh

Heliodora (Spanish) loves
sun

Helki (Native American)
tender
Helkie, Helky

Hella (Greek) form of Helen:
beautiful; light
Helle

Helma (German) helmet;
well protected

Helmina (German) form of
Wilhelmina: staunch
protector

Heloise (German) hearty
*Hale, Haley, Heley, Heloese,
Heloyse*

Helsa (Scandinavian)
God-loving
Helse, Helsie

Helynne (French) moon

Hema (Indian) gold child

Henda (English) form of
Henna: mehndi
Hende, Hendel, Heneh

Hender (American)
embraced
Hendere

Henia (English) form of
Henrietta: home-ruler
Henna, Henie, Henye

Henia (Spanish) well-
groomed

Henley (American) sociable
*Hendlee, Hendly, Henli,
Henlie, Hinlie, Hynlie*

Henna (Hindi) mehndi
*Hena, Hannah, Hennuh,
Henny*

Henrietta (English/German)
home-ruler
*Harriet, Hattie, Henny, Hetta,
Hettie*

Henriette (French) leads the
home

Hensley (American)
ambitious
Henslee, Henslie, Hensly

Henton (Last name used as
first name) open arms

Hera (Greek) wife of Zeus;
radiant

Heraclea (Biblical) place
name; of Hercules

Herdis (Scandinavian) army
woman

Herendira (Invented) tender
and dear
Heren

Herise (Invented) warm
Heree, Hereese, Herice

Herleen (American) quiet
*Herlee, Herlene, Hurleen,
Herley, Herline, Herly*

Herliza (Spanish) sweet

Hermaina (Spanish) speedy

Hermelinda (Spanish) earthy

Hermilla (Spanish) fighter
Herm, Hermila, Hermille

Hermina (Greek) of the earth
Hermine

Hermione (Greek) sensual
Hermina, Hermine

Hermosa (Spanish) beautiful
Ermosa

Hernanda (Spanish)
feminine form of Hernando:
daring

Herra (Greek) earth girl
Herrah, Hera

Hersala (Spanish) lithe and
lovely
Hers, Hersila, Hersilia, Hersy

Hersilia (Spanish) delicate

Hertha (English) earth
*Erta, Ertha, Eartha, Erda,
Herta*

Hertnia (English) earth
Herrntia

Herwena (Slavic) winner

Hesna (Arabic) star

Hesper (Greek) night star
Hespera, Hespira

Hest (Greek) form of Hester:
starlike; literary
Hessie, Hesta, Hetty

Hesta (Greek) starlike
Hestia

Hester (American) starlike
literary
*Esther, Hestar, Hesther, Hett,
Hettie, Hetty*

Hestia (Greek) hearth

Heti (English) form of
Henrietta: home-ruler

Hetta (German) ruler
Hedda, Heta, Hettie, Hetty

Hetty (English) form of
Henrietta: home-ruler

Heven (American) pretty
*Hevan, Hevin, Hevon, Hevun,
Hevven*

Hewaida (Indian) gift

Heydee (German) form of
Heidi: noble; watchful; perky

Heyzell (American) form of
Hazel: powerful
Hayzale, Heyzel, Heyzelle

Hezekiah (Biblical) pleases

Hiah (Korean) form of Heija:
bright
Hia, Hy, Hya, Hye

Hiatt (English) form of Hyatt:
high gate; worthwhile
Hi, Hye

Hibernia (Place name) Latin
word for Ireland

Hibiscus (Botanical) pretty

Hicks (Last name as first
name) saucy
Hicksee, Hicksie

Hidee (American) form of
Heidi: noble; watchful; perky
*Hidey, Hidie, Hidy, Hydee,
Hydeey*

Hideko (Japanese) excellence

Hidie (German) lively

Hila (Hebrew) angelic

Hilan (Greek) happy

Hilaria (Latin/Polish)
merrymaker
Hilarea, Hilareeah, Hilariah

Hilary (Latin) cheerful and
outgoing
*Hilaire, Hilaree, Hilari,
Hilaria, Hillarree, Hillary,
Hillerie, Hillery*

Hilda (German) protector
*Hild, Hilde, Hildi, Hildie,
Hildy*

Hildar (Scandinavian) feisty

Hildebrand (German) strong

Hildegard (German) battle
*Hilda, Hildagarde, Hildegarde,
Hildred, Hillie*

Hildegunde (Last name as
first name) princess

Hildemar (German) strong

Hildreth (German) struggles

Hilina (Hawaiian) celestial

Hilja (Finnish) silence

Hilma (German) helmet;
protects herself
Helma

Hilmah (Scandinavian) form
of Hilja: silence

Hilton (American) wealthy
Hillie, Hilltawn, Hillton, Hilly

Himalaya (Place name)
mountain range; upwardly
mobile
Hima

Hina (Scandinavian) leads the
home

Hinda (Hebrew) held high

Hindal (Hebrew) form of
Hinda: held high

Hinton (American) affluent
*Hintan, Hinten, Hintun,
Hynton*

Hirani (Indian) gold child

Hiroko (Japanese) giving; wise

Hisa (Japanese) forever
Hissa, Hysa, Hyssa

Hisaye (Japanese) longlasting

Hoa (Southeast Asian) flowers

Hodalla (Jewish) queenly

Hodel (German) stern
Hodi

Hodge (Last name as first name) confident
Hodj

Hoku (Hawaiian) starlike

Holda (German) secretive

Holden (English) willing
Holdan, Holdun

Holder (English) beautiful voice
Holdar, Holdur

Holiday (American) jazzy
Holidae, Holidaye, Holladay, Holliday, Holly

Holine (American) special
Hauline, Holinn, Holli, Holyne

Hollah (German) hides much

Holland (Place name) expressive
Hollan, Hollyn, Holyn

Hollander (Dutch) form of Holland: expressive
Holander, Holender, Holynder, Hollender, Hollynder

Hollis (English) smart; girl by the holly
Hollice, Hollyce

Hollisha (English) ingenious; Christmas-born; holly
Holicha, Hollice, Hollichia, Hollise

Holly (Anglo-Saxon) Christmas-born; holly tree
Hollee, Holleigh, Holley, Holli, Hollie, Hollye

Holsey (American) laidback
Holsee, Holsie

Holton (American) whimsical
Holt, Holten, Holtun

Holyn (American) fresh-faced
Holan, Holen, Holland, Hollee, Hollen, Holley, Hollie, Holly, Hollyn, Hollyn

Homer (American) tomboyish
Homar, Home, Homera, Homie, Homir, Homma

Honesty (American) truthful
Honeste, Honestee, Honesti, Honestie, Honestye

Honey (Latin) sweet-hearted
Honie, Hunnie

Honeyblossom (American) sweet

Honeylee (American) sweet

Honor (Latin) ethical
Honer, Honora, Honour

Honora (Latin) honorable
Honorah, Honoree, Honoria, Honoura

Honorata (Polish) respected woman

Honoreen (American) has honor

Honoria (Spanish) of high integrity; a saint
Honoreah

Honorina (Spanish) honored
Honor, Honora, Honoryna

Hope ♀ (Anglo-Saxon) optimistic

Hopkins (American) perky
Hopkin

Hopsey (American) lively

Horatia (Latin) keeps time;
careful
Horacia

Horiya (Japanese) gardens

Hortencia (Spanish) green
thumb
*Hartencia, Hartense,
Hartensia, Hortence, Hortense,
Hortensia*

Hortense (Latin) caretaking
the garden
Hortence, Hortensia, Hortinse

Hosanna (Greek) time to
pray; worshipping
Hosana, Hosanah, Hosannah

Hoshi (Japanese) shines

Houston (Place name) leader
Houst, Houstie, Huston

Hoyden (Last name as first
name) having high spirits
Hoydin, Hoydyn

Huberta (German) brilliant

Hud (American) tomboyish
Hudd

Huda (Arabic) the right way
Hoda

Hudalia (Spanish) leads

Hudel (Scandinavian) lovable

Hudi (Arabic) the right way

Hudson (English) explorer;
adventuresome
Hud, Huds

Hueline (German) smart
*Hue, Huee, Huel, Huela,
Huelene, Huelette, Huelyne,
Huey, Hughee, Hughie*

Huella (American) joyous
Huela, Huelle

Hueretta (American) smart

Huette (German) intellectual
Hughette, Huetta, Hugette

Hulda (Scandinavian)
sweetheart
Huldy, Huldie, Huldah

Hum (Indian) togetherness

Humairaa (Asian) generous

Humla (Polish) humble

Hun (American) form of
Hunny; form of Honey:
sweetness
Hon

Hunni (American) form of
Honey: sweet-hearted

Hunter (English) searching;
jubilant
*Hun, Huner, Hunner, Hunt,
Huntar, Huntter*

Hunting (English) hunts

Hurd (Last name used as first
name) herds cattle

Hurley (English) fit
Hurlee, Hurlie, Hurly

Hutton (English) right
Hutten, Huttun

Huxlee (American) creative
Hux, Huxleigh, Huxley, Huxly

Hyacinth (Greek) flower
Hy, Hycinth, Hyacinthe

Hyatt (English) high gate;
worthwhile
Hyat

Hyde (American)
tough-willed
Hide, Hydie

Hydia (German) form of
Heidi: noble; watchful; perky

Hydie (American) spirited
Hidi, Hydee, Hydey, Hydi

Hylaine (American) form of Elaine: dependable girl

Hypatia (Greek) tops

I

Iadanna (Biblical) place name

Iana (Greek) form of Iantha: flowering
Iann

Ianeke (Hawaiian) believer in a gracious God
Ianete, Iani

Ianthe (Greek) flowering
Ianthina, Ian, Iantha, Ianthiria

Ibeth (Spanish) form of Elizabeth: God's promise

Ibleam (Biblical) place name

Ibsen (Scandinavian) scholarly

Ida (German) heroine; warrior
Idah, Iduh

Idaa (Hindi) earth woman

Idahlia (Greek) sweet
Idali, Idalia, Idalina, Idaline, Idalis

Idalia (Italian) sweet

Idam (American) feminine form of Adam: original

Idarah (American) social
Idara, Idare, Idareah

Idasia (English) joyful

Ide (Irish) thirsty

Ideh (German) form of Ida: heroine; warrior
Idit

Idelle (Celtic) generous
Idele

Idetta (German) serious worker
Ideta, Idettah, Idette

Idil (Latin) pleasant
Idee, Idey, Idi, Idie, Idyll

Idola (German) worker
Idolah, Idolia

Idolina (American) idolizes
Idol, Idolena

Idolyne (Spanish) idolizes

Idoma (American) form of Idona: fresh

Idona (Scandinavian) fresh
Idonea, Idonia, Iduna, Idonah, Idonia, Idonna

Idonie (Scandinavian) loving

Idony (Scandinavian) reborn

Idoris (Greek) adores

Idowu (African) baby after twins

Idra (Aramaic) rich; fig tree; flourishes

Idriya (Hebrew) duck; rich
Idria

Idumea (Biblical) place name

Iduna (Scandinavian) fresh
Idun

Iduvina (Spanish) dedicated
Iduvine, Iduvynna, Vina

Ieesh (Arabic) feminine
Ieasha, Ieesha, Iesha, Yesha

Ierne (Irish) form of Ireland: vibrant

Iesha (Arabic) feminine

Ieshia (English) form of Iesha: feminine

Ifama (African) well being

Ife (African) loving

Ifigenia (Spanish) form of
Effie: well-spoken

Ignacia (Latin) passionate
Ignatia, Ignatzia, Ignacy

Ihab (Arabic) gift

Iheoma (Hawaiian) lifted by
the Lord

Ihsan (Arabic) good will
Ihsana, Ihsanah

Iianena (Slavic) form of
Ileana: soaring

Iilia (English) form of Ileana:
soaring

Ijada (Spanish) jade; beauty

Ikabela (Hawaiian) form of
Isabella: consecrated to God
Ikapela

Ikea (Scandinavian) smooth
Ikee, Ikeah, Ikie

Ikeida (Invented)
spontaneous
Ikae, Ikay

Iku (Japanese) nurturing

Ila (Hindi) of the earth; lovely

Ilaisaane (Asian) bright

Ilamay (French) sweet; from
an island
*Ila May, Ilamae, Ila-May,
Ilamaye*

Ilana (Hebrew) tree; gorgeous
*Elana, Ilaina, Ilane, Ilani,
Illana, Lainie, Lanie*

Ilaria (Greek) girl with a good
attitude

Ilda (German) warring; feisty

Ildiko (Hungarian)
contentious; warrior

Ileannah (American) soaring
*Ileana, Ileanna, Ilene, Iliana,
Ilianna, Illeana, Illiana*

Ilena (Greek) regal
Ileena, Ilina

Ilene (American) svelte
Ileen, Ilenia

Ilesha (Hindi) loves the Lord
of the earth

Ilfa (American) ecstatic

Ilia (Greek) from ancient city
Ilion; traditional

Iliana (Greek) woman of Troy
Ileanai, Illeana

Ilima (Hawaiian) oahu flower

Ilka (Hungarian) beauty

Ilkee (Slavic) form of Ilka:
beauty

Ilkka (Slavic) form of Ilka:
beauty

Illana (Hebrew) tree

Illiana (Spanish) form of
Helen: beautiful; light

Ilma (American) stubborn

Ilon (Biblical) place name

Ilona (Hungarian) form of
Helen: beautiful; light

Ilonka (Slavic) lovely

Ilsa (Scottish) glowing
*Elyssa, Illisa, Illysa, Ilsah, Ilse,
Lissie*

Ilse (German) form of
Elizabeth: God's promise

Ilyse (English) charms

Ilyssa (English) form of
Alyssa: flourishing

Ima (Japanese) now; the
present
Imah

Imagine (Word as name)
imaginative

Imaine (Arabic) form of
Iman: living in the present
Imain, Iman, Imane

Imala (Native American)
strongwilled

Iman (Arabic/African) living
in the present
Imen

Imana (Arabic) faithful; true

Imani (Arabic) faithful

Imanuela (Spanish) faithful

Imara (Hungarian) ruler

Imari (Japanese) today's girl

Imelda (German) contentious
Imalda

Imena (African) dreamy

Imin (Arabic) loyal

Immaculada (Spanish)
spotless

Imogen (Gaelic) maiden
Emogen, Imogene

Imperia (Latin) imperial;
stately

In (Arabic) generous

Ina (Latin) small
Inah

Inaki (Asian) generous spirit

Inam (Arabic) generous

Inanna (Mythology) goddess

Inas (Arabic) friendly

Inca (Indian) adventurer
Incah

Inda (Place name) lady

India (Place name) woman of
India
*Indeah, Indee, Indie, Indy,
Indya*

Indiana (Place name) salt-of-
the-earth; U.S. state
Inda, India, Indiana

Indiece (American) capable
Indeece, Indeese

Indigo (Latin) eyes of deep
blue
Indego, Indigoh

Indira (Hindi) ethereal; God
of heaven and thunderstorms
Indra

Indra (Hindi) goddess of
thunder and rain; powerful
Indee, Indi, Indira, Indre

Indranee (Hindi) sky God's
wife

Indrani (Indian) wife of
Indra; Excellent

Indray (American) outspoken
Indrue, Indee, Indree

Indre (Hindi) splendor

Indya (Place name) form of
India: woman of India

Ineesha (African American)
sparkling
Inesha, Ineshah, Inisha

Ineke (Japanese) nurtures

Ines (Spanish) chaste
Inez, Innez, Ynez

Inessa (Russian) pure
Inesa, Nessa

Inessae (Spanish) form of
Ines: chaste

Inetha (Slavic) pure

Inez (Spanish) lovely
Ines

Infinity (American) lasting
*Infinitee, Infinitey, Infiniti,
Infinitie*

Inga (Scandinavian) hero's
daughter

Ingalill (Scandinavian) fertile

Ingalls (American) peaceful

Inge (Scandinavian) fertile
Inga

Ingeborg (Scandinavian) fertile

Ingegerd (Scandinavian) form of Ingrid: beautiful

Inger (Scandinavian) lovely

Inglesa (Spanish) english girl

Ingrad (American) form of Ingrid: beautiful
Inger, Ingr

Ingrid (Scandinavian) beautiful
Inga, Inge, Inger, Ingred

Ingrida (Scandinavian) form of Ingrid: beautiful

Iniguez (Spanish) good
Ina, Ini, Niqui

Inka (Scandinavian) abundant

Inna (Slavic) little girl

Innocence (American) pure
Innoce, Innocents, Inocence, Inocencia, Inocents

Inoa (Hawaiian) named

Inocencia (Spanish) innocent
Inocenta, Inocentia

Inola (Greek) form of Iola: dawn

Integrity (American) truthful
Integritee, Integritie

Ioannis (Greek) believer

Iola (Greek) dawn
Iole

Iolana (Hawaiian) violet; pretty

Iolanthe (English) violet; delicate
Iole, Iola

Iona (Place name) for the Isle of Iona in Scotland
Ione, Ionia

Ioni (English) place name; innocent

Ionica (Biblical) place name

Iosepine (Hawaiian) form of Josephine: blessed

Ira (Hebrew) contented; watchful
Irah

Ireland (Place name) vibrant
Irelan, Irelande, Irelyn, Irelynn

Irene (Greek) peace-loving; goddess of peace
Irine

Ireta (Greek) serene
Iretta, Irette

Irina (Greek/Russian) comforting
Ireena, Irena, Irenah, Irene, Irenia, Irenya

Iris (Greek) bright; goddess of the rainbow

Irisal (Greek) form of Iris: bright; goddess of the rainbow

Iriseene (American) iris flower; rainbow

Irish (American) Irish girl

Irma (Latin) realistic
Irmah

Irmaletta (Spanish) noble; complete

Irmgard (Latin) form of Irma: realistic

Irnee (Scandinavian) growth

Irodell (Invented) peaceful
Irodel, Irodelle

Irra (Greek) serene

Irvette (English) friend of the sea

Isa (Spanish) dark-eyed
Isah

Isabel ✪ (Spanish) God-loving
Isabela, Isabella, Isabelle, Issie, Iza

Isabella ✪ ✪ (Spanish/
Italian) consecrated to God
Isabela, Izabella

Isadora (Greek) beautiful; gift
of Isis; fertile
Dora, Dori, Dory, Isidora

Isairis (Spanish) lively
Isa, Isaire

Isamu (Japanese) high-energy

Isandra (Spanish) form of
Sandra: helpful; protective

Isatas (Native American)
snow
Istas

Isaura (Greek) Asian country

Isela (American) giving
Iselah

Iselderine (Invented) loyal

Iseult (Irish) lovely

Isha (Hindi) protected

Ishana (Hindi) sheltered

Ishi (Japanese) rock; safe
Ishie

Ishiko (Japanese) rock;
dependable

Ishtar (Biblical) mother-
goddess; faithful

Isis (Egyptian) goddess
supreme of moon and
fertility

Isla (Place name) river in
Scotland; flows

Isleana (Latin) sun girl; jolly
Islean, Isleen, Isaeileen

Ismaela (Hebrew) feminine
form of Ishmael: God hears
Isma, Mael, Maella

Ismat (Arabic) protective

Ismene (French) form of the
name Esme: much loved
Isme, Ismyne

Ismenia (Place name) region
of Mars; loyal

Ismey (French) form of
Esme: much loved

Isobelette (American)
believes in God

Isoka (African) given by God
Isoke, Soka

Isoke (African) God's gift

Isola (Spanish) lovely

Isolde (Welsh) beautiful
*Iseult, Isolda, Isolt, Izette,
Yseult*

Isotta (Irish) princess

Isra (Arabic) night mover

Issa (English) form of Isabel:
God-loving
Isa

Issus (Biblical) place name; wise

Istvan (Hungarian) crowned

Ita (Irish) thirsts for
knowledge

Italia (Italian) girl from Italy

Iti (Irish) form of Ita: thirsts
for knowledge

Itiah (Hebrew) God comforts
her
Itia, Itiya

Itica (Spanish) eloquent
Itaca, Iticah

Itidal (Arabic) cautious

Itinsa (Hawaiian) waterfall

Itka (Irish) form of Ita: thirsts for knowledge

Ito (Japanese) thread; delicate

Ituha (Native American) sturdy oak; white stone

Itzel (Spanish) form of Isabel: God-loving
Itz

Itzelle (Native American) earth goddess

Itzy (American) lively
Itsee, Itzee, Itzie

Iuana (Welsh) believes in gracious God

Iudita (Hawaiian) praises; affectionate

Iuginia (Hawaiian) highborn
Iugina

Iulaua (Hawaiian) eloquent

Iulia (Irish) form of Juliana: youthful; Jove's child

Iunia (Hawaiian) good victory

Iusitina (Hawaiian) justice

Iva (Slavic) dedicated
Ivah

Ivania (Russian) feminine form of Ivan: believer in a gracious God; reliable one

Ivaniah (Russian) feminine form of Ivan: believer in a gracious God; reliable one

Ivanna (Russian) gracious gift from God
Iva, Ivana, Ivanka, Ivie, Ivy

Iverem (African) lucky girl

Ives (French) form of Yves: clever

Ivet (Spanish) athletic

Iveta (French) athletic

Ivette (French) clever and athletic
Ivet, Ivett

Ivey (English/American) a climbing evergreen ornamental plant
Ivee, Ivie, Ivy

Iviannah (American) adorned
Iviana, Ivianna, Ivie, Ivy

Ivisse (American) graceful
Ivice, Iviece, Ivis, Ivise

Ivnia (Russian) feminine form of Ivan: believer in a gracious God; reliable one

Ivon (Spanish) light
Ivonie, Ivonne

Ivona (Slavic) gift
Ivana, Ivanna, Ivannah, Ivonah, Ivone, Ivonne

Ivonne (French) athlete
Ivonn

Ivory (Latin) white
Ivoree, Ivori, Ivorie

Ivria (Hebrew) from Abraham's country
Ivriah, Ivrit

Ivrie (English) form of Ivory: white

Ivy (English) growing
Iv, Ivee, Ivey, Ivie

Iwa (Japanese) strong character

Iwalani (Hebrew) heavenly girl

Iwilla (African American) i will rise

Iwona (Polish) archer; athletic; gift
Iwonna

Iyabo (African) her mother is home

Iyana (Hebrew) sincere

Izabella (American) form of Isabella: consecrated to God
Iza, Izabela, Izabelle, Izabell

Izanne (American) calming
Iza, Izan, Izann, Izanna, Ize

Izdihar (Arabic) blossoming

Izebe (African) staunch supporter

Izegbe (African) baby who was wanted

Izena (Slavic) gracious

Izene (Slavic) gracious

Izolde (Greek) philosophical
Izo, Izolade, Izold

Izusa (Native American) white rock; unique

Izzy (American) zany
Izzee, Izzie

J

J'Netta (American) form of Jeanetta: impish
J'netta, J'Nette, Janetta, Janny

Jaala (Arabic) seeks clarity

Jabinea (Biblical) sees

Jacalyn (American) form of Jacqueline: supplanter; substitute
Jacelyn, Jacelyne, Jacelynn, Jacilyn, Jacilyne, Jacilynn, Jacolyn, Jacolyne, Jacolynn, Jacylyn, Jacylyne, Jacylynn

Jacey (Greek) sparkling
J.C., Jace, Jacee, Jaci, Jacie, Jacy

Jacinda (Greek) attractive girl
Jacenda, Jacey, Jaci, Jacinta

Jacinta (Spanish) hyacinth; sweet
Jace, Jacee, Jacey, Jacinda, Jacinna, Jacintae, Jacinth, Jacinthia, Jacy, Jacynth

Jacinth (Greek) beauty

Jackalyn (American) form of Jacqueline: supplanter; substitute
Jackalene, Jackalin, Jackaline, Jackalynn, Jackalynne, Jackelin, Jackeline, Jackelyn, Jackelynn, Jackelynne, Jackilin, Jackilyn, Jackilynn, Jackilynne, Jackolin, Jackoline, Jackolyn, Jackolynn, Jackolynne

Jackie (French) form of Jacqueline: supplanter; substitute
Jackee, Jacki, Jacky, Jaki, Jaky

Jacklyn (American) careful
Jacklin, Jackline, Jackline, Jacklyne, Jacklynn, Jacklynne

Jackquel (French) watchful
Jackquelin, Jackqueline, Jackquelyn, Jackquelynn, Jackquilin, Jackquiline, Jackquilyn, Jackquilynn, Jackquilynne

Jackson (Last name as first name) swaggering
Jacksen, Jaksin, Jakson

Jaclyn (French) form of Jacqueline: supplanter; substitute
Jacalyn, Jackalene, Jackalin, Jackalyn, Jackeline, Jackolynne, Jacleen, Jaclin, Jacline, Jaclyne, Jaclynn

Jacoba (Hebrew) replaces

Jacobi (Hebrew) stand-in
Cobie, Coby

Jacomine (Dutch) best girl

Jacoy (French) form of Jackie:
supplanter; substitute

Jacqua (American)
replacement

Jacqueline (French)
supplanter; substitute
*Jacki, Jackie, Jacklin, Jacklyn,
Jaclyn, Jacqualin, Jacqualine,
Jacqualyn, Jacqualyne, Jacquel,
Jacquelyn, Jacquelynn, Jacqui,
Jacquie, Jakie, Jakline, Jaklinn,
Jaklynn, Jaqueline, Jaquie*

Jacquelyn (French) form of
Jacqueline: supplanter;
substitute
Jacquelyne, Jacquelynn

Jacquet (Invented) form of
Jacqueline: supplanter;
substitute
*Jackett, Jackwet, Jacquee,
Jacquie, Jakkett*

Jacquetta (American)
replacement

Jacqui (French) form of
Jacquline: supplanter;
substitute
*Jacquay, Jacque, Jacquee,
Jacquie, Jakki, Jaki, Jaquay,
Jaqui, Jaquie*

Jacynth (Spanish) hyacinth;
flower

Jada ☼ ☉ (Spanish)
personable; precious
Jadah

Jade (Spanish) green
gemstone; courageous;
adoring
*Jada, Jadah, Jadda, Jadea,
Jadeann, Jadee, Jaden, Jadera,
Jadi, Jadie, Jadielyn, Jadienne,
Jady, Jadzia, Jadziah, Jaeda,
Jaedra, Jaida, Jaide, Jaiyde,
Jaiden*

Jaden (Hebrew) God has
heard
*Jadi, Jadie, Jadin, Jadyn,
Jaeden, Jaiden, Jadan*

Jadie (Spanish) jade stone

Jadine (Spanish) jade stone

Jadran (American) jade stone

Jadwiga (Polish) religious
Jad, Jadwig, Wiga

Jadwin (American) friend of
Jade

Jadza (Spanish) jade

Jae (Latin) small; jaybird
Jaea, Jay, Jayjay

Jael (Hebrew) high-climbing
Jaela, Jaelee, Jaeli, Jaelie, Jaelle

Jaela (Hebrew) bright
Jael, Jaell, Jayla

Jaelyn (African American)
ambitious
*Jaela, Jaelynne, Jala, Jalyn,
Jaylyn*

Jaenesha (African American)
spirited
*Jacey, Jae, Jaeneisha, Jaeniesha,
Janesha, Jaynesha, Nesha*

Jae-Sun (Japanese) sun's bird

Jaffa (Hebrew) lovely

Jagan (American) form of
Jaden: God has heard
Jag, Jagann, Jagen, Jagun

Jagger (English) cutter
Jaeger, Jag, Jager

Jagodah (Slavic) little berry
Jagoda, Jagada, Jago, Jaga

Jaguar (American) runner
Jag, Jaggy, Jagwar, Jagwor

Jahel (Hebrew) moves upward

Jahnea (Scandinavian)
feminine form of John: God
is gracious

Jahnika (Scandinavian)
believes in God

Jahnny (American) feminine
form of Johnny: God is
gracious
*Jahnae, Jahnay, Jahnie,
Jahnnee, Jahnney, Jahnnie,
Jahny*

Jaidan (American) golden
child
*Jaedan, Jai, Jaide, Jaidee, Jaidi,
Jaidon, Jaidun, Jaidy, Jaidyn,
Jaydan, Jaydyn*

Jaime (French) girl who loves
*Jaeme, Jaemee, Jaima, Jaimee,
Jaimey, Jaimi, Jaimie, Jaimy,
Jamie, Jaymee*

Jaime-Day (American) loving

Jaimela (Spanish) lovely

Jainil (English) form of Janel:
exuberent

Jairia (Spanish) taught by
God's lessons

Jakira (Arabic) warmth

Jakisha (African American)
favored
Jakishe

Jakki (American) form of
Jackie: supplanter; substitute
Jakea, Jakia, Jakkia

Jalalynne (Combo of Jala and
Lynne) important

Jalila (Arabic) excellent
Jalile

Jalit (American) sparkling
Jal, Jalitt, Jalitte, Jallit

Jalona (Spanish) excellence

Jalou (Scandinavian) form of
Jaela: bright

Jamaica (Place name)
Caribbean island
*Jama, Jamaika, Jamaka,
Jamake, Jamana, Jamea,
Jameca, Jameka, Jamica,
Jamika, Jamiqua, Jamoka,
Jemaica, Jemika, Jemyka*

Jamais (French) ever
Jamay, Jamaye

Jamalita (Invented) feminine
form of James: supplanter
Jama

Jamar (African American)
strong
*Jam, Jamara, Jamareah,
Jamaree, Jamarr, Jamarra,
Jammy*

Jamashia (African American)
soulful
Jamash, Jamashea

Jame (Hebrew) feminine
form of James: supplanter

Jameah (African American)
bold
Jamea, Jameea, Jamiah

Jamecka (African American)
studious
*Jamecca, Jameeka, Jameka,
Jameke, Jamekka, Jamie,
Jamiea, Jamieka*

Jameelah (Arabic) lovely

Jameia (Arabic) lovely

Jamelae (American) smart

Jamesetta (American) feminine form of James: supplanter
Jamesette

Jamesha (African American) outgoing
Jamece, Jamecia, Jumeciah, Jameisha, James, Jamese, Jameshia, Jameshyia, Jamesia, Jamesica, Jamesika, Jamesina, Jamessa, Jamie, Jamisha, Jay

Jami (Hebrew) replacement
Jamay, Jamia, Jamie, Jamy

Jamie (Hebrew) supplants; fun-loving
Jami, Jamee, James, Jaymee

J'Amie (French) form of Jamie: supplants; fun-loving
Friend

Jamika (African American) buoyant
Jameeka, Jamey, Jamica, Jamicka, Jamie

Jamila (Arabic) beautiful female
Jahmela, Jahmilla, Jam, Jameela, Jami, Jamie, Jamil, Jamilah, Jamile, Jamilla, Jamille, Jamilya, Jammell, Jammie

Jan (English) form of Janet: small; forgiving
Jani, Jania, Jandy, Jannie, Janny

JaNa (American) form of Jane: believer in a gracious God

Jana (Slavic/Scandinavian) God's gracious gift
Janna, Janne

Janae (American) giving
Janea, Jannay, Jennae, Jannah, Jennay

Janaina (Arabic) soulful

Janaki (Indian) seeta

Janalyn (American) giving
Jan, Janalynn, Janelyn, Janilyn, Jannalyn, Jannnie, Janny

Janan (Arabic) soulful
Jananee, Janani, Jananie, Janann, Jannani

Janara (American) generous
Janarah, Janerah, Janira, Janirah

Janay (American) forgiving
Janae, Janah, Janai

Janaya (American) form of Janae: giving

Jancy (American) risk-taker
Jan, Jance, Jancee, Jancey, Janci, Jancie, Janny

Jandy (American) fun
Jandee, Jandey, Jandi

Jane (Hebrew) believer in a gracious God
Jaine, Jan, Janelle, Janene, Janeth, Janett, Janetta, Janey, Janica, Janie, Jannie, Jayne, Jaynie

Janeana (American) sweet
Janea, Janean, Janeanah, Janine

Janeer (American) heartfelt

Janel (French) form of Janelle: exuberant
Janell, Jannel, Jaynel, Jaynell

Janelle (French) exuberant
J'Nel, J'nell, Janel, Janell, Jannel, Jenelle, Nell

Janene (American) form of Jane: believer in a gracious God
Janeen, Jenean, Janine, Jenine

Janessa (American) forgiving
*Janesha, Janeska, Janessah,
Janie, Janiesa, Janiesha,
Janisha, Janissa, Jannesa,
Jannesha, Jannessa, Jannisa,
Jannisha, Jannissa, Janyssa*

Janet (English) small;
forgiving
*Jan, Janett, Janetta, Janette,
Jannet, Jannett, Janot, Jessie,
Jinett, Johnette, Jonetta, Jonette*

Janeth (American)
fascinating
Janith

Jania (American) heart's
delight

Janice (Hebrew) knowing
God's grace
*Genese, Jan, Janece, Janecia,
Janeese, Janeice, Janiece,
Jannice, Janyce, Jynice*

Janida (Spanish) gracious

Janie (English) form of Jane:
believer in a gracious God
Janey, Jani, Jany

Janiece (American) devout;
enthusiastic
*Janece, Janecia, Janeese, Janese,
Janesea, Janesse, Janneece,
Jeneece, Jeneese*

Janiecia (African American)
sporty
*Janesha, Janeisha, Janeshah,
Janisha, Jan, Jannes, Jannesa*

Janielle (English) form of
Janelle: exuberant

Janier (French) gracious

Janika (Scandinavian) form of
Jane: believer in a gracious
God
*Janica, Janicah, Janik, Jannike,
Janikka*

Janina (Scandinavian) devout

Janine (American) kind
*Janean, Janeen, Janene, Janey,
Janie, Jannine, Jannyne,
Janyne, Jenine*

Janineata (American) form
of Janine: kind

Janique (Scandinavian)
believer; smart

Janis (English) form of Jane:
believer in a gracious God
*Janees, Janeesa, Janes, Jenice,
Jenis, Janise*

Janisse (American) elegant

Janitza (American) form of
Juanita: believer in a gracious
God; forgiving

Janiya (American) believer

Janiyah (American) believer

Janiyal (American) pious

Janjan (Last name as first)
sweet; believer
*Jan Jan, Jange, Janja, Jan-Jan,
Janje, Janni, Jannie, Janny*

Janke (Scandinavian) believer
in God
Jankee, Jankey, Jankie

Janna (Hebrew) form of
Johana: believer in gracious
God

Janneke (Scandinavian)
smart; believer

Jannette (American) lovely
*Jan, Janette, Jannett, Jannie,
Janny*

Jannie (English) form of Jane:
believer in a gracious God;
form of Jan: small; forgiving;
knowing God's grace
Janney, Janny, Jannye

Janoah (Biblical) place name

Jansen (Scandinavian)
smooth
*Jan, Jannsen, Jans, Jansie,
Janson, Jansun, Jansy*

Janteya (Dutch) form of
Jantine: giving

Jantine (Dutch) giving
*Janteen, Jantene, Jantee, Janty,
Jantie*

Jantje (Scandinavian) believer

Japana (American) form of
Japan

Japha (Biblical) place name

Jaqueline (French) form of
Jacquelyn: supplanter;
substitute
*Jaqlinn, Jaqlyn, Jaqlynn, Jaqua,
Jaquaeline, Jaqualine,
Jaqualyn, Jaquelina, Jaquelyn,
Jaquelynne, Jaquie, Jaqulene*

Jaquonna (African
American) spoiled
*Jakwona, Jakwonda,
Jakwonna, Jaqui, Jaquie,
Jaquon, Jaquona, Jaquonne*

Jaranescia (Scandinavian)
magnificent

Jardana (American) gardener
Jardana, Jarde, Jardee, Jardy

Jardena (French) gardens
*Jardan, Jardane, Jarden,
Jardenia, Jardine, Jardyne*

Jarenda (American) lovely

Jarene (American) bright
*Jare, Jaree, Jareen, Jaren,
Jareni, Jarine, Jarry, Jaryne,
Jerry*

Jariesha (India) clear-headed

Jarita (Arabic) carries water;
befriends
*Jara, Jari, Jaria, Jarica, Jarida,
Jarietta, Jarika, Jarina, Jaritta,
Jaritza*

Jariya (Arabic) form of Jarita:
carries water; befriends

Jarmila (Czech) beautiful
spring

Jarone (American) optimistic
Jaron, Jaroyne, Jerone, Jurone

Jaroslava (Czech) glorious
spring

Jarren (American) lovable
Jaren, Jarran, Jarre

Jas (American) form of
Jasmine: fragrant; sweet
Jass, Jaz, Jazz, Jazze, Jazzi

Jasalin (American) devoted
*Jasalinne, Jasalyn, Jasalynn,
Jaselyn, Jasleen, Jaslene, Jass,
Jassalyn, Jassy, Jazz, Jazzy*

Jasia (Slavic) hopeful

Jasira (Polish) form of Jane:
believer in a gracious God

Jasmine ✿ (Persian/
Spanish) fragrant; sweet
*Jas'mine, Jasamine, Jasime,
Jasimen, Jasimin, Jasimine,
Jasmaine, Jasman, Jasme,
Jasmie, Jasmina, Jasminah,
Jasminen, Jasminne, Jasmon,
Jasmond, Jasmone, Jasmyn,
Jasmynn, Jasmynne, Jazie,
Jazmaine, Jazman, Jazmeen,
Jazmein, Jazmen, Jazmin,
Jazmine, Jazmon, Jazmond,
Jazmyn, Jazmyne, Jazs,
Jazsmen, Jazz, Jazza,
Jazzamine, Jazzee, Jazzi,
Jazzmeen, Jazzmin, Jazz-
Mine, Jazzmun, Jazzy*

Jasna (American) talented
Jas, Jazna, Jazz

Jasper (French) gemstone

Jaspreet (Punjabi) pure
*Jas, Jaspar, Jasparit, Jasparita,
Jasper, Jasprit, Jasprita, Jasprite*

Jasvina (Spanish) form of
Jasmine: fragrant; sweet

Ja-Tawn (African American)
tawny
J'Tawn, Ja Tawn, Jatawn

Jatsue (Spanish) lively
Jat, Jatsey

Jatumn (American) form of
Autumn: joy of changing
seasons

Jautanza (American) creative

Javalin (American) thrower

Javana (Asian) girl from Java;
dancer
*Javanna, Javanne, Javon,
Javonda, Javonna, Javonne,
Javonya, Jawana, Jawanna,
Jawn*

Javette (American) lively

Javiera (Spanish) owns a
home
Javeera, Viera

Jawanda (African) bejeweled

Jawara (Arabic) true gem

Jaya (Hindi) winning
Jaea, Jaia, Jay, Jayah

Jayal (Sanskrit) special

Jayanti (Indian) winning

Jayare (African) winner

Jayatissa (Indian) wins

Jayci (American) vivacious
*Jacee, Jacey, Jaci, Jacie, Jacy,
Jaycee, Jaycey, Jayci, Jaycie*

Jayden (American)
enthusiastic
*Jaden, Jay, Jaydeen, Jaydon,
Jaydyn, Jaye*

Jaydie (American) lively
*Jadie, Jady, Jay-Dee, Jaydeye,
Jaydie*

Jaydra (Spanish) treasured
jewel; jade
Jadra, Jay, Jaydrah

Jaye (Latin) small as a jaybird
Jae, Jay

Jayla (American) smiling
Jaila, Jaylah, Jayle, Jaylee

Jayleena (English) wins
Jaylena, Jaylenna

Jaylen ♂ (English) wins

Jaylene (American) feminine
form of Jay: colorful
*Jayelene, Jayla, Jaylah, Jaylan,
Jayleana, Jaylee, Jayleen*

Jaylynn (American) feminine
form of Jay: colorful
*Jaelin, Jaeline, Jaelyn, Jaelyne,
Jaelynn, Jaelynne, Jalin, Jaline,
Jalyn, Jalyne, Jalynn, Jalynne,
Jaylin, Jayline, Jaylyn, Jaylyne,
Jaylynne*

Jayma (English) dedicated

Jayme (English) feminine
form of James: supplanter
*Jami, Jamie, Jaymee, Jaymi,
Jaymia, Jaymie*

Jayna (Hindi) winner
Jaynae

Jayne (Hindi) victorious
*Jane, Janey, Jani, Jayn, Jaynee,
Jayni, Jaynie, Jaynita, Jaynne*

Jaynille (American) form of
Janelle: exuberent

Jayrette (American) dear

Jazael (American) form of
Giselle: a promise

Jazel (American) form of
Giselle: a promise

Jazl (American) zany

Jazz (American) rhythmic
*Jas, Jassie, Jaz, Jazzi, Jazzie,
Jazzle, Jazzy*

Jazza (American) quirky

Jazzell (American)
spontaneous
*Jazel, Jazell, Jazz, Jazzee,
Jazzie*

Jean (Scottish) God-loving
and gracious
*Jeana, Jeanie, Jeunne, Jeannie,
Jeanny, Jena, Jenay, Jenna*

Jeana (American) form of
Gina: wellborn
Jeanna

Jeanane (French) religious

Jeanetta (American) impish
*Janetta, Jeannet, Jeannette,
Jeanney, Jen, Jenett, Jennita*

Jeanette (French) lively
*Janette, Jeanette, Jeanett,
Jeanetta, Jeanita, Jeannete,
Jeannett, Jeannetta, Jeannette,
Jeannita, Jenet, Jenett, Jenette,
Jennett, Jennetta, Jennette,
Jennita, Jinetta, Jinette*

Jeanie (Scottish) devout;
outspoken
Jeani, Jeannie, Jeanny, Jeany

Jeanine (Scottish)
peace-loving
*Jeanene, Jeanina, Jeannina,
Jeannine, Jenine, Jennine*

Jeanisha (African American)
pretty
*Jean, Jeaneesh, Jeanise, Jeanna,
Jeannie, Jenisha*

Jearlean (American) vibrant
*Jearlee, Jearlene, Jearley, Jearli,
Jearline, Jearly, Jerline*

Jebel (Origin unknown) form
of Jezebel: wanton woman

Jeca (Slavic) untainted
Jeka

Jecelyn (Invented) form of
Jocelyn: joyful
Jece, Jecee, Jeselyn, Jess

Jedid (Biblical) loving

Jeena (American) bold

Jeffrey (German) peaceful;
sparkling personality
*Jef, Jeff, Jeffa, Jefferi, Jeffery,
Jeffie, Jeffre, Jeffrie, Jeffy, Jefry*

Jefjun (Scandinavian) rich

Jekemea (Slavic) my Jeka

Jelana (Russian) form of
Helen: beautiful; light

Jelane (Russian) light heart
*Jelaina, Jelaine, Jelanne, Jilane,
Julane*

Jelani (American) pretty sky
*Jelaney, Jelani, Jelanie, Jelainy,
Jelanni*

Jele (Slavic) light

Jelee (Slavic) moon child

Jelena (Slavic) moon child

Jelene (Slavic) moon

Jelka (Slavic) sturdy

Jelline (French) robust

Jemiccia (Italian) treasured

Jemima (Hebrew) dove-like
*Jamima, Jem, Jemi, Jemimah,
Jemm, Jemma, Jemmi, Jemmia,
Jemmiah, Jemmy, Jemora*

Jemine (American) treasured
Jem, Jemmy, Jemyne

Jemma (Hebrew) form of
Gemma: gem; jewel
Jem

Jems (American) treasured
*Gemas, Jemma, Jemmey,
Jemmi, Jemmy*

Jena (Arabic; small)
Jenaa, Janae, Jenaeh, Jenah,
Jenai, Jenal, Jenay, Jenna

Jenaseth (English) bird

Jenavieve (American) form
of Genevieve: generous

Jenaya (African) hospitable

Jene (English) form of Jane:
believer in a gracious God

Jenea (English) form of Jane:
believer in a gracious God

Jenell (American) form of
Janelle: exuberant
Janele, Jen, Jenaile, Jenalle,
Jenel, Jenella, Jennelle, Jenny

Jenesia (Latin) newcomer

Jenette (English) form of
Jeanette: lively

Jeniece (American) form of
Janice: knowing God's grace

Jenifer (Welsh) form of
Jennifer: white wave
Gennefer, Gennifer, Ginnifur,
Ginnipher, Jay, Jenefer, Jenifer,
Jenjen, Jenna, Jenni, Jennifer,
Jenny

Jenika (English) blonde

Jenille (English) believes in
gracious God

Jenis (Hebrew) the start
Jenesis

Jenna ⊙ (English) form of
Jean: God-loving and gracious
Jena, Jennah, Jennat, Jennay,
Jhenna, Jynna

Jennah (English) form of
Jennifer: white wave
Jena, Jenna, Genna

Jennell (English) form of
Janelle: exuberant

Jennelle (English) form of
Janelle: exuberant

Jenni (Welsh) form of
Jennifer: white wave
Jeni, Jenica, Jenie, Jenisa,
Jenka, Jenne, Jennee, Jenney,
Jennia, Jennier, Jennita,
Jennora, Jensine

Jennifer ⊙ (Celtic) white wave
Gennefur, Ginnifer, Jen, Jenefer,
Jenife, Jenifer, Jeniferr, Jeniffer,
Jenipher, Jenn, Jenna, Jennae,
Jennafer, Jennefer, Jenni,
Jenniffe, Jenniffer, Jenniffier,
Jennifier, Jenniphe, Jennipher,
Jenniphur, Jenny, Jennyfer,
Jennypher

Jennings (Last name as first
name) pretty
Jen, Jenny

Jennis (American) white;
patient
J, Jay, Jen, Jenace, Jenice, Jenis,
Jenn, Jennice

Jennison (American) form of
Jennifer: white wave
Gennison, Jenison, Jennisyn,
Jenson

Jenny (English) form of
Jennifer: white wave
Jen, Jenae, Jeni, Jenjen, Jenney,
Jenni, Jennie, Jennye, Jeny,
Jinny

Jennys (American) white

Jeno (Greek) heavenly

Jenova (Italian) form of
Genoa: playful

Jensen (Scandinavian)
athletic

Jenvie (American) lovely
Jennvey, Jenvee, Jenvy

Jenz (Scandinavian) feminine form of Johannes: God is gracious
Jen, Jens

Jeolle (American) fair

Jerdin (English) grows a garden

Jeredine (English) grows a garden

Jerett (English) rules well

Jergen (Dutch) earthy

Jeri (American) hopeful
Geri, Jere, Jerhie, Jerree, Jerri, Jerry, Jerrye

Jeriesha (Biblical) owned

Jerikah (American) sparkling
Jereca, Jerecka, Jeree, Jeri, Jerica, Jerik, Jeriko, Jerrica, Jerry

Jerin (American) daring
Jere, Jeren, Jeron, Jerinn, Jerun

Jerina (Slavic) loyal

Jermaina (American) form of Germaine: important

Jermaine (French) form of Germaine: important
Germaine, Jermain, Jerman, Jermane, Jermanee, Jermani, Jermany, Jermayne

Jernina (English) form of Jemima: dove-like

Jeroen (Scandinavian) strong

Jerrett (American) spirited
Jerett, Jeriette, Jerre, Jerret, Jerrette, Jerrie, Jerry

Jerrica (American) free spirit
Jerrika

Jerusha (Hebrew) wealthy

Jesa (Indian) flowers

Jesaren (English) form of Jessie: Giving

Jesenia (Spanish) witty
Jesene, Jess, Jessenia, Jessie, Jessie, Jisenia, Yesenia

Jessa (American) spontaneous
Jessah

Jessamine (French) form of Jasmine: fragrant; sweet
Jesamyn, Jess, Jessamin, Jessamon, Jessamy, Jessamyn, Jessemin, Jessemine, Jessie, Jessmine, Jessmon, Jessmy, Jessmyn

Jesse (Hebrew) friendly
Jesie, Jessey, Jessi, Jessy

Jessenia (Arabic) flowering
Jescenia, Jesenia

Jessica ✪ (Hebrew) rich
Jesica, Jess, Jessa, Jessie, Jessika, Jessy, Jezika

Jessie (Scottish) casual
Jescie, Jesey, Jess, Jesse, Jessee, Jessi, Jessye

Jessika (Hebrew) rich
Jesika, Jessieka, Jessika, Jessyka, Jezika

Jesusa (Spanish) feminine form of Jesus: saved by God

Jesusa (Spanish) loves Jesus

Jesusita (Spanish) little Jesus

Jett (American) high-flying
Jettie, Jetty

Jetta (English) black gem; knowing
Jette, Jettie

Jette (Dutch) black as coal
Jet, Jeta, Jetia, Jetta, Jette, Jettee, Jettie

Jeudi (French) born on Thursday

Jeune-Fille (French) young girl

Jevae (Spanish) desired
Jevaie, Jevay

Jevonne (African American)
kind
*Jev, Jevaughan, Jevaughn, Jevie,
Jevon, Jevona, Jevonn, Jevvy*

Jewel (French) pretty
*Jeul, Jewelia, Jewelie, Jewell,
Jewelle, Jewels, Juel, Jule*

Jewelina (Spanish) jewel

Jezana (Slavic) womanly

Jezbelline (Spanish) form of
Jezebel: wanton woman

Jeze (Biblical) form of Jezebel:
wanton woman

Jezebel (Hebrew) wanton
woman
*Jessabel, Jessebel, Jessebelle, Jez,
Jezabel, Jezabella, Jezahelle,
Jeze, Jezebell, Jezel, Jezell,
Jezybel, Jezzie*

Jezenya (American)
flowering
Jesenya, Jeze, Jezey

Jhamesha (African
American) lovely; soft
Jamesha, Jmesha

Jharna (Hindi) springtime

Jhonsi (Scandinavian)
feminine form of John: God
is gracious

Jianna (Italian) trusts in God
Jiana, Jianina, Jianine

Jigna (Hindi) intellectual

Jignasa (Hindi) curious

Jila (American) energetic;
Young
Young

Jilan (American) mover
*Jilyn, Jillan, Jillyn, Jylan,
Jylann*

Jilana (Slavic) moon child
Moon child

Jilen (American) young girl

Jill (English) form of Jillian:
youthful
Jil, Jilee, Jilli, Jillie, Jilly

Jillaine (Latin) young-hearted
*Jilaine, Jilane, Jilayne, Jillana,
Jillane, Jillann, Jillanne,
Jillayne*

Jilleen (American) energetic
*Jil, Jileen, Jilene, Jiline, Jill,
Jillain, Jilline, Jlynn*

Jillian (Latin) youthful
*Giliana, Jill, Jillaine, Jillana,
Jillena, Jilliane, Jilliann, Jillie,
Jillion, Jillione, Jilly, Jilyan*

Jillit (English) form of Jillian:
youthful

Jills (Scandinavian) young

Jillyn (American) high-energy;
Young

Jimi (Hebrew) replaces;
reliable
Jimae

Jimmi (American) assured
Jim, Jimi, Jimice, Jayjay

Jimmye (English) replaces; in
pain

Jimye (English) replaces; in
pain

Jin (Chinese) golden; gem
Jinn, Jinny

Jina (Italian) form of Gina:
wellborn
*Jena, Jinae, Jinan, Jinda,
Jinna, Jinnae*

Jinger (American) form of
Ginger: ginger plant
Jin, Jinge

Jini (American) form of Jenny:
white wave

Jinkie (American) bouncy
Jinkee, Jynki, Jinky

Jinny (Scottish) form of
Jenny: white wave
*Jin, Jina, Jinae, Jinelle, Jinessa,
Jinna, Jinnae, Jinnalee, Jinnee,
Jinney, Jinni, Jinnie*

Jinte (Hindi) patient

Jinx (Latin) a spell
Jin, Jinks, Jinxie, Jinxy, Jynx

Jinxia (Latin) form of Jinx: a
spell
Jinx, Jynx, Jynxia

Jirina (Czech) works the earth

Jisola (African) affluent

Jitendea (Indian) good

Jnae (American) darling
J'Nay, Jenae, Jnay, Jnaye

J'Neane (American) form of
Jeannine: peace-loving

J-Nyl (American) flirtatious

Jo (American) form of
Josephine: blessed
Joey, Jojo

Joan (Hebrew) heroine; God-
loving
*Joane, Joane, Joani, Joanie,
Joanni, Joannie, Jonie*

Joana (Hebrew) kind
*Joanah, Joanna, Joannah,
Jonah*

Joanie (Hebrew) kind
*Joanney, Joanni, Joannie,
Joanny, Joany, Joni*

Jo-Ann (French) believer;
gregarious
*Joahnn, JoAn, JoAnn, Joann,
Joanna, Joanne, Jo-Anne,
Joannie*

Joanna (English) kind
*Jo, Joana, Joandra, Joananna,
Joananne, Joannah, Joeanna,
Johannah, Josie*

Joanne (English) form of
Joan: heroine; God-loving
*JoAnn, Joann, Jo-Ann, JoAnne,
Joeanne*

Joannie (Hebrew) forgiving
Joani, Joany, Joanney, Joanni

Joappa (Origin unknown)
noisy

Joaquina (Spanish) form of
Joaquin: God helps

Jobi (Hebrew) misunderstood;
inventive
Jobee, Jobey, Jobie, Joby

Jobina (Hebrew) hurting
Jobey, Jobie, Joby, Jobye, Jobyna

Jobine (Biblical) friend

Jocasta (Italian) light

Jocelyn ✿ (Latin) joyful
*Jocelie, Jocelin, Jocelle, Jocelyne,
Jocelynn, Joci, Joclyn, Joclynn,
Jocylan, Jocylen, Joycelyn*

Jochebal (Biblical) glory to
God

Joci (Latin) happy
Jocee, Jocey, Jocie, Jocy, Josi

Jocosa (Latin) laughs; jokes

Jocquice (French) blessed

Jodase (American) brilliant
Jo, Jodace, Jodasse, Jodie, Jody

Jode (American) form of
Jodie: happy girl

Jodie (American) happy girl
Jo, Jodee, Jodey, Jodi, Jody

Joedy (American) jolly
Joedey, Joedi, Joedie

Joelle (Hebrew) willing
Jo, Joel, Joela, Joele, Joelee,
Joeleen, Joelene, Joeli, Joeline,
Joell, Joella, Joelle, Joellen, Joelly

Joelly (American) kindhearted
Joelee, Joeli, Joely

Joely (Hebrew) believer; lively
Jo, Joe, Joey

Joey (American) easygoing
Joe, Joeye

Joezee (American) form of
Josey: blessed
Jo, Joe, Joes, Joezey, Joezy

Johanna (German) believer
in a gracious God
Johana, Johanah, Johanna,
Jonna

Johnay (American) steadfast
Johnae, Jonay, Jonaye, Jonnay

Johnette (Hebrew) feminine
form of John: God is gracious

Johnica (American) feminine
form of John: God is gracious
Jonica

Johnna (American) upright
Jahna, John, Johna, Johnae,
Jonna, Jonnie

Johnnell (American) happy
Johnelle, Jonell, Jonnel

Johnnetta (American) joyful
Johneta, Johnete, Johnetta,
Johnette, Jonetta, Jonette,
Jonietta

Johnnisha (African
American) steady
Johnisha, Johnnita, Johnny,
Jonnisha

Johnson (Last name as first
name) confident
Johns

Johntell (African American)
sweet
Johna, Johntal, Johntel,
Johntelle, Jontell

Johntria (Hebrew) believer

Johppa (Origin unknown)
different
Johppah

Joi (Latin) joyful
Joicy, Joie, Jojo, Joy

Joice (American) form of
Joyce: joyous

Joji (English) form of JoJo:
joyful

Jo-Kiesha (African American)
vibrant
Joekiesha

Jola (Greek) violet flower

Jolan (Latin) violet

Jolanda (Italian) a violet
flower
Jola, Jolan, Jolana, Jolande,
Jolander, Jolane, Jolanka,
Jolantha, Jolanthe, Joli

Jolanta (Greek) lovely girl

Jolene (American) jolly
Jo, Joeleane, Joeleen, Joelene,
Joelynn, Joleen, Joleene, Jolen,
Jolena, Joley, Jolie, Joline, Jolyn,
Jolynn

Joletta (American) happy-go-
lucky
Jaletta, Jolette, Joley, Joli, Jolie,
Jolitta

Jolia (English) joyful girl

Jolie (French) pretty
Jo, Jole, Jolea, Jolee, Joleigh,
Joley, Joli, Jollee, Jollie, Jolly,
Joly

Jolienne (American) pretty
Joliane, Jolianne, Jolien, Jolina,
Joline

Jolina (English) joyful girl

Joline (English) blessed

Jolivette (French) jubilant

Jolly (English) jolly

Jolyane (American) sweetheart
Joliane, Jollyane, Jolyan, Jolyann, Jolyanne

Jomonia (American) loyal

Jona (English) peaceful

JonBenet (French) with God's benediction

Jones (American) saucy

Jonette (American) peaceful

Joni (American) form of Joan: heroine; God-loving
Joanie, Jonie, Jony

Jonica (American) sweet soul

Jonice (American) casual
Joneece, Joneese, Jonni, Jonise

Jonille (English) believer

Jonina (Hebrew) sweetheart
Jona, Jonika, Joniqua, Jonita, Jonnina

Jonita (Hebrew) pretty little one
Janita, Jonati, Jonit, Jonite, Jonta, Jontae

Jonna (Scandinavian) believer
Johnna

Jonquill (American) flower
Jonn, Jonque, Jonquie, Jonquil, Jonquille

Jontelle (American) musical
Jahntelle, Jontaya, Jontel, Jontell, Jontelle, Jontia, Jontlyl

Joone (American) form of June: born in June
Joon

Jophery (American) feminine form of Christopher: the bearer of Christ

Joplin (Last name as first name) wild girl

Jorah (Hebrew) fresh as rain
Jora

Jordan ✿ (Hebrew) excellent descendant
Johrdon, Jordaine, Jordane, Jorden, Jordenne, Jordeyn, Jordi, Jordie, Jordin, Jordon, Jordyn, Jordynne, Joudane, Jourdan

Jordana (Hebrew) smart; departs; lonely
Giordanna, Jordain, Jordana, Jordane, Jordann, Jordanna, Jordanne, Jordannuh, Jorden, Jordenne, Jordi, Jordin, Jordine, Jordon, Jordona, Jordonna, Jordyn, Jordyne, Jori, Jorie, Jourdana, Jourdann, Jourdanna, Jourdanne

Jordy (American) quick
Jordee, Jordey, Jordi, Jordie, Jorey

Jorene (American) wanted

Joretta (English) pretty girl

Joretta (English) wanted

Jorgina (Spanish) nurturing
Jorge, Jorgine, Jorgy, Jorgie, Jorgi, Georgina, Georgeena

Jorie (Hebrew) form of Jordan: excellent descendant
Joree, Jorey, Jorhee, Jorhie, Jori, Jorre, Jorrey, Jorri, Jory

Jorja (American) smart
Georgia, Jorge, Jorgia, Jorgie, Jorgy

Jorunn (American) loved by God

Josany (American) joyful girl

Joscelin (Latin) happy girl
Josceline, Joscelyn, Joscelyne, Joscelynn, Joscelynne, Joselin, Joseline, Joselyn, Joselyne, Joselynn, Joselynne, Joshlyn

Josee (American) delights
Joesee, Joesell, Joesette, Joselle, Josette, Josey, Josi, Josiane, Josiann, Josianne, Josielina, Josina, Josy, Jozee, Jozelle, Jozette, Jozie

Josefat (Spanish) feminine form of Joseph: he will add
Fata, Fina, Josef, Josefa, Josefana, Josefenna, Josefita, Joseva, Josey, Josie

Josefina (Hebrew) fertile
Jose, Josephina, Josey, Josie

Joselita (Spanish) joyful girl

Joselito (Spanish) joyful girl

Joselyn (German) pretty
Josalene, Joselene, Joseline, Josey, Josiline, Josilyn, Joslyn, Josselen, Josseline, Josselyne, Josslyn, Josslynn, Josylynn

Josephine (French) blessed
Fena, Fifi, Fina, Jo, Joes, Josefina, Josephene, Josie, Jozaphine

Josetta (French) she trusts in God

Josette (French) little Josephine

Josey (American) form of Josephine: blessed
Josee, Josi, Josie, Jozie

Josezaldy (Spanish) joyful girl

Joshi (Hebrew) God loves

Joshlyn (Latin) saved by God
Joshalin, Joshalyn, Joshalynn, Joshalynne, Joshann, Joshanna, Joshanne, Joshleen, Joshlene, Joshlin, Joshline, Joshlyne, Joshlynn, Joshlynne

Josie (American) thrills
Josee, Josey, Josi, Josy, Josye

Josien (American) joy

Josilin (Latin) form of Jocelyn: joyful
Josielina, Josiline, Josilyn, Josilyne, Josilynn, Josilynne, Joslin, Josline, Joslyn, Joslyne, Joslynn, Joslynne

Joslyn (Latin) jocular
Joclyn, Joslene, Joslinn, Josslin, Josslyn, Josslynn

Jossalin (Latin) form of Jocelyn: joyful
Jossaline, Jossalyn, Jossalynn, Jossalynne, Josseline, Jossellen, Jossellin, Jossellyn, Josselyn, Josselyne, Josselynn, Josselynne, Jossie, Josslin, Jossline, Josslyn, Josslyne, Josslynn, Josslynne

Jostin (American) adorable
Josten, Jostun, Josty, Jostyn

Joubyne (American) joy

Joudn (American) diplomatic
Joy

Jour (French) day

Jourbine (French) doer

Journey (Word as name) adventurer

Jovan (Slavic) feminine form of John: God is gracious

Jovana (Slavic) feminine form of John: God is gracious

Jovannah (Latin) regal
*Jeovana, Jeovanna, Jouvan,
Jouvanna, Jovan, Jovana,
Jovanee, Jovani, Jovanie,
Jovann, Jovanna, Jovanne,
Jovannie, Jovena, Jovon,
Jovonna, Jovonne, Jowanna*

Joverne (Slavic) challenges

Jovernita (Slavic) challenges

Jovi (Latin) jovial

Jovita (Latin) glad
*Joveeda, Joveeta, Jovena, Joveta,
Jovetta, Jovi, Jovida, Jovie,
Jovina, Jo-Vita, Jovitta, Jovy*

Jowannah (American) happy
Jowanna, Jowanne, Jowonna

Joy (Latin) joyful
Joi, Joie, Joya, Joye

Joyalle (American) joy

Joyce (Latin) joyous
*Joice, Joy, Joycey, Joyci, Joycie,
Joysel*

Joyceen (American) form of
Joyce: joyous

Joycela (American) form of
Joyce: joyous

Joycey (American) form of
Joyce: joyous

Joyous (American) joyful
Joy, Joyus

Joyria (American) of the Lord

Joyslyn (American) form of
Jocelyn: joyful
Joycelyn, Joyslin, Joyslinn

Joysteen (American) joy

Jozel (American) joy

Jualle (American) young girl

Juandali (African) believer

Juanisha (African American)
delightful
*Juanesha, Juaneshia,
Juannisha*

Juanita (Spanish) believer in
a gracious God; forgiving
*Juan, Juana, Juaneta, Juanika,
Juanna, Juanne, Juannie,
Juanny, Wanita*

Juanitra (Spanish) ill-fated

Juba (Hebrew) ram;
strongwilled

Jubal (Biblical) flowing
Jubilant

Jubelka (African American)
jubilant
Jube, Jubi, Jubie

Jubilee (Hebrew) jubilant
Jubalie

Jubini (American) grateful;
jubilant
Jubi, Jubine

Jucinda (American) relishing
life
Jucin, Jucindah, Jucinde

Judalon (Hebrew) merry
Judalonn, Juddalone, Judelon

Jude (French) confident
Judea, Judee, Judde

Judit (Hebrew) Jewish
Jude, Judi, Juditt

Judith (Hebrew) woman
worthy of praise
*Judana, Jude, Judi, Judie,
Judine, Juditha, Judy, Judyth,
Judythe*

Judy (Hebrew) form of Judith:
woman worthy of praise
Judi, Judie, Joodie, Judye, Jude

Juel (American) dependable
Jewel, Juelle, Juels, Jule, Juile

Jueta (Scandinavian) form of
Judith: woman worthy of
praise
Juetta, Juta

Juiby (Asian) flower girl

Juirl (American) careful
Ju, Juirll

Jula (American) form of Julia:
forever young

Juleen (American) sensual
Jule, Julene, Jules

Julenett (American) form of
Julia: forever young

Jules (American) brooding
Jewels, Juels

Juleva (Spanish) young

Julia ✪ (Latin) forever young
*Jula, Juliann, Julica, Julina,
Juline, Julisa, Julissa, Julya,
Julyssa*

Julian (Latin) effervescent
*Jewelian, Julean, Juliann,
Julien, Juliene, Julienn, Julyun*

Juliana (Latin) youthful;
Jove's child
*Juleanna, Julianna, Juliannah,
Julie-Anna, Jullyana*

Julice (American) feminine
form of Julius: attractive

Julie (English) young and
vocal
*Juel, Jule, Julee, Juli, Juliene,
Jullie, July, Julye*

Juliet (Italian) loving

Juliette (French) romantic
Julie, Jules, Juliet, Julietta

Juling (American) form of
Julia: forever young

Julisan (American) young

Julissa (Latin) universally
loved
Jula, Julessa, Julisa, Julisha

Julita (Spanish) adorable;
young
Juli, Julitte

Juliza (Latin) form of Julia:
forever young

Julo (American) form of Julia:
forever young

Juluette (American) adorable;
young
*Jule, Jules, Julett, Julette, Julie,
Julu, Julue, Juluett, Julu-Ette,
LuLu*

July (Latin) month; warm

Jumoke (African) most
popular

Jun (Chinese) honest

Jundt (Scandinavian) hopeful

June (Latin) born in June
*Juneth, Junie, Junieth, Juney,
Juny*

Junelle (American) form of
June: born in June

Junia (Biblical) warm

Junieth (Latin) from the
month June; heavenly
Juney, Juni, Junie, Juniethe

Junko (American) form of
June: born in June

Juno (Latin) queenly
Juna, June

Juntese (American) form of
June: born in June

Juokaka (Asian) pure

Juqwanza (African
American) bouncy
Jukwanza, Juqwann, Qwanza

Juraj (American) moves fast

Jurgan (Scandinavian)

Jus (American) fair

Justice (Latin) fair-minded
Just, Justise, Justy

Justika (American) dancing-girl
Justeeka, Justica, Justie, Justy

Justille (American) fair

Justina (Latin) honest
Jestena, Jestina, Justeena, Justena, Justinna, Justyna

Justinan (American) fair

Justine (Latin) fair; upright
Jestine, Justa, Juste, Justean, Justeen, Justena, Justene, Justi, Justie, Justina, Justinn, Justinna, Justy, Justyne, Justynn, Justynne, Juzteen

Jutta (American) ebullient
Juta

Juttah (Biblical) place name

Juturna (Mythology) trickling water

Juvelia (Spanish) young
Juvee, Juvelle, Juvelya, Juvie, Juvilia, Velia, Velya

Juven (Mythology) young girl

Juwanne (African American) lively
Juwan, Juwann, Juwanna, Juwon, Jwanna, Jwanne

Jyneice (American) form of Janeese: devout; enthusiastic

Jyneisce (American) form of Janeese: devout; enthusiastic

Jynx (American) form of Jinx: a spell

Jyoti (Indian) bright light

Jyotsna (Indian) moonlight

Jzquelyn (Slavic) form of Jacqueline: little Jacquie; small replacement

Kacey (Irish) daring
Casey, Casie, K.C., K.Cee, Kace, Kacee, Kaci, Kacy, Kasey, Kasie, Kaycee, Kaycie, Kaysie

Kachina (Native American) sacred dancer; doll-like
Kacia Cachina, Kachena, Kachine

Kacia (Greek) form of Acacia: everlasting; tree
Kaycia, Kaysia

Kacondra (African American) bold
Condra, Connie, Conny, Kacon, Kacond, Kaecondra, Kakondra, Kaycondra

Kaden (American) charismatic
Caden, Kadenn

Kadenza (Latin) cadence; dances
Cadenza, Kadena, Kadence

Kadie (American) virtuous
Kadee

Kady (English) sassy
Cady, K.D., Kadee, Kadie, Kaydie, Kaydy

Kaela (Arabic) sweet
Kaelah, Kayla, Kaylah, Keyla, Keylah

Kaelin (Irish) pure; impetuous
Kaelan, Kaelen, Kaelinn, Kaelyn, Kaelynn, Kaelynne, Kaylin

Kagan (American) form of Keagan: melodious

Kai (Hawaiian) the sea
Kaia

Kailah (Greek) virtuous
Kail, Kala, Kalae, Kalah

Kaileen (American) sweet

Kailey (American) spunky
Kalee, Kaili, Kailie, Kaylee, Kaylei

Kaimi (American) form of Cammy: wonderful

Kairen (French) pure heart

Kaitlin ♀ (Irish) purehearted
Caitlin, Caitlyn, Kaitlan, Kaitland, Kaitlinn, Kaitlyn, Kaitlynn, Kalyn, Katelyn, Katelynn, Katelynne, Kathlin, Kathlinne, Kathlyn

Kaiulania (Hawaiian) sea and heavens

Kajasa (Asian) forgiving

Kakay (American) pure

Kakiesta (Hawaiian) unblemished

Kala (Hindi) black; royal

Kalan (American) celestial

Kalani (Hawaiian) leader
Kalauni, Kaloni, Kaylanie

Kalavati (Indian) creates

Kalb (German) willful

Kalea (Arabic) sweet
Kahlea, Kahleah, Kailea, Kaileah, Kallea, Kalleah, Kaylea, Kayleah, Khalea, Khaleah

Kalei (American) sweetheart
Kahlei, Kailei, Kallei, Kaylei, Khalei

Kaleigh (Sanskrit) energetic; dark
Kalea

Kalele (Hawaiian) pure

Kalena (Hawaiian) chaste
Kaleena

Kalet (French) beautiful energy
Kalay, Kalaye

Kaley (Sanskrit) energetic
Kalee, Kaleigh, Kalleigh

Kali (Greek) beauty
Kala, Kalli

Kalidas (Greek) most beautiful
Kaleedus, Kali

Kalila (Arabic) sweet; lovable
Cailey, Cailie, Caylie, Kailey, Kaililah, Kaleah, Kalela, Kalie, Kalilah, Kaly, Kay, Kaykay, Kaylee, Kayllie, Kyle, Kylila, Kylilah

Kalina (Hawaiian) unblemished
Kalinna, Kalynna

Kalinda (Hindi) mythical mountains; goal-oriented
Kaleenda, Kalindi, Kalynda, Kalyndi

Kalindee (Indian) river
Kalindi

Kaliyan (Southeast Asian) excellent

Kallan (American) loving
Kall, Kallen, Kallun

Kallie (Greek) beautiful
Callie, Kalley, Kali, Kalie, Kally

Kalliope (Greek) beautiful voice
Calli, Calliope, Kalli, Kallyope

Kallista (Greek) pretty; bright-eyed
Cala, Calesta, Calista, Callie, Callista, Cally, Kala, Kalesta, Kalista, Kalli, Kallie, Kally, Kallysta, Kalysta

Kalota (Hawaiian) vivacious

Kalpana (Indian) dream

Kalyana (Indian) lucky

Kalyani (Indian) lucky
Kalni

Kalyn (Arabic) loved
Calynn, Calynne, Kaelyn, Kaelynn, Kalen, Kalin, Kalinn, Kallyn

Kama (Sanskrit) beloved

Kama (Sanskrit) beloved; Hindu god of love
Kam, Kamie

Kamala (American) interesting
Camala, Kam, Kamali, Kamilla, Kammy

Kamala (Arabic) perfection
Kamalah

Kamaria (African) moonlike
Kamara, Kamaarie

Kambria (Latin) girl from Wales
Kambra, Kambrie, Kambriea, Kambry

Kambrin (American) form of Cambria: the people

Kamea (Hawaiian) adored
Kameo

Kamea (Hawaiian) precious darling
Cammi, Kam, Kammie

Kameko (Japanese) turtle girl; hides

Kamela (Italian) form of Camilla: wonderful
Kam, Kamila, Kammy

Kameron (American) form of Cameron: popular; crooked nose
Cam, Cameron, Cami, Cammie, Kamreen, Kamrin, Kamren, Kamron

Kamethia (American) divine

Kami (Japanese) perfect aura
Cami

Kami (Italian) spiritual little one
Cami, Cammie, Cammy, Kammie, Kammy

Kamiah (Slavic) form of Kamila: desires

Kamilah (Hindi) desires
Kamila, Kamilla, Kamillah

Kamilah (North African) perfect

Kamilia (Polish) perfect character
Kam, Kamila, Kammy, Milla

Kamilia (Polish) pure

Kamini (Indian) woman

Kamna (Indian) desired

Kamoya (Asian) focused

Kamyra (American) light
Kamera

Kanaka (Indian) golden child

Kanara (Hebrew) tiny bird; lithe
Kanarit, Kanarra

Kanda (Native American) magical

Kandace (Greek) charming; glowing
Candace, Candie, Candy, Dacie, Kandace, Kandi, Kandice, Kandiss, Kandy

Kandi (American) form of
Kandace: charming; glowing
Candi, Kandie, Kandy

Kandra (American) light
Candra

Kanear (American) talented

Kaneesha (American) dark-
skinned
*Caneesha, Kaneesh, Kaneice,
Kaneisha, Kanesha, Kaneshia,
Kaney, Kanish, Nesha*

Kanel (Spanish) yellow hair

Kanesha (African American)
spontaneous
*Kaneesha, Kaneeshia,
Kaneisha, Kanisha, Kannesha*

Kanga (Australian) form of
kangaroo: jumpy

Kanik (Egyptian) darkness

Kanisha (American) pretty
*Kaneesha, Kanicia, Kenisha,
Kinicia, Kinisha, Koneesha*

Kannitha (Vietnamese)
angelic

Kanoa (Hawaiian) freedom

Kansas (Place name) U.S.
state
Kanny

Kanthi (Asian) angelic

Kanti (Indian) lovely

Kanya (Hindi) virginal
Kania

Kaori (Asian) free

Kaprece (American)
capricious
*Caprice, Kapp, Kappy,
Kapreece, Kapri, Kaprise,
Kapryce, Karpreese*

Kapuki (African) first girl in
the family

Kara (Danish) form of Cara:
beloved friend
*Cara, Carina, Carita, Kar,
Karah, Kari, Karie, Karina,
Karine, Karita, Karrah, Karrie,
Kera*

Karbie (American) energetic
Karbi, Karby

Karelle (French) joyful singer
Carel, Carelle, Karel

Karen (Greek/Irish)
purehearted
*Caren, Carin, Caron, Caronn,
Carren, Carrin, Carron,
Carryn, Caryn, Carynn,
Carynne, Kare, Kareen,
Karenna, Kari, Karin, Karina,
Karna, Karon, Karron, Karryn,
Karyn, Keren, Kerran, Kerrin,
Kerron, Kerrynn, Keryn,
Kerynne, Taran, Taren, Taryn*

Karenina (Literature) purest

Karenz (English) form of
Kerenza: loveable
Karence, Karens, Karense

Karhime (Arabic) giving

Kari (Scandinavian) pure
Cari, Karri, Karrie, Karry

Kariah (American) form of
Mariah: sorrowful singer

Karian (American) daring
Kerian

Karianne (Scandinavian)
pure
*Kariane, Kariann, Kari-Ann,
Karianna, Kerianne*

Karida (Arabic) pure
Kareeda, Karita

Karima (Arabic) giving
*Kareema, Kareemah, Kareima,
Kareimah, Karimah*

Karin (Scandinavian) kindhearted
Karen, Karine, Karinne

Karina (Russian) form of Karen: purehearetd
Kare, Karinda, Karine, Karinna, Karrie, Karrina, Karyna

Karine (Russian) pure
Kaarrine, Karryne, Karyne

Karineh (Italian) form of Chiarina: clear

Karise (Greek) graceful woman
Karis, Karisse, Karyce

Karissa (Greek) longsuffering
Carissa, Karessa, Karisa

Karitina (Spanish) pure

Karizma (African) hopeful
Karisma

Karla (German) well-loved
Carla, Karlah, Karlie, Karlla, Karrla

Karlea (German) form of Karla: well-loved

Karlee (Slavic) form of Karla: well-loved

Karlin (American) winning; daring

Karlotta (German) form of Charlotte: little woman
Karlota, Karlotte, Lotta, Lottee, Lottey, Lottie

Karly (German) womanly; strength
Carly, Karlee, Karlie, Karlye

Karma (Hindi) destined for good things
Karm, Karmie, Karmy

Karmel (Hebrew) garden
Carmel, Karmela, Karmelle

Karmen (Hebrew) loving songs
Carmen, Karmin, Karmine

Karmiaso (Italian) garden girl

Karmilita (Spanish) form of Carmelita: in the garden

Karmille (Spanish) form of Carmel: garden

Karmit (Native American) nature

Karnesha (American) spicy
Carnesha, Karnisha, Karny

Karnit (American) gem

Karolina (Polish) form of Caroline: little; womanly
Karaline, Karalyn, Karalynna, Karalynne, Karla, Karleen, Karlen, Karlena, Karlene, Karli, Karlie, Karlina, Karlinka, Karo, Karolina, Karolline, Karolinka, Karolyn, Karolyna, Karolyne, Karolynn, Karolynne, Leena, Lina, Lyna

Karoline (German) feminine form of Karl: forceful
Kare, Karola, Karolah, Karolina, Lina

Karolyn (American) friendly
Carolyn, Kara, Karal, Karalyn, Karilynne, Karolynn

Karre (English) form of Carrie: womanly; little

Karri (American) form of Karen: purehearetd
Kari, Karie, Karrie, Karry

Karrington (Last name as first name) admired
Carrington, Kare, Karring

Karryoun (American) form of Caroline: little; womanly

Karuenne (American)
sweetness

Karwa (African) independent

Karwanna (African)
independent

Karwey (African)
independent

Karyn (American) sweet
Caren, Karen

Karynn (English) pure

Kasalya (Indian) clever

Kasandrae (English) shines

Kasandrah (English) shines

Kascade (Italian) water

Kasey (American) spirited
Casey, Kacey, Kasie, Kaysie

Kasha (Greek) form of
Katherine: pure

Kashmir (Place name) a
region near India and
Pakistan; fertile
*Cahmere, Cashmir, Kash,
Kashmere*

Kashonda (African
American) dramatic
*Kashanda, Kashawnda
Koshonda*

Kashondra (African
American) bright
*Kachanne, Kachaundra,
Kachee, Kashandra,
Kashawmdra, Kashee, Kashon,
Kashondrah, Kashondre,
Kashun*

Kasi (American) form of
Cassie: insightful
Kass, Kassi, Kassie

Kasia (Polish) form of
Katarzyna: creative

Kasmira (Slavic) peacemaker

Kassandra (Greek)
capricious
*Cassandra, Kass, Kasandra,
Kassandrah, Kassie*

Kassidy (Irish) clever
*Cassidy, Cassir, Kasadee, Kass,
Kassie, Kassy, Kassydi*

Kassie (American) clever
Kassee, Kassi, Kassy

Kat (American) outrageous
Cat

Katalin (American) pure
heart

Katalin (American) smart

Katana (English) form of
Catina: pure

Kataniya (Hebrew) little girl

Katarina (Greek) pure
*Katareena, Katarena,
Katarinna, Kataryna,
Katerina, Katryna*

Katarzyna (Origin unknown)
creative
Katarzina

Katchen (Greek) virtuous
Kat, Katshen

Katchi (American) sassy
*Catshy, Cotchy, Kat, Kata,
Katchie, Kati, Katshi, Katshie,
Katshy, Katty, Kotchee, Kotchi,
Kotchie*

Kate (Greek) form of
Katherine: pure
*Cait, Caitie, Cate, Catee, Catey,
Catie, Kait, Kaite, Kaitlin,
Katee, Katey, Kathe, Kati,
Katie, Katy, Kay-Kay*

Katelyn ☼ (Irish)
purehearted
*Caitlin, Kaitlin, Kaitlynne, Kat,
Katelin, Katelynn, Kate-Lynn,
Katline, Katy*

Katera (Origin unknown)
celebrant
Katara, Katura

Katherine ✿ ❂ ❸ (Greek) pure
*Kat, Katharin, Katherin,
Katwin, Katharine, Kathy,
Kathyrn, Kaykay*

Kathlaya (American)
fashionable

Kathleen (Irish) brilliant;
unflawed
*Cathaleen, Cathaline, Cathleen,
Kathaleen, Kathaleya,
Kathaleyna, Kathaline,
Kathelina, Katheline, Kathlene,
Kathlin, Kathline, Kathlynn,
Kathlyn, Kathie, Kathy*

Kathryn (English) powerful
and pure
*Kathreena, Kathren, Kathrene,
Kathrin, Kathrine, Kathryne*

Kathy (English/Irish) form of
Katherine: pure
*Cathie, Cathy, Kath, Kathe,
Kathee, Kathey, Kathi, Kathie*

Katia (French) stylish
Kateeya, Kati, Katya

Katie ✿ (English) lively
*Kat, Katy, Kay, Kaykay, Kate,
Kaytie*

Katina (American) form of
Katrina: melodious
Kat, Kateen, Kateena

Katlynn (Greek) pure
Kat, Katlinn, Katlyn

Katrice (American) graceful
*Katreese, Katrese, Katrie,
Katrisse, Katry*

Katrina (German) melodious
*Catreena, Catreina, Catrina,
Kaitrina, Katreena, Katreina,
Katryna, Kay, Ketreina,
Ketrina, Ketryna*

Katrine (German/Polish)
form of Kate: pure
*Catrene, Kati, Katrene,
Katrinna, Kati*

Katy (English) lively
*Cady, Katie, Kattee, Kattie,
Kaytee*

Kau (Indian) princess
Kaur

Kaulana (Hawaiian) well-
known girl
Kaula, Kauna, Kahuna

Kaulene (American) famed

Kavinli (American) feminine
form of Kevin: pretty; gentle
*Cavin, Kaven, Kavin, Kavinlee,
Kavinley, Kavinly*

Kavita (Hindi) poem
Kaveta, Kavitah

Kavitha (Indian) poetic
Kavita

Kawana (African) certain

Kay (Latin/Welsh) happy;
rejoicing
Cay, Caye, Kaye, Kaykay

Kaya (Native American)
intelligent
Kaja, Kayia

Kaycie (American)
merrymaker
*CayCee, K.C., Kaycee, Kayci,
Kaysie*

Kaydence (American) in
cadence

Kayla ✿ (Greek) pure
*Cala, Cayla, Caylie, Kala,
Kaela, Kaila, Kaylah, Kaylyn,
Keyla*

Kaylan (Irish) form of Caitlin:
virginal

Kaylee ✪ (American) open
*Cayley, Kaelie, Kaylea, Kaylie,
Kayleigh*

Kayleen (Hebrew/American)
sweet
*Kaileen, Kalene, Kay, Kaylean,
Kayleene, Kaykay*

Kayley (Irish) form of Kaylee:
open
*Caleigh, Cayleigh, Cayley,
Kaeleigh, Kailee, Kaileigh,
Kailey, Kaili, Kaleigh, Kaley,
Kaylea, Kaylee, Kaylie,
Kaylleigh, Kaylley*

Kaylin (American) form of
Kaylee: open
*Kailyn, Kaylan, Kaylanne,
Kaylen, Kaylinn, Kaylyn,
Kaylynn, Kaylynne*

Kaylina (English) slim girl

Kaylon (Hebrew) crowned
*Kaylan, Kayln, Kaylond,
Kaylon, Kalonn, Kaylen,
Kaylun*

Kayterly (American)
delightful

Kazuya (Asian) lovely

Keahs (Unknown) optimist

Keane (American) keen
Kanee, Keanie, Keany, Keen

Keani (Asian) bold

Keanna (American) curious
Keana, Keannah

Keara (Irish) darkness
*Kearia, Kearra, Keera, Keerra,
Keira, Keirra, Kera, Kiara,
Kiarra, Kiera, Kierra*

Kearney (Irish) winning
Kearne, Kearni, KeKe, Kerney

Keatha (American) feminine
form of Keith: witty

Kechia (African) determined

Kecia (American) focused

Keekee (American) dancing
Keakea, Kee-Kee

Keeley (Irish) noisy
*Kealey, Kealy, Keeley, Keeli,
Keelia, Keelie, Keely, Keighley,
Keighly, Keili, Keilie, Keylee,
Keyley, Keylie, Keylley, Keyllie*

Keelian (Irish) pretty

Keena (Irish) courageous
Keenya, Kina

Keenan (Irish) small
Keanan, Keen, Keeny

Keesee (American) joyous

Kefira (Hebrew) lioness
*Kefeera, Kefeira, Kefirah,
Kefirra*

Kehohtee (Invented)
alternate spelling for Quixote

Kei (Japanese) respectful

Keidra (American) form of
Kendra: ingenious
Kedra, Keydra

Keija (Slavic) rapport

Keiki (Hawaiian) child

Keiko (Hawaiian) child of joy
Kei

Keila (Hebrew) crowned
Keilah

Keilani (Hawaiian) graceful
leader
Kei, Lani, Lanie

Keira (Irish) dark-skinned
Keera, Kera

Keisha (American) dark-eyed
*Keasha, Keesha, Keeshah,
Keicia, Keishah, Keshia,
Keysha, Kicia*

Keishla (American) dark

Keishonna (English) form of
Keysha: dark-eyed

Keita (Scottish) lives in the
forest
Keiti

Keitha (Scottish) from the
forest
Keithana

Kekoa (Hawaiian) happy

Kelby (English) lives in a
farmhouse
Kelbea, Kelbeigh, Kelbey, Kellbie

Kelda (Scandinavian) spring
of youth
Kellda

Keledi (African) sorrows

Kelila (Hebrew) regal woman
*Kayla, Kayle, Kaylee, Kelula,
Kelulah, Kelulla, Kelylah, Kyla,
Kyle*

Kelinda (American) form of
Melinda: honey; sweetheart

Keller (Irish) daring
Kellers

Kellia (American) form of
Kelly: brave

Kelly (Irish) brave
Keli, Kellie, Kelley, Kellye

Kellyn (Irish) brave heart
*Kelleen, Kellen, Kellene, Kellina,
Kelline, Kellynn, Kellynne*

Kelsey (Scottish) opinionated
*Kelcey, Kelcie, Kelcy, Kellsey,
Kellsie, Kelsea, Kelsee, Kelseigh,
Kelsi, Kelsie, Kelsy*

Keltoriah (American) brave

Kember (American) zany
Kem, Kemmie, Kimber

Kemeel (American) form of
Camille: swift runner; great
innocence

Kemeelah (American) form
of Camille: swift runner;
great innocence

Kemelah (American) form of
Camille: swift runner; great
innocence

Kemella (American) self-
assured
Kemele, Kemellah, Kemelle

Kemicia (American) form of
Kim/Kem: sharp

Kempley (English) from a
meadowland: rascal
*Kemplea, Kempleigh, Kemplie,
Kemply*

Kenda (English) aware
*Kendi, Kendie, Kendy, Kennda,
Kenndi, Kenndie, Kenndy*

Kendall (English) quiet
*Kendahl, Kendal, Kendell,
Kendelle, Kendie, Kendylle*

Kendella (English) form of
Kendall: quiet

Kendra (American) ingenious
*Ken, Kendrah, Kenna, Kennie,
Kindra, Kinna, Kyndra*

Kendrelle (English) rules
quiet place

Kendry (English) rules quiet
place

Kenia (African) giving; from
the place name Kenya
Ken, Keneah

Kenichi (American) feminine
form of Kenneth: good-
looking

Kenine (Scottish) pretty

Kenith (American) feminine
form of Kenneth: good-
looking

Kenna (English) brilliant
*Kenina, Kennah, Kennina,
Kennette, Kynna*

Kenna (Scottish) creative

Kennae (Irish) feminine
form of Ken: good-looking
Kenae, Kenah

Kennedy (Irish) formidable
Kennedie, Kenny

Kenner (Scottish) feminine
form of Kenneth: good-
looking

Kennice (English) beauty
*Kanice, Keneese, Kenese,
Kennise*

Kensington (English) brash
Kensingtyn

Kenta (English) feminine
form of Kent: fair-skinned

Kentucky (Place name) u.s.
state
Kentuckie

Kenya (Place name) country
in Africa
Kenia, Kennya

Kenyatta (African) form of
Kenya: country in Africa

Kenyetta (Place name) form
of Kenya: country in Africa

Kenyie (Place name) form of
Kenya: country in Africa

Kenzie (Scottish) pretty
Kensey, Kinsey

Keoshawn (African
American) clever
Keosh, Keoshaun

Kerdonna (African
American) loquacious
*Donna, Kerdy, Kirdonna,
Kyrdonna*

Kerensa (English) lovable
Karensa, Karenza, Kerenza

Keri-Gee (English) awesome

Kerla (American) curly-haired

Kern (Irish) darkness

Kerra (American) bright
Cara, Carrah, Kara, Kerrah

Kerry (Irish) dark-haired
*Carrie, Kari, Kera, Keree, Keri,
Kerrey, Kerri, Kerria,
Kerridana, Kerrie*

Kerst (American) form of
Kerstin: a Christian

Kerstin (Scandinavian) a
Christian
Kersten, Kerston, Kerstyn

Kerthia (American) giving
Kerth, Kerthea, Kerthi, Kerthy

Kesha (American) laughing
Kecia, Kesa, Keshah

Keshla (American) bouncy
*Kecia, Keishia, Keschia, Kesia,
Kesiah, Kessiah*

Keshon (African American)
happy
*Keshann, Keshaun, Keshonn,
Keshun, Keshawn*

Keshondra (African
American) joy-filled
*Keshaundra, Keshondrah,
Keshundra, Keshundrea,
Keshundria, Keshy*

Keshonna (African
American) happy
*Keshanna, Keshauna,
Keshaunna, Keshawna,
Keshona, Keshonna*

Kesi (African) baby born in
hard times

Kessie (African) fat baby
cheeks
*Kess, Kessa, Kesse, Kessey, Kessi,
Kessia, Kessiah*

Ketrina (German) musical

Keturah (African) long-suffering
Katura, Ketura

Kevine (Irish) lively
Kevina, Kevinne, Kevyn, Kevynn, Kevynne

Kevyn (Irish) form of Kevin: lovely face
Keva, Kevan, Kevina, Kevone, Kevonna, Kevynn

Kew (English) form of Cue and Cumale: personality

Keydy (American) knowing
Keydee, Keydi, Keydie

Keyla (Irish) form of Kelia: crowned

Keynny (American) feminine form of Kenneth: good-looking

Keynshalli (Invented) form of Keysha: dark-eyed

Keyonna (African American) energetic

Keyshawn (American) lively
Keyshan, Keyshann, Keyshaun, Keyshaunna, Keyshon, Keyshona, Keshonna, Keykey, Kiki

Kezettea (African) form of Kezia: confident

Kezia (Hebrew) form of Cassis: confident
Kazia, Kessie, Kessy, Ketzia, Ketziah, Keziah, Kezzie, Kissie, Kizzie, Kizzy

Keziane (African) form of Kezia: confident
Kezi, Kezian

Khadijah (Arabic) sweetheart
Kadija, Kadiya, Khadiya, Khadyja

Khai (American) unusual
Ki, Kie

Khaki (American) personality-plus
Kakee, Kaki, Kakie, Khakee, Khakie

Khali (Origin unknown) lively
Khalee, Khalie, Koli, Kollie

Khalida (Hindi) eternal
Khali, Khalia, Khalita

Khalilah (Arabic) friendly

Khalique (African) lasting

Kharol (American) form of Carol: feminine; joyful song

Khasha (American) brash

Khawaja (American) excitable

Khawla (African) enthusiastic

Khiana (American) different
Kheana, Khianah, Khianna, Ki, Kianah, Kianna, Kiannah

Khloe (English) form of Chloe: flowering

Khonesa (Indian) able

Khorus (Greek) musical

Khyra (English) form of Kira: sunny; lighthearted

Ki (Korean) born again

Kia (American) form of Kiana: graceful
Keeah, Kiah

Kiana (American) graceful
Kia, Kiah, Kianna, Kiannah, Quiana, Quianna

Kiani (Hawaiian) form of Kiana: graceful

Kiantyne (Invented) laughs

Kiara (Irish) dark-skinned
Chiara, Chiarra, Keearah, Keearra, Kiarra

Kibibi (African) small girl

Kidre (American) loyal
Kidrea, Kidrey, Kidri

Kiele (Hawaiian) aromatic
flower; gardenia
Kiela, Kieley, Kieli, Kielli, Kielly

Kienalle (American) light
Kieana, Kienall, Kieny

Kienna (Origin unknown)
brash
Kiennah, Kienne

Kiera (Irish) dark-skinned
Keara, Keera, Kierra

Kiersten (Greek) blessed
*Kerston, Kierstin, Kierstn,
Kierstynn, Kirst, Kirsten,
Kirstie, Kirstin, Kirsty*

Kiersty (American) spiritual

Kihae (Asian) fragrant

Kijana (American) form of
Kiana: graceful

Kiki (Spanish/American)
form of names beginning
with K: vivacious
Keiki, Ki, Kiekie, Kikee

Kiko (Japanese) lively
Kiki, Kikoh

Kiku (Japanese) flower mum
Kiko

Kilday (American) pretty

Kiley (Irish) pretty
*Kilea, Kilee, Kili, Kylee, Kyley,
Kylie*

Kiliki (Mythology) feminine

Killie (English) returns

Kim (Vietnamese) sharp
Kimey, Kimmi, Kimmy, Kym

Kima (American) bright

Kimalida (Spanish) hopes

Kimana (American) form of
Kim: sharp

Kimaya (Asian) golden child

Kimberly ☺ (English) leader
*Kim, Kimber-Lea, Kimberlee,
Kimberleigh, Kimberley,
Kimberli, Kimberlie, Kimmy,
Kymberly, Kimmie*

Kimbra (English) fortified

Kimbrell (African American)
smiling
*Kim, Kimbree, Kimbrel,
Kimbrele, Kimby, Kimmy*

Kimeo (American) form of
Kim: sharp
Kim, Kime, Kimi

Kimetha (American) form of
Kimberly: leader
Kimeth

Kimi (Japanese) spiritual

Kimo (Asian) strong

Kimone (Origin unknown)
darling
Kimonne, Kymone

Kimthy (Asian) form of
Timothy: reveresGod

Kimula (Invented) strength

Kimya (American) form of
Kim: sharp

Kina (Hawaiian) girl from
China

Kindrah (American) form of
Kendra: ingenious

Kineisha (American) form of
Keneisha: gorgeous woman
*Keneesha, Keneisha, Kineasha,
Kinesha, Kineshia, Kiness,
Kinisha, Kinnisha, Kinny*

Kineta (Greek) energetic
Kinetta

Kini (American) form of
Kenny: formidable

Kinneta (Greek) kinetic energy

Kinsey (English) child
Kensey, Kinnsee, Kinnsey, Kinnsie, Kinsee, Kinsey, Kinsie, Kinzee

Kinshasa (Asian) child

Kinsley (Origin unknown) familiar
Kingslea, Kingslee, Kingslie, Kinslea, Kinslee, Kinslie, Kinsly, Kinzlea, Kinzlee, Kinzley, Kinzly

Kintra (American) joyous
Kentra, Kint, Kintrey

Kinza (American) relative

Kioko (Japanese) happy baby
Kiyo, Kiyoko

Kiona (Native American) girl from the hill

Kionea (Native American) interesting

Kip (Literature) naive

Kipling (Last name as first name) energetic
Kiplin

Kippareen (American) humorous; Young

Kipple (American) form of Kipling: energetic

Kira (Russian) sunny; light-hearted
Keera, Kera, Kiera, Kierra, Kiria, Kiriah, Kirya, Kirra

Kiran (Indian) light

Kiran (Irish) pretty
Kiara, Kiaran, Kira, Kiri

Kirby (Anglo-Saxon) right
Kirbee, Kirbey, Kirbie

Kiriath (Biblical) place name

Kirima (Eskimo) hill child; high aspirations

Kirsta (Scandinavian) Christian

Kirsten (Scandinavian) form of Christine: follower of Christ
Karsten, Keerstin, Keirstin, Kersten, Kerstin, Kiersten, Kierstin, Kiersynn, Kirsteen, Kirstene, Kirsti, Kirstie, Kirstin, Kirston, Kirsty, Kirstynn, Kristen, Kristin, Kristyn, Krystene, Krystin

Kirstie (Scandinavian) irrepressable
Kerstie, Kirstee, Kirsty

Kirti (Indian) famous

Kirtrina (American) form of Katrina: melodious

Kischchan (American) tries hard

Kisha (Russian) ingenious
Keshah

Kishala (English) form of Kisha: delights

Kishi (Japanese) eternal

Kishori (Indian) young

Kismet (Hindi) destiny; fate
Kismat, Kismete, Kismett

Kissa (African) a baby born after twins

Kit (American) strong
Kitt

Kita (Japanese) northerner

Kithos (Greek) worthy

Kitten (English) form of Katherine: pure

Kitty (Greek) form of Katherine: pure
Kit, Kittee, Kittey, Kitti, Kittie

Kiva (Origin unknown) bright
Keva

Kiwa (Origin unknown) lively
Kiewah, Kiwah

Kiya (Australian) form of
Kylie: always returning; pretty
girl
Kya

Kizzie (African) energetic
*Kissee, Kissie, Kiz, Kizzee,
Kizzi, Kizzie, Kizzy*

Klara (Hungarian) bright
*Klari, Klarice, Klarika,
Klarissa, Klarisza, Klaryssa*

Klarissa (German) bright-
minded
Clarissa, Klarisa, Klarise

Klarybel (Polish) beauty
Klaribel, Klaribelle

Klaudia (Polish) lame

Klea (American) bold
Clea, Kleah, Kleea, Kleeah

Klementina (Polish)
forgiving
*Clemence, Clementine,
Klementine, Klementyna*

Kleta (Greek) form of
Cleopatra: Egyptian queen
Cleta

Klotild (Hungarian) famous
*Klothild, Klothilda, Klothilde,
Klotilda, Klotilde*

Klyra (Slavic) noble

Knoi (American) annoys

Koa (Hawaiian) seaside

Kobi (American) california
girl
Cobi, Kobe

Kobra (Indian) form of cobra

Koche (American) bright

Koffi (African) friday-born
Kaffe, Kaffi, Koffe, Koffie

Kogan (Last name as first
name) self-assured
Kogann, Kogen, Kogey, Kogi

Koichi (Asian)

Kokan (American) real

Kokkie (Dutch) horn

Koko (Japanese) the stork
comes

Kolleen (Irish) form of
Colleen: young girl

Kona (Hawaiian) feminine
Koni, Konia

Konia (Hawaiian) bright light

Konki (American) constant

Konstance (Latin) loyal
*Constance, Kon, Konnie,
Konstanze, Stanze*

Kora (Greek) practical
Cora, Koko, Korey, Kori

Koren (English) form of
Corinne: maiden; protective

Kori (Greek) little girl; popular
Cori, Corrie, Koree, Korey, Kory

Korina (Greek) maiden
*Corinna, Koreena, Korena,
Korinna, Koryna*

Kornelia (Latin) straight-laced
*Cornelia, Kornelya, Korney,
Korni, Kornie*

Kortney (American) form of
Courtney: domain of Curtis
*Courtney, Kortnee, Kortni,
Kourtney, Kourtnie*

Koshatta (Native American)
diligent
*Coushatta, Kosha, Koshat,
Koshatte, Koshee, Koshi, Koshie,
Koushatta*

Koska (American) loose cannon

Kosta (Latin) form of Constance: loyal
Kostia, Kostusha, Kostya

Koto (Japanese) harp; musical

Koverne (Last name used as first name) homebody

Krenie (American) capable
Kren, Kreni, Krenn, Krennie, Kreny

Kresenz (German) crescent

Kris (American) form of Kristina: follower of Christ
Kaykay, Krissie, Krissy

Krishen (American) talkative
Crishen, Kris, Krish, Krishon

Krissa (German) form of Krista: follower of Christ

Krissen (American) feminine form of Christian: follower of Christ

Krissy (American) friendly
Kris, Krisie, Krissey, Krissi

Krista (German) form of Christina: follower of Christ
Khrista, Krysta

Kristanie (American) Christian

Kristeen (German) form of Christine: follower of Christ

Kristeenea (English) form of Christina: follower of Christ

Kristen (Greek) form of Christine: follower of Christ
Christen, Cristen, Kristin, Kristyn

Kristian (Greek) Christian woman
Kristiana, Kristianne, Kristyanna

Kristie (American) saucy
Christi, Christy, Kristi

Kristin (Scandinavian) high-energy
Kristen, Kristyne

Kristina (Scandinavian) form of Christina: follower of Christ
Christina, Krista, Kristie, Krysteena, Tina

Kristine (Swedish) form of Christine: follower of Christ
Christine, Kristee, Kristene, Kristi, Kristy

Kristy (American) form of Kristine: follower of Christ
Kristi, Kristie

Krysta (Polish) clear
Chrsta, Krista

Krystal (American) clear and brilliant
Cristalle, Cristel, Crysta, Crystal, Crystalle, Khristalle, Khristel, Khrystle, Khrystalle, Kristel, Kristle, Krys, Krystalle, Krystalline, Krystelle, Krystie, Krystle, Krystylle

Krystyna (Polish) Christian

Kuawanna (African) fragrant

Kubbae (American) wanderer

Kue (Biblical) place name

Kukan (Scandinavian) blossoms

Kumiko (Japanese) long hair in braids
Kumi

Kumud (Indian) lotus flower; Bright

Kundany (Indian) golden child

Kunday (Invented) form of
Sunday: day of the week;
sunny

Kurara (Japanese) peaceful

Kurene (American) monied

Kwanita (African) form of
Juanita: believer in a gracious
God; forgiving

Kyan (American) lively
Beginnings

Kyatana (American) vivacious
Beginnings

Kyishia (American) form of
Keisha: dark-eyed
Delightful

Kyla (Irish) pretty
Kiela, Kila, Ky

Kyle (Irish) pretty
Kyall, Kyel, Kylee, Kylie, Kyll

Kylee (Irish) form of Kylie:
graceful
*Kielie, Kiely, Kiley, Kye, Kyky,
Kyleigh, Kylie*

Kyleighan (English) form of
Kylie: graceful

Kylene (American) cute
Kyline

Kylera (English) feminine
form of Kyler: peaceful
On target

Kylern (English) feminine
form of Kyler: peaceful
On target

Kylie ○ (Irish) graceful
Keyely, Kilea, Kiley, Kylee, Kyley

Kylynne (American)
fashionable
Kilenne, Kilynn, Kyly

Kym (American) favorite
*Kim, Kymm, Kymmi, Kymmie,
Kymy*

Kyna (African) diamond

Kynci (American) form of
Kinsey: child

Kynthia (Greek) goddess of
the moon
Cinthia, Cynthia

Kyoko (Japanese) sees herself
in a mirror

Kyra (Greek) feminine
*Kaira, Keera, Keira, Kira,
Kyrah, Kyreena, Kyrene, Kyrha,
Kyria, Kyrie, Kyrina, Kyrra,
Kyry*

Kyria (Greek) form of Kyra:
feminine
Kyrea, Kyree, Kyrie, Kyry

L

L'Amour (French) love
*Amor, Amour, Lamore,
Lamour, Lamoura*

La Verta (American) truth

Laarni (American) honest

Labe (American) slow-moving
Labie

Lace (American) delicate
Lacee, Lacey, Laci, Lacie, Lase

Lacey (Greek) cheery
Lacee, Laci, Lacie, Lacy

Lachelle (African American)
sweetheart
*Lachel, Lachell, Laschell,
Lashelle*

Lachesis (Mythological) one
of the Greek Fates; the
measurer

Lachina (African American)
fragile

Lacole (American) sly
Lucole

Lacreta (Spanish) form of
Lacretia: efficient
Lacrete, LaLa

Lacretia (Latin) efficient
*Lacracia, Lacrecia, Lacrisha,
Lacy*

LaDaune (African American)
the dawn
Ladaune, LaDawn

Ladda (American) open
Lada

Ladey (American) form of
Lady: feminine
Feminine

LaDorna (Spanish) adorned

Ladrenaan (Invented)
likeable

Ladrenda (African American)
cagy
*Ladee, Ladey, Ladren,
Ladrende, Lady*

Lady (American) feminine
Ladee, Ladie

Laela (Hebrew) form of Leila:
beauty of the night

Laetitia (Latin) joy
*Leticia, Lateaciah, Lateacya,
Latycia, Letisia, Letyziah*

Laheelah (American) gifted

Laila (Scandinavian) dark
beauty
*Laili, Laleh, Layla, Laylah,
Leila*

Lainil (American) softhearted
Lainie, Lanel, Lanelle

Laitalin (American) secure

Laith (Scottish) princess

Lajean (French) soothing;
steadfast
L'Jean, LaJean, Lajeanne

LaJoyce (English) la and
Joyce

Lakanel (American) hurt

Lake (Astrology) graceful
dancer

Lakeisha (African American)
the favorite; combo of La and
Keisha

Lakeita (American) caring

Lakela (Hawaiian) feminine
Lakla

Lakendrae (American) great
hopes

Lakeny (American) superb

Lakesha (African American)
favored
*Keishia, Lakaisha, Lakeesha,
Lakeishah, Lakezia, Lakisha,
LaKisha*

Lakeyshia (African-
American) crafty

Lakiesta (English) form of
Lakesha: favored

Lakiya (English) form of
Lakesha: favored

Lakya (Hindi) born on
Thursday

Lakysha (English) form of
Lakesha: favored

Lala (Slavic) pretty flower girl;
tulip

Lalage (Greek) talkative
Lal, Lallie, Lally

Lalaney (American) form of
Leilani: heavenly girl
Lala, Lalanee, Lalani

Laleema (Spanish) devoted
Lalema, Lalima

Lalena (Indian) girlish
Lalana

Lalita (Sanskrit) charmer
*Lai, Lala, Lali, Lalitah, Lalite,
Lalitte*

Lalita (Indian) charmer

Lalitha (Spanish) form of
Lalita: charmer

Lally (English) babbling
Lalli

Lalmani (American) sociable

Lalya (Latin) eloquent
Lalia, Lall, Lalyah

Lama (Muslim) dark lips

Lamarian (American)
conflicted
Lamare, Lamarean

Lambda (Greek)

Lamercie (French) forgiving

Lamia (Egyptian) calm
Lami

Lamiena (Spanish) calming

Lamika (African American)
form of Tamika: lively

Lana (Latin) pretty;
peacemaker
Lan, Lanna, Lanny

Lanai (Hawaiian) heavenly
Lenai

Lanalee (Combo of Lana and
Lee)

Land (American) word as
name; confident
Landd

Landa (American) blonde
beauty
Landah

Landra (American) form of
Landa: pretty; peacemaker

Landry (American) leader
Landa, Landree

Landy (American) confident
Land, Landee, Landey, Landi

Lane (Last name as first
name) precocious
*Laine, Lainey, Laney, Lanie,
Layne, Laynie*

Lanee (Asian) graceful

Laneedy (English) form of
Laney: precocious

Lanette (American) healthy
La-Net, LaNett, LaNette

Langley (American) special
Langlee, Langli, Langlie, Langly

Lani (Hawaiian) form of
Leilani: heavenly girl
Lannie

LaNiece (Invented) form of
Lenice: delightful

Lanigill (American) happy

Lanilee (American) heaven

Lanitia (Slavic) unique

Lanle (African) enriched

Lannea (American) mobile

Lannette (American) form of
Lynnette: small and fresh

Lanola (American) generous

Lanonre (American) of the
sea

Lanora (Italian) form of
Leonora: bright light

Lansing (Place name)
hopeful
Lanseng

Lantana (Botanical) flowering
Lantanna

Laperonita (Spanish) upward

Laquanna (African American) outspoken
Kwanna, LaQuanna, LaQwana, Quanna

Lara (Russian) lovely

Larae (Slavic) form of Lara: lovely
Grace

Laraine (Latin) pretty
Lareine, Larene, Loraine

Larante (Last name used as first name) shares

Laray (American) form of Lara: lovely

Larby (American) form of Darby: a free woman
Larbee, Larbey, Larbi, Larbie

Larch (American) full of life

Lareina (Greek) seagull; flies over water
Larayna, Larayne, Lareine, Larena, Larrayna, Larreina

Larenya (English) form of Laraine: pretty

Laressia (English) form of Larissa: giving cheer

Lariesha (English) form of Larissa: giving cheer

Larinda (American) smart
Lare, Larin, Larine, Lorinda

Larissa (Latin) giving cheer
Laressa, Larisse, Laryssa

Lark (American) pretty
Larke

Larkin (American) pretty
Larken, Larkun

Larklee (Combo of Lark and Lee) birdlike

Larkly (American) form of Larklee: birdlike

Larkspur (Botanical) tall and stately

Larla (American) deserving

Larlett (American) winner

Larni (American) form of Marni: storyteller

LaRobin (English) la and Robin

Larrie (American) tomboyish
Larry

Larsa (Biblical) place name

Larsen (Scandinavian) laurel-crowned
Larson, Larssen, Larsson

Laruthenne (American) la and Ruthenne

Lasa (American) complex

Lasalle (French) explorer

Lasea (Biblical) place name

Lasha (Spanish) forlorn
Lash, Lass

Lashanda (American) brassy
Lala, Lasha, LaShanda, LaShounda

Lashauna (American) happy
Lashona, Leshauna, Lashawna

LaShea (American) sparkling
Lashay, La-Shea, Lashea

Lashoun (African American) content
Lashaun, Lashawn, Lashown

Lassie (American) lass
Lass

Lastashtia (American) form of Latasha: lovely Christian girl

Lastenia (Spanish) lovely Christian girl

Lata (Hindi) lovely vine; entwines

Latash (American) form of
Latasha: glorious; born on
Christmas

Latasha (American) born on
Christmas
*Latacha, LaTasha, Latayshah,
Latisha*

LaTeasa (Spanish) tease
*Latea, Lateasa, LaTease,
LaTeese*

Lateefah (African) gentle;
pleasant
*Lateefa, Latifa, Latifah,
Lotifah, Tifa, Tifah*

Latesha (American) form of
Letitia: joy
*Lateesha, Lateisha, Lateshah,
Laticia, Latisha*

Lathenia (American) verbose
Lathene, Lathey

Latice (American) form of
Letitia: joy

Latifah (Muslim) gentle
Lateefa, Latifa, Latiffe, Latifuh

Latiki (Indian) small
Latika

Latina (Spanish) spanish girl

Latisa (English) form of
Latasha: born on Christmas

Latisehsha (African
American) happy; talkative
Lati, Latise, Latiseh, Latisha

Latochia (English) form of
Latasha: born on Christmas

Latona (Latin) goddess

Latonia (African American)
rich
Latone, Latonea

Latosha (African American)
happy

Latoyia (English) watchful

Latoyra (American)
circumspect

Latreece (American) go-
getter
*Latreese, Latrice, Letrice, Lettie,
Letty*

Latrelia (Spanish) of the
trellis

Latrelle (American) laughing
Lettie, Letrel, Letrelle, Litrelle

Latrice (Latin) noble
Latreece, Latreese

Latricia (American) happy
*Latrecia, Latreesha, Latrisha,
Latrishah*

Latrisha (African American)
prissy
Latrishe

Latroa (American) athletic

Latunga (African) athletic

Latunya (American) form of
Latonya: birdlike

Latyffanie (American) la and
Tyfannie

Lauda (Latin) praised

Laudette (American) lauded

Laudomia (Italian)
praiseworthy

Laufeia (Scandinavian)
thriving

Launa (American) ideal

Launie (American) heavenly

Laura (Latin) laurel-crowned;
joyous
Lara, Lora

Laurain (English) graceful

Laurdina (American) form of
Laurinda; Pretty

Laureen (American) old-fashioned
Laurie, Laurine, Loreen

Laureens (Scandinavian) wins laurels

Laurel (Latin) the laurel plant
Laurell, Lorel, Lorell, Laural, Laurell, Laurella, Laurelle, Lorel, Lorella, Lourelle

Lauren ✿ (Latin) laurel-crowned
Laren, Laurene, Lauryn, Laryn, Loren

Laurencia (Latin) laurel-crowned
Laurenciah, Laurens, Laurentana

Laurenne (Scandinavian) wins laurels

Laurent (French) graceful
Lorent, Laurente

Laurentine (French) bright

Lauretta (American) graceful
Laureta, Laurettah, Lauritta, Lauritte, Loretta

Laurette (American) form of Laura: laurel-crowned; joyous
Etta, Ette, Laure, Laurett, Lorette

Laurette (English) form of Laurita: victorious

Laurettean (English) form of Laurita: victorious

Laurid (Welsh) form of Laura: laurel-crowned; joyous

Laurie (English) careful
Lari, Lauri, Lori

Laurima (Spanish) form of Laura: laurel-crowned; joyous

Laurinda (Spanish) the laurel plant

Laurissaa (Greek) pleased

Laurita (Spanish) victorious

Lavanda (Spanish) pure

Laveda (Latin) pure
Lavella, Lavelle, Laveta, Lavetta, Lavette

LaVeeda (Spanish) alive

Lavena (Celtic) joy
Lavi, Lavie, Lavina

Lavender (Latin) pale purple flowers; peaceful

Laverne (Latin) breath of spring
Lavern, Lavirne, Verna, Verne

Laveta (American) vibrant

Lavette (Latin) pure; natural
Laveda, Lavede, Lavete, Lavett

Lavigne (French) vineyard

Lavilla (Spanish) gathers

Lavina (Latin) woman of Rome

Lavinia (Greek) ladylike
Lavenia

Lavinia (Latin) cleansed
Vin, Vina, Vinnie, Vinny

Lavita (American) charmer
Laveta, Lavitta, Lavitte

Lawanda (American) sassy
LaWanda, Lawonda

Lawenna form of Lawan: lovely

Lawrencetta (American) feminine form of Lawrence: honored

Layce (American) spunky

Layine (Scandinavian) loves the sea

Layla (Arabic) dark
Laela, Laila, Lala, Laya, Laylah, Laylie, Leila

Layli (American) form of
Layla: dark

Layne (French) from the
meadow
Laine, Lainee, Lainey

Laynn (American) form of
Lane: precocious

Layoce (American) form of
Loyce: delightful

Layouce (American) form of
Loyce: delightful

Laysha (American) form of
Letitia: joy

Lazette (American) form of
Lizette: lively

Lazine (Dutch) joyful
Lazina, Lazee

Le Etta (American) small

Lea (Hawaiian) goddess-like

Leacille (American) form of
Lucille: bright-eyed

Leaf (Botanical) hip

Leah ✪ (Hebrew) tired and
burdened
Lea, Lee, Leeah, Leia, Lia

Leala (French) steadfast

Leandra (Greek) lionine
*Leandrea, Leanndra, Leeandra,
Leedie*

Leanette (English) form of
Lynnette: small and fresh

Leanna (English) leaning
Leana, Leelee, Liana

Leanne (English) sweet
*Lean, Leann, Lee, Leelee,
Lianne*

Leanona (English) form of
Leona: bravehearted

Leanora (Greek) light
Lenora, Lanora, Lanoriah

Leanore (Greek) form of
Eleanor: lighthearted
Lanore

Leatha (English) form of
Alethea: truthful

Leatrice (American)
charming
Leatrise

Leatricea (English) leader

Lebonah (Biblical) place name

Lecia (Latin) form of Letitia:
joy
Leecia, Leesha, Lesha, Lesia

Lectricia (English) form of
Leatrice: charming

Leda (Greek) feminine
Ledah, Lida, Lita

Lee
(English/American/Chinese)
light-footed
Lea, Leelee, Leigh

Leeannette (Greek) form of
Leandra: lionine
*Leann, Lee Annette, Leeanett,
Lee-Annette, Leiandra*

Leelee (American/Slavic)
form of Leanne: sweet
Lee-Lee, Lele, Lelee

Leena (Latin) temptress
Lina, Lena

Leene (Scandinavian) form of
Lena: siren

Leeo (American) sunny
Leo

Leesha (English) form of
Lisha: dark

Leeuwen (Dutch) dear friend

Leeza (American) gorgeous
Leesa, Leeze, Liza, Lize

Legend (American) memorable
Legen, Legende, Legund

Legia (Spanish) bright
Legea

Lehava (Hebrew) flaming

Lei (Hawaiian) form of Leilani: heavenly girl
Leilei

Léi (Chinese) open; truthful

Leigh (English) light-footed
Lee, Leelee

Leila (Arabic) beauty of the night
Layla, Leela, Leilah, Lelah, Leyla, Lila

Leilani (Hawaiian) heavenly girl
Lanie

Leisa (English) form of Lisa: dedicated and spiritual

Leith (Scottish) from the river; nature-loving
Leithe, Lethe

Lejoi (French) joy
Joy, Lejoy

Leka (Indian) graphic proof
Lehka

Leland (American) special
Lelan, Lelande

Lelann (Greek) faithful

Lelia (Greek) articulate
Lee, Leelee

Lemetria (American) perfection

Leminda (American) mindful

Lemon (Botanical) zany

Lemtraia (American) sporty

Lemuela (Hebrew) loyal
Lemuelah, Lemuella, Lemuellah

Lena (Latin) siren
Leena, Lenette, Lina

Lendez (Spanish) form of Linda: pretty girl

Lendorah (English) form of Linda: pretty girl

Lendtra (English) form of Linda: pretty girl

Lenesha (African American) smiling
Leneisha, Lenisha, Lenni, Lennie, Neshie

Lenetta (English) form of Lynnette

Lenice (American) delightful
Lenisa, Lenise

Lenikka (American) roving

Lenita (Latin) gentle spirit
Leneeta, Leneta, Lineta

Lenka (Slavic) cleansed

Lenkan (Slavic) excellent

Lenna (Hebrew) shy

Lenoa (Greek) form of Lenore: lighthearted
Len, Lenor, Lenora

Lenore (Greek) form of Eleanor: lighthearted

Leoda (German) popular
Leota

Leola (Latin) fierce; lionine
Lee, Leo, Leole

Leolan (Last name used as first name) lionlike

Leolia (English) form of Leola: lionine

Leoma (American) form of Leona: bravehearted

Leona (Greek/American)
bravehearted
Liona

Leonarda (German)
lionhearted
*Lenarda, Lenda, Lennarda,
Leonarde*

Leondrea (Greek) strong
Leondreah, Leondria

Leonetta (English) feminine
form of Leon: tenacious

Leonie (Latin) lionlike; fierce
*Leola, Leonee, Leoni, Leoney,
Leontine, Leony*

Leonila (Spanish) lioness

Leonora (English) bright
light
*Leanor, Leanora, Leanore,
Lenora, Lenore, Leonore*

Leonore (Greek) glowing
light
Lenore, Leonor, Leonora

Leonsio (Spanish) feminine
form of Leon: tenacious
Leo, Leonsee, Leonsi

Leopoldina (Invented)
feminine form of Leopold:
brave
*Dina, Leo, Leopolde,
Leopoldyna*

Leora (Greek) lighthearted
Liora, Leorah

Leoycey (Invented) sassy

Lequita (Spanish) bright;
clear

Lera (Russian) strong
Lerae, Lerie, Lira

Leretta (American) form of
Loretta: large-eyed beauty
Lere, Lerie, Loretta

Leria (Italian) brave

Lerita (Spanish) gives joy

Leritha (Spanish) gives joy

Lesha (Italian) kind

Leshia (Italian) feminine

Leslie (Scottish) fiesty;
beautiful; smart
Les, Lesli, Lesley

Leslin (American) form of
Lesley: fiesty, beautiful; smart

Lessie (Scottish) form of
Lesley: fiesty, beautiful; smart

Lesstene (American) form
of Lesley: fiesty, beautiful;
smart

Lesvia (Slavic) spiritual

Leszlee (American) form of
Lesley: fiesty, beautiful;
smart

Leta (Latin) happy
Leeta, Lita

Letai (Latin) glad

Letha (Greek) ladylike
Litha

Letian (Latin) glad

Letichel (American) happy;
important
*Chel, Chelle, Leti, Letichell,
Letishell, Lettichelle, Lettychel*

Leticia (Spanish) form of
Letitia: joy
*Letecia, Leticia, Letisha, Letitia,
Lettice, Lettie, Letty, Tiesha*

Letina (Spanish) latina

Letitia (Latin) joy

Leto (Greek) mother of Apollo

Letricia (Spanish) happy

Letsey (American) form of
Lettie: happy
Letsee, Letsy

Lettice (American) sweet
Letty

Lettie (Latin/Spanish) happy
Lettee, Letti, Letty, Lettye

Letycee (Invented) insightful

Leutricia (Spanish) form of
Letricia: happy

Leutu (Asian)

Levana (Hebrew) fair
Lev, Liv, Livana

Leverah (American) form of
Deborah: prophetess

Leverne (French) grove of
trees

Levina (Latin) lightning

Levitt (American)
straightforward
Levit

Levity (American) humorous

Levora (American) home-
loving
*Levorah, Levore, Livee, Livie,
Livora, Livore*

Lewana (Hebrew) moon
bright

Lexa (American) cheerful
Lex, Lexah

Lexandra (Slavic) bold

Lexi (Greek) helpful;
sparkling
Lex, Lexie, Lexsey, Lexsie, Lexy

Lexine (Scottish) helper

Lexus (American) rich
*Lexi, Lexorus, Lexsis, Lexuss,
Lexxus*

Lexy (Scottish) helper

Leya (Spanish) true blue

Leysa (Spanish) loyal

Lez (American) form of
Lesley: fiesty; beautiful; smart

Lezena (American) smiling
Lezene, Lezina, Lyzena

Lez'lee (American) form of
Lesley: fiesty; beautiful; smart

Li (Chinese) plum

Li (Chinese) strong

Lia (Greek/Russian/Italian)
singular
Li, Liah

Liadin (Irish) sad

Lial (Italian) form of Leah:
tired and burdened

Lialeh (Italian) form of Leah:
tired and burdened

Lian (Latin/Chinese) graceful
Leane, Leanne, Liane

Liana (Greek) flowering;
complicated
Leanna, Lee, Liane

Liani (Hawaiian) caressed

Lianna (Italian) sunny

Lianne (English) light
Leann, Leanne, Leeann

Libba (Biblical) place name;
desired

Libby (Hebrew) form of
Elizabeth: God's promise
Lib, Libbi, Libbie

Liber (American) from the
word liberty; free
Lib, Libby, Lyber

Liberty (Latin) free and open
Lib, Libbie

Libnah (Biblical) place name; white

Librada (Spanish) free
Libra, Libradah

Libva (Biblical) place name; white

Liceth (American) form of Lysette

Licia (Greek) outdoorsy
Lisha

Licona (Spanish)

Lida (Greek) beloved girl
Leedah, Lyda

Liddan (Irish) form of Liadin: sad

Lidia (Greek) pleasant spirit
Lydia

Lidiya (Russian) form of Lydia: musical, unusual

Liese (German) given to God

Liesel (German) pretty
Leesel, Leezel

Lieselotte (Hebrew/French) charming woman

Light (American) light-hearted
Li, Lite

Ligia (Greek) talented musician
Ligea, Lygia, Lygy

Lignon (French) clarity

Liguria (Greek) music lover

Likiana (Invented) likeable
Like, Likia

Lila (Arabic) playful
Lilah, Lyla, Lylah

Lilac (Botanical) tiny blossom
Lila

Lilah (Sanskrit) playful

Lila-Lee (American) lily

Lilavati (Hindi) goddess

Lileah (Latin) lily-like
Lili, Liliah, Lill, Lily, Lylya

Lilette (Latin) little lily; delicate
Lill, Lillette, Lillith, Lilly, Lylly

Lilia (American) flowing
Lileah, Lyleah, Lylia

Lilian (Latin) pure beauty

Liliana (Italian) pretty
Lilianah, Lylianah

Lilias (Hebrew) night
Lilas, Lillas, Lillias

Liliash (Spanish) lily; innocent
Lil, Lileah, Liliosa, Lilya, Lyliase, Lylish

Lilith (Arabic) nocturnal
Lilis, Lilita, Lill, Lilli, Lillie, Lillith, Lilly, Lilyth, Lilythe

Lillian ○ (Latin) pretty as a lily
Lila, Lileane, Lilian, Liliane, Lill, Lilla, Lillah, Lillie, Lillyan, Lillyann, Lilyanne, Liyan

Lillias (Hebrew) night

Lily ○ (Latin/Chinese) elegant
Lil, Lili, Lilie

Limor (Hebrew) myrrh; treasured
Leemor

Lin (English/Chinese) beautiful
Linn, Lynn

Lina (Greek/Latin/Scottish) light of spirit; lake calm
Lena, Lin, Linah, Lynn

Linda (Spanish) pretty girl
Lind, Lindy, Lynda

Linden (American)
harmonious
*Lindan, Lindun, Lynden,
Lynnden*

Lindsay (English/Scottish)
calming; bright and shining
*Lindsee, Lindsey, Lindsi, Lindz,
Lyndsie, Lyndzee, Lynz*

Lindse (Spanish) form of
Lindsay: calming; bright and
shining
Linds, Lindz, Lindze, Lyndzy

Lindy (American) music-lover
*Lind, Lindee, Lindi, Lindie,
Linney, Linnie, Linse, Linz,
Linze*

Linette
(French/English/American)
graceful and airy
Lanette, Linet, Linnet, Lynette

Ling (Chinese) delicate

Linga (American) form of
Ling: delicate

Lingga (Scandinavian)

Linji (English) form of Linzi:
bright spirit

Lin-Lin (Chinese) beauty of a
tinkling bell
Lin, Lin Lin

Linna (Scandinavian) flower

Linnea (Swedish) statuesque
*Lin, Linayah, Linea, Linnay,
Linny, Lynnea*

Linnesh (American) form of
Lindsay: calming, bright and
shining

Linnz (American) form of
Lindsay: calming, bright and
shining

Lino (American) form of
Lindsay: calming, bright and
shining

Linsey (English) bright spirit
Linsie, Linsy, Linzi, Linzie

Linsley (English) bright

Linsley (English) form of
Lindsay: calming; bright and
shining

Linzetta (American) form of
Linzey: calming; bright and
shining
Linze, Linzette, Linzey

Linzey (American) form of
Lindsay: calming; bright and
shining

Lio (Jewish) form of Liora:
light

Liora (Hebrew) light
Leeor, Leeora, Lior, Liorit

Lioren (Jewish) form of Liora:
light

Liotta (Italian) of the bay

Lioudmila (Slavic) loved

Lisa (Hebrew/American)
dedicated and spiritual
*Lee, Leelee, Leesa, Leesah,
Leeza, Leisa, Lesa, Lysa*

Lisanne (English/Dutch) God
is my oath; favor; grace

Lisbet (Scandinavian) sweet

Lisbeth (Hebrew) form of
Elizabeth: God's promise

Lise (German) form of Lisa:
dedicated and spiritual
Lesa

Lisen (Dutch) form of
Lisanne;: God is my oath;
favor; grace

Lisette (French) little
Elizabeth
Lise, Lisete, Lissette, Liz

Lisha (Hebrew) form of
Elisha: God-loving
Lish, Lishie

Lissa (Greek) sweet
Lyssa

Lissandra (Greek) defends
others

Lisset (French) form of
Elizabeth: God's promise

Lisseth (Hebrew) form of
Elizabeth: God's promise
*Liseta, Liseth, Lisette, Lisith,
Liss, Lisse, Lissi*

Lissie (American) form of
Elise: concecrated to God
Lis, Lissi, Lissey, Lissy

Liszt (Hungarian) musical

Lita (Latin) life-giving
Leta

Lithyia (Mythology) prepared

Litisha (Spanish) form of
Letitia: joy

Litzy (Spanish) form of
Letitia: joy

Liv (Latin/Scandinavian) lively
Leev

Livia (Hebrew) lively
Levia, Livya

Liviu (Spanish) lively

Livona (Hebrew) vibrant
Levona, Liv, Livvie, Livvy

Liya (Russian) lily; lovely
Leeya

Liz (English) form of
Elizabeth: God's promise
Lis, Lissy, Lizy, Lizzi, Lizzie

Liza (American) smiling
*Leeza, Liz, Lizah, Lizzie,
Lizzy, Lyza*

Lizabeth (English) abundant
in God

Lizeth (Hebrew) ebullient
Liseth, Lizethe

Lizette (Hebrew) lively
Lizet, Lizett

Lizset (Spanish) form of
Lysette

Lizzie (American) devout
*Liz, Liza, Lizae, Lizette,
Lizzee, Lizzey, Lizzi, Lizzy*

Lizzine (American) form of
Elizabeth: God's promise

Llewwllyn (Welsh) shines
brightly

Lo (American) spunky
Loe

Loa (English) form of Louise:
hardworking and brave

Loelia (Arabic) nocturnal
Leila

Loen (Spanish) lovely

Loey (Mythology) kind
Louhi

Logan (English) climbing
Lo, Logun

Logana (Scottish) form of
Logan: climbing

Loganah (Scottish) form of
Logan: climbing

Logred (Welsh) dedication

Loicy (American) delightful
*Loice, Loisee, Loisey, Loisi, Loy,
Loyce, Loycy, Loyse, Loysie*

Loire (Place name) river in
France; lovely wonder
Loir, Loirane

Lois (Greek) good
Lo, Loes

Loise (English) form of Louise: hardworking and brave

Lola (Spanish) pensive
Lo, Lolah, Lolita

Loleatha (Spanish) sad

Loleen (American) jubilant
Lolene

Loleta (Spanish) sad

Lo-Lin (Asian) sure

Lolita (Spanish) sad
Lo, Lola, Loleta, Lita

Lolly (English) candy; sweet

Loma (Spanish) lucky

Lomita (Spanish) good

Lona (Latin) lionlike
Lonee, Lonie, Lonna, Lonnie

Lona (Indian) lovely

Londa (American) shy
Londah, Londe, Londy

London (Place name) calming
Londen, Londun, Londy, Loney, Lony

Loni (American) beauty
Loney, Lonie, Lonnie, Loney

Lonise (American) form of Denise: wine-lover

Lonjeana (Spanish) tall

Lonnecke (American) lone

Lonnette (American) pretty
Lonett, Lonette, Lonnie, Lonn

Lonzine (French) alone

Lopa (Spanish)

Loperena (Spanish)

Lora (Latin) regal
Laura, Lorah, Lorea, Loria

Lorain (English) sad

Loranden (American) ingenious
Lorandyn, Lorannden, Luranden

Lordena (Spanish) form of Lourdes: a girl from Lourdes, France; hallowed

Lordyn (American) enchanting
Lorden, Lordin, Lordine, Lordun, Lordynn

Loreen (American) variation on Lauren: crowed with laurel
Lorene

Lorel (German) tempting
Loreal

Lorela (German) attracts

Lorelei (German) siren
Loralee, Lorilie, LoraLee, Lurleen, Lurlene

Lorelle (American) lovely
Lore, Loreee, Lorel, Lorey, Lori, Lorie, Lorille, Lorel, Lorille

Loren (American) form of Lauren: laurel-crowned
Lorren, Lorri, Lorrie, Lorron, Lorryn, Lory, Loryn, Lourie

Lorena (English) form of Loren: laurel-crowned
Loreen, Lorene, Lorrie, Lorrine

Lorenia (English) form of Lorena: laurel-crowned

Loreniana (English) given laurels

Lorenza (Latin) form of Laura: laurel-crowned; joyous
Laurenza

Loreto (Italian) miraculous; honored

Loretta (English) large-eyed beauty
Lauretta

Lori (Latin) laurel-crowned and nature-loving
Laurie, Loree, Lorie, Lory

Lorinthe (American) form of Laura: laurel-crowned; joyous

Loris (Greek/Latin) fun-loving
Lorice, Lauris

Loriz (American) form of Loris: fun-loving

Lorna (Latin) laurel-crowned; natural
Lorenah

Lorola (Origin unknown) family

Lorraine (Latin/French) sad-eyed
Laraine, Lauraine, Lorain, Loraine, Lorrie, Lors

Lorril (American) praise-worthy

Lorya (American) form of Laura: laurel-crowned; joyous

Lotta (Swedish) sweet

Lottie (American) old-fashioned
Lottee, Lotti, Lotty

Lotus (Greek) flowery
Lolo, Lotie

Lou (American) form of Louise: hardworking and brave
Loulou, Lu

Louella (English) elf
Loella, Loellah, Loelle, Luella, Luela

Louie (American) strong

Louisa (English) patient
Lou, Loulou, Luisa, Luizza, Lu

Louise (German) hardworking and brave
Lolah, Lou, Loulou, Luise

Louiseine (American) intimidating

Louiselle (French) form of Louise: hardworking and brave

Loura (Catalan) laurels

Louray (English) enchants

Lourdes (French) girl from Lourdes, France; hallowed
Lourd, Lordes, Lordez

Louria (American) form of Laura: laurel-crowned; joyous

Loutan (English) released

Love (English/American) loving
Lovey, Lovi, Luv

Loveada (Spanish) loving
Lova, Lovada

Lovella (Native American) soft spirit
Lovela

Lovely (American) loving
Lovelee, Loveley, Loveli, Lovey

Lovie (American) warm
Lovee, Lovey, Lovi, Lovy

Lovina (American) warm
Lovena, Lovey, Lovinah, Lovinnah

Lovisa (Scandinavian) aggressor

Loway (Last name used as first name) wolf; free

Lowe (English) sly; pretty

Lowell (American) lovely
Lowel

Lowena (American) form of Louise: hardworking and brave
Lowenek, Lowenna

Loy (English) adoring

Loyalty (American) loyal
Loyaltie

Loycie (English) adoring

Loydia (Spanish) form of
Lydia: musical; unusual

Ltanya (American) form of
Latonya: birdlike

Ltaya (American) form of
Latonya

Lu Verna (English) form of
Laverne: breath of spring

Lualla (American) adoring;
graceful

Luba (Yiddish) dear
Liba, Lubah, Lyuba

Luberda (Spanish) light; dear
Luberdia

Luberta (Slavic) form of
Luba: dear

Lubica (Slavic) form of Luba:
dear

Lublain (Slavic) form of Luba:
dear

Luca (Italian) light
Luka

Lucasta (Spanish) bringer of
light

Luceil (French) light; lucky
Luce, Lucee, Lucy

Lucelle (French) sheds light

Lucellene (French) sheds
light

Lucerne (Latin) born into the
light
Lucerna

Lucero (Italian) light-hearted
Lucee, Lucey, Lucy

Lucetta (English) radiating
joy

Lucette (French) pale light

Lucia (Italian/Greek/Spanish)
light; lucky in love
*Chia, Luceah, Lucey, Lucey,
Luci*

Luciana (Italian) fortunate
Louciana, Luceana, Lucianah

Lucie (French/American)
lucky girl
Lucy

Lucienne (French) lucky
*Lucien, Lucianne, Lucienn,
Lucy-Ann*

Lucilla (English) form of
Lucille: bright-eyed
*Loucilla, Loucilah, Loucilla,
Lucilah, Lucylla, Lusyla, Luzela*

Lucille (English) bright-eyed
*Loucil, Loucile, Loucille, Lucyl,
Lucie, Lucile, Lucy*

Lucillea (French) sheds light

Lucillet (French) sheds light

Lucina (American) happy
*Lucena, Lucie, Lucinah, Lucy,
Lucyna*

Lucinda (Latin) prissy
*Cinda, Cindie, Lu, Luceenda,
Lucynda, Lulu*

Lucindia (English) form of
Lucinda: prissy

Lucine (Scandinavian) lucid

Lucinea (Spanish) lucid

Lucita (Spanish) light
Lusita, Luzita

Lucja (Polish) light
Luscia

Luckette (Invented) lucky
Luckett

Lucretia (Latin) wealthy
woman
*Lu, Lucrecia, Lucreesha,
Lucritia*

Lucy (Latin/Scottish/Spanish)
lighthearted
Lu, Luca, Luce, Luci, Lucie

Ludivina (Slavic) loved

Ludmilla (Slavic) beloved one
*Lu, Ludie, Ludmila, Ludmylla,
Lule, Lulu*

Ludne (French) loved

Ludora (Spanish) loved

Lue (English) cheering

Lue-Ella (English) form of
Ella: beautiful and fanciful
Louel, Luella, Luelle

Luella (German) conniving
*Loella, Louella, Lu, Lula,
Lulah, Lulu*

Luenetter (American)
egotistical
Lou, Lu, Luene, Luenette

Lugene (American) form of
Eugene: blue-blood

Luicia (Spanish) light

Luisa (Spanish) smiling
Louisa

Luisana (Place name) from
Louisiana
Luisanna, Luisanne, Luisiana

Luisito (Spanish) light

Luke (American) bouncy
Luc, Luka, Lukey, Lukie

Lula (German) all-
encompassing
Lulu

Lulani (Polynesian)
heaven-sent
Lula, Lani, Lanie

Lular (English) bounty of
heaven

Lulu (German/English) kind
Lou, Loulou, Lu, Lulie

Lulua (English) comforts

Lulunena (German) comforts

Luminosa (Spanish)
luminous

Luna (Latin) moonstruck
Loona

Luna-Coco (American)
coconut moon

Lunan (Latin) moon

Lund (German) genius
Lun, Lunde

Lundria (Slavic) smart; from
the grove

Lundy (Scottish) grove by an
island
Lundea, Lundee, Lundi

Lundyn (American) different
Lundan, Lunden, Lundon

Luned (Welsh) moonlike

Lunell (American) luminous

Lunette (French) of the moon

Lunwonda (African) moon
child

Lupe (Spanish) enthusiastic
*Loopy, Loopey, Lupeta, Lupey,
Lupie, Lupita*

Luquitha (African American)
fond
Luquetha, Luquith

Lur (Spanish) earth

Lura (American) loquacious
Loora, Lur, Lurah, Lurie

Luree (German) lures

Luretta (German) lures

Lurissa (American) beguiling
*Luresa, Luressa, Luris, Lurisa,
Lurissah, Lurly*

Lurlaine (German) alluring

Lurlene (German) tempting
Lura, Lurleen, Lurlie, Lurline

Lushea (American) form of
Lucia: light; lucky in love

Lutee (German) of the people

Lutherene (American)
feminine form of Luther:
reformer

Luticha (Spanish) form of
Letitia: joy

Luvelle (American) light
Luvee, Luvell, Luvey, Luvy

Luvy (American) spontaneous
Lovey, Luv

Lux (Latin) light
Luxe, Luxee, Luxi, Luxy

Luz (Spanish) lighthearted
Lusa, Luzana, Luzi

Luzille (Spanish) light
Luz, Luzell

Lyanna (English) fierce

Lyanne (Greek) melodious
*Liann, Lianne, Lyan, Lyana,
Lyaneth, Lyann*

Lyawonda (African
American) friend
Lyawunda, Lywanda, Lywonda

Lycia (Biblical) place name

Lycoris (Greek) twilight

Lyda (American) unique

Lydda (Biblical) place name

Lydia (Greek) musical;
unusual
*Lidia, Lidya, Lyddie, Lydie,
Lydy*

Lydie (Slavic) girl of Lydia

Lyfe (American) life

Lyla (French) island girl
Lila, Lilah, Lile

Lyle (English) strident
Lile

Lymekia (Greek) form of
Lydia: musical; unusual
Lymekea

Lynda (Spanish) form of
Linda: pretty girl
*Linda, Lindi, Lynde, Lyndie,
Lynn*

Lyndsay (Scottish) bright and
shining
Lindsay, Lindsey

Lynelle (English) pretty girl;
bright as sunshine
Linelle, Lynel, Lynie, Lynn

Lynette (French) small and
fresh
*Lyn, Lynet, Lynnet, Lynette,
Lynnie*

Lynita (English) form of
Lynnette: small and fresh

Lynn (English) fresh as spring
water
Lin, Linn, Linnie, Lyn, Lynne

Lynna (English) by the lake

Lynnaia (English) lake girl

Lynona (American) form of
Wynona: firstborn girl

Lynsey (American) form of
Lindsay: calming; bright and
shining
Linzie, Lyndsey, Lynze, Lynzy

Lynzeen (American) form of
Lindsay: calming; bright and
shining

Lyonda (American) form of
Lynda: pretty girl

Lyra (Greek) musical
Lyre

Lyric (Greek) musical
Lyrec

Lyrics (English) lyrical

Lyris (Greek) plays the lyre
Liris, Lirisa, Lirise

Lys (German) form of
Elizabeth: God's promise

Lysa (Hebrew) God-loving
Leesa, Lisa

Lysalette (English) form of
Lisette: little Elizabeth

Lysandra (Greek) liberator;
she frees others
Lyse, Lysie

Lysanne (Greek) helpful
Lysann

Lysbeth (English) form of
Elizabeth: God's promise

Lysett (American) pretty little
one
Lyse, Lysette

Lysle (Spanish) pretty

Lyssan (Greek) form of
Alexandra: defender of
mankind
*Liss, Lissan, Lissana, Lissandra,
Lyss*

Lyssette (English) form of
Lisette: little Elizabette

Lystra (Biblical) place name

Lytanisha (African
American) scintillating
*Litanisha, Lyta, Lytanis,
Lytanish, Lytanishia, Nisa,
Nisha*

Lyttle (Last name used as first
name) small

Lyudmilea (Slavic) beloved

M

Maacah (Biblical) place name

Maarath (Biblical) place name

Mab (Literature)
Shakespearean queen of
fairies

Mabel (Latin) well-loved
*Mabbel, Mabil, Mable, Mabyl,
Maybel, Maybie*

Mabellee (Asian) beauty

Maben (Welsh) child

Mablee (Welsh) pretty

Macallister (Irish) confident

Macander (Biblical) place
name

Macarena (Spanish) name of
a dance; blessed
*Macarene, Macaria, Macarria,
Rena*

Macaria (Spanish) blessed
*Maca, Macarea, Macarie,
Maka*

Macey (American) upbeat;
happy
Mace, Macie, Macy

Machelle (Hebrew) thinks of
God

Mackenzie ✪ ✆ (Irish) leader
*Mac, Mackenzee, Mackenzey,
Mackenzi, Mackenzie,
Mackenzy, Mackie, Mackinsey,
Mckenzie, McKinsey, McKinzie*

Macress (American) thankful

Mada (American) helpful
Madah, Maida

Madai (Biblical) place name

Madalena (Greek) form of Madeline: jaunty
Madalayna, Madaleyna, Madelyna, Madalayna, Madelena, Madeleyna

Madalyn (Greek) high goals
Madelyn

Madchen (German) girl
Madchan, Madchin, Maddchen

Maddie (English) form of Madeline: strength-giving
Mad, Maddee, Maddey, Maddi, Maddy, Mady

Maddox (English) giving
Maddax, Maddee, Maddey, Maddie, Maddux, Maddy

Maddye (English) form of Madeleine: cleansed

Madeleine (French) high-minded
Madelon

Madeleinea (English) form of Madeleine: cleansed

Madeline ○ (Greek) strength-giving
Madaleine, Maddie, Maddy, Madelene, Madi

Madelyn (Greek) strong woman
Madalyn, Madlynne, Madolyn

Madge (Greek/American) spunky
Madgie, Madg

Madgie (English) form of Madge: spunky; form of Margaret: treasured pearl; pure-spirited

Madhur (Hindi) sweet girl

Madina (Greek) form of Madeline: strength-giving
Mada, Maddelina, Maddi, Maddy, Madele, Madena, Madlin

Madine (American) form of Nadine: dancer

Madis (English) form of Madison: popular

Madison ○ ○ (English) good-hearted
Maddie, Maddison, Maddy, Madisen, Madysin

Madlyina (English) form of Madeleine: cleansed

Madonna (Latin) my lady; spirited

Madora (Place name) from Madeira, Spain: volcanic
Madorra

Madrigal (Word as name)

Madrina (Spanish) godmother
Madra, Madreena, Madrine

Madrona (Spanish) mother; maternal
Madrena

Mae (English) bright flower
May

Maegan (Irish) a gem of a woman
Megan

MaElena (Spanish) light
Elena, Lena

Maeli (English) great; form of Maez
Maelee, Maeley, Maelie, Maely, Maylee, Mayley, Mayli, Maylie, Mayly

Maeve (Irish) queen
Maive, Mave, Mayve

Maevey (Irish) exciting

Mafe (Italian) strong

Magadan (Biblical) place name

Magali (French) treasured pearl

Magan (Greek) heavy-hearted
Mag, Magen, Maggie

Magany (Greek) doleful

Magda (Scandinavian)
believer
Mag, Maggie

Magdala (Greek) girl in the
tower
Magdalla

Magdalene
(Greek/Scandinavian)
spiritual
*Mag, Magda, Magdalena,
Magdaline, Magdalyn,
Magdelin, Magdylena Maggie*

Magella (Slavic) starry-eyed

Maggie
(Greek/English/Irish)
priceless pearl
Mag, Maggee, Maggi

Magina (Russian)
hardworking
Mageena, Maginah

Magli (French) treasured
pearl

Maglie (French) treasured
pearl

Magnolia (Latin) flowering
and flourishing
*Mag, Maggi, Maggie, Maggy,
Magnole, Nolie*

Magryta (Slavic) desired

Mahal (Filipino) loving
woman
Mah, Maha

Mahala (Hebre/Native
American) tender femal
*Mah, Mahalah, Mahalia,
Mahla, Mahlie*

Mahelia (Arabic) form of
Mahala: tenderness
Maheelia, Maheelya, Mahelya

Mahina (Hawaiian)
moonbeam

Mahira (Hebrew) vibrant

Mahogany (Spanish) rich as
wood
Mahagonie, Mahogony

Mahoney (American) high
energy
*Mahhony, Mahonay, Mahonie,
Mahony*

Mai (Scandinavian/Japanese)
treasure; flower; singular
Mae, May

Maia (Greek) fertile; earth
goddess
Maya, Mya

Maida (Greek) shy girl
Mady, Maidie, May, Mayda

Maidie (Scottish) maiden;
virgin
Maidee, Maydee, Maydie

Maija (Scandinavian) form of
Mary: star of the sea; sea of
bitterness

Maike (German) form of
Maria: desired child

Mailanna (Hawaiian) lei of
Anna

Maileen (Hawaiian) lei

Mailene (Hawaiian) lei

Mailie (Scottish) virtuous

Mainan (American) guesses

Mair (Irish) form of Mary:
star of the sea; sea of
bitterness
Maire

Maira (Hebrew) bitter; saved
Mara, Marah

Maired (Irish) pearl;
treasured
Mairead, Mared

Mairin (Irish) form of Mary: star of the sea; sea of bitterness

Maisha (Arabic) proud

Maisie (Scottish) treasure
Maesee, Maesey, Maesi, Maesie, Maesy, Maisee, Maisey, Maisi, Maisy, Maizie, Mazee

Maitland (American) form of Maitlyn: kind
Maitlande, Mateland, Matelande, Maytland, Maytlande

Maitlin (American) form of Maitlyn: kind
Maitlyn, Matelin, Matelyn, Maytlin, Maytlyn

Maj (Slavic) star

Maja (Scandinavian) fertile

Majella (Slavic) star

Majidah (Arabic) slendid

Majula (Slavic) star

Maka (Hawaiian) face

Makala (Hawaiian) natural outdoors
Makal, Makie

Makani (Hawaiian) in the wind

Makay (American) charming

Makayla ♥ (American) magical
Makaila, Makala, Michaela, Mikaela, Mikayla, Mikaylah

Makeda (African) excellent

Makena (African) wisdom's child

Makkedah (African) lovely

Makula (American) exacting

Makyll (American) innovative
Makell

Makynna (American) friendly
Makenna, Makinna

Malah (Indian) garland
Mala

Malak (Arabic) angelic

Malatha (Biblical) place name

Malati (Indian) Jasmine flower

Malay (Place name) from Malaysia; softspoken
Malae

Malaya (Filipino) free and open
Malea

Maleah (Hawaiian) sad

Malendita (Spanish) royal

Malene (Scandinavian) in the tower
Maleen, Maleene, Malyne

Malha (Hebrew) queenlike and regal

Mali (Thai) flowering beauty
Malee, Maley, Mali, Malie, Malley, Mallie, Maly

Malia (Hawaiian) thoughtful
Maylia

Maliaval (Hawaiian) peaceful

Malika (Hungarian) hardworking and punctual
Maleeka

Malikian (Hawaiian) of the queen

Malin (Native American) comfort-giver
Malen, Maline, Mallie

Malina (Scandinavian) in the tower
Maleena, Maleenah, Malinah, Malyna, Malynah

Malinda (Greek/American)
honey
Melinda

Malinee (American) sweet

Malini (Indian) river

Malisa (English) loyal

Malissa (Greek) honey bee
Melissa

Maliyah (Hawaiian) form of
Malia: thoughtful

Malla (Indian) adorned with
necklace

Mallika (Indian) watchful;
tending the garden
Malika

Mallory
(French/German/American)
tough-minded; spunky
*Mal, Malery, Mallari, Mallery,
Mallie, Mallorey, Mallori,
Mallorie, Maloree, Malorey,
Malori, Malorie, Malory*

Malu (Hawaiian) peaceful
Maloo

Malvika (Slavic) darkness

Malvina (Scottish) romantic
Malv, Malva, Malvie, Melvina

Mame (American) form of
Margaret: treasured pearl;
pure-spirited
Maime, Mayme

Mamie (American) form of
Margaret: treasured pearl;
pure-spirited
Mamee, Mamey, Mami, Mamy

Manasa (Asian) lovely

Mancie (American) hopeful
Manci, Mansey, Mansie

Manda (American) form of
Amanda: fit to be loved
*Amand, Mandee, Mandi,
Mandy*

Mandana (African)
combative

Mandeece (African) loved

Mandeen (American) form
of Amanda: fit to be loved

Mandia (Indian) beloved

Mandisa (African) kind

Mandy (Latin) lovable
*Manda, Mandee, Mandey,
Mandi, Mandie*

Mane (American) top
Main, Manie

Manee (Korean) peace giving
Mani, Manie

Manessa (Sanskrit) wise

Manilow (Last name as first
name) musical

Manisha (Hindi) sharp
intellect

Manju (Hindi) sweetheart

Manna (Hawaiian) perceptive
Mana, Manah, Mannah

Manolita (Spanish) girl who
lives in God

Manon (French) exciting

Mantae (Slavic) form of
Maria: desired child

Mantill (American) guarded
Mant, Mantell, Mantie

Manuela (Spanish)
sophisticated girl
Manuella

Manya (Spanish) form of
Maria: desired child

Manzie (Native American) flower
Mansi

Mappie (American) zany

Maquila (Spanish) stubborn

Mara (Greek) thoughtful believer
Marah, Marra

Maralys (American) devout

Maranda (Latin) wonderful
Marandah, Miranda

Marat (American) form of Merit: deserving

Marbell (American) pretty

Marbella (Spanish) pretty
Marb, Marbela, Marbelle

Marbury (American) substantial
Mar, Marbary

Marcelina (Latin) form of Marcella: dedicated to Mars
Marceleena, Marcelyna, Marcileena, Marcilina, Marcilyna, Marcyleena

Marceline (Latin) form of Marcella: dedicated to Mars
Marceleene, Marcelyne, Marcileene, Marcilyne, Marcyleene, Marcelline

Marcella (Latin) dedicated to Mars
Marce, Marcela, Marci, Marcie, Marse, Marsella

Marcellette (French) staunch

Marcellita (Spanish) desired; feisty
Marcel, Marcelita, Marcelite, Marcelle, Marcelli, Marcey, Marci

Marcellyn (English) form of Marceline: dedicated to Mars

Marcena (Latin/American) spirited
Marce, Marceen, Marcene, Marcie

March (American) month of March; spring girl

Marcia (Latin/American) dedicated to Mars
Marcie, Marsha

Marciana (Spanish) warring

Marcie (English) chummy
Marcee, Marcey, Marci, Marcy, Marsi, Marsie

Marcine (American) bright
Marceen, Marceene

Marconi (Italian) creates

Marcy (English/American) opinionated
Marci, Marsie, Marsy

Mardi (French) Tuesday

Mardjaneh (Indian) of the meadow

Mardonia (American) approving
Mardee, Mardi, Mardone, Mardonne, Mardy

Mare (American) living by the ocean

Mareane (Irish) form of Mary: star of the sea; sea of bitterness

Marelly (French) form of Mary: star of the sea; sea of bitterness

Maren (American) ocean-lover
Marin, Marren, Marrin

Marenz (Slavic) of the sea

Maret (English) form of
Mary: star of the sea; sea of
bitterness
*Marett, Marit, Maritt, Maryt,
Marytt*

Marete (English) pearl girl

Marfelia (Spanish) form of
Martha: lady

Marfo (Russian) form of
Martha: lady

Marg (American) tenacious
Mar

Margaret
(Greek/Scottish/English)
treasured pearl; pure-spirited
*Mag, Maggie, Marg, Margerite,
Margie, Margo, Margret, Meg,
Meggie*

Margaretta (Spanish) pearl

Margarita (Italian/Spanish)
winning
*Marg, Margarit, Margarite,
Margie, Margrita, Marguerita*

Margarite (Greek/German)
form of Margaret: treasured
pearl; pure-spirited
*Gretal, Marga, Margareeta,
Margaryta, Margereeta,
Margerita, Margeryta, Margit,
Margot*

Margaux (French) form of
Margaret: treasured pearl;
pure-spirited

Marge (English/American)
form of Marjorie: bittersweet;
pearl
Marg, Margie

Margery (English) form of
Marjorie: bittersweet; pearl
Marge, Margie

Marghanita (Spanish) pearl

Margherita (Italian/Greek)
form of Margaret: treasured
pearl; pure-spirited
Marg

Margia (American) form of
Margie: friendly
Marge, Margea, Margy

Margie (English) friendly
Margey, Margy, Marjie

Margina (American)
centered

Margoletta (French) little
Margo; spunky

Margot (French) lively
Margaux, Margo

Margrit (Spanish) treasured

Margrita (Spanish) treasure
Margreeta, Margrytaa

Margrite (Dutch) form of
Margaret: treasured pearl;
pure-spirited

Margrune (Slavic) form of
Margaret: treasured pearl;
pure-spirited

Marguerite (French) stuffy
*Maggie, Marg, Margerite,
Margie, Margina, Margurite*

Margyd (Welsh) pearl-like

Mari (Japanese) ball; round

Maria ✪
(Latin/French/German/Italian/
Polish/Spanish) desired child
*Maja, Malita, Mareea, Marica,
Marike, Marucha, Mezi, Mitzi*

Mariah ✪ (Hebrew) God is
my teacher
*Marayah, Mariahe, Marriah,
Meriah, Moriah*

Marial (Spanish) embittered

Mariama (Hebrew) form of Mariam: bitter

Mariamne (French) form of Miriam: living with sadness
Mariam, Marianne

Marian (English) thoughtful
Mariane, Marianne, Maryann, Maryanne

Mariana (Spanish) quiet girl
Maryanna

Marianda (Combo of Mari and Rianda)

Maribel
(French/English/American) star of the sea; beautiful
EmBee, Marabel, Maribela, Merrybelle

Maricruz (Combo of Maria and Emma) Maria of the cross

Marid (English) form of Maria: desired child

Marie (French) form of Mary: star of the sea; sea of bitterness
Maree, Marye

Mariea (English) form of Maria: desired child

Mariel (German) spiritual
Mari, Mariele, Marielle

Mariella (Italian) form of Maria: desired child

Marielos (Spanish) form of Mariel: spiritual

Mariene (Spanish) devout
Mari, Marienne

Mariet (French) form of Marie: dignified and spiritual
Mariett, Mariette, Maryet, Maryett, Maryette

Marigene (Dutch) embittered

Marigold (Botanical) sunny
Maragold, Marigolde, Marigole, Marrigold, Marygold, Marygolde

Marijana (Slavic) aggressive

Marijonna (Slavic) aggressive

Marika (Slavic/American) thoughtful and brooding
Mareeca, Mareecka, Mareeka, Marica, Maricka, Maryca, Marycka, Maryka, Merica, Merika, Merk, Merkie

Marikae (Slavic) bitter

Marilan (American) form of Marilyn: fond-spirited

Marilyn (Hebrew) fond-spirited
Maralynne, Mare, Marilin, Mariline, Marilinn, Marilynn, Marrie, Marrilyn, Marylyn, Marylynn, Merilyn, Merrilyn

Marin (Latin) sea-loving
Mare, Maren

Marina (Latin) lover of the ocean
Mareena, Marena, Marina, Maryna

Marinaea (American) form of Marin: sea-loving

Marinalla (American) of the sea

Marine (French) of the sea

Marinen (Mythology) sea

Marineuza (Spanish) sea child

Marioara (Indian) delicate

Marion (French) form of Mary: star of the sea; sea of bitterness
Mare, Marien, Marrion, Mary, Maryen, Maryian, Maryon

Mariposa (Spanish) butterfly
Mari, Mariposah, Maryposa

Mariquita (Spanish) form of
Margaret: treasured pearl;
pure-spirited
*Marikita, Marrikita,
Marriquita*

Maris (Latin) sea-loving
Mere, Marice, Meris, Marys

Marisa ✪ (Latin) sea-loving
*Marce, Maressa, Marissa,
Marisse, Mariza Marsie,
Marysa, Maryssa, Merisa*

Marisela (Spanish) hearty
Marisella, Marysela

Mariska (American)
endearing
Mareska, Marisca, Mariskah

Marisol (Spanish) stunning
*Mare, Mari, Marizol, Marrisol,
Marzol, Merizol*

Marisse (French) beloved

Maritala (Scandinavian) pearl

Maritel (Scandinavian) pearl

Maritza (Place name) for St.
Moritz, Switzerland

Marixa (Spanish) endearing

Marixbel (Spanish) pretty
Marix

Marizu (Spanish) blessed

Marjetta (Slavic) form of
Margaret: treasured pearl;
pure-spirited

Marjie (Scottish) form of
Marjorie: bittersweet; pearl
Marji, Marjy

Marjolein (Dutch) spice

Marjorie
(Greek/English/Scottish)
bittersweet; pearl
*Marg, Marge, Margerie,
Margery, Margorie, Marjie,
Marjori*

Marketa (Slavic) form of
Margaret: treasured pearl;
pure-spirited
Marketta

Marky (American)
mischievous
Marki, Markie

Marla (German) believer;
easygoing
Marlah, Marlla

Marlaina (American) form of
Marlene: child of light; bitter
Marlaine, Marlane

Marlake (Slavic) of the lake

Marlam (American) wanted

Marlana (Hebrew/Greek)
vamp
Marlanna

Marleal (American) form of
Mary: star of the sea; sea of
bitterness
Marle, Marleel, Marly

Marlee (Greek) guarded
*Marleigh, Marley, Marli,
Marlie, Marly*

Marlen (American) desired
Marl, Marla, Marlin

Marlena (German) pretty;
bittersweet
*Marla, Marlaina, Marleena,
Marlina, Marlyna, Marlynne,
Marnie*

Marlene (German) child of
light; bitter
*Marlean, Marlee, Marleen,
Marleene, Marley, Marline,
Marly, Marlyne*

Marlette (English) form of Merlette: magical

Marley (English) form of Marlene: child of light; bitter
Mar, Marlee, Marlie, Marly

Marliece (Spanish) desirable

Marlinn (German) form of Mary: star of the sea; sea of bitterness

Marlise (English) considerate
Marlice, Marlis, Marlys

Marlo (American) vivacious
Marloe, Marloh, Marlow, Marlowe

Marlona (German) form of Mary: star of the sea; sea of bitterness

Marlonene (German) form of Mary: star of the sea; sea of bitterness

Marluce (German) form of Marlis: religious

Marlycia (Spanish) desired
Lycia, Marly, Marlysia

Marlys (English) form of Marlis: religious

Marna (French) form of Marlene: star of the sea

Marnelle (Hebrew) form of Marnie: celebrates

Marnie (Hebrew) storyteller
Marn, Marnee, Marney, Marni, Marny

Marnina (French) form of Marlene: star of the sea
Marneena, Marnyna

Marnita (American) worrier
Marneta, Marni, Marnite, Marnitta, Marny

Marolyn (Invented) form of Marilyn: fond-spirited
Maro, Marolin, Marolinne

Marqeen (American) form of Marquees: noble-spirited

Marquetisha (Spanish) form of Marquita: happy leader

Marquise (French) noble-spirited
Markeese, Marquees, Marquisa, Mars

Marquisha (African American) form of Marquise: noble-spirited
Marquish

Marquista (Spanish) form of Marquita: happy leader

Marquita (Spanish) happy girl
Marqueda, Marquitta, Marrie

Marquittaian (Spanish) form of Marquita: happy leader

Marrea (American) form of Maria: desired child

Marri (American) form of Mary: star of the sea; sea of bitterness

Marrie (American) form of Mary: star of the sea; sea of bitterness
Marry

Mars (Roman) warring

Marsala (Italian) seaport in Sicily
Marse, Marsela, Marsie

Marschelle (Scottish) form of Marsail: happy

Marselle (Spanish) happy

Marsha (Latin) form of Marcia: dedicated to Mars
Marcia, Mars, Marsie

Marshay (American) exuberant
Marshae, Marshaya

Marshaye (French) difficult

Marshette (French) difficult

Marta (Danish) treasure
Mart, Marte, Marty, Merta

Martcia (Spanish)
unmanageable

Marterrell (American)
changeable
Marte, Marterill, Martrell

Martha (Aramaic) lady
Marta, Marth, Marti, Marty,
Mattie

Marthe (Aramaic) ladylike

Marti (English) form of
Martha: dreamy
Martee, Martey, Martie, Marty

Martijn (Dutch)
unmanageable

Martina (Latin/German)
combative
Marteena, Martene, Marti,
Martinna, Martyna, Tina

Martine (French) combative

Martivanio (Italian) form of
Martina: combative
Mart, Marti, Tivanio

Martonette (American)
feminine form of Martin:
warlike
Martanette, Martinette,
Martonett

Martreece (American)
unmanageable

Marty (English) form of
Martha: lady
Marti

Maruja (Slavic) soft heart

Marusya (Slavic) softhearted

Marvel (French) astounding;
marvelous

Marvella (French) marvelous
woman
Marva, Marvelle, Marvie,
Mavela

Marvis (American) form of
Mavis: singing bird

Marwyn (Welsh) beautiful

Mary ☉ (Latin/Hebrew) star
of the sea; sea of bitterness
Maire, Mara, Mare, Maree,
Mari, Marie, Mariel, Marlo,
Marye, Merree, Merry, Mitzie

Marya (Arabic) white and
bright
Marja

Maryam (Arabic) form of
Miriam: living with sadness

Maryann (English) form of
Mary: star of the sea; sea of
bitterness
Mariann, Marianne, Muryan,
Maryann, Maryanne

Maryina (Spanish) little Mary

Maryke (Dutch) kind; desired
Mairek, Marika, Maryk,
Maryky

Mary-Marg (American)
dramatic
Marimarg

Maryon (American) form of
Marian: thoughtful

Marzel (Italian) form of
Marzia: blessed

Marzia (Italian) form of
Mary: star of the sea; sea of
bitterness

Marzol (Spanish) form of
Marisol: stunning

Masailda (American)
supportive

Masha (Russian) child who
was desired

Mashayl (Slavic) form of Mary: star of the sea; sea of bitterness; form of Masha: child who was desired

Mashella (Slavic) form of Mary: star of the sea; sea of bitterness; form of Masha: child who was desired

Mashonda (African American) believer
Masho, Mashonde

Masi (African) star

Masina (Last name as first) charming; delightful

Mason (French) diligent; reliable

Massey (German) confident
Massi, Massie

Massiel (American) giving
Masie, Masiel, Massey, Massielle

Massim (Latin) great
Massima, Maxim, Maxima

Matia (Hebrew) a God-given gift
Matea, Mattea, Mattie

Matild (Hungarian) strong

Matilda (German) powerful fighter
Mat, Mathilda, Mattie, Tilda, Tillie, Tilly

Matina (Scandinavian) morning child

Matney (American) born in the morning

Mattanah (Biblical) place name; God's child

Mattie (English) most honored
Matt, Matte, Mattey, Matti, Matty

Matus (Slavic) essential

Matusea (Slavic) essential

Matylda (Polish) strong fighter
Matyld

Maude (English) old-fashioned
Maud, Maudie

Maudeen (American) countrified
Maudie, Mawdeen, Mawdine

Maudella (English) mighty

Maudest (French) modest

Maudette (English) mighty

Maudisa (African) sweet
Maudesa, Maudesah

Mauline (English) strong

Mauna (American) attractive
Maune, Mawna, Mon

Maupassant (French) writes

Maura (Latin/Irish) dark
Moira, Maurie

Mauree (Spanish) dark

Maureen (Irish/French) night-loving
Maura, Maurene, Maurine, Moreen, Morene

Maureena (Irish) form of Mary: star of the sea; sea of bitterness

Maurelle (French) petite
Maure, Maurie, Maurielle

Mauricea (Spanish) form of Mary: star of the sea; sea of bitterness

Maurilia (Spanish) dark beauty

Maurise (French) dark
Morise, Maurice

Maurshia (Slavic) form of
Marsha: dedicated to Mars

Mauve (French) gentle
Mauvey, Mauvie

Mave (French) bird; melodic

Mavi (French) sings

Mavis (French) singing bird
Mauvis, Mav, Mave

Maxcie (English) best

Maxcien (English) best

Maxeeme (Latin) form of
Maxime: maximum

Maxence (English) best

Maxie (Latin) fine
Maxee, Maxey, Maxy

Maxien (English) best

Maxilla (English) best

Maxime (Latin) maximum
Maxey, Maxi, Maxim

Maxine (Latin) greatest of all
*Max, Maxeen, Maxene, Maxie,
Maxy*

May (English) the fifth month
Mae, Maye

Maya ✿
(Spanish/Hindi/Russian)
industrious; one of a kind;
bitter
*Maia, Maiya, Mayah, **Mya**,
Myah, Mye*

Mayada (English) form of
May: the fifth month

Maybelline (Latin) variation
of Mabel: well-loved
*Mabie, May, Maybeline,
Maybie, Maybleene*

Maybelyn (Spanish) form of
Mabel: loved girl

Mayeta (Native American)
fruitful

Mayghaen (American)
fortunate

Mayim (Origin unknown)
special
Mayum

Maykaylee (American)
ingenious
*Maykayli, Maykaylie,
Maykayly*

Mayo (Place name) a county
in Ireland; vibrant
Mayoh

Mayphous (American)
imaginative

Mayra (Spanish) flourishing;
creative
Mayrah

Mayrallea (Spanish) form of
May: the fifth month

Mayrant (Spanish)
industrious
Maya, Mayrynt

Maytra (English) form of
Myra: fragrant

Mayuri (Indian) hen

Mayya (Slavic) lovely

Mazeka (Slavic) form of May:
the fifth month

Mazel (Hebrew) luck
Masel, Mazil, Mazal

Mazella (English) form of
May: the fifth month

Mazen (English) form of
May: the fifth month

Mazie (Scottish) form of
Maisie: treasure

Mazu (Chinese) goddess of
the sea

McCanna (American)
ebullient
Maccanna, McCannah

McCauley (Irish) feisty
Mac, McCuuly, McCawlie

McCay (Irish) creative
Mackaylee, McCaylee

McCormick (Irish) last name
as first name
MacCormack, Mackey

McGown (Irish) sensible
*Mac, MacGowen, Mackie,
McGowen*

McKenna (American) able
Mackenna, Makenna

McKenzie (Scottish) form of
Mackenzie: leader
Mackie, McKinzie, Mickey

McMurtry (Irish) last name
as first name
Mac, McMurt

Mead (Greek) honey-wine-
loving
Meade, Meed, Meede

Meadhoh (Irish) joyful

Meador (Irish) righteous;
form of the meadow

Meadow (English) open
land; calm
Meadoh

Meagan (Irish) joyous;
precious
*Maegan, Meaghan, Meegan,
Meg, Meganne, Meggie,
Meggye, Meghan*

Meagara (Mythology) first

Meanda (Invented) models

Meanne (American) models

Meara (Irish) happy girl

Meashley (American)
charmer
Meash, Meashlee

Meatah (American) athletic
Mea, Mia, Miata, Miatah

Meatra (American) models

Meave (Irish) sings

Mecjhelle (Slavic) form of
Michelle: like the Lord

Mecoline (American) form of
Nicole: winning

Medal (Word as name)

Medalla (Spanish) lovely

Medalle (American) pretty
Medahl, Medoll

Medardo (Spanish) pretty

Medea (Greek) ruling; cruel
Medeia

Medeba (Biblical) place name

Medes (Biblical) place name

Media (Greek) form of
Medea: ruling; cruel

Mediatrix (Greek) ingenious

Medilyn (American) gift

Medina (Place name)

Medisyn (American) gift

Medusa (Greek) contriver;
temptress

Medy (American) gift

Meeleen (Irish) excites

Meena (Hindi) fish

Meeno (Sanskrit) form of
Meena: fish

Meera (Hindi) rich

Meg (Greek) able; lovable
Megs

Megan ♀ ☿ (Irish) precious;
joyful
*Meagan, Meaghen, Meggi,
Meghan, Meghann*

Meggie (Greek) best
Meggey, Meggi, Meggy

Megha (Indian) cloudy

Megha (Welsh) pearl

Meghan (Welsh) pearl
Meghen, Meghyn

Mehetabel (Hebrew) won by
faith
Mehitabel

Mehul (Hindi) rain girl

Meirion (Hebrew) light

Meissa (Hindi) form of
Mesha: born in lunar month;
moon-loving
Meisa, Meysa, Meyssa

Mejia (Slavic) flowers

Mekeba (Invented) jubilant

Mel (Greek) sporty
Mell

Melada (Greek) form of
Melanie: dark beauty; sweet
Mel, Melli

Melaina (Greek) dark;
generous

Melana (Greek) giving; dark

Melancon (French) dark
beauty; sweet
*Mel, Melance, Melaney,
Melanie, Melanse, Melanson,
Melonce, Melonceson*

Melangel (Welsh) darling
angel

Melania (Italian) giving;
philanthropic
Mel, Melly

Melanie ✪ (Greek) dark; sweet
*Melanee, Melaney, Melani,
Melany, Meleni, Melenie,
Meleny*

Melanna (Greek) dark

Melantha (Greek) dark-
skinned; sweet
Melanthah

Melaynee (Greek) dark;
sweet

Melb (Greek) mellow

Melba (Australian) talented;
light-hearted
Melbah

Melbal (Greek) mellow

Melea (German) diligent

Melecio (Spanish) mild

Meleda (Spanish) sweet
Meleeda, Melida, Melyda

Melete (Greek) effective

Melezio (Spanish) mild

Melia (German) dedicated
Meelia, Meleea, Melya, Melyah

Melicent (English) form of
Millicent: softhearted
Melisent

Melina (Greek) honey; sweet
*Meleena, Melena, Melinah,
Melyna*

Melinane (Greek) honey
sweetness

Melinda (Latin) honey;
sweetheart
*Linda, Linnie, Linny, Lynda,
Mellie, Melynda, Milinda,
Mindy, Mylinde*

Melisande (French) strong
Melisenda

Meliss (American) honey bee

Melissa (Greek) honey
*Melisa, Melysa, Melyssa,
Melyssuh*

Melita (Biblical) place name

Melitene (Biblical) place name

Melize (English) nymph; Bee

Melizza (English) form of
Melissa: honey

Mellicent (German) form of
Millicent: soft-hearted
Melicent, Mellycent, Melycent

Mellie (Greek) bee; busy

Mellony (English) form of
Melanie: dark; sweet

Melnie (English) dark

Melody (Greek) song;
musical
*Mel, Mellie, Melodee, Melodey,
Melodie*

Melona (English) dark

Meloney (American) form of
Melanie: dark; sweet
Mel, Melone, Meloni

Melora (Latin) good
Meliora, Melorah, Melourah

Melosa (Greek) form of
Melissa: honey
Melossa

Melotta (English) form of
Melissa: honey

Melrose (English) honey of
roses; sweet girl
Mellrose, Melrosie

Melua (Unknown) rising

Melusine (Mythology) honey
bee

Melvia (American) leader;
dark
Mel, Mell, Melvea

Melvina (Irish) prepared to
lead
Malvina

Mena (Egyptian) pretty
Meenah, Menah

Menaka (Indian) heavenly
girl

Mencina (Place name)
serious

Mendee (American) form of
Melinda: honey; sweetheart

Meng (Asian) shines

Mengline (Asian) shines

Menon (French) form of
Mariel: spiritual

Menzalah (Biblical) place
name

Meosha (African American)
talented
Meeosha, Meoshe, Miosha

Merah (Biblical) abundant

Merary (American) merry
Marary, Meraree, Merarie

Mercadel (Spanish) mirth

Merce (Asian) merciful

Mercedes (Spanish)
merciful; rewarded
*Mercedez, Mercides, Mersadez,
Mersaydes*

Mercer (English) mercy

Mercia (English) form of
Marcia: dedicated to Mars

Mercilite (American) mercy

Mercy (English) forgiving
*Merce, Mercee, Mercey, Merci,
Mercie*

Meredith (Welsh) protector
*Mer, Meredithe, Meredyth,
Merridith, Merry, Merydith,
Merydithe*

Meredythe (English)
excellent

Merel (Scandinavian) sea

Meri (Irish) by the sea
Merrie

Meria (Scandinavian) sea

Meribah (Biblical) place
name

Meridian (American) perfect posture
Meredian, Meridiane

Merie (French) secretive; blackbird
Mer, Meri, Myrie

Meriel (Irish) girl who shines like the sea
Meri, Merial, Merri, Merriyl, Merry

Meris (Latin) form of Merissa: ocean-loving
Meriss, Merris, Merrys, Merys

Merissa (Latin) ocean-loving
Merisa, Meryssa

Merit (American) deserving
Merite, Meritt, Meritte, Meryt, Merytt, Mirit

Merithian (American) sea girl

Merka (Slavic) connives

Merle (Irish) shining girl
Merl, Murl, Murle

Merlette (English) magical

Merlin (English) magical

Merlina (English) magical

Merlyn (Spanish) sea child

Merney (American) form of Marnie: celebrates

Merolina (American) form of Carolina: well-loved

Merom (Biblical) place name

Meroth (Biblical) place name

Merribeth (English) cheerful
Merri-Beth, Merrybeth

Merridy (American) form of Meredith: protector

Merrience (American) merry child

Merrill (Irish) shines
Merril

Merry (English) cheerful
Mer, Meri, Merie, Merree, Merrey, Merri, Merrie, Mery

Mersaydes (Invented) form of Mercedes: merciful; rewarded
Mercy, Mersa, Mersy

Mersey (English) river Mersey; rich
Merce, Merse

Mersia (Hebrew) princess
Mercy, Mers, Mersea, Mersy

Mertha (American) joyful

Mertie (American) famed

Meryl (Irish) shining sea
Mer, Merel, Merri, Merrill, Merryl, Meryll

Meryletta (American) form of Mary: star of the sea; sea of bitterness

Merylette (American) form of Mary: star of the sea; sea of bitterness

Merynda (American) form of Marin: sea-loving

Merzi (American) mercy

Mesa (Place name) earthy
Mase, Maysa, Mesah

Mesembria (Biblical) place name

Mesha (Hindi) born in lunar month; moon-loving
Meshah

Meshalle (French) leader

Meshawnda (Invented) oblivious

Meshelle (French) leader

Messana (Biblical) place name

Meta (Scandinavian) form of Margaret: treasured pearl; pure-spirited

Metchie (Scandinavian) odd

Metta (Scandinavian) unique

Meverly (American) form of Beverly: beavers by the stream; friendly

Mexill (Invented) self-involved

Mhari (Scottish) form of Mary: star of the sea; sea of bitterness
Mhairi

Mi (Chinese) obsessive
My, Mye

Mia ○ (Scandinavian/Italian) blessed; girl of mine
Me, Mea, Meah, Meea, Meya, Mya

Miaka (Japanese) influential

Mialinda (Italian) my sweet beauty

Miami (Place name)

Miano (Italian) my sweet

Micaela (Italian) form of Michael: like the Lord

Micah (Hebrew) religious
Mica, Mika, My, Myca

Micala (Hebrew) form of Michaela: magical
Micalah, Michala, Michalah, Mikala, Mikalah, Mycala, Mycalah, Mychala, Mychalah, Mykala, Mykalah

Michaela (Hebrew) God-loving
Meeca, Micaela, Micela, Michael, Michal, Michala, Michalla, Michela, Mikaela, Mikala, Mikela, Mycaela, Mycaela, Mycela, Mychaela, Mychela, Mykaela, Mykela

Michaele (Hebrew) loving God

Michaeleen (Italian) feminine form of Michael: like the Lord

Michaelena (Italian) feminine form of Michael: like the Lord

Michelin (American) lovable
Michalynn, Mish, Mishelin

Micheline (French) form of Michelle: like the Lord
Mishelinne

Michelle ○ (Italian/French/American) feminine form of Michael: like the Lord
Machele, Machelle, Mechele, Mia, Michell, Michele, Mischel, Mischell, Mischelle, Mish, Mishell, Mishelle

Mickellette (Slavic) feminine form of Michael: like the Lord

Mickey (American) quirky
Mick, Mickee, Micki, Micky, Miki, Mikie, Mycki

Mickley (American) form of Mickey: fun-loving; quirky
Mick, Mickaella, Micklee, Mickley, Mickli, Miklea, Miklee, Mikleigh, Mikley, Myk, Mykkie

Mid (American) middle child
Middi, Middy

Middy (American) middle

Midge (English) form of Margaret: treasured pearl; pure-spirited

Midian (Biblical) place name

Mie (Dutch) form of Mary: star of the sea; sea of bitterness

Mienna (Dutch) form of Mary: star of the sea; sea of bitterness

Migdaluy (Spanish) form of Miguel; form of Michael: like the Lord

Mignon (French) cute
Migonette, Mim, Mimi, Minyon, Minyonne

Migon (American) precious
Mignonne, Migonette, Migonn, Migonne

Mika (Hebrew) wise and pious
Micah, Mikah, Mikie

Mikaela (Hebrew) God-loving
Mik, Mikayla, Mike, Mikhaila, Miki

Mikan (Slavic) child of God

Mikelle (Slavic) loves God

Mikenzi (American) form of Mackenzie: leader

Mila (Russian; Italian) form of Camilla: wonderful
Milah, Milla, Millah, Mimi

Milagros (Spanish) miracle
Mila, Milagro

Milagros (Spanish) miracle

Milana (Slavic) hospitable

Milandi (Italian) form of Milan: city in Italy; smooth

Milantia (Panamanian) calm
Mila

Milcah (Biblical) direct

Milda (Slavic) love goddess

Mildred (English) gentle
Mil, Mildread, Mildrid, Millie, Milly

Mildredena (Slavic) favorite

Milena (Greek) loving girl
Mela, Mili, Milina

Miley (Invented) form of Smiley: radiant

Miliani (Hawaiian) one who caresses
Mil, Mila

Milind (Slavic) favorite

Milinea (Slavic) favorite

Milissa (Greek) softspoken
Melissa, Missy

Miliulva (Slavic) loved

Milla (Polish) gentle; pure
Mila, Millah

Millay (Literature) for poet Edna St. Vincent Millay; soft

Millea (English) mild

Millice (French) favored

Millicent (Greek/German) softhearted
Melicent, Melly, Milicent, Millie, Millisent, Milly, Millycent, Milycent, Missy

Millie (English) form of Mildred: gentle and Millicent: soft-hearted
Mil, Mili, Millee, Milley, Milli, Milly

Millimaci (Spanish) softhearted

Milu (Asian) lovely

Mim (American) form of Miriam: living with sadness
Mimm, Mym, Mymm

Mima (Burmese) feminine

Mimi (French) form of
Camilla: wonderful
Meemee, Mim, Mims, Mimsie

Mimosa (Botanical) sensitive;
tree

Min (Chinese) sensitive;
softhearted

Mina (German/Polish)
resolute protector; willful
*Meena, Mena, Min, Minah,
Myna, Mynah*

Minal (German) kind

Minda (American) form of
Melinda: honey; sweetheart

Minda (Hindi) wise

Minden (American) form of
Melinda: honey; sweetheart

Mindy (Greek) form of
Melinda: honey; sweetheart
*Mindee, Mindey, Mindi,
Mindie, Myndee, Myndi*

Minelle (English) pretty

Minerv (English) form of
Minerva: bright; strong

Minerva (Latin/Greek)
bright; strong
Menerva, Min, Minnie, Myn

Minette (French) loyal
woman
Min, Minnette, Minnie

Mineya (American) form of
Minerva: bright; strong

Ming (Chinese) shiny; hope
of tomorrow

Minhtu (Asian) light and
clear

Mini (Scandinavian) mine

Miniver (English) assertive
Meniver, Minever, Miniverr

Minn (German) form of
Minnie: bright; strong

Minna (German) sturdy
Mina, Minnie, Mynna

Minnae (American) form of
Minnie: bright; strong

Minnie (German) form of
Minerva: bright; strong
Mini, Minni, Minny

Minnifer (American) form of
Jennifer: white wave

Minstie (American) amiable

Minsue (Asian) paradise

Minta (English) memorable
Minty

Mira (Latin/Spanish)
wonderful girl
Meara, Mirror

Mirabel (Latin) marvelous;
beautiful reflection
*Marabelle, Mira, Mirabell,
Mirabelle*

Mirabella (Italian) marvelous
*Mira, Mirabellah, Mirabelle,
Mirabell, Myrabell, Myrabelle*

Miracle (American) miracle
baby
Merry, Mira, Mirakle, Mirry

Miraflor (Spanish) flower girl

Miranda (Latin) unique and
amazing
*Maranda, Meranda, Mira,
Mirrie, Myranda*

Mirella (Spanish) wonderful
*Mira, Mirel, Mirela, Mirell,
Mirelle, Myrela, Myrella*

Mirelle (Latin) wonder
Mirell, Myrell, Myrelle

Mireya (Hebrew) form of
Miriam: living with sadness

Mireyli (Spanish) wondrous; admirable
Mire, Mirey

Miri (Gypsy) bittersweet
Meeri, Miree, Mirey, Mirie, Miry

Miriam (Hebrew) living with sadness
Mariam, Maryam, Meriam, Miri, Miriame, Miriem, Mirriam, Miryam, Miryem, Mitzi, Myriam, Myriem, Myryam, Myryem

Mirinse (American) form of Marin: sea-loving

Mirit (English) form of Merit: deserving
Miritt, Miryt, Mirytt

Mirka (Polish) glorious
Mira, Mirk

Mirtha (Greek) burdened
Meert, Meerta, Mirt, Mirta

Mirthe (Dutch) mirth

Miryana (American) form of Mariana: quiet girl

Mischanna (Hebrew) form of Miriam: living with sadness
Misch, Mischana, Mish, Mishanna, Mishke

Miselsa (Spanish) form of Michael: like the Lord

Misha (Russian) feminine form of Michael: like the Lord
Mischa

Mishelene (French) form of Micheline: like the Lord
Mish, Mishlene

Mishna (Slavic) form of Misha; form of Michale: like the Lord

Missy (English) form of Melissa: honey
Miss, Missee, Missey, Missi, Missie

Misty (English) dreamy
Miss, Missy, Mistee, Mistey, Misti, Mistie, Mysti

Misty-Kyd (American) child in the mist

Mistyne (American) form of Misty: dreamy

Mita (Slavic) the day

Mitola (American) hopeful

Mitri (American) feminine form of Dimitri: fertile; flourishing

Mitten (American) cuddly
Mitt, Mittun, Mitty

Mittie (American) form of Matilda: fighter and Mitten: cuddly
Mittee, Mittey, Mitti, Myttie

Mitylene (Biblical) place name

Mitzi (German) dancer
Mitsee, Mitzee, Mitzie, Mitzy

Miya (Japanese) peaceful as a temple
Miyah

Mizpah (Biblical) place name

Mnemosyne (Greek) goddess of memory

Mo (Irish) form of Maureen: night-loving

Moana (Hawaiian) from the ocean

Mobley (Last name as first name) beauty queen
Moblee, Mobli, Moblie, Mobly

Mocha (Arabic) coffee with chocolate
Mo, Moka, Mokka

Modena (American) modest

Modesty (Latin) modest
Modesti, Modestie

Modestyne (French) modest
Modestine, Modie

Moema (Native American) sweetness

Moeshea (African American) talented
Moesha, Moeesha, Moeshia, Moisha, Mosha, Moysha

Mohana (Hindi) enchants; siren

Mohini (Indian) bewitches

Moina (Hawaiian) ocean-loving
Moyna

Moira (English/Irish) pure; great one
Maura, Moir, Moirah, Moire, Moyrah

Moire (Irish) great girl

Moirin (Irish) excellent

Mokysha (African American) dramatic
Kisha, Kysha, Mokesha, Mokey

Moladah (Biblical) place name

Moll (Literature) for Daniel Defoe's Moll Flanders; outgoing
Mol, Molly

Mollo (Italian) form of Molly: jovial

Molly ○ (Irish) jovial
Moli, Moll, Molley, Molli, Mollie

Momo (Japanese) peaches

Mona (Greek) form of Ramona: beautiful protector
Monah, Mone

Monael (American) form of Monet: artistic

Moncita (Spanish) alone

Monday (American) born on Monday; hopeful
Mondae

Mondra (American) of the world

Monecha (English) alone

Moneek (Invented) form of Monique: saucy; advisor
Moneeke

Monet (French) artistic
Mon, Monae, Monay

Monge (Spanish) thoughtful

Monica (Greek) seeking company of others
Mon, Mona, Monicka, Monika, Monike, Monique

Monicke (Spanish) form of Monique: saucy; advisor

Monika (Polish) advisor

Monina (American) alone

Monique (French) saucy; advisor
Mon, Mone, Monee, Moneeqe, Moneeque, Moni, Moniqe

Monita (Spanish) regal

Monroe (Last name as first) orderly
Monro, Monrow, Monrowe

Monserrat (Latin) tall
Monserat

Montana (Place name) U.S. state
Montayna, Montie, Monty

Montenia (Spanish) climber
Monte, Montenea, Montynia

Montoyia (Spanish) of the mountain

Monya (American) confident
Mon, Monyeh

Monyka (American) moon

Moon (American) dreamy
*Monnie, Moone, Moonee,
Mooney, Moonny, Moonnye*

Moon Unit (Invented)
universal appeal
Moon-Unit

Moonbeam (American)
moon child

Moonbee (American) moon
bee

Moonstone (American)
gemstone

Mor (Irish) sweet

Mora (Spanish) sweet as a
blueberry

Morag (Scottish) goddess
Morrag

Moraima (Spanish) forgiving
Mora, Morama

Moran (French) dark

Morayma (Spanish) lovely;
forgiving

More (American) bonus
Moore, Morie

Moreen (English) good
friend

Moreh (Biblical) place name

Morena (Irish) dark

Moreshath (Biblical) place
name

Morettlia (American) royal

Morgan ❂ ❂ (Welsh) girl on
the seashore
*Mor, Morey, Morgane,
Morgannna, Morgen, Morgyn*

Morgander (American)
soft-spoken; divine

Moriah (French/Hebrew)
dark girl; God-taught
*Mareyeh, Mariah, Moorea,
More, Moria, Morie, Morria,
Morya*

Morigan (Mythology) queenly

Morimasa (Asian) mermaid

Morimosa (Spanish)
mermaid

Morine (American) form of
Maureen: night-loving
Morri

Morinette (Irish) lush mane

Moritza (Place name) st.
Moritz, Switzerland

Morla (American) form of
Marla: believer; easygoing
Morley, Morly

Morna (French) dark

Morta (Mythological) one of
the Roman Fates; the cutter

Morteza (Spanish) mortal

Morven (American) magical
Morvee, Morvey, Morvi

Morwenna (Welsh)
seamaiden
Mo, Morwen

Morwyn (Welsh) maiden
*Morwen, Morwenn, Morwynn,
Morwynna*

Moselle (Hebrew) uplifted
Mose, Mozelle, Mozie

Motumia (African) desirable

Mouna (Arabic) wanted

Moxie (American)
determined

Moya (Scandinavian) mother
Moiya, Moy

Moyra (Irish) excellent

Mrina (Indian) lotus girl

Muadhnait (Irish) little
noble girl

Mudeana (Spanish) glowing

Mudiwa (African) beloved
Mudewa

Muirne (Irish) affectionate

Muna (Arabic) hopes
Moona

Munashe (African) believer

Mundee (Irish) in demand

Munder (American) in
demand

Mundy (Irish) in demand

Munira (Irish) wishful

Murali (Irish) seagoing

Murdina (Slavic) dark spirit
Murdi, Murdine

Mureann (Irish) pale

Mureen (Irish) form of
Muriel: shining

Muriel (Celtic) shining
*Meriel, Mur, Murial, Muriele,
Muriell, Murielle, Muryel,
Muryell, Muryelle*

Murieliette (Irish) little
Muriel; of the sea

Murieline (French) form of
Muriel: shining

Murla (American) form of
Merle: shining girl

Murle (American) form of
Merle: shining girl

Murleance (American)
blackbird; secretive

Murma (American) whispers

Murphy (Irish) spirited
*Murphee, Murphey, Murphi,
Murphie*

Murray (Last name as first
name) brisk
Muray, Murraye

Musa (African) child; muse

Musetta (French)
instrument; musical
Museta

Musette (French)
instrument; musical
Musett

Musette (American) musical

Musique (French) musical
Museek, Museke, Musik

Mussie (American) musical
Muss, Mussi, Mussy

Muthanna (Biblical) gifted

Muyka (American) form of
Michael: like the Lord

Mwazi (Israeli) type of fig

My (Scandinavian) dear

Myalinda (American) my
beauty

Myana (American) my Ana

Myeshande (American) my
Shande

Myeshia (African American)
giving
Meyeshia, Mye, Myesha

Myfanwy (Welsh) water baby

Myisha (American) form of
Moesha: talented

Mykala (Scandinavian) giving
Mykaela, Mykela, Mykie

Mykelle (American) generous
Mykell

Mykenya (American) form of
Michaela: like the Lord

Myla (English) forgiving
Miela, Mylah

Mylee (American) forgives

Mylene (Greek) dark-skinned
girl
Myleen

Mylie (German) forgiving
Miley, Mylee, Myli

Myliki (Mythology)
changeable

Myna (English) talkative
Mina, Minah

Myndee (American) form of
Melinda: honey; sweetheart

Mynola (Invented) smart
*Minola, Monoa, Mynolla,
Mynolle*

Myra (Latin) fragrant
Mira, Myrah

Myralette (American) form
of Myra: fragrant

Myreka (American) form of
Myra: fragrant

Myriam (French) bittersweet
life

Myrisa (Spanish) fragrant

Myrischa (African American)
fragrant doll
*Myresha, Myri, Myrish,
Myrisha, Rischa*

Myrna (Irish) loved
Merna, Mirna, Murna

Myrnatte (Irish) adored

Myrtle (Greek) loving
Mertle, Mirtle, Myrt, Myrtie

Mysha (Russian) form of
Misha: like the Lord
Mischa, Mish, Misha, Mysh

Mysta (Invented) mysterious
Mista, Mystah

Mystique (French) intriguing
woman
*Mistie, Mistik, Mistique, Misty,
Mystica*

Myteen (American) girl

Mythi (American) loved

Mythiah (American) loved

Mythili (Slavic) most

Naama (Hebrew) sweet
Naamah, Naamit

Naamah (Biblical) sweet
Nanay, Nayamah, Naynay

Naarah (Aramaic) bright
light
Naara

Naava (Hebrew) delightful
girl
Naavah, N'Ava

Nabiha (Arabic) noble
Naihah

Nabila (Arabic) noble
Nabeela, Nabilah, Nabilia

Nabulungi (African) of
nobility

Nacarena (Spanish) reborn

Nacey (Spanish) born

Nachaka (African) born
leader

Naci (Spanish) born

Nada (Arabic) morning dew;
giving

Nadaka (American) gives

Nadara (American) gives

Nadasen (American) gives

Nadelie (American) form of Natalie: born on Christmas
Nadey

Nadeline (Invented) born on Christmas
Nad, Nadelyne

Nadera (Indian) gives

Nadette (French) darling girl

Nadezda (Russian) hopeful
Nadeia

Nadia (Slavic) hopeful
Nada, Nadea, Nadeen, Nadene, Nadi, Nadie, Nadina, Nadine, Nady

Nadidaa (Slavic) hopes
Nadidah

Nadine (Russian/French) dancer
Nadeen, Nadene, Nadie, Nadyne, Naidyne

Nadinia (Slavic) optimist

Nadira (Arabic) precious gem
Nadirah, Nadra

Nadya (Russian) optimistic; life's beginnings

Nadyan (Hebrew) pond; reflective
Nadian

Nadzieja (Greek) water nymph
Nadzia, Nata, Natia, Natka

Naeemah (African) breathtaking

Nafisa (Arabic) treasure

Nafshiya (Persian) precious girl

Nagara (Indian) flourishes

Nagida (Hebrew) thrives
Nagia, Nagiah, Nagiya, Najiah, Najiya, Najiyah, Negida

Nagisa (Japanese) from the shore

Nahara (Aramaic) light
Nehara, Nehora

Nahida (Hebrew) rich
Nahid

Nahla (Arabic) succeeds

Nahtanha (African) warm

Nai (Japanese) intelligent
Nayah

Naia (Hawaiian) water nymph

Naida (Greek) nymph-like
Naiad, Naya, Nayad, Nyad

Nailah (African) successful
Naila

Naimah (Arabic) happy
Naeemah, Naima

Naimaina (American) sweet

Naja (Greek) form of Nadia: hopeful

Najat (Arabic) safe
Nagat

Najiba (Arabic) safe
Nagiba, Nagibah, Najibah

Najla (Arabic) large-eyed

Najwa (Arabic) confidante
Nagwa

Nakecia (American) pure

Nakeya (Arabic) pure

Nakeylia (American) pure

Nakia (Arabic) purest girl
Nakea

Nakita (Russian) precocious
*Nakeeta, Nakeita, Nakya,
Naquita, Nikita*

Nala (African) loved
Nalah, Nalo

Nalani (Hawaiian) calming
Nalanie, Nalany

Nalin (Native American)
serene maiden

Nalinee (Indian) lotus girl
Nalini

Nalini (American) form of
Nalani: calming

Nallely (Spanish) friend
Nalelee, Naleley, Nallel

Nalukea (Hawaiian) sky girl

Nami (Japanese) rides a wave
Namiko

Namisha (African) content
with life

Namono (African) twin

Nampeyo (Native American)
female snake; sly
Nampayo, Nampayu

Namrata (Indian) demure

Nan (German/Scottish/English)
bold; graceful
Na, Nana, Nannie, Nanny

Nana (Hebrew) form of Ann:
loving; hospitable

Nanabah (Hebrew) form of
Ann: loving; hospitable

Nanala (Hebrew) form of
Ann: loving; hospitable

Nanalie (American) form of
Natalie: born on Christmas
Nan, Nana, Nanalee

Nance (American) giving
Nans

Nancy (English/Irish)
generous woman
*Nan, Nancee, Nanci, Nancie,
Nansee, Nonie*

Nandana (Hindi) delightful;
challenges
Nandini, Nandita

Nandini (Indian) gives
happiness

Nanek (Hebrew) form of
Nancy: generous woman
Naneka, Naneki, Naneta

Nanette (French) giving and
gracious
Nanet

Nani (Greek) charming
beauty
Nan, Nannie

Nanice (American) open-
hearted
*Nan, Naneece, Naneese,
Naniece*

Nanie (Hawaiian) charismatic
beauty

Nanise (American) form of
Nan: bold; graceful

Nanna (Scandinavian) brave
Nana

Nanon (French) slow to
anger
Nan, Nanen

Nanvah (African) God's gift;
an infant

Nao (Japanese) truthful;
pleasing

Naola (American) form of
Naomi: beautiful woman

Naoma (Hebrew) lovely

Naomi (Hebrew) beautiful
woman
*Naoma, Naomia, Naomie,
Naomy, Naynay, Nene, Neoma,
Noami, Noemi, Noemie, Noma,
Nomah, Nomi*

Naone (Hawaiian) fragrant

Naora (Native American)
happy

Naoya (Asian) happy

Nara (Greek/Japanese)
happy; dreamy
Narah, Nera

Narbata (Biblical) place name

Narbona (Spanish) place
name

Narcedalia (Spanish) dark
flower

Narcisista (Spanish) self-
absorbed

Narcissa (Greek) narcissistic
*Narcisa, Narcisse, Narkissa,
Nars*

Narcisse (French) self-
absorbed

Narcissie (Greek) conceited;
daffodil
*Narci, Narcis, Narcissa,
Narcisse, Narcissey, Narsee,
Narsey, Narsis*

Narcy (French) self-absorbed

Narda (Latin) fragrant

Narelle (Australian) of the
sea

Narendara (Indian) form of
Narendra man of Indra:
goddess of thunder and rain;
powerful

Naresha (Hindi) ruler; wise

Nari (Japanese) thunders
loudly

Narilla (Gypsy) boisterous
Narrila, Narrilla

Naroline (American) form of
Caroline: little; womanly

Narses (American) self-
absorbed

Nartlyn (American) self-
conscious

Nasaria (Spanish) miracle

Nascha (Native American)
owl; watchful

Naseem (Hindi) breezy

Nasha (Spanish) miracle

Nashae (American) miracle

Nashan (Origin unknown)
miracle child

Nashota (Native American)
second twin

Nasia (Hebrew) miraculous
child
*Naseea, Naseeah, Nasiah,
Nasya, Nsayah*

Nasnan (Native American)
miracle child; mystical

Naspa (Hebrew) form of
Nasia: miraculous child
Nasia, Nasya

Nasrin (Hindi) wild rose
Nasreen

Nastasia (Greek/Russian)
gorgeous girl
Nas, Nastasha, Natasie

Nasya (Hebrew) God's
miracle
Nasia

Nat (American) form of
Natalie: born on Christmas
Natt

Nata (Latin) saving

Natalia (Russian) form of
Natalie: born on Christmas
*Nat, Nata, Natala, Natalea,
Natalee, Natalie, Natalya,
Nati, Nattie, Nattlee, Natty*

Natalie ○ ❶ (Latin) born on
Christmas
*Natala, Natalee, Natalene,
Natalia, Natalina, Nataline,
Natalka, Natalya, Natelie,
Nathalia, Nathalie*

Natane (Native American)
daughter; giving

Nataniah (Hebrew) God's
gift
*Natania, Nataniela,
Nataniella, Natanielle,
Natanya, Nathania,
Nathaniella, Nathanielle,
Netana, Netanela, Netania,
Netaniah, Netaniela,
Netaniella, Netanya, Nethania,
Nethanisah, Netina*

Natarsha (American)
splendid
Natarsh, Natarshah

Natasha (Russian) form of
Natalie: born on Christmas
*Nastasia, Nastassia, Nastassja,
Nastassya, Nastasya, Natacha,
Natashah, Natashia, Natassia,
Nitasha, Tashi, Tashia, Tasis,
Tassa, Tassie*

Natesa (Hindi) goddess

Nathadria (Hebrew)
feminine form of Nathan:
God's gift to mankind
*Natania, Nath, Nathe, Nathed,
Nathedrea, Natty, Thedria*

Nathalie (French) form of
Natalie: born on Christmas
Natalie

Nathitfa (Arabic) unflawed
*Nathifa, Nathifah, Natifa,
Natifah*

Nation (American) spirited;
patriotic
Nashon, Nayshun

Natividad (Spanish)
Christmas baby

Natka (Polish) hope for
tomorrow

Natka (Russian) wonders;
hopes

Natosha (African American)
form of Natasha: born on
Christmas
Nat, Natosh, Natoshe, Natty

Natsu (Japanese) summer's
child
Natsuko, Natsuyo

Nauasia (Latin) kind
princess in *The Odyssey*

Navaira (Spanish) lovely girl

Naveen (Spanish) snowing

Navita (Hindi) new
Nava, Navite

Navy (American) daughter of
a member of the Navy; dark
blue

Nawal (Arabic) gifted

Nayana (Irish) form of Neala:
spirited

Nayeli (African) of
beginnings

Nayo (African) joy baby

Nazihah (Arabic) truthful

Nazira (Arabic) equality
Nazirah

Nazly (American) idealistic
Nazlee, Nazli, Nazlie

Neal (Irish) spirited
Neale, Neel, Neil

Neala (Irish) spirited
*Neal, Nealie, Nealy, Neeli,
Neelie, Neely, Neila, Neile,
Neilla, Neille*

Nealy (Irish) winner
Nealee, Nealey, Neali, Nealie

Neapolis (Biblical) place name

Neary (English) form of
Nerissa: snail; movves slowly
*Nearee, Nearey, Neari, Nearie,
Neeree, Neerey, Neeri, Neerie,
Neery*

Neasa (Irish) sweet

Neata (Russian) born on
Christmas
Neeta

Neba (Latin) misty
Neeba, Niba, Nyba

Necati (Spanish) sad

Necedah (Native American)
yellow hair

Nechama (Hebrew) comforts
others
*Nachmi, Necha, Neche,
Nehama*

Neche (Spanish) pure

Nechona (Spanish) pure

Neci (Hungarian) intense

Necie (Hungarian) intense
Neci

Necolae (Spanish) form of
Nicole: spontaneous; winning

Necole (French) winning

Neda (Slavic) sunday baby
Nedda, Neddie, Nedi

Nedaviah (Hebrew)
generous girl
Nedavia, Nedavya, Nediva

Nedda (English) born to
money
Ned, Neddy

Nedra (English) secretive
Ned, Nedre

Nedwyn (American) ned's
friend

Nedya (American) flourishes

Neeka (American) flourishes

Neelima (Indian) flourishes;
sapphire
Neelam, Neela

Neely (Irish) sparkling smile
Nealy, Neelee, Neilie, Nelie

Neema (Hebrew) melodious

Neenah (Native American)
flowing water

Neevay (American) gives

Nefertari (Egyptian) beautiful
queen

Nefris (Spanish) glamorous
Nef, Neff, Neffy, Nefras, Nefres

Neh (Hebrew) form of
Nehara: light

Neha (Hindi) loves
Nehali, Nehi

Neha (Indian) rainy

Nehanda (Hebrew)
comforter

Neia (African) promising

Neiana (Slavic) winning

Neidy (Spanish) winning

Neiley (Irish) winner
*Neelee, Neeley, Neeli, Neelie,
Neely, Neilee, Neili, Neilie,
Neily*

Neilytta (American) winning

Neima (Hindi) growing; tree

Neith (Egyptian) feminine
Neit, Neithe

Neka (Native American) wild

Nekeisha (African American) bold spirit
Nek, Nekeishah, Nekesha, Nekisha, Nekkie

Nekia (Arabic) unblemished

Nekoma (Native American) uninhibited; new moon

Neld (American) blonde

Nelda (American) friend
Neldah, Nell, Nellda, Nellie

Nelemita (Spanish) honest

Nelia (Spanish) form of Cornelia: practical
Neelia, Neely, Nela, Nelie, Nene

Nelida (Spanish) honest

Nelka (Spanish) yellow hair
Nela

Nell (English) sweet charmer
Nelle, Nellie

Nellena (American) honest

Nellie (English) form of Cornelia: practical; form of Eleanor: lighthearted
Nel, Nela, Nell, Nelle, Nelli, Nelly

Nelliene (American) form of Nellie: practical; lighthearted
Nell, Nelli, Nellienne

Nelvia (Greek) brash
Nell, Nelvea

Nelwynette (American) nell's friend

Nemera (Hebrew) leopard; exotic

Nemesis (Mythological) goddess of justice and retribution

Nemoria (American) crafty
Nemorea

Nenan (American) sea child

Nenet (Egyptian) sea goddess

Nenita (Spanish) of the sea

Neola (Greek) new baby
Neolah

Nepa (Arabic) talented

Nera (Hebrew) candlelight
Neria, Neriah, Neriya

Nereida (Spanish) sea nymph
Nere, Nereide, Nereyda, Neri, Nireida

Neressa (Greek) coming from the sea
Narissa, Nene, Nerissa, Nerisse

Nerida (Greek) sea nymph
Nerice, Nerina, Nerine, Nerisse, Neryssa, Rissa

Nerissa (English) snail; moves slowly
Nerisa, Nerise

Nerizza (Spanish) slow

Nerthus (Scandinavian) masterful

Nerys (Welsh) ladylike
Neris, Neriss, Nerisse

Neshalinda (Spanish) peak of beauty

Nesiah (Greek) lamb; meek
Nesia, Nessia, Nesya, Nisia, Nisiah, Nisva

Nessa (Irish) devout
Nessah

Nessie (Greek) form of Vanessa: flighty
Nese, Nesi, Ness

Nest (Welsh) pure
Nesta

Nestora (Spanish) she is leaving
Nesto, Nestor

Neta (Hebrew) growing and flourishing

Netania (Hebrew) form of Nathaniel: God's gift

Netia (Hebrew) form of Neta: growing and flourishing

Netira (Spanish) flourishing

Netis (Native American) worthwhile

Netra (American) maturing well
Net, Netrah, Netrya, Nettie

Netta (Scottish) champion
Nett, Nettie

Nettie (French) gentle
Net, Neta, Netta, Netti, Nettia, Netty

Neva (English) new child

Neva (Russian/English) the newest; snow
Neeva, Neve, Niv

Nevada (Spanish) girl who loves snow
Nev, Nevadah

Nevaeh ✪ (American) heaven spelled backward

Neve (Irish) promising princess

Neviah (Irish) form of Nevina: she worships God
Nevia

Nevina (Irish) she worships God
Nev, Niv, Nivena, Nivina

Newlin (Last name as first name) healing
Newlinn, Newlinne, Newlyn, Newlynn

Neya (Spanish) wishful

Neyda (Spanish) pure
Ney

Neza (Slavic) form of Agnes: pure
Neysa

Ngabile (African) aware; knowing

Ngozi (African) fortunate

Ngu (African) peaceful

Nguyet (Vietnamese) moon child

Nia (Greek) priceless
Niah

Niabi (Native American) fawn; docile

Niamh (Irish) promising

Niandrea (Invented) form of Diandro: special
Andrea, Nia, Niand, Niandre

Niani (Spanish) icon

Nibal (Arabic) completed

Nibedita (Spanish) nubile

Nicaea (Biblical) place name

Nicelda (American) industrious
Niceld, Nicelde, Nicey

Nichole (French) light and lively
Nichol

Nichols (Last name as first name) smart
Nick, Nickee, Nickels, Nickey, Nicki, Nickie, Nicky, Nikels

Nick (American) form of Nicole: winning
Nik

Nicki (French) form of Nicole: winning
Nick, Nickey, Nicky, Niki

Nicks (American) fashionable
Nickee, Nickie, Nicksie, Nicky, Nix

Nico (Italian) victorious
Nicco, Nicko, Nikko, Niko

Nicola (Italian) lovely singer
Nekola, Nick, Nikkie, Nikola

Nicolasa (Spanish)
spontaneous; winning
Nico, Nicole

Nicole ✪ (French) winning
*Nacole, Nichole, Nick, Nickie,
Nikki, Nikol, Nikole*

Nicolette (French) a tiny
Nicole; little beauty
*Nettie, Nick, Nickie, Nicoline,
Nikkolette, Nikolet*

Nicolie (French) sweet
Nichollie, Nikolie

Nicomedia (Biblical) place
name

Nicopolis (Biblical) place
name

Nida (Greek) sweet girl

Nidhi (Indian) beloved gift

Nidia (Latin) home-loving
Nidie, Nidya

Niecy (Spanish) pure

Niemi (Origin unknown)
beauty
Nyemi

Niesha (African American)
virginal
Neisha, Nesha, Nesia, Nessie

Nieves (Spanish) snow
maiden

Nieves (Spanish) snows
Neaves, Ni, Nievez, Nievis

Nihal (Greek) form of Nicole:
spontaneous; winning

Nika (Scandinavian) God's
child

Nike (Greek) goddess of
victory; fleet of foot; a winner

Nikeesha (American) form
of Nikita: daring
*Niceesha, Nickeesha, Nickisha,
Nicquisha, Nykesha*

Niki (American) form of
Nicole: winning and Nikita:
daring
*Nick, Nicki, Nicky, Nik, Nikki,
Nikky*

Nikita (Russian) daring
Nakeeta, Niki, Nikki, Niquitta

Nikithia (African American)
winning; frank
Kithi, Kithia, Nikethia, Niki

Niko (Greek) form of Nikola:
lovely singer
Neeko, Nyko

Nikole (Greek) winning
Nik, Niki

Nilana (Combo) nila and
Lana

Nilanjana (Indian) girl of
Nile

Nile (Biblical) place name;
form of the Nile River

Niles (American) of the Nile
River

Nili (Hebrew) plant;
flourishes

Nilima (Indian) blue

Nilsine (Scandinavian) wine;
ages well

Nima (Arabic) blessed
*Neema, Neemah, Nema,
Nimah*

Nimfa (Spanish) blessed

Nina
(Russian/Hebrew/Spanish)
bold girl
Neena, Nena, Ninah

Ninel (Spanish) girlish

Ninelle (Spanish) girlish

Ninetta (American) form of
Nanette: giving and gracious
Nineta

Ninette (American) form of
Nanette: giving and gracious

Nineveh (Biblical) place name

Nini (Hungarian) forgiving
*Ninee, Niney, Ninie, Ninnee,
Ninney, Ninni, Ninnie, Niny*

Ninon (French) feminine
Ninen

Ninoska (Russian) form of
Nina: bold girl

Niobe (Greek) vain

Nipa (Hindi) stream

Nira (Hindi) night
Neera, Nyra

Niranjana (Hindi) full moon

Nirel (Hebrew) light of
knowledge

Nirvana (Hindi) completion;
oneness with God
Nirvahna, Nirvanah

Nirveli (Hindi) water babe

Nisha (Hindi) nighttime
Nishi

Nishi (Japanese) from the
west; sincere
Nishie, Nishiko, Nishiyo

Nisibis (Biblical) place name;
feminine

Nissa (Hebrew) symbolic
Nisa, Niss, Nissah, Nissie

Nissie (Scandinavian) pretty;
elf
Nisse, Nissee

Nita (Hebrew) form of
Juanita: believer in gracious
God; forgiving
Neeta, Nitali, Nite, Nittie

Nitalooma (American) moral

Nitara (Hindi) well grounded

Niteen (American) growing

Nitsa (Greek) form of Helen:
beautiful; light

Nituna (Native American)
sweet daughter

Niu (Chinese) girlish;
confident

Niva (Spanish) form of Neva:
new child
Neva

Nivaeh (Spanish) form of
Nieves: snow maiden

Nivea (Spanish) reborn

Nixi (German) mystical
Nixee, Nixie

Niy (American) lively
Nye

Nizana (Hebrew) form of
Nitzana: budding beauty
Nitza, Nitzana, Zana

Noa (Hebrew) chosen
Noah

Noami (Hebrew) form of
Naomi: beautiful woman
*Noamee, Noamey, Noamie,
Noamy*

Nobantu (African) able

Noel (Latin) born on
Christmas
Noela, Noelle, Noellie, Noli

Noelan (Hawaiian)
Christmas girl

Noelani (Hawaiian)
Christmas child

Noelle (French) Christmas
baby
Noel, Noell

Noemian (Spanish) pleases

Noga (Hebrew) light of day

Noheali (Hawaiian)
Christmas

Nohelia (Hispanic) kind
Nohelya

Noicha (African) light heart
Nolcha

Noirin (Irish) form of Norin:
acknowledging others

Nokomis (Native American)
moon child

Noksu (African) princess

Nola (Latin) sensual
Nolah, Nolana, Nole, Nolie

Nolan (Latin) bell; form of
Nola: sensual
Nolen, Nolyn

Noleen (Irish) known

Noleta (Latin) reluctant
Nolita

Nolia (American) known

Nolina (Spanish) reticent

Nomalanga (Hawaiian)
lingers

Nombeko (African) honored
child

Nombese (African) wonder
girl

Nomble (African) beautiful
Nombi

Nomita (Spanish) wins

Nomusa (African)
goodhearted

Nona (Latin) ninth; knowing
*Nonah, Noni, Nonie, Nonn,
Nonna, Nonnah*

Noni (Latin) ninth child

Nonie (Spanish) ninth child

Noor (Hindi) lights the world
Noora

Nora
(Greek/Scandinavian/Scottish)
light
Norah, Noreh

Norazah (Malaysian) light

Norberta (German) famous
girl from the north

Noreen (Latin)
acknowledging others
*Noreena, Norene, Noire, Norin,
Norine, Norinne, Nureen*

Norell (Scandinavian)
northern girl
Narelle, Norelle

Norena (American) leads

Nori (Japanese) normal

Norika (Japanese) athletic
Nori, Norike

Noriko (Japanese) follows
tradition

Norita (Spanish) form of
Nora: light

Norlaili (Asian) northern

Norlita (Spanish) knowing

Norma (Latin) gold standard
*Noey, Nomah, Norm, Normah,
Normie*

Norna (Scandinavian) time
goddess

Norrie (Asian) traditional
Nori

Norris (English) serious
Nore, Norrus

Nota (American) negative
Na, Nada, Not

Notaku (Asian) dealing with
grief

Noula (Irish) form of Nuala:
white
Noulah

Noura (Arabic) light girl
Nourah

Nourbese (African)
wonderful

Nouvel (French) new

Nova (Latin) energetic; new
Noova, Novah, Novella, Novie

Novak (Last name as first
name) emphatic
Novac

Novella (Latin) new

Novena (Latin) blessing;
prayerful
Noveena, Novina, Novyna

Novia (Spanish) girlfriend

Novia (Spanish) sweetheart
Nov, Novie, Nuvia

Nowell (American) form of
Noelle: Christmas baby
Nowel, Nowele, Nowelle

Noyola (Spanish) knowing

Nu (Vietnamese) confident
Niu

Nuala (Irish) white

Nubia (Egyptian) white

Nudar (Arabic) golden girl

Nueva (Spanish) new; fresh
Nue, Nuey

Nuha (Arabic) great mind

Numa (Spanish) delightful
Num

Nuna (Native American) girl
of the land

Nunia (Native American) girl
of the land

Nunu (Vietnamese) friendly

Nur (Arabic) bright light
Nura, Nuri, Nurya

Nura (Aramaic) light-footed
Noora, Noura, Nurrie

Nuria (Arabic) light
*Noor, Noura, Nur, Nuriah,
Nuriel*

Nurit (Hebrew) form of
Nurita: flower
Nurice, Nurita

Nurlene (American)
boisterous
Nerlene, Nurleen

Nuru (African) light of day

Nusi (Hungarian) form of
Hannah: merciful; God-
blessed

Nutan (Native American)
heart

Nuvia (American) new
Nuvea

Nyasia (Greek) starts life

Nyckillan (American) form
of Nicky: smart

Nydia (Latin) nest-loving;
home and hearth woman
*Nidia, Nidiah, Ny, Nydiah,
Nydie, Nydya*

Nyla (Arabic) successful;
astounding
Nila

Nylee (American) girl of Nile

Nylene (American) shy
*Nyle, Nylean, Nyleen, Nyles,
Nyline*

Nyque (American) sea child

Nyra (American) sea child

Nyree (Asian) seagoing

Nysa (Greek) life-starting
*Nisa, Nissa, Nissie, Nysa,
Nyssa*

Nyura (African) light

Nyx (Greek) lively
Nix

Oak (Botanical) sturdy

Oakene (Botanical) sturdy

Oanna (Hawaiian) oceanic

Oba (Mythology) river goddess

Obala (African) form of Oba: river goddess
Oballa, Obla, Obola

Obdulia (Spanish) comforts

Obede (English) obedient
Obead

Obedience (American) obedient
Obey

Obelia (Greek) needle; cautious
Obellia, Obel, Obiel

Obey (American) obedient

Obioma (African) kind

Oceana (Greek) ocean-loving; name given to those with astrological signs that have to do with water
Oceonne, Ocie, Oh

Ocin (Origin unknown) comes into life

Octavia (Latin) eighth child; born on eighth day of the month; musical
Octave, Octavie, Octivia, Octtavia, Ottavia, Tave, Tavi, Tavia, Tavie

Oda (Hebrew) praises the Lord

Odalis (Spanish) humorous
Odales, Odallis, Odalous, Odalus

Oddrun (Scandinavian) secret love
Oda, Odd, Oddr

Oddveig (Scandinavian) woman with spears

Ode (African) born on a road

Odeda (Hebrew) strength of character

Odeen (Hebrew) praises

Odele (Hebrew/Greek) melodious
Odela, Odelle, Odie

Odelette (Greek) melodic; rich
Odelet, Odette

Odelia (Hebrew/Greek) singer of spiritual songs
Odele, Odelle, Odie, Odila, Odile, Othelia

Odelimpia (Spanish) melodic; wealthy

Odelinda (Hebrew) praises

Odelita (Spanish) vocalist
Odelite

Odera (Hebrew) works the soil

Odessa (English) traveler on an odyssey
Odessah, Odie, Odissa

Odette (French) good girl
Oddette, Odet, Odetta

Odhairnait (Irish) little and green; elfin-like

Odile (French) sensuous
Odyll

Odilia (Spanish) wealthy
Eudalia, Odalia, Odella,
Odylia, Othilia

Odina (Native American)
mountain girl

Odine (Scandinavian) rules

Odiya (Hebrew) God's song

Odra (English) affluent

Odrenne (American) rich

Ofa (Polynesian) loving

Ofira (Hebrew) golden girl

Ogin (Native American) rose

Ohara (Japanese) meditative
Oh

Ohela (Hebrew) tent; nature-
loving

Oheo (Native American)
beauty

Oira (Latin) form of Ora:
glowing

Okalani (Hawaiian) heavenly
child

Okei (Japanese) form of Oki:
born mid-ocean; loves the
water

Oki (Japanese) born mid-
ocean; loves the water

Oksana (Russian) praise to
God
Oksanah, Oksie

Ola (Scandinavian) bold
Olah

Olabisi (African) joy

Olaide (American) lovely;
thoughtful
Olai, Olay, Olayde

Olaug (Scandinavian) loves
her ancestors; loyal

Olda (Spanish) snow child

Oldriska (Czech) ruling
noble
Olda, Oldra, Oldrina, Olina,
Oluse

Oleda (Spanish) audacious

Oleia (Greek) smooth

Olena (Russian) generous
Olenya

Olenka (Russian) form of
Helen: beautiful; light

Olenta (Origin unknown)
sweet

Olesia (Greek) regal

Oleta (Greek) true
Oletta

Olga (Russian) holy woman
Ola, Olgah, Ollie

Olgicia (Scandinavian) holy
child

Oliana (Polynesian) oleander;
beautiful

Olida (Spanish) lighthearted
Oleda

Olidie (Spanish) light
Oli, Olidee, Olydie

Olina (Hawaiian) joy
Oleen, Oline

Olinda (Latin) fragrant

Oline (Hawaiian) happy
Olina

Olino (Spanish) scented
Olina, Oline

Olisa (African) loves God

Olive (Latin) subtle
Olyve

Olivia ✪ ✫ (English)
flourishing
Alivia, Olive, Olivea, Oliveah,
Oliviah, Ollie

Olubayo (African) resplendent

Olufemi (African) God loves her

Olva (Latin) form of Olivia: flourishing

Olvyen (Welsh) footprint in white; lasting impression

Olwen (Welsh) magical; white
Olwynn

Olwyn (Welsh) holy friend

Olya (Latin) perfect
Olyah

Olympia (Greek) heavenly woman
Olimpia, Ollie, Olympe, Olympie

Olynda (Invented) form of Lynda: pretty girl
Lyn, Lynda, Olin, Olinda, Olynde

Oma (Hebrew) reverant
Omah

Omana (Hindi) womanly

Omani (African) devout

Omanie (Origin unknown) exuberant
Omanee

Omari (African) believer

Omayra (Latin) fragrant
Oma, Omyra

Omega (Greek) last is best

Omemee (Native American) dove; peaceful

Omesha (African American) splendid
Omesh, Omie, Omisha

Omie (Italian) homebody
Omee

Ominotago (Native American) sweet sound

Omolara (African) birth timed well; welcome baby

Omora (Arabic) red-haired

Omorose (African) lovely

Omri (Arabic) red-haired

Omusa (African) adored

Omusupe (African) precious baby

Ona (Latin) the one
Oona

Onamwa (Native American) from the river

Onatah (Native American) earth child

Onawa (Native American) alert

Ondina (Latin) water spirit
Ondi, Ondine, Onyda

Ondrea (Czech) form of Andrea: feminine
Ondra

Ondreja (Czech) form of Andrea: feminine

Oneida (Native American) anticipated
Ona, Oneeda, Onida, Onie, Onyda

Oni (African) desired child

Onia (Latin) one and only

Onie (Latin) flamboyant
Oh, Oona, Oonie, Una

Onita (American) holy

Onora (Latin) honorable
Onoria, Onorine

Ontina (Origin unknown) an open mind
Ontine

Onyx (Latin) pretty shine

Oona (Latin) one alone
Oonagh, Oonah

Opa (Native American) owl;
stares

Opal (Hindi) the opal;
precious
Opale, Opalle, Opie

Opalina (Sanskrit) gem
Opaline

Ophelia (Greek) helpful
woman; character from
Shakespeare's *Hamlet*
*Ofelia, Ofilia, Ophela, Ophelie,
Ophlie, Phelia, Phelie*

Ophira (Hebrew) fawn;
lovable
Ofira

Ophrah (Biblical) place name;
helpful

Opportina (Italian) sees
opportunity; successful
Opportuna

Oprah (Hebrew) one who
soars; excellent
*Ophie, Ophrie, Opra, Oprie,
Orpah*

Ora (Greek) glowing
Orah, Orie

Orabel (Latin) believes in
prayer
*Orabelle, Oribel, Oribella,
Oribelle*

Oraleyda (Spanish) light of
dawn
Ora, Oraleydea, Oralida

Oralie (Hebrew) light of
dawn
Oralee, Orali, Orla

Orange (English) warm

Oranna (Australian) sought
after

Orbelina (American) excited;
dawn
*Lina, Orbe, Orbee, Orbeline,
Orbey, Orbi, Orby*

Orchard (American) fruitful

Ordan (American) form of
Jordan: excellent descendant

Ordella (Latin) form of Ora:
glowing

Orea (Latin) form of Ora:
glowing

Oreille (Latin) form of Oriel:
golden light

Orela (Latin) form of Oriole:
golden light

Orella (Latin) golden girl
Oralla

Orelle (Italian) feminine

Orenda (Place name) orinda,
California; lovely gold

Orene (French) nurturing
Orane, Orynne

Oresty (Greek) form of
Orestes: leader

Orestynna (Greek) form of
Orestes: leader

Oreun (Greek) star

Orfelinda (Spanish) pretty
dawn
Orfelinde, Orfelynda

Orgina (Greek) origins

Orianettea (Italian) form of
Orianna: sunny; dawn

Orianna (Latin) sunny; dawn
*Oria, Orian, Oriana, Oriane,
Orianna, Oriannah, Orie*

Orin (Irish) dark-haired
Oren, Orinn

Oringa (Invented) golden

Orino (Japanese) works
outside
Ori

Oriole (Latin) golden light
*Oreilda, Oreole, Oriel, Oriella,
Oriol, Oriola*

Orit (Spanish) dawn

Orita (Spanish) dawn

Oritha (Greek) motherly

Orithna (Greek) natural

Orla (Irish) gold

Orlain (French) famed

Orlaith (Irish) golden lady

Orlanda (German) celebrity

Orlena (Russian) sharp-eyed

Orlenda (Russian)
eagle-eyed
Orlinda

Orly (French) busy
Orlee

Ormanda (Latin) noble
Ormie

Ormey (German) sea child

Orna (Irish) dark-haired
Ornah, Ornas, Ornie

Ornice (Irish) pale face

Oropeza (Spanish) peaceful

Orpah (Hebrew) escapes;
fawn
*Ophra, Ophrah, Orpa, Orpha,
Orphy*

Orrilla (Spanish) gold

Orrine (French) golden

Orsa (Greek) form of Ursula:
little female bear

Orseline (Latin) bearlike

Orshan (American) of stars

Ortega (Spanish) nettles

Ortensia (Italian) form of
Hortense: caretaking the
garden

Orthia (Greek)
straightforward

Ortia (Spanish) golden child

Ortrud (Scandinavian) form
of Gertrude: beloved
Ortrude

Orva (French) golden girl
Or, Orvan, Orvah

Orwenn (Welsh) waves

Orya (Origin unknown)
forthcoming

Osa (American) praises God

Osana (Latin) praises the
Lord

Osarma (Origin unknown)
sleek

Osbely (Spanish) lovely you

Osen (Japanese) one in a
thousand

Oseye (African) happy

Osithe (Place name) form of
Ostia, Italy: together
Osyth

Osni (Spanish) bearlike

Osroene (Biblical) place name

Ostia (Biblical) place name

Osyka (Native American)
eagle-eyed

Otellia (Spanish) form of
Othelia: singer of spiritual
songs

Otha (German) excels

Otha (Spanish) form of
Othelia: singer of spiritual
songs

Otilia (Slavic) fotrunate

Otilie (Czech) fortunate girl

Otina (Origin unknown) fortunate

Ottavia (English) form of Octavia: eighth child; born on the eighth day of the month; musical

Otthild (German) prospers
Ottila, Ottilia, Ottilie, Otylia

Ottilie (Czech) lucky omen

Otylia (Polish) rich
Oteelya

Ouida (Literature) for the Victorian author Ouida; romantic

Ourania (Greek) heavenly

Ovalia (Spanish) helpful
Ova, Ove, Ovelia

Ovanna (Italian) feminine form of Ivan: believer in a gracious God; reliable one

Ovida (Hebrew) worships

Ovidea (German) sheep herder; believer

Ovyena (Spanish) helps

Owen (Welsh) wellborn

Owena (Welsh) feisty
Oweina, Owina, Owinne

Oya (Africa) invited to earth

Oyama (African) called out

Oza (African) strong

Ozara (Hebrew) treasured
Ozarah

Ozelina (Spanish) strong

Ozera (Hebrew) of merit

Ozioma (Origin unknown) strength of character

Ozmeen (American) prepared

Ozora (Hebrew) rich

Paavani (Hindi) purity of the river

Paavna (Hindi) pure

Pabiola (Spanish) small girl
Pabby, Pabi, Pabiole

Paca (Spanish) free girl

Pace (Last name as first name) charismatic
Pase

Pacifica (Spanish) peaceful
Pacifika

Pacita (Spanish) free

Pacita (Spanish) peaceful

Paden (American) pious

Padgett (French) growing and learning; lovely-haired
Padge, Padget, Paget, Pagett, Pagette

Padilla (Spanish) loving

Padma (Hindi) lotus blossom

Page ○ (French) sharp; eager
Pagie, Paige, Paje, Payge

Pageant (American) theatrical
Padg, Padge, Padgeant, Padgent, Pagent

Paigene (American) youth

Paili (Irish) wished-for child

Paisha (Slavic) wise

Paisley (Scottish) patterned
Paislee, Pazley

Paiton (English) from a warring town; sad

Paiva (Scandinavian) sun goddess

Paiz (Spanish) peaceful

Paka (African) kitty cat

Pal (American) friend; buddy

Pala (Native American) water

Palacia (Spanish) palace

Palakika (Hawaiian) much loved

Palanis (American) water child

Palcey (American) wise

Palemon (Spanish) kind
Palem, Palemond

Paley (Last name as first name) wise
Palee, Palie

Palila (Polynesian) bird; free flight

Palla (Greek) form of Pallas: wise woman

Pallas (Greek) wise woman
Palace, Palas

Pallavi (Indian) new growth

Palma (Latin) successful
Palmah, Palmeda, Palmedah

Palmer (Latin) palm tree; balmy

Palmira (Spanish) palm-tree girl
Palmyra

Palom (Spanish) dove

Paloma (Spanish) dove
Palloma, Palometa, Palomita, Peloma

Palomaelle (Spanish) dove

Palomares (Spanish) dove

Pamela (Greek) sweet as honey
Pam, Pamala, Pamalia, Pamalla, Pamee, Pamelia, Pamelina, Pamelinn, Pamella, Pamelyn, Pamilla, Pammee, Pammela, Pammi, Pammie, Pammy, Pamyla, Pamylla

Pana (Native American) partridge; small

Panchett (American) freedom

Panda (Greek) all-knowing

Pandita (Hindi) learned

Pandora (Greek) a gift; curious
Pan, Pand, Panda, Pandie, Pandorah, Pandorra, Panndora

Panea (Biblical) place name; open

Panfila (Greek) befriends all

Pang (Chinese) innovative

Panga (Native American) nature

Pangiota (Greek) all is holy

Panna (Hindi) emerald; knowing

Pannonia (Biblical) place name; friend of all

Panola (Greek) all

Panphila (Greek) all loving
Panfila, Panfyla, Panphyla

Panse (Greek) pansy flower

Pansee (Greek) pansy flower

Pansy (Greek) fragrant
Pan, Pansey, Pansie, Panze, Panzee, Panzie

Pantea (Indian) all-loving of gods

Pantelis (Greek) happy with all

Panthea (Greek) loves all
gods

Panther (Greek) wild; all
gods
*Panthar, Panthea, Panthur,
Panth*

Panya (Greek) she is crowned

Panyin (African) the older
twin

Paola (Italian) firebrand

Paolabella (Italian) lovely
firebrand

Papina (African) vine; clings

Paradise (Word as name)
dream girl

Parenth (American)

Parima (Indian) perfection

Paris (French) capital of
France; graceful woman
*Pareece, Parie, Parice, Parisa,
Parris, Parrish*

Parissa (Spanish) form of
Paris: capital of France;
graceful woman

Pariste (American) of Paris

Paristeen (American) of
Paris

Park (Last name as first name)
of the park

Parker (English) noticed; in
the park
Park, Parke, Parkie

Parminder (Hindi) attractive

Parnelle (French) small stone
Parn, Parnel, Parnell, Parney

Paronda (Indian) good

Parslee (Botanical)
complementary
Pars, Parse, Parsley, Parsli

Partha (Greek) pure; full

Parthenia (Greek) from the
Parthenon; virtuous
*Parthania, Parthe, Parthee,
Parthena, Parthene, Parthenie,
Parthina, Parthine, Pathania,
Pathena, Pathenia, Pathina,
Thenia*

Parthenope (Greek) siren

Parthia (Biblical) place name;
pure; full

Parvani (Hindi) full moon
Parvina

Parvati (Hindi) mountain
child

Parvati (Indian) mountain
girl

Parvin (Hindi) star
Parveen

Pascale (French) born on a
religious holiday
*Pascal, Pascalette, Pascaline,
Pascalle, Paschale, Paskel,
Paskil*

Pascasia (French) born on
Easter
Paschasia

Pascha (Slavic) easter baby

Paschel (African) spiritual
Paschell

Pash (French) clever
Pasch

Pasha (Greek) lady by the sea
Passha

Pasionne (Spanish) passion

Pasqualina (Spanish) Easter
baby

Passion (American) sensual
Pashun, Pasyun, Pass, Passyun

Pasua (French) Easter child

Pat (Latin) form of Patricia:
woman of nobility;
unbending
Patt, Patty

Patara (Biblical) place name

Paterekia (Hawaiian)
patrician
Pakelekia

Pati (African) gathers fish

Patia (Latin) form of Patricia:
woman of nobility;
unbending

Patience (English) woman of
patience
Pacience, Paciencia, Pat, Pattie

Patric (American) form of
Patricia: woman of nobility;
unbending

Patrice (French) form of
Patricia: woman of nobility;
unbending
*Pat, Patreas, Patreece, Pattie,
Pattrice, Trece, Treecc*

Patricia (Latin) woman of
nobility; unbending
*Pat, Patreece, Patreice, Patria,
Patric, Patrica, Patrice,
Patricka, Patrizia, Patrisha,
Patsie, Patsy, Patti, Pattie,
Patty, Tricia, Trish, Trisha*

Patriena (Slavic) form of
Patrice: woman of nobility;
unbending

Patrika (Slavic) form of
Patrice: woman of nobility;
unbending

Patrina (American) noble;
patrician
*Patryna, Patrynna, Tryna,
Trynnie*

Patriz (Italian) noble

Patsy (Latin) form of Patricia:
woman of nobility;
unbending
*Pat, Patsey, Patsi, Patsie, Patti,
Patty*

Patty (English) form of
Patricia: woman of nobility;
unbeding and Patrice: svelte
Pat, Pati, Patti, Pattie

Paula (Latin) small and
feminine
*Paola, Paolina, Paulah, Paule,
Pauleen, Paulene, Pauletta,
Paulette, Paulie, Paulina,
Pauline, Paulita, Pauly,
Paulyn, Pavla, Pavlina,
Pavlinka, Pawlah, Pawlina,
Pola*

Paulee (American) small

Paulette (French) form of
Paula: small and feminine
*Paula, Paulett, Paulie,
Paullette*

Paulina (Latin/Italian) small;
lovely
Paula, Paulena, Paulie

Pauline (Latin) form of Paula:
small and feminine
Pauleen, Paulene

Paulisee (American) small

Pausha (Hindi) lunar month;
moonlike

Pavana (Origin unknown)
form of Paulina: small and
feminine
Pavani

Pavana (Indian) holy

Pax (Latin) peace goddess

Paxton (Latin) peaceful
Pax, Paxten, Paxtun

Payton ❶ (Last name as first name) aggressive
Pay, Paye, Payten, Paytun, Peyton

Paz (Hebrew/Spanish) sparkling; peaceful
Paza, Pazia, Paziah, Pazice, Pazit, Paziya, Pazya

Paza (Hebrew) golden child
Paz

Pazzy (Latin) peaceful
Paz, Pazet

Peace (English) peaceful woman
Pea, Peece

Peaches (American) outrageously sweet
Peach, Peachy

Peakalika (Hawaiian) happiness

Pearl (Latin) jewel from the sea
Pearla, Pearle, Pearaleen, Pearlena, Pearlette, Pearley, Pearlie, Pearline, Pearly, Perl, Perla, Perle, Perlette, Perley, Perlie, Perly

Pearlette (American) treasured pearl

Pearline (American) treasured pearl

Pecola (American) brash
Pekola

Pedzi (Origin unknown) gold

Pefilia (Spanish) profile

Pega (Greek) form of Peggy: pearl; princess

Peggy (Greek) pearl; priceless
Peg, Peggi, Peggie

Pegma (Greek) happy

Pehel (Biblical) place name

Pei (Place name) village; from Tang Pei, China

Peigi (Scottish) pearl; priceless

Peigo (American) athletic

Peisha (American) lovely

Peke (Hawaiian) form of Bertha: bright

Pela (Polish) loves the sea; special

Pelagia (Polish) sea girl
Pelage, Pelageia, Pelagie, Pelegia, Pelgia, Pellagia

Pelagla (Greek) girl of the sea
Pelagie, Pelagi, Pelagia, Pelagias, Pelaga

Pele (Hawaiian) volcano; conflicted

Pele (Polish) weaves dreams

Peleka (Hawaiian) strong; marvel

Pelham (English) thoughtful
Pelhim, Pellam, Pellham, Pellie

Pelia (Hebrew) marvelous
Peliah, Pelya, Pelyia

Pelika (Hawaiian) strong

Pelipa (African) loves horses
Phillipa

Pella (Biblical) place name; weaves dreams

Pelulio (Hawaiian) sea treasure

Pelusium (Biblical) place name

Pemba (African) powerful

Pemelia (American) form of Pamela: sweet as honey

Penda (African) beloved

Pendant (French) necklace; adorned
Pendan, Pendanyt

Penelope (Greek) patient;
weaver of dreams
*Pela, Pelcia, Pen, Penalope,
Penelopa, Penina, Penine,
Penna, Pennelope, Penni,
Pennie, Penny, Pinelopi, Popi*

Peni (Greek) thinker

Peninah (Hebrew) pearl;
lovely
*Peni, Penie, Penina, Penini,
Peninit, Penny*

Peninia (Biblical) precious
girl

Penn (Last name as first
name) loyal

Pennelle (American) loyal

Penny (Greek) form of
Penelope: patient; weaver of
dreams
Pen, Penee, Penni, Pennie

Penthea (Spanish) orchid;
lovely
*Fentheam, Fentheas, Pentha,
Pentheam, Pentheas*

Peony (Greek) flowering;
giving praise
Pea, Peoni, Peonie

Peoria (Place name) city in
Illinois; poised

Pepita (Spanish) high-energy
Pepa, Peppita, Peta

Pepper (Latin) spicy
Pep, Peppie, Peppyr

Peppy (American) cheerful
Pep, Peppey, Peppi, Peps

Pequita (Spanish) form of
Pepita: high-energy

Perach (Hebrew) flowering
*Perah, Pericha, Pircha, Pirchia,
Pirchit, Pirchiya, Pirha*

Perano (Spanish) wanders

Perciella (Greek) great excess

Perdita (Latin) wanders away

Perea (Biblical) place name

Perel (Latin) tested
Perele

Perfecta (Spanish) perfection
Perfekta

Perga (Biblical) place name

Peridot (Arabic) green gem;
treasured
Peri

Peril (Latin) victor

Perita (Spanish) treasure

Periwinkle (Botanical) blue-
eyed; flower girl

Perla (Latin) substantial
Perlah

Perlace (Spanish) small pearl
Perl, Perlahse, Perlase, Perly

Perlette (French) pearl;
treasured
*Pearl, Pearline, Peraline, Perl,
Perle, Perlett*

Perlie (Latin) form of Pearl:
jewel from the sea
Perli, Purlie, Perly

Perlina (American) small
pearl
Pearl, Perl, Perlinna, Perlyna

Pernella (Scandinavian) rock;
dependable
Pernelle, Parnella, Pernilla

Pernille (Scandinavian) rock;
safe

Peron (Latin) travels

Perouze (Armenian)
turquoise gemstone
Perou, Perous, Perouz, Perry

Perpetua (Spanish) lasting

Perri (Greek/Latin) outdoorsy
Peri, Perr, Perrie, Perry

Perri (English) wanderer

Perrinada (American) generous

Persephone (Greek) breath of spring
Pers, Perse, Persefone, Persey

Persevera (Spanish) persevers

Pershella (American) philanthropic
Pershe, Pershel, Pershelle, Pershey, Persie, Persy

Persia (Place name) colorful
Persha, Perzha

Persis (Latin) form of Persia: colorful
Perssis

Perusia (Biblical) place name

Pesha (Hebrew) flourishing
Peshah, Peshia

Peshe (Hebrew) saved

Pessim (Native American)

Peta (English) saucy
Pet, Petra, Petrice, Petrina, Petrona, Petty

Petila (Slavic) adored

Petra (Slavic) glamorous; capable
Pet, Peti, Petrah, Pett, Petti, Pietra

Petri (Scandinavian) form of Peter: dependable; rock

Petrine (Scandinavian) rock

Petrona (Italian) reliable

Petronilla (Greek) form of Peter: dependable; rock
Petria, Petrina, Petrine, Petro, Petrone, Petronela, Petronella, Pett

Petru (Slavic) able

Petula (Latin) petulant song
Pet, Petulah, Petulia

Petunia (American) flower; perky
Pet, Petune

Pfeiffer (Last name as first name) lovely blonde; talented

Phaedra (Greek) bright
Faydra, Faydrah, Padra, Phae, Phedra

Phalba (American) offspring

Phalin (Asian) sapphire

Phan (Asian) shares

Phaselis (Biblical) place name

Phashestha (American) decorative
Phashey, Shesta

Pheakkley (Vietnamese) faithful

Pheba (Greek) smiling
Phibba

Phedella (American) lasting; loyal

Phedra (Greek) bright child
Faydra, Fedra, Phadra, Phaedra, Phedre

Phelisa (American) form of Felicity: friendly; happy

Phemia (Greek) language

Phenice (Origin unknown) enjoys life
Phenicia, Pheni, Phenica, Venice

Pheodora (Greek) God's gift to mankind

Pheresa (Spanish) form of Theresa: gardener

Phernita (American) articulate
Ferney, Phern

Phia (Irish) saint

Phila (Greek) loving
Phil, Philly

Philadelphia (Greek) loving
one's fellow man
Fill, Phil, Philly

Philana (Greek) loving
Filana, Filly, Philly

Philantha (Greek) loves
flowers

Philberta (English)
intellectual

Philene (Greek) loving others

Philenet (American) loving

Philia (American) loving

Philida (Greek) loving others
Philina, Phillada, Phillida

Philippa (Greek) horse lover
*Feefee, Felipa, Phil, Philipa,
Philippe, Phillie, Phillipina,
Phillippah, Pippa, Pippy*

Philippitta (American) loves
horses

Philise (Greek) loving
Felece, Felice, Philese

Philistia (Biblical) place name

Philly (Place name) from
Philadelphia, Pennsylvania:
loving one's fellow man
Filly, Philee, Phillie

Philma (Greek) loves others

Philomena (Greek) beloved
*Filomena, Filomina, Mena,
Phil, Phillomenah, Philomen,
Philomene, Philomina*

Philoteria (Biblical) place name

Philtherian (Greek) loving

Phiona (Scottish) form of
Fiona: fair-haired
Phionna

Phira (Greek) loves music

Phoebe (Greek) bringing
light
*Febe, Fee, Feebe, Feebs, Pheabe,
Phebe, Phebee, Pheby, Phobe,
Phoeb, Phoebey, Phoebie, Phoebs*

Phoenicia (Biblical) place
name

Phoenix (Greek) rebirth
*Fee, Fenix, Fenny, Phenix,
Phoe*

Phonsa (Origin unknown)
jubilant

Phosa (Biblical) delicate girl

Photina (Origin unknown)
fashionable

Phrgia (Biblical) place name

Phylicia (Greek) fortunate
girl
Felicia, Phillie, Phyl, Phylecia

Phyllida (Greek) lovely; leafy
bough
Filida, Phyll, Phyllyda

Phyllis (Greek) beautiful;
leafy bough; articulate;
smitten
*Fillice, Fillis, Phil, Philis,
Phillis, Philliss, Phillisse, Phyl,
Phylis, Phyllys*

Phynise (American)

Phyrus (Greek) form of
Zephyrus: breezy

Pia (Latin) devout
Peah, Piah

Picabo (Place name) city in
Idaho; swift
Peekaboo

Piedad (Spanish) devout

Pier (Greek) feminine form of
Peter: dependable; rock
Peer

Pierette (Greek) reliable
Perett, Perette, Piere

Pierina (Greek) dependable
Peir, Per, Perina, Perine, Pieryna

Pierrette (French) little rock

Piers (French) little rock

Piki (Hindi) little cuckoo

Pilar (Spanish) worthwhile;
pillar of strength

Pili (Spanish) pillar; strength

Pililani (Hawaiian) strong one

Pilisi (Hawaiian) simple life

Piluki (Hawaiian) little leaf;
small

Pilvi (Italian) cheerful
Pilvee

Pineki (Hawaiian) peanut;
tiny girl

Pinga (Hindi) dark

Pingjarje (Native American)
shy; little doe

Pingla (Hindi) goddess

Pink (American) blushing
*Pinkee, Pinkie, Pinky, Pinkye,
Pynk*

Pinquana (Native American)
fragrant girl

Piper (English) player of a
pipe; musical

Pippa (English) ebullient;
horse-lover
Pip, Pipa

Pippi (English/French)
blushing; loving horses
Pip, Pippie, Pippy

Pirene (French) rock;
dependable

Pirouette (French) ballet
term
Piro, Pirouet, Pirouetta

Pisidia (Biblical) place name;
of the water

Pita (English) comforting

Pitana (Origin unknown)
accented

Pitarra (American)
interesting
Pitarr Peta, Petah

Pity (American) sad
Pitee, Pitey, Pitie

Pixie (American) small; perky
Pixee, Pixey, Pixi

Pixie (English) zany

Placida (Latin) serenity
Plasida

Platinum (English) from the
Spanish platinal; fine metal
Plati, Platnum

Platona (Spanish) good
friend
*Pleasance, Pleasant, Pleasants,
Pleasence*

Playla (Place name)

Pleshette (American) plush
Plesh

Pleun (Origin unknown)
wordsmith

Plina (Spanish) full

Plum (Botanical) fruit;
healthy

Po (Italian) effervescent
Poe

Pocahontas (Native
American) joyful
Poca, Poka

Poe (Last name as first name)
mysterious

Poetry (Word as name)
romantic
Poe, Poesy, Poet

Polete (Hawaiian) small; kind
Poleke, Polina

Policia (Spanish) guards

Polina (Russian) small
Po, Pola, Polya

Poliquin (Last name as first
name) all-encompassing

Polishia (Slavic) smooth

Polly (Irish) devout; joyous
*Pauleigh, Paulie, Pol, Pollee,
Polley, Polli, Pollie*

Pollyanna (English) heroine
of Eleanor Porter's novel
*Polianna, Polliana, Pollie-
anna, Polly*

Polymnea (Mythology)
songstress for all

Polyxena (Mythology) very
hospitable

Pomona (Latin) apple of my
eye
Pomonah

Pomona (Mythology) bears
fruit

Pompa (Last name as first
name) pompous
Pompy

Pompey (Place name) lavish
Pomp, Pompee, Pompei, Pompy

Poni (African) second
daughter

Ponise (Spanish) sets aside
Pomice

Pony (American) wild west
girl
Poney, Ponie

Poodle (American) sweet;
curly-haired
Poo, Pood, Poodly

Poonam (Hindi) kind soul

Poppy (Latin) flower; bouncy
girl
Pop, Poppi, Poppie

Poppy-Honey (American)
sweet girl

Pora (Hebrew) fertile

Porsche (Latin) giving; high-
minded
*Porsh, Porsha, Porshe, Porshie,
Portia*

Porsha (German) giving
Porshea

Portia (Latin) a giving woman
*Porcha, Porscha, Porsh, Porsha,
Porshuh*

Posala (Native American)
good-bye to spring

Posh (American) fancy girl
Posha

Posy (American) sweet
Posee, Posey, Posie

PoupÈe (French) doll
Pou

Powder (American) gentle;
light
*Pow, Powd, Powdy, Powdyr,
PowPow*

Poweline (American) ready

Pragyata (Hindi)
knowledgeable

Prancey (American)
rambunctious

Prancine (American) form of
Francine: beautiful

Prarthana (Hindi) prays

Prasanna (Indian)
unswerving

Pratibha (Hindi)
understanding

Precia (Latin) important
*Preciah, Presha, Presheah,
Preshuh*

Preciliano (Spanish) precious

Precious (English) beloved
*Precia, Preciosa, Preshie,
Preshuce, Preshus*

Predenita (Spanish)
pretentious

Prema (Hindi) love

Premlata (Hindi) loving

Prentice (Last name as first
name) learns
Prentiss

Prescilian (Hispanic)
fashionable
Pres, Priss

Prescilline (Spanish) form of
Priscilla: wisdom of the ages

Presencia (Spanish) presents
well

Presley (English) talented
*Preslee, Preslie, Presly, Prezlee,
Prezley, Prezly*

Prestha (Hindi) dearest girl

Pretice (American) form of
Prentice: learns

Pribislava (Polish) glorifed;
helpful
Pribena, Pribka, Pribuska

Price (Welsh) loving
Pri, Prise, Pry, Pryce, Pryse

Prima (Latin) first; fresh
*Primalia, Primetta, Primia,
Primie, Primina, Priminia,
Primma, Primula*

Primalia (Spanish) prime;
first

Primavera (Italian) spring
child

Primola (Botanical) flower;
from primrose; first
Prim, Prym, Prymola

Primrose (English) rosy;
fragrant
Prim, Primie, Rosie, Rosy

Princelle (American) princess

Princess (English) precious
*Prin, Prince, Princesa,
Princessa, Princie, Prinsess*

Princy (American) form of
Princess: precious

Prisca (Latin) old spirit

Prisciliana (Spanish) wise;
old
Cissy, Priscili, Priss, Prissy

Priscilla (Latin) wisdom of
the ages
*Cilla, Precilla, Prescilla,
Pricilla, Pris, Priscella, Priscila,
Prisilla, Priss, Prissie, Prissilla,
Prissy, Prysilla*

Prisisima (Spanish) wise and
feminine
Priss, Prissy, Sima

Prisma (Hindi) cherished
baby

Prissy (Latin) form of
Priscilla: wisdom of the ages
Prisi, Priss, Prissie

Pristina (Latin) pristine

Priti (Hindi) lovely

Priya (Hindi) sweetheart
Preeya, Preya, Priyah

Prizela (Spanish) form of
Priscilla: wisdom of the ages

Prochora (Latin) leads

Promise (American) sincere
Promis

Proserpine (Mythology)
queen of the underworld;
secretive

Prospera (Latin) does well

Protima (Hindi) dancing girl

Prova (Place name) provence,
France
Pro, Proa, Provah

Pru (Latin) form of Prudence:
wise; careful
Prudie, Prue

Prudence (Latin) wise;
careful
*Perd, Pru, Prudencia, Prudie,
Prudince, Pruds, Prudu, Prudy,
Prue*

Prunella (Latin) shy
Pru, Prue, Prune, Prunie

Pryor (Last name as first
name) wealthy
Prieyer, Pryar, Prye, Pryer

Psyche (Greek) soulful
Sye, Sykie

Pua (Hawaiian) flower

Pulcheria (Italian) chubby;
curvy
Pulchia

Puma (American) cougar;
wild spirit
*Poom, Pooma, Poomah,
Pumah, Pume*

Punita (Indian) unblemished

Punsey (American) form of
Pansy: fragrant

Purity (English) virginal
Puretee, Puritie

Purnima (Hindi) full moon
baby

Pyera (Italian) sturdy;
formidable; rock
Pyer, Pyerah

Pyllyon (English) enthusiastic
Pillion, Pillyon, Pillyun

Pyrena (Greek) fiery temper

Pyria (Origin unknown)
cherished
Pyra, Pyrea

Pyrrha (Latin) fire

Pythia (Greek) prophet

Qadira (Arabic) wields power
Kadira

Qamra (Arabic) moon girl
Kamra

Qing (Origin unknown) quick

Qitarah (Arabic) aromatic

Qiturah (Arabic) aromatic
Qeturah, Quetura, Queturah

Q-Malee (American) form of
Cumale: open-hearted
*Cue, Q, Quemalee, Quemali,
Quemalie*

Quan (Chinese) goddess of
compassion

Quanda (English) queenly
*Kwanda, Kwandah, Quandah,
Qwanda*

Quanella (African American)
sparkling
Kwannie, Quanela

Quanesha (African American) singing
Kwaeesha, Kwannie, Quaneisha, Quanisha

Quantina (American) brave queen
Kwantina, Kwantynna, Quantinna, Quantyna, Tina

Qubilah (Arabic) easygoing

Queen (English) regal; special
Quanda, Queena, Queenette, Queenie

Queendiosa (American) queenly

Queenie (English) royal and dignified
Kweenie, Quee, Queen, Queeny

Queisha (American) contented child
Queysha, Queshia

Quenby (Swedish) feminine
Quenbee, Quenbey, Quenbi, Quenbie, Quinbee, Quinbie, Quinby

Quenna (English) feminine
Kwenna

Queosha (American) soulful

Querida (Spanish) dear one

Questa (French) looking for love
Kesta

Queta (Spanish) head of the house
Keta

Quiana (Origin unknown) form of Hannah: merciful; God-blessed
Qiana, Qianna, Quianna, Quiyanna

Quilla (English) writer
Kwila, Kwilla, Quila, Quillah, Quyla, Quylla

Quillee (Spanish) high spirits

Quina (African) fifth baby

Quinby (Scandinavian) living like royalty
Quenby, Quin, Quinbie, Quinnie

Quinceanos (Spanish) fifteenth child
Quin, Quince, Quincy

Quincy (French) fifth
Quince, Quincey, Quinci, Quincie, Quincy, Quinsy

Quincylla (American) popular; fifth child
Cylla, Quince, Quincy

Quindelin (American) form of Gwendolyn: mystery goddess; bright

Quinella (Latin) a girl who is as pretty as two
Quinn

Quinetra (American) fifth baby

Quinise (American) fifth baby

Quinitka (American) fifth baby

Quinn (English/Irish) smart
Quin, Quinnie

Quinta (Latin) fifth day of the month

Quintana (Latin) fifth; lovely girl
Quentana, Quinn

Quintessa (Latin) essential goodness

Quintessen (American) fifth baby

Quintilla (Latin) fifth girl
Quintina

Quintina (Latin) fifth child
*Quentina, Quintana,
Quintessa, Quintona,
Quintonetta, Quintonice*

Quintona (Latin) fifth

Quintwana (American) fifth
girl in the family
Quintuana

Quinyette (American)
likeable; fifth child
Kwenyette, Quiny

Quirina (Latin) contentious

Quisagna (Slavic) sister

Quisha (African American)
beautiful mind
Keisha, Kesha, Key

Quita (Latin) peaceful
Keeta, Keetah

Raah (Greek) saved

Rabab (Origin unknown)
different

Rabbah (Biblical) place name

Rabbit (American) lively;
energetic
Rabit

Rabia (Arabic) wind

Rabiah (Arabic) breezy

Rachael (Hebrew) form of
Rachel: peaceful as a lamb
*Rach, Rachaele, Rachal,
Rachel, Rachie, Rae, Raechal,
Rasch, Ray, Raye*

Rache (American) form of
Rachel: peaceful as a lamb

Rachel ✪ (Hebrew) peaceful
as a lamb

Rachelle (French) calm
*Rach, Rachell, Rashell,
Rashelle, Rochelle, Rachella*

Rachen (Slavic) peaceful

Rachene (French) peaceful

Rachna (Indian) organized

Racinda (Slavic) peaceful

Racquel (French) friendly
Racquelle, Raquel

Rada (Polish) glad

Radha (Indian) excels

Radha (Hindi) successful
Radhika

Radia (Slavic) happy

Radmilla (Slavic) glad;
hardworking

Rae (English) raving beauty
Raedie, Raena, Ray, Raye

Raegan (French) delicate
Reagan, Regan, Regun

Raelan (American) simple
beauty

Rafa (Arabic) joyful girl
Rafah

Rafaela (Hebrew) spiritual
Rafayela

Rafeline (French) happy

Raffaella (French) happy

Rafferty (Irish) prospering
Raferty, Raff, Raffarty, Rafty

Rageana (Spanish) form of
Regina: queen

Ragnild (Scandinavian)
goddess of war
*Ragnhild, Ragnhilda,
Ragnhilde, Ragnilda, Ranillda,
Reinheld, Renilda, Renilde,
Reynilda, Reynilde*

Raheel (Hebrew) form of Rachel: peaceful as a lamb
Raheela

Rahela (Hawaiian) lamb

Rahil (Hebrew) form of Rachel: peaceful as a lamb

Rahima (Pakistani) loving
Raheema, Raheema

Rain (English) falling water
Rainie, Reign

Raina (German) dramatic
Raine, Rainna, Rayna

Rainbow (American) bright
Rain, Rainbeau, Rainbo, Rainie

Raine (Latin) helpful friend
Raina, Rainie, Rana, Rane, Rayne

Rainey (Last name as first name) giving
Rainee, Rainie, Raney

Raisa (Russian) embraced
Rasa

Raissa (Russian) form of Rose: rose; blushing beauty

Raja (Arabic) optimist

Rajani (Hindi) dark; hopeful

Rajata (Hindi) silver

Rajata (Indian) silver; queen

Rajeana (Slavic) form of Regina: queen

Raji (Hindi) royal

Rajni (Hindi) dark night

Raka (Hindi) royal

Raleigh (Irish) admirable
Raileigh, Railey, Raley, Rawleigh, Rawley

Ralphenne (American) form of Ralph: advisor to all

Ralphina (American) form of Ralph: advisor to all
Ralphine

Rama (Hindi) godlike; good

Ramah (Biblical) place name

Ramani (Indian) lovely

Ramba (African) high goals

Ramilia (Slavic) strong

Ramina (German) lovely

Ramona (Teutonic) beautiful protector
Rae, Ramonah, Ramonna, Raymona

Ramonda (American) form of Ramona: beautiful protector

Ramsay (English) from the isle of rams; country girl
Ramsey

Ramsee (English) from the rams' land

Ramsie (English) from the rams' land

Rana (Hindi) royal

Ranchel (American) range girl

Randa (Latin) admired
Ran, Randah

Randall (English) protective of her own
Rand, Randal, Randi, Randy

Randella (American) sheltered

Randelle (American) wary
Randee, Randele

Randi (English) audacious
Randee, Randie, Randy

Rane (Scandinavian) queen-like
Rain, Raine, Ranie

Rani (Sanskrit) a queen
Rainie, Ranie

Rania (Sanskrit) regal
Ranea, Raneah, Raney, Ranie

Ranielle (French) royal; frank

Ranita (Hebrew) musical
Ranit, Ranite, Ranitra, Ranitta

Raoule (Spanish) form of
Raoul: wild heart
Raoula, Raula

Rapa (Hawaiian) lovely by
moonlight

Raphaela (Hebrew) helping
to heal
Rafaela, Rafe

Raphenn (American) dreamy

Raphia (Biblical) place name

Raphina (German) exciting

Raquel (Spanish) sensual
Racuell, Raquelle, Raqwel

Raquita (Spanish) aggressive

Rasa (Slavic) morning dew

Rasheeda (Hindi) pious
Rashee, Rashida, Rashie, Rashy

Rashidah (Arabic) on the
right path
Rashida

Rashinique (African
American) rash
Rash, Rashy

Ratna (Indian) beauty

Raula (French) advises

Ravada (Spanish) raven

Raven (English) blackbird
Ravan, Rave, Ravin

Ravenna (English) blackbird

Ravette (English) special

Ravistene (American) raven

Rawn (American) ambitious

Rawnie (Slavic) ladylike
Rawani, Rawn, Rawnee

Ray (American) simplistic
approach
Rae, Raymonde

Rayleen (American) popular
Raylene, Raylie, Rayly

Rayna (Scandinavian) strong
girl

Raynee (Scandinavian) strong

Raynekka (Slavic) raven

Raynelle (American) giving
hope; combo of Ray and Nelle
Nellie, Rae, Raenel, Raenelle

Raynette (American) ray of
hope; dancer
Raenette, Raynet

Rayola (Spanish) hopeful

Razia (Hebrew) secretive
Razeah, Raziah

Raziella (Italian) graceful

Razina (African) nice

Rea (Polish) flowing
Raya

Reagan ♀ (Last name as first
name) strong
Regan, Reganne, Reggie

Reanika (American) happy

Reanne (American) happy
Reann, Rennie, Rere, Rianne

Reason (Word as name)

Reba (Hebrew) fourth-born
Rebah, Ree, Reeba

Rebazar (Spanish) fourth
child

Rebecca ♀ (Hebrew) loyal
*Becca, Becki, Beckie, Becky,
Rebeca, Rebeka, Rebekah*

Rebi (Hebrew) friend who is steadfast
Reby, Ree, Ribi

Rebop (American) zany
Reebop

Redettea (American) righteous

Redita (Slavic) peaceful

Redonna (American) peaceful

Ree (Asian) mannered

Reed (English) red-haired
Read, Reade, Reid, Reida

Reem (Arabic) antelope; graceful

Reena (Arabic) antelope

Reenie (Greek) peace-loving
Reena, Reeni, Reeny, Ren, Rena

Reese (American) style-setting
Ree, Reece, Rees, Rere

Reeve (Last name as first name) strong

Regan (Irish) queenly
Reagan

Reganean (American) form of Regan: strong

Regeana (American) form of Regina: thoughtful
Rege, Regeanah, Regeane

Regene (Latin) queen

Regina (English/Latin) queen
Gina, Rege, Regena, Reggie, Regine

Regine (Latin) royal
Regene, Rejean

Reginia (American) queen

Regne (Slavic) leader

Rehema (African) well-grounded
Rehemah, Rehemma, Rehima

Reidee (American) red hair

Reidnilda (German) form of Reynalda: wise

Reiko (Japanese) appreciative

Rein (German) advises

Reina (Spanish) a thinker
Rein, Reinie, Rina

Reine (Spanish) form of Reina: queen

Reith (American) shy
Ree, Reeth

Rejena (Slavic) queen

Rejunda (Slavic) queen

Rekha (Hindi) focuses

Rela (German) everything
Reila, Rella

Relin (German) kind

Rella (Origin unknown) rogue

Remah (Hebrew) pale beauty
Rema, Remme, Remmie, Rima, Ryma

Remaliah (American) helps

Remata (German) helps

Remedios (Spanish) helpful

Remember (American) memorable
Remi, Remmi, Remmie, Remmy

Remi (French) woman of Rheims; jaded
Remee, Remie, Remy

Remille (French) helps

Remolda (Slavic) strong

Remonia (Slavic) strong

Ren (Asian) flower

Rena (Hebrew) joyful singer
Reena, Rinah, Rinne

Renae (French) form of
Renee: born again
Renay, Rennie, Rere

Renard (French) fox; sly
Ren, Renarde, Rynard, Rynn

Renata (French) reaching out
Renie, Renita, Rennie, Rinata

Renatha (Slavic) born again

Rene (Greek) hopeful
Reen, Reenie, Reney

Renea (French) form of
Renee: born again
Renny

Renee (French) born again
Rene, Rennie, Rere

Renetta (French) reborn
Ranetta, Renette

Renie (Latin) renewal

Renis (American) welcomed

Renita (Latin) poised
Ren, Renetta, Rennie

Renite (Latin) stubborn
Reneta, Renita

Reniti (English) upward

Renna (English) reborn

Rennyll (French) form of
Renee: born again
Renelle

Renshaw (Last name as first
name) directed

Renuka (Slavic) calm

Renzia (Greek) form of
Renee: born again
Renze

Reonne (Welsh) maiden

Resa (Greek) productive;
laughing
Reesa, Reese, Risa

Reseda (Latin) healing
Res, Reseta

Reseme (American) fragrant

Resenetta (Spanish) fragrant
flower

Reshea (American) girlish

Reshma (African)
compassionate

Reshma (Indian) sun

Resie (German) form of
Theresa: gardener

Reta (African) shakes up
*Reda, Reeda, Reeta, Rheta,
Rhetta*

Retanica (American) chaotic

Retha (German) form of
Aretha: virtuous; vocalist

Retrola (American)
retrospective

Reva (Hebrew) rainmaker
Ree, Reeva, Rere

Revada (American) revival

Reveca (Spanish) form of
Rebecca: loyal
Reba, Rebeca, Reva

Revelina (American) revival

Reveriana (Spanish) of the
river

Rew (Australian) of the spring

Rexie (American) confident
Rex, Rexi, Rexy

Reyna (Filipino) queen
Raina, Rayna, Rey

Reynalda (German) wise
Raynalda, Rey, Reyrey

Reynee (English) peaceful

Reynolds (Scottish) wispy
Rey, Reye, Reynells, Reynold

Reza (Czech) form of
Theresa: gardenerl
Rezi, Rezka, Riza

Rezeda (Spanish) prayerful

Rhea (Greek) earthy; mother
of gods; strong
Ria

Rheta (American) form of
Rita: precious pearl

Rhiall (Welsh) nymph

Rhianna (Welsh) pure
Rheanna

Rhiannon (Welsh) goddess;
intuitive
*Rhian, Rhiane, Rhianen,
Rhiann, Rhianon, Rhyan,
Rhye, Riannon*

Rhilla (Slavic) nymph

Rhoda (Greek) rosy
*Rhodie, Roda, Rodi, Rodie,
Rody, Roe*

Rhodanthe (Greek) form of
Rhodes: lovely
Rhodante

Rhodette (American) rose
girl

Rhodora (Spanish) rose girl

Rhogean (French) form of
Regine: royal

Rhola (Slavic) form of Rachel:
peaceful as a lamb

Rhon (Welsh) blessing

Rhona (Scottish) power-
wielding
Rona, Ronne

Rhonda (Welsh) vocal;
quintessential
Rhon, Ron, Ronda, Ronnie

Rhondie (American) perfect
Rond, Rondie, Rondy

Rhonella (American) form of
Ronald: kind

Rhonetta (American)
maximum

Rhonni (American) form of
Ronnie: energetic

Rhonwen (Welsh) lovely
Rhonwenne, Rhonwin, Ronwen

Rhuenette (American) great

Rhyan (Welsh) magical

Rhyannah (Greek) nymph

Ria (Spanish) water-loving;
river
Reah, Riah

Riah (Biblical) river

Riana (Irish) frisky
Reana, Rere, Rianna, Rinnie

Rianda (American) river

Riane (American) attractive
Reann, Reanne

Riannah (Irish) sweet

Riannon (Irish) free spirit
Rianna

Rica (Spanish) celestial
*Ric, Ricca, Rickie, Rieka, Rika,
Ryka*

Ricarda (German) has power

Richelle (French) strong and
artistic
*Chelle, Chellie, Rich, Richel,
Richele, Richie*

Richenda (German) rules

Richesse (French) wealthy
Richess

Richilda (American) sainted

Ricielle (African) beauty

Ricki (American) sporty
Rici, Rick, Rickie, Ricky, Rik, Riki, Rikki

Rickiann (Combo of Ricki and Ann) sporty

Rickma (Hindi) golden

Rico (Italian) sexy
Reko, Ricco

Rida (Arabic) satisfied
Ridah

Rierla (Scandinavian) helpful

Rieshanda (American) nymph

Rihana (Irish) pretty

Rihanna (Scandinavian) nymph

Rijana (Slavic) nymph

Rikina (Hawaiian) Christian

Rilena (English) lively

Riley ♂ ♀ (Irish) courageous; lively
Reilly, Rylee, Ryleigh, Ryley, Rylie

Rilla (German) lives by the brook

Rima (Arabic) graceful; antelope
Rema, Remmee, Remmy, Rimmy, Ryma

Rimona (Hebrew) pomegranate; small

Rina (Hebrew) joy
Renah

Rinda (Scandinavian) loyal
Rindah

Ring (American) magical
Ringe, Ryng

Riona (Irish) regal
Rina, Rine, Rionn, Rionna, Rionne

Ripley (American) unique
Riplee, Ripli, Riplie

Riquette (French) feminine form of Richard: wealthy leader

Risen (Last name as first name) rysen
Ryzenne

Rish (American) born in religion

Risingsun (Native American) sun child

Rissa (Latin) laughing
Resa, Risa, Riss, Rissah, Rissie

Rita (Greek) precious pearl
Reda, Reita, Rida

Ritsa (Greek) form of Alexandra: defender of mankind

Ritz (American) rich
Rits

Riva (Hebrew) joining; sparkling
Reva, Revi, Revvy

River (Latin) woman by the stream
Riv

Rivernne (American) water child

Rivers (American) trendy

Riya (American) excited

Riza (Greek) dignified
Reza, Rize

Rizalin (American) form of Theresa: gardener

Rizalina (American) form of Theresa: gardener

Rizalinne (American) form of Theresa: gardener

Rizalyne (American) form of Theresa: gardener

Roanna (Spanish) brown
skin
*Ranna, Roanne, Ronni,
Ronnie, Ronny*

Roberta (English) brilliant
mind
Robbie, Robby, Robertah, Robi

Robertia (English) form of
Robert: brilliant; renowned

Robertz (French) form of
Robert: brilliant; renowned

Robin (English) taken by the
wind; bird
*Robbie, Robby, Robinn,
Robinne, Robyn*

Robina (Scottish) birdlike;
robin
Robena

Robitaille (French) girl of
grace

Rocheen (French) sturdy

Rochelle (French/Hebrew)
small and strong-willed;
dreamlike beauty
*Roch, Roche, Rochel, Rochi,
Rochie, Rochy, Roshelle*

Rockella (Invented) rocker
Rockell, Rockelle

Rocky (American) tomboy
Rock, Rockee, Rockey, Rockie

Roda (Polish) intelligent

Roddy (German) well-known
*Rod, Roddee, Roddey, Roddi,
Roddie*

Roderica (German) princess
*Rica, Roda, Roddie, Rodericka,
Rodrika*

Roelina (German) famous

Rogelim (Biblical) place name

Rogeria (American) form of
Roger: famed warrior

Rogertha (American)
feminine form of Roger:
famed warrior
Rodge

Rohan (Hindi) sandalwood;
pretty

Rohana (Hindi) sandalwood;
textured
Rohanna

Roi Anne (American) royal

Roisin (Irish) rose

Roksana (Polish) dawn
Roksanna, Roksona

Rolanda (German) rich
woman
Rolane, Rollande, Rollie

Rolandan (German)
feminine form of Roland:
renowned
Roland, Rolanden, Rollie, Rolly

Roldyn (Spanish) famed

Roline (German) destined for
fame
*Roelene, Roeline, Rolene,
Rollene, Rolleen, Rollina,
Rolline, Rolyne*

Rolleen (Italian) famed

Rollettea (Italian) rolling

Roma (Italian) girl from
Rome; adventurous
Romy

Romaine (French) daredevil
*Romain, Romane, Romayne,
Romi*

Romalice (American) form
of Rome: city in Italy

Roman (Italian) adventurous
*Romi, Romie, Rommie,
Rommye, Romyn*

Romana (Italian) distinct;
Roman

Romey (Latin) sea-loving
Romy

Romilda (Latin) striking
Romelda, Romey, Romie, Romy

Romilla (Latin) form of
Rome: city in Italy
Romella, Romi, Romie, Romila

Romilly (Latin) wanderer
Romillee, Romillie, Romily

Romina (Spanish) form of
Rome: city in Italy

Romney (Welsh) winding
river

Romola (Latin) form of
Rome: city in Italy

Romona (Spanish) form of
Ramona: beautiful protector
Mona, Rome, Romie, Romy

Romy (French) form of
Romaine: daredevil
Roe. Romi, Romie

Rona (Scandinavian/Scottish)
powerful
Rhona, Ronne, Ronni

Ronallia (Scottish) smart

Ronat (Scandinavian) form of
Rhona: power-wielding

Ronda (Welsh) form of
Rhonda: vocal; quintessential
Ronni

Rondra (American) form of
Rhonda: vocal; quintessential

Ronea (American) form of
Rona: powerful

Roneathea (American) good
face

Ronelle (English) winner
Ronnie

Ronette (English) form of
Rona: powerful

Roney (Scandinavian) form of
Rona: powerful
Roneye, Roni

Ronia (Scandinavian) lake

Ronis (English) image of
beauty

Ronna (Slavic) image of
beauty

Ronneta (English) go-getter
*Roneda, Ronnete, Ronnette,
Ronnie*

Ronni (American) energetic
*Ron, Ronee, Roni, Ronnie,
Ronny*

Rooki (American) sharp
novice

Roopa (Hindi) beauty

Roquia (Spanish) royal

Rori (Irish) spirited; brilliant
Rory

Ros (English) form of
Rosalind: lovely rose
Roz

Rosa (Italian/German) rose;
blushing beauty
Rose, Rossah, Roza

Rosa-Adriana (Spanish)
exotic rose

Rosaire (French) rosary

Rosalba (Latin) glorious as a
rose
*Rosalbah, Rosey, Rosi, Rosie,
Rosy*

Rosalia (Italian) hanging
roses
*Rosa, Rosalea, Rosaleah,
Rosaliah, Roselia, Rosey, Rosi,
Rosie, Rossalia, Rosy*

Rosalie (English) striking dark beauty
Leelee, Rosa, Rosalee, RosaLee, Rosa-Lee, Rosie, Rossalie, Roz, Rozalee, Rozalie

Rosalind (Spanish) lovely rose
Lind, Ros, Rosa, Rosalyn, Rosalynde, Rosie, Roslyn, Roslynn, Roz

Rosalinda (Spanish) lovely rose
Rosa-Linda, Rosalynda

Rosaline (Spanish) a rose
Rosalyn, Rosalynne, Roslyn

Rosallie (Italian) fair rose

Rosalvo (Spanish) rosy-faced
Rosa, Rosey

Rosamond (English) beauty
Rosa, Rosamun, Rosamund, Rose, Rosemond, Rosie, Roz

Rosanna (English) lovely
Rosannah

Rosau (Spanish) rosary

Rosaura (Spanish) rosary

Rose (Latin) rose; blushing beauty
Rosa, Rosey, Rosi, Rosie, Rosy, Roze, Rozee

Rosebud (Latin) flowering

Roselle (Latin) rose

Rosellen (English) pretty
Roselinn, Roselyn

Rosena (American) form of Rose: rose; blushing beauty
Roze, Rozenna, Rozena

Rosenda (Spanish) rosy
Rose, Rosend, Rosende, Rosey, Rosie, Senda

Rosetta (Italian) longlasting beauty
Rose, Rosy, Rozetta

Rosette (Latin) flowering; rosy
Rosett, Rosetta

Roshall (African American) form of Rochelle: small and strong-willed; dreamlike beauty
Rochalle, Roshalle

Rosheen (Latin) rose

Roshell (French) form of Rochelle: small and strong-willed; dreamlike beauty
Rochelle, Roshelle

Roshi (Indian) bright
Roshni

Roshni (Sanskrit) light

Roshumba (African American) gorgeous
Rosh, Roshumbah

Roshunda (African American) flamboyant
Rosey, Roshun, Roshund, Rosie, Roz

Rosie (English) bright-cheeked
Rose, Rosi, Rosy

Rosina (English) rose

Rosita (Spanish) pretty
Roseta, Rosey, Rosie, Rositta

Ross (Scottish) peninsula is home
Rosse

Rossana (Italian) rose

Rosshalde (Welsh) rosary

Rossian (American) rosary

Roszl (Scottish) rose

Rotella (American) smart
Rotel, Rotela

Roth (American) studious
Rothe

Rotnei (American) bright
Rotnay

Roula (Scandinavian) secret

Rowan (Welsh) blonde
Rowanne

Rowena (Scottish) blissful;
beloved friend
Roe, Roenna, Rowina

Rowenta (Slavic) highborn

Roxanna (Persian) bright
Roxana, Roxie

Roxanne (Persian) lovely as
the sun
Roxane, Roxann, Roxie, Roxy

Roxy (American) sunny
Rox, Roxi, Roxie

Royal (English) royal

Royale (English) of royal
family
*Royalla, Royalene, Roayalina,
Royall, Royalle, Royalyn,
Royalynne*

Royce (English) king's child
Roice

Roynale (American)
motivated
Roy, Royna, Roynal

Roysee (English) royal

Roz (French) form of
Rosalind: lovely rose
Ros, Rozz, Rozzie

Rozanne (Slavic) rose

Rozen (Native American) rose

Rozettaline (American) rose

Rozina (Indian) pretty rose

Rozonda (American) pretty
Rosonde, Rozon, Rozond

Rubaina (Hindi) bright

Rube (Hawaiian) ruby; gem

Rubena (Hebrew) sassy
Rubyn, Rubyna, Rueben

Rubicela (Spanish) ruby

Rubina (Pakistani) gem
Rubi

Rubra (French) form of Ruby:
precious jewel
Rube, Rue

Ruby (French) precious jewel
Rubi, Rubie, Rue

Ruchi (German) brash

Rudelle (English) ruddy skin
Rudella

Rudy (German) sly
Rudee, Rudell, Rudie

Rue (English/German)
looking back
Ru

Ruʃaro (African) happy

Rufina (Italian) red-haired
*Rufeena, Rufeine, Ruffina,
Ruphyna*

Rujona (Slavic) form of
Regina: queen

Rujula (Indian) rich

Rujuta (Hindi) truthful

Rula (American) wild-spirited
Rue, Rulah, Rewela

Rulia (English) ruler

Rumah (Biblical) place name

Rumer (English) unique
Ru, Rumor

Rumiko (Asian)

Runa (Scandinavian) secret

Rupli (Hindi) beautiful

Ruri (Japanese) emerald
Rure, Rurrie, RuRu

Rusbel (Spanish) beautiful girl with reddish hair
Rusbell, Rusbella

Ruselle (French) red hair

Rushenda (Slavic) red hair

Russine (French) red hair

Russo (American) happy
Russoh

Rusty (English) red-haired girl
Rustee, Rusti

Ruta (Lithuanian) practical
Rue, Rudah, Rutah

Rutanya (Slavic) friend

Ruth (Hebrew) loyal friend
Rue, Ruthie, Ruthy

Rutha (Hebrew) friend

Ruthian (American) friend

Ruthie (Hebrew) friendly and young
Ruth, Ruthey, Ruthi, Ruthy

Ryan (Irish) royal; assertive
Ryann, Ryen, Ryunn, Rian

Ryanna (Irish) leader
Rianna, Rianne, Ryana, Ryanne, Rynn

Ryba (Hebrew) traditional
Reba, Ree, Riba, Ribah

Ryenline (American) ruler

Ryenni (American) ruler

Rylee (Irish) brave
Rilee, Rili, Ryelee, Ryley, Ryli, Ryly

Ryleen (American) brave

Ryn (American) form of Wren: flighty girl; bird
Ren, Rynn

Ryne (Irish) form of Ryan: royal; assertive
Rynea, Ryni, Rynie

Rynie (American) loves the woods
Rinnie, Ryn

Rynn (American) outdoorsy woman
Rin, Rynna, Rynnie, Wren

Rynnea (American) sun-lover
Rynnee, Rynni, Rynnia

Saba (Arabic) morning star
Sabah

Sabella (English) spiritual
Bella, Belle, Sabela, Sabell, Sabelle, Sebelle

Sabeth (American) form of Elisabeth: God's promise

Sabina (Latin) desirable
Sabeena, Sabine, Sabinna, Sabyna, Say

Sabine (Latin) tribe in ancient Italy
Sabeen, Sabienne, Sabin, Sabyne

Sabirah (Arabic) young

Sabla (Arabic) young

Sable (English) chic
Sabelle, Sabie

Sablette (American) luxurious
Sable, Sablet

Sabra (Hebrew) substantial
Sabe, Sabera, Sabrah

Sabrina (Latin) passionate
Breena, Brina, Brinna, Sabe, Sabreena, Sabrinna

Sabrinus (English) princess

Sabry (American) worthwhile

Sacha (Greek) helpful girl
Sachie, Sachy

Sachen (Slavic) lucky

Sachi (Japanese) girl
*Sachee, Sachey, Sachie, Sachy,
Sashi, Shashie*

Sachika (Japanese) happy

Sachin (Slavic) lucky

Sadawn (American) pure

Sadhana (Hindi) loyal

Sadiah (Arabic) good omen

Sadie (Hebrew) charmer;
princess
*Sade, Sadee, Sady, Sadye,
Shaday*

Safe (Word as name)

Safeenah (Muslim) ship at
sea

Saffron (Indian) spice
Saffrone, Safron

Safia (Arabic) pure

Saga (Scandinavian) sensual
Sagah

Sagal (American) action-
oriented
Sagall, Segalle

Sagartia (Biblical) place name

Sage (Latin) wise
Saige

Sahara (Place name) desert;
wilderness
Saharra

Sahare (American) loner

Sahila (Hindi) guides others

Sahri (Arabic) giving

Saiby (American) gifted

Saida (Hebrew) happy girl
Sada, Sadie

Saige (English) wise

Sailor (American) outdoorsy
Sail, Saile, Sailer, Saylor

Sairsha (Indian) defends

Sajah (Hindi) meritorious
Sajie, Sayah

Sajida (Arabic) lady

Sakura (Japanese) wealthy

Sal (Spanish) savior

Salacia (Mythology) earthy

Salama (African) safe

Salamis (Biblical) place name

Salecah (Biblical) place name

Salena (Latin) needed; basic
Salene, Sally

Saletta (American) earthy

Salia (American) esoteric

Salih (Arabic) virtuous

Saliha (Arabic) correct

Salila (Indian) water child

Salima (Arabic) healthy
Salma

Salima (Arabic) safety

Salina (French) quiet and
deep
Sale, Salena

Sally (Hebrew) princess
Sal, Salli, Sallie

Salma (Hebrew; Spanish)
peaceful; ingenious
*Sal, Sali, Sallee, Salley, Salli,
Sally, Salmah, Salwah*

Salmone (Biblical) place name

Salome (Hebrew) sensual;
peaceful
Sal, Salohme, Salomey, Salomi

Salonae (Biblical) place name

Saloni (Indian) peaceful

Salonna (American) peaceful

Salowmee (Invented) form of Salome: peaceful; sensual
Sal, Salomee, Salomie, Salomy, Slowmee

Salvadora (Spanish) saved
Sal, Salvadorah

Salvia (Spanish) healthy

Salwa (Indian) healthy

Sam (Hebrew) God leads

Samalyn (American) God-loving

Samantha (Hebrew) good listener
Sam, Samath, Sammi, Sammie

Samara (Hebrew) God-led; watchful
Sam, Samora

Samaria (Biblical) place name

Samatha ✪ (American) form of Samantha: hears

Sami (Hebrew) insightful
Sam, Sammie, Sammy

Samia (Hindi) joyful
Sameah, Samee, Sameea, Samina, Sammy

Samimah (Hebrew) praised

Samine (Hindi) happy

Samira (Arabic) charismatic

Samona (Hebrew) form of Simone: wise and thoughtful

Samosata (Biblical) place name

Samothrace (Biblical) place name

Samuela (Hebrew) selected
Samm, Sammi, Sammy, Samula

Samyrah (African American) music-loving
Samirah, Samyra

Sana (Arabic) quintessential beauty

Sanaa (Arabic) excellent

Sancha (Spanish) sacred child
Sanchia

Sanchine (Italian) aware

Sandal (Word as name)

Sandhya (Indian) night

Sandhyn (Indian) night

Sandi (Greek) defends others
Sand, Sanda, Sandee, Sandie, Sandy

Sandip (Hindi) knowing

Sandra (Greek) helpful; protective
Sandrah, Sandy

Sandrea (Greek) selfless
Sandreea, Sandie, Sanndria

Sandreen (American) great
Sandrene, Sandrin, Sandrine

Sandy (American) playful
Sandee, Sandey, Sandi, Sandie

Sanella (Indian) golden

Saniata (Spanish) praised

Sanika (Spanish) old

Sanila (Indian) full of praise
Sanilla

Sanimora (Asian) good health

Sanita (Spanish) twilight

Saniyya (Hindi) a special moment in time

Sanjuana (Spanish)
God-loving
Sanwanna

Sanjuanita (Spanish) form of
San Juan; combo of San Juan
and Juanita: believer
Juanita, Sanjuan

Sanna (Scandinavian)
truthful
Sana

Sanne (Persian) regal

Sanqueneta (Spanish) saint

Santa (Latin) saint

Santana (Spanish) saintly
San, Santanne, Santie, Santina

Sante (Spanish) healthy

Santeene (Spanish)
passionate
*Santeena, Santene, Santie,
Santina, Santine, Satana*

Santi (Spanish) saint

Santia (African) lovable
Santea

Santina (Italian) loves life

Santine (Italian) loves life

Santonina (Spanish) ardent

Sanya (Slavic) dreamer

Sanyu (African) joy

Saper (American) dancer

Sapphira (Greek) blue gem

Sapphire (Greek) precious
gem
*Safire, Saphire, Sapphie,
Sapphyre*

Sapphireen (Greek) blue
gem

Sappho (Greek) blue

Saqqarah (Biblical) place
name

Sarafina (Hebrew) angelic
Seraphina

Sarah ✪ ❶ (Hebrew) God's
princess
Sae, Sara, Saree, Sarrie

Sarai (Hebrew) contentious
Sari

Saraid (Irish) best

Saralyn (American) Combo
of Sara and Lyn

Saree (Hebrew) woman of
value
Sarie, Sary

Sarepta (Biblical) place name

Saretta (Indian) river
Sarita

Sari (Hebrew; Arabic) noble
*Saree, Sarey, Sarie, Sarree,
Sarrey, Sarri*

Sariah (English) form of
Sarah: God's princess

Sarika (Hindi) thrush; sings

Sarilla (Spanish) princess
Sarella, Sarill, Sarille

Sarina (Hebrew) strong
Sareena, Sarena, Sarrie

Sarit (Hebrew) form of Sarah:
God's princess
Saritt, Saryt, Sarytt

Sarita (Spanish) regal
Sareeta, Sarie, Saritah

Sarmila (Indian) comforts

Sarolyn (English) form of
Sharilyn: dear

Sarria (Arabic) superb

Sarun (Indian) valued

Sarva (Indian) river

Sash (Indian) moon child
Sashhi

Sasha (Russian) beautiful
courtesan; helpful
*Sacha, Sachie, Sascha,
Sasheen, Sashy*

Sashay (American) defends

Sasi-Ann (American)
dramatic

Sasily (American) form of
Cecile: blind

Saskia (Dutch) armed with a
knife

Saskia (Dutch) dramatic
Saskiah

Saskie (Dutch) saxon girl

Sasmita (Hindi) laughter

Sassy (Irish) saxon girl;
flirtatious
Sass, Sassi, Sassie

Sata (Spanish) princess

Satchel (American) unusual
Satchal

Satha (Hindi) untruthful

Satin (French) shiny
Saten

Satomi (Indian) sweet

Saturine (American) from
planet Saturn; melancholy
*Saturenne, Saturinne, Saturn,
Saturyne*

Satya (Arabic) lucky

Sauda (African) darkness

Saumet (French) good
advisor

Saundra (Greek) defender
Sandi, Sandra, Sandrah

Saundrall (American) form
of Saundra: defender

Sauni (Arabic) genius
Sani

Sauri (Hebrew) princess

Savannah ○ (Spanish) open
heart
*Sava, Savana, Savanah,
Savanna, Seven*

Savarne (Indian) ocean

Savea (Scandinavian) global
view

Savedra (Indian) sun love

Saveen (Indian) morning

Savina (Latin) form of
Sabina: desirable
Saveena, Savyna

Savone (Italian) morning

Savonna (American)
morning

Savy (American) morning

Sawyer (Last name as first
name) industrious
*Sawya, Sawyar, Sawyhr,
Sawyie, Sawyur*

Say (Asian) night

Sayde (American) form of
Sadie: charmer; princess
Saydey, Saydie

Sayleem (Arabic) safe haven

Saylem (Arabic) safe haven

Sayo (Japanese) born at night
Saio, Sao

Sayuri (Hindi) blooms

Sazana (African) princess

Scally (Last name as first)
introspective
Scalley, Scalli

Scarlett (English) red
Scarlet, Scarletta, Scarlette

Schae (Irish) variation of
Shea: soft beauty
Schay

Scharissea (American) form
of Cherise: cherry

Schelunda (American)
invented

Schemika (African
American) form of Shameka:
loving
Schemi, Schemike

Scheree (American) form of
Sherry: outgoing

Scherry (American) form of
Sherry: outgoing
Scherri, Scherrie

Schmoopie (American)
baby; sweetie
*Schmoopee, Schmoopey,
Schmoopy, Shmoopi*

Schulyer (Dutch) form of
Skyler: protective; sheltering
Schulyar, Sky, Skye

Schunetta (American)
invented

Schylar (Dutch) sheltering
*Schylarr, Schyler, Schylerr,
Schylur, Schylurr*

Scodra (Biblical) place name

Scooter (American) wild-
spirit
Scooder, Scoot

Scottia (Scottish) form of
Scotland

Scotty (Scottish) girl from
Scotland
Scota, Scotti, Scottie

Scout (French) precocious
Scouts

Scully (Irish) strong
*Scullee, Sculleigh, Sculley,
Sculli, Scullie*

Scupi (Biblical) place name

Scylla (Greek mythology)
monstrous

Scyllaea (Greek) mythological
monster; menace
Cilla, Scylla, Silla

Scythian (Biblical) place name

Sea (American) sea-loving;
flowing
Cee, See

Sealy (Last name as first
name) fun-loving
Celie, Seal, Sealie

Sean (Hebrew/Irish) God is
giving

Seana (Irish) giving
Seane, Seanna, Suannea

Seandra (American) form of
Deandra: divine
Seandre, Seandreah, Seanne

Season (Latin) special;
change
*Seas, Seasee, Seasen, Seasie,
Seasun, Seazun, Seezun*

Seaton (English) from the
coast
*Seaten, Seeten, Seeton, Seten,
Seton*

Sebaste (Biblical) place name

Sebastiana (French)
respected

Sebastiane (Latin) respected
female
Sebastian, Sebbie

Seely (English) bright
*Sealee, Sealey, Seali, Sealie,
Sealy, Seelee, Seeley, Seeli,
Seelie*

Seema (Hebrew) treasured;
softhearted
Seem

Sehba (Indian) form of
Shobha: smart and pretty

Sehria (American) form of
Sarah: God's princess

Seine (French) river; flowing
Sane

Seire (Irish) form of Sierra:
peaks; outdoorsy

Sejal (Hindi) good character

Sejal (Origin unknown)
together

Sela (Hebrew) form of
Cecilia: blind
Cela, Celia, Selah, Selia

Selahkiyah (Indian) girl of
mountain

Selame (Biblical) place name

Selanne (American) of the
moon

Selannotta (American) of the
moon

Selda (German) sure-footed
*Seda, Seldah, Selde, Seldee,
Seldey, Seldi, Seldie*

Selena (Greek) like the
moon; shapely
*Celina, Sela, Seleene, Selene,
Selina, Sylena*

Selene (Greek) goddess of the
moon
Seleene, Seline, Selyne

Seleucia (Biblical) place name

Selfina (Spanish) moon child

Selima (Hebrew) peacemaker
Selema, Selemmah

Selin (Turkish) calm

Selina (Greek) moon
Celina

Sella (English) form of
Selena: like the moon;
shapely
Sela

Selma (German) fair-minded
female
*Selle, Sellma, Selmah, Zele,
Zelma*

Selona (Greek) form of
Selena: like the moon
Celona, Sela, Seli, Selo, Selone

Selsa (Hispanic) enthusiastic
Sel, Sels

Sema (Greek) earthy
Semah, Semale, Semele

Semane (Biblical)

Semele (Mythology) needs
proof

Semele (Latin) number one

Semilia (Latin) number one

Semilla (Spanish) earth
mother
*Samilla, Sem, Semila,
Semillah, Semmie, Semmy,
Sumilla*

Semira (Indian) divine

Semiramis (African) meets
goals

Semone (American)
sentimental
Semonne

Semora (English) form of
Samara: God-led; watchful

Semra (Arabic) earthy

Senay (Italian) happy

Sendy (American) form of
Cindy: moon goddess
Sendee, Sendie

Seneca (Native American)
name of a tribe that is part of
the Iroquis confederacy
Seneka

Senell (American) serene

Sennabis (Biblical) place
name

Senone (Spanish) energetic

Senora (Spanish) old soul

Senorah (Spanish) old soul

Senovian (American) high-energy

Senta (German) crescent

Senza (Spanish) sensation

Senzala (Spanish) sensation

Seone (Scottish) sweet

Sephene (American) form of Stephanie: regal

Sepphoris (Biblical) place name

September (Latin) serious; month
Seppie, Sept

Septima (Latin) seventh child
Septimma, Septyma

Sequoia (Cherokee) giant redwood; formidable
Sekwoya

Serafina (Hebrew) ardent
Serafeena, Serafeenah, Serafinah, Serafyna, Serafynah, Serifina, Seraphina, Seraphine

Seraphina (Latin) angel
Serapheena, Serapheenah, Seraphinah, Seraphyna, Serphynah

Seraphine (French) treasure

Seren (Latin) serene
Ceren, Seran

Serena (Latin) calm
Sarina, Sereena, Serenah, Serina

Serendipity (Invented) mercurial; lucky
Sere, Seren, Serendipitee, Serin

Serene (American) word as name; calm

Serenity (American) serene
Sera, Serenitee, Serenitie

Seriah (Spanish) smooth

Serida (Spanish) aggressive

Serpina (Mythology) form of Proserpine: queen of the underworld; secretive

Sesame (American) inventive
Sesamee, Sezamee

Sesha (Hindi) snake

Sesiti (Italian) sixth sextus

Seta (Hindi) form of Sita: divine

Seth (Hebrew) set; appointed; gentle
Sethe

Severia (Spanish) severe

Seville (Place name) from Seville, Spain
Sevill, Sevyll, Sevylle

Sevrea (American) severe

Sexton (English) church worker

Seymoura (Invented) feminine form of Seymour: prayerful
Seymora

Shade (English) cool
Shadee, Shadi, Shady

Shadi (Iranian) happy

Shadow (English) mysterious
Shado, Shadoh

Shady (English) in shade

Shae (Hebrew) shy
Shay

Shaela (Irish) pretty
Shae, Shaelie, Shala

Shaelin (Irish) pretty
Shae, Shaelyn, Shaelynn, Shalyn

Shaeterral (African American) well-shaped
Shatey, Shatrell, Shayterral

Shafiqa (Arabic) loves fellow man

Shahira (Arabic) famed

Shahla (Afghani) pretty girl

Shail (American) pretty
Shale

Shaila (Indian) laughter

Shailendra (Jewish) lovely

Shailesh (Jewish) lovely

Shaina (Hebrew) beauty

Shaina (Jewish) lovely

Shaine (Hebrew) pretty girl
Shanie, Shay, Shayne

Shainel (African American) animated
Shainell, Shainelle, Shaynel

Shajara (Muslim) tree

Shajee (Muslim) brave

Shakila (Arabic) beauty

Shakira (Arabic/Spanish) grateful
Shak, Shakeera, Shakeerah, Shakeira, Shakie, Shakyra, Skakarah

Shakonda (African American) lovely

Shalanda (African American) vivid
Shalande, Shally, Shalunda

Shaleah (Hebrew) weary
Shalea, Shalee, Shaleeah

Shaleina (Turkish) humorist
Shalina, Shalyna, Shalyne

Shalene (Hindi) giving

Shalimar (Polish) peace and glory

Shalina (Indian) form of Selena: like the moon; shapely

Shalini (Indian) modest

Shallan (American) humorous

Shalonda (African American) enthusiastic
Shalie, Shalondah, Shalonna, Shelonda

Shamara (Arabic) assertive
Shamarah, Shemera

Shamarie (American) form of Shamara: assertive

Shameccah (American) form of Shameka: loving

Shameena (Arabic) beautiful
Shamee, Shameenah, Shamina, Shaminna

Shameka (African American) loving
Shameika, Shamika, Shamekah, Shamika, Shemeca

Shamica (American) form of Shameka: loving

Shamilia (American) form of Shameka: loving

Shamine (Hindi) pretty

Shamiyk (African) believer

Shamsa (Pakistani) adorable

Shan (Chinese) coral

Shana (Hebrew) pretty girl
Shaina, Shan, Shanah, Shane, Shannah, Shanni, Shannie, Shanny, Shayna, Shayne

Shanae (Irish) generous
Shan, Shanea, Shanee

Shanan (American) believes in a gracious God

Shanasita (Spanish) wishful

Shanaye (American) form of Shay: spirited

Shanda (American)

Shandee (English) hopeful
Shandi, Shandie, Shandy

Shandel (American)

Shandilyn (American) not forsaken
Shandi, Shandy

Shandon (American)

Shandra (American) fun-loving
Chandra, Shan, Shandrie

Shane (Irish) soft-spoken
Shain, Shaine, Shanee, Shanie, Shayne

Shaneka (African American) perky; pretty
Chuneka, Shan, Shanekah, Shanie, Shanika

Shanelle (African American) form of Chanel: fashionable; designer name
Shanel, Shannel, Shannell, Shanny

Shaney (African) fabulous

Shani (African) great

Shania (African) ambitious; bright-eyed
Shane, Shaniah, Shanie, Shaniya, Shanya

Shanian (American) form of Shania: ambitious; bright-eyed

Shanice (African American) bright-eyed
Chaniece, Shaneese, Shani, Shaniece

Shaniga (American) believer

Shanigan (Last name used as first name)

Shaniger (Last name as first name)

Shanika (African American) pretty; optimistic
Shan, Shane, Shanee, Shaneeka, Shaneika, Shaneikah, Shanequa, Shaney, Shaneyka

Shaniqua (African American) outgoing
Shane, Shaneekwa, Shaneequa, Shanequa, Shanie, Shanikwa, Shaniquah, Shanneequa

Shanique (African American) pretty; optimistic

Shanique (American) form of Shanika: pretty; optimistic

Shanisha (African American) bright
Chaneisha, Chanisha, Shan, Shanecia, Shaneisha, Shanie

Shaniya (American) form of Shania: ambitious; bright-eyed

Shaniyer (American)

Shanna (Irish) lovely
Shanah, Shanea, Shannah

Shannon (Irish) smart
Shann, Shanna, Shannen, Shannyn, Shanon

Shanny (Irish) bubbly
Shannee, Shanni, Shannie

Shanta (Indian) peace

Shanta (French) singing
Shantah, Shante, Shantie

Shantara (French) bright-eyed
Shantay, Shantera, Shantie

Shante (French) form of Chantal: singer of songs
Shantae, Shantay

Shantell (American) bright
singer
Chantel, Shantal, Shantel

Shanti (Hindi) calm

Shantinel (American) form
of Shantel: bright singer

Shaphane (American)

Shaqi (American) form of
Shaqua: fine

Shaquan (American) fine
*Shak, Shaq, Shaquanda,
Shaquanna, Shaquie,
Shaquonda*

Shaquita (African American)
delight
*Shaq, Shaqueita, Shaqueta,
Shaquie*

Shara (Hebrew) form of
Sharon: open heart; desert
plain
Sharah, Sharra, Sherah

Sharada (Indian) knowledge

Sharath (Slavic) protects

Shardae (Arabic) wanderer
*Chardae, Sade, Shaday,
Sharday, SharDay*

Shar-Dae (African) generous

Sharee (American) dear
Sharie

Sharel (Spanish) princess

Shari (French) beloved girl
*Shar, Sharee, Sharree, Sher,
Sherri*

Sharice (French) graceful
Cherise, Shar, Shareese, Shares

Sharif (Russian) mysterious
*Shar, Shareef, Sharey, Shari,
Sharrey, Shary*

Sharil (American) form of
Cheryl: beloved

Sharine (Hebrew) form of
Sharon: open heart; desert
plain
Shareen, Shareene, Sharyne

Sharissa (Hebrew) flat plain;
quiet

Sharita (French) charitable
Shar, Shareetah, Shareta

Sharla (American) friendly
Sharlah

Sharlena (French) strong

Sharlene (German) form of
Charlene: petite and beautiful
*Charleen, Charlene, Shar,
Sharl, Sharleen, Sharline,
Sharlyne*

Sharlette (American) form of
Charlotte: little woman

Sharlott (American) form on
Charlotte: little woman
Charlotte

Sharmaine (American) form
of Charmaine: bountiful
orchard

Sharmanah (American)
form of Sharmaine: feminine

Sharmeal (African
American) exhilarating
*Sharm, Sharma, Sharme,
Sharmele*

Sharna (Hebrew) broad-
minded
Sharn, Sharnah

Sharnam (American) form of
Sharmaine: feminine

Sharnea (American) quiet
Sharnay, Sharnee, Sharney

Sharnelle (African American)
spiritual
Sharnel, Sharnie, Sharny

Sharnette (American) fighter
*Chanet, Charnette, Shanet,
Sharn, Sharnett, Sharney*

Sharon (Hebrew) open heart;
desert plain
*Shar, Sharen, Shari, Sharin,
Sharren, Sharron, Sharry,
Sharyn, Sheron, Sherron*

Sharona (Hebrew) form of
Sharon: open heart; desert
plain
*Sharonah, Sharonna,
Sharonnah*

Sharonda (African
American) open
Sharondah, Sheronda

Sharonett (American) form of
Sharon: open heart; desert plain

Sharonetta (American) form
of Sharon: open heart; desert
plain

Sharr (Hebrew) vigilant

Sharrona (Hebrew) open
*Sharona, Sharonne, Sherona,
Shironah*

Sharterica (African
American) beloved
*Sharter, Sharterika, Shartrica,
Sharty*

Sharuhen (Biblical) place
name

Shashee (Hindi) luminous

Shashi (Indian) giving

Shasta (American) majestic
mind
Shastah

Shatoya (African American)
spirited
Shatoye, Shay, Shaytoya, Toya

Shauhna (Irish) form of
Shauna: giving heart

Shauna (Hebrew/Irish)
giving heart
*Shauhna, Shaunie, Shaunna,
Shawna*

Shaundra (American) giving

Shaune (American) wide
smile
Shaun, Shaunie, Shawn

Shauneice (American)
excitable

Shaunelle (American)
excitable

Shaunta (American) sings

Shauntee (Irish) dancing
eyes
*Shaun, Shawntey, Shawntie,
Shawnty*

Shauntrie (American) sings

Shavon (Irish) devout;
energetic
*Chavon, Chavonne, Shavaun,
Shavon, Shavonne*

Shawana (African American)
dramatic
*Shavaun, Shawahna,
Shawanna, Shawnie*

Shawandreka (African
American) gutsy
*Shawan, Shawand,
Shawandrika, Shawann,
Shawuan*

Shawn (American) smiling
*Shawne, Shawnee, Shawnie,
Shawny*

Shawna (Hebrew/Irish)
feminine form of Sean: God
is gracious
Shawnna

Shawnda (Irish) helpful
friend
Shaunda, Shaundah, Shona

Shawneequa (African American) loquacious
Shauneequa, Shawneekwa

Shawnel (African American) audacious
Shaune, Shaunel, Shaunelle, Shawn, Shawnee, Shawnelle, Shawney, Shawni

Shawnet (American) feminine form of Sean: God is gracious

Shawnie (American) playful
Shaunie, Shawni

Shawyne (American) feminine form of Sean: God is gracious

Shay (Irish) fairy place
Shaye

Shayla (Irish) fairy palace

Shayleen (Greek) moon

Shaylie (Latin) playful
Shaleigh, Shaylea, Shaylee, Shealee

Shayna (Hebrew) beauty

Shayne (Hebrew) form of Shane: soft-spoken
Shaine, Shane, Shay, Sheyne

Shayni (Hebrew) beauty

Shayonda (African American) regal
Shay, Shaya, Shayon, Shayonde, Sheyonda, Yona, Yonda

Shayter (American) friend of fairies

Shea (Irish) soft beauty
Shae, Shay

Sheaden (French) lovely

Sheba (Hebrew) form of Bathsheba: beautiful; daughter of Sheba
Chebah, Sheeba, Sheebah

Sheconna (American) of fairies

Sheddreka (African American) dynamo
Shedd, Sheddrik, Shedreke

Shedy (American) of fairies

Sheela (Hindi) gentle spirit
Sheelah, Sheeli, Sheila

Sheelyah (Irish) form of Shelia: woman; gorgeous
Sheel, Sheil

Sheem (Native American) believer

Sheena (Hebrew) shining
Sheen, Sheenah, Shena

Shefalia (American)

Shehagh (Irish)

Sheila (Irish) vivacious; divine woman
Shaylah, Sheela, Sheilia, Sheilya, Shel

Shelagh (Irish) fairy princess

Shelby (English) dignified
Chelby, Shel, Shelbee, Shelbi, Shelbie

Sheldon (English) farm on the ledge
Shelden

Sheleatha (American) shy

Shelia (Irish) woman; gorgeous
Shelya, Shelyah, Shillya

Shelita (Spanish) little girl
Chelita, Shelite, Shelitta

Shell (English) meadow
Shel

Shelley (English) outdoorsy; meadow
Shelee, Shelli, Shelly

Shelline (French) form of Shelley: outdoorsy; meadow

Shelton (English) farm on a ledge
Shelten

Shemari (American) sheltered

Shemelia (American) sheltered

Shemina (American) sheltered

Shemira (American) sheltered

Shena (Irish) shining
Shenae, Shenea, Shenna

Shenease (Hebrew) believer

Sheneda (Hebrew) believer

Sheneeka (African American) easygoing
Shaneeka, Shaneka, Sheneecah, Sheneka

Shepard (English) vigilant
Shep, Sheperd, Shepherd, Sheppie

Shephelah (Biblical) place name

Shera (Hebrew) lighthearted
Sheera, Sheerah, Sherah

Sherael (American) form of Sherry: outgoing
Sheraelle, Sherelle, Sherryelle

Sheray (French) saucy
Cheray, Sherayah

Sheree (French) dearest girl
Sheeree, Sher, Shere

Shereen (Indian) sheen

Shereitta (Spanish) effervescent

Sherele (French) bouncy
Sher, Sherell, Sherrie

Sheresa (American) dancer
Sher, Sherisa, Sherissa, Sherri

Shereth (American) loved

Sheretta (American) sparkling
Shere, Sherette

Sheri (French) sparkling eyes
Sher, Sherri, Sherrie

Sherice (French) artistic
Cherise, Sher, Shereece, Sherisse

Sheridan (Irish) free spirit; outstanding
Cheridan, Cheridyn, Sheridyn, Sherridan

Sherika (Arabic)

Sherine (American) shines

Sherita (French) stylish
Cherita, Sheretta

Sheritt (French) form of Sherry: outgoing

Sherleen (American) easygoing
Sherl, Sherlene, Sherline, Sherlyn, Shirline

Sherlie (English) form of Shirley: bright meadow; cheerful girl

Sherlitha (Spanish) feminine
Sherl, Sherli

Sherlotta (American) form of Charlotte: little woman

Sherolynna (American) lovely
Cherolina, Sher, Sheralina, Sherrilina

Sherrill (English) bright
Cheril, Cherrill, Sherelle, Sheril, Sherrell, Sheryl

Sherrone (Hebrew) form of Sharon: open heart; desert plain

Sherrunda (African American) free spirit
Sharun, Sharunda, Sherr, Sherrunde, Sherunda

Sherry (French) outgoing
Sher, Sheri, Sherreye, Sherri, Sherrie, Sherye

Sheryl (French) beloved woman
Cheryl, Sharal, Sher, Sheral, Sheril, Sherill

Shevonne (Gaelic) ambitious
Shavon, Shevaune, Shevon

Sheyenne (Native American) form of Cheyenne: Native American tribe
Shey, Shianne, Shyann, Shyanne, Shyenne

Sheyn (Hebrew) beauty

Shiaray (Native American)

Shibhan (Irish) variation of Siobhan: believer; lovely
Shiban, Shibann, Shibhann

Shiela (Irish) blind

Shiffawn (American) pretty

Shifra (Hebrew) beautiful woman
Sheefra, Shifrah

Shikendra (African American) spirited
Shiki, Shikie, Skikend

Shiloh (Hebrew) gifted by God
Shilo, Shy

Shilpa (Indian) in synch

Shilpa (Indian) rock

Shimchi (Asian) good

Shinae (American) shines

Shine (American) shining example
Shena, Shina

Shinea (Asian) good

Shinetta (American) shines

Shiney (American) glowing
Shine, Shiny

Shinikee (African American) glorious
Shinakee, Shinikey, Shynikee

Shira (Hebrew) song; singer
Shirah, Shiree

Shireen (English) charmer
Shareen, Shiree, Shireene, Shirene, Shiri, Shiry, Shoreen, Shureen, Shurene

Shirenzio (American) form of Sharon: open heart; desert plain

Shirince (American) form of Sharon: open heart; desert plain

Shirleen (American) nature-loving
Shirlene, Shirline

Shirlei (English) form of Shirley: bright meadow; cheerful girl

Shirleth (American) form of Shirley: bright meadow; cheerful girl

Shirley (English) bright meadow; cheerful girl
Sherlee, Sherley, Sherly, Shir, Shirl, Shirly

Shiyama (African) believer in God

Shlomith (Jewish) peaceful

Shlonda (African American) bright
Londa, Schlonda, Shodie

Shobby (American) smart

Shobha (Indian) smart and pretty

Shola (Hebrew) spirited
Sholah

Sholia (American) form of
Salih: virtuous

Shon (Irish) form of Shona:
open-hearted
Shonn

Shona (Irish) open-hearted
Shonah, Shonie

Shonda (Irish) runner
*Shondah, Shonday, Shondie,
Shounda, Shoundah*

Shondra (Irish) pretty

Shonta (Irish) fearless
*Shauntah, Shawnta, Shon,
Shontie*

Shony (Irish) shining
Shona, Shonee, Shoni, Shonie

Shoshana (Hebrew)
beautiful; lily
*Shoshanna, Shoshannah,
Shoshauna*

Shreya (Indian) good fortune

Shrill (American) word as
name; Ingenious

Shrilla (Hindi) beauty
Shrila

Shryl (American) ingenious

Shu Jane (Asian) kind

Shuchi (Hindi) pure

Shue (Asian) kind

Shula (Arabic) flaming

Shulamit (Hebrew) serene

Shulondia (African
American) dynamic
*Shulee, Shuley, Shuli,
Shulonde, Shulondea,
Shulondiah*

Shumay (Muslim) eloquent

Shun (Irish) form of Jane:
believer in a gracious God

Shuna (Irish) form of Jane:
believer in a gracious God

Shunta (Irish) form of Jane:
believer in a gracious God

Shuntay (African American;
Irish) form of Shonta:
goodness
Shuntae

Shuntele (Irish) energetic

Shura (Greek) protective

Shuranda (American) kind

Shurkela (American) kind

Shurla (American) fun

Shushan (Biblical) place name

Shyama (Native American)
form of Cheyenne: Native
American tribe

Shyanne (Native American)
form of Cheyenne: Native
American tribe
Shy

Shyla (English) creative
Shila, Shy, Shylah

Shyne (American) standout
Shine

Shyree (Native American)
cheyenne

Sia (Welsh) calm; believer
Cia, Seea

Sian (Welsh) believer

Siana (Welsh) ebullient
Sian, Siane

Sianoee (Welsh) believer

Sib (Anglo-Saxon) form of
Sibley: related
Sibb

Sibila (Greek) form of Sybil:
future-gazing

Sibley (Anglo-Saxon) related
Siblee, Sibly

Sibmah (Biblical) place name

Sibyl (Greek) intuitive
*Cibyl, Cyb, Cybil, Cybill, Cybyl,
Sib, Sibbi, Sibbie, Sibby,
Sibella, Sibil, Sibill, Sibyll,
Sibylla, Sybela, Sybil, Sybyl*

Sicily (Biblical) place name

Sid (Place name) form of
Sidney: from Saint-Denis,
France
Sidd

Sidelia (Spanish) stars

Sidhi (Indian) excels

Sidnah (American) form of
Sidney: from Saint-Denis,
France

Sidney (Place name) from
Saint-Denis, France
Sidnee, Sidni, Sidny

Sidonia (French) spiritual
Sid, Sidoneah, Sydonya

Sidonie (French) appealing
Sidonee, Sidony, Sydoni

Sidra (Latin) star
*Cidra, Siddey, Siddie, Siddy,
Sidi, Sidrie, Sydra*

Siely (American) form of
Sealy: fun-loving

Sienna (English) delicate;
reddish-brown
Siena, Siene

Sierra (Place name) peaks;
outdoorsy
*Cierra, Searah, Searrah, Siera,
Sierrah, Sierre*

Sigfrid (German) peacemaker
Sig, Sigfred, Sigfreid, Siggy

Signe (Latin) symbol
Sig, Signie, Signy

Signet (Scandinavian) form
of Signe: symbol

Sigourney (English) leader
who conquers
*Sig, Siggie, Signe, Signy,
Sigournay, Sygourny*

Sigrid (Scandinavian) lovely
Segred, Sig, Siggy, Sigrede

Sigrun (Scandinavian)
winning
Cigrun, Segrun

Sikita (American) active
Sikite

Sila (Native American)
flowers

Sile (Turkish) misses home

Silenceia (Spanish) quiet

Siline (Greek) form of Selene:
like the moon; shapely
Sileen, Sileene, Silyne

Silke (German) divine
spirituality

Silvanna (Spanish) nature-
lover
*Sil, Silva, Silvana, Silvane,
Silvanne, Silver*

Silver (Anglo-Saxon) light-
haired
Silva, Silvar, Sylver

Silvia (Latin) deep; woods-
loving
Sill, Silvy, Siviah, Sylvia

Sima (Indian) wise

Simcha (Hebrew) joyful
Simchah

Simi (Lebanese) soft
Sim

Simica (American) tender
Sim, Simika, Simmy

Simoli (American) energy

Simona (American) form of Simone: wise and thoughtful
Sim, Simon, Sims

Simone (French) wise and thoughtful
Sim, Simonie, Symone

Simonetta (French) form of Simon: good listener; thoughtful

Simonias (Biblical) place name

Sinaflor (Spanish) flowers

Sinai (Place name) Mt. Sinai

Sinclair (French) person from St. Clair; admired
Cinclair, Sinclare, Synclair, Synclare

Sinden (English) form of Cindy: moon goddess

Sindy (American) left behind
Cindy

Sine (Irish) God's gift

Sinead (Irish) singer; believer in a gracious God
Shanade

Sinforosa (Spanish) bad luck

Singrid (Scandinavian) form of Sigrid: lovely

Sinope (Biblical) place name

Sinue (Spanish)

Siobhan (Irish) believer; lovely
Chevon, Chevonne, Chivon, Shavonne, Shevon

Siphronia (Greek) sensible
Ciphronia, Sifronea, Sifronia, Syfronia

Sippar (Biblical) place name

Sirbonis (Biblical) place name

Siren (Greek) enchantress
Syren

Sirena (Greek) temptress
Sireena, Sirenah, Sirine, Sisi, Sissy, Syrena

Sirene (Greek) enchantress
Sireen, Sireena, Siryne

Siri (Scandinavian) lovely

Siriny (Greek) spellbinding

Sirmium (Biblical) place name

Sirneicsa (Sanskrit) immortal

Siscia (Biblical) place name

Sisely (American) form of Cicely: clever

Sisley (Last name as first name) able

Sissy (Latin) form of Cecilia or little sister: immature; ingenue
Cissee, Cissey, Cissy, Sis, Sissi, Sissie

Sistene (Italian) spiritual
Sisteen, Sisteene

Sita (Hindi) divine
Seeta, Seetha

Sitiveni (Slavic) high esteem

Siv (Scandinavian) kinship; wife of Thor
Sive

Sivana (Irish) form of Sivney: satisfied
Sivanah

Siwa (Biblical) place name

Siyona (Hindi) graceful

Sjanie (Scandinavian) energetic

Skayla (Slavic) smart

Skudra (Biblical) place name

Skye (Scottish) high-minded; head in the clouds

Skyler (Dutch) protective; sheltering
Schuyler, Skieler, Skilar, Skiler, Skye, Skyla, Skylar, Skylie, Skylor

Slane (Irish) form of Sloane: strong
Slaine

Slaney (Last name as first name) selective

Slava (Russian) glory

Sloane (Irish) strong
Sloan, Slone

Sloni (Latin) clarity

Sly (American) form of Slyvestra: forest-dweller; heavy duty

Slyvestra (American) feminine form of Slyvester: forest-dweller; heavy duty

Smera (Hindi) smiles

Smiley (American) radiant
Smile, Smilee, Smiles, Smili, Smily

Smirna (American) refined

Smisha (American) form of Smith: crafty; blacksmith

Smita (Indian) grinning

Smyrna (Biblical) place name

Snooks (American) sweetie
Snookee, Snookie

Snow (American) quiet
Sno, Snowy

Snowdrop (Botanical) white flower

Sochia (American) form of Sasha: beautiful courtesan; helpful

Socoh (Biblical) place name

Socorro (Spanish) helpful
Socoro

Socra (Greek) form of Socrates: philosophical; brilliant

Sofie (Greek) wise

Sofina (Spanish) form of Sophia: wise one

Sofonias (Greek) form of Sophia: wise one

Sofya (Russian) wise
Sofi, Sofie, Sofiya

Sohanne (Hindi) lovely

Soheila (Indian) sun

Sohella (Arabic) form of Saliha: correct

Sohni (Hindi) lovely

Sohni (Hindi) lovely

Sokan (Native American)

Solada (Asian) attentive

Solana (Spanish) sunny
Solanah, Soley, Solie

Solange (French) sophisticated
Solie

Soledad (Spanish) solitary woman
Saleda, Solada, Solay, Sole, Solee, Solie, Solita

Soleil (French) sun

Soli (Biblical) place name

Solida (Spanish) alone

Soline (French) solemn
Solen, Solenne, Souline

Solita (Latin) alone
Soleeta, Solyta

Soloma (Hindi) lunar

Somansh (Hindi) half-moon

Somayeh (Indian) moon

Somers (Last name as first name) summer girl

Somilla (Hindi) calm

Sommai (American) summer

Sommer (English) warm
Sommie, Summer, Summi

Sona (Hindi) form of Sonal: golden girl of the sun

Sona (Indian) golden

Sonal (Hindi) golden girl of the sun

Sonali (Hindi) golden

Sonay (Asian) bright-eyed
Sonnae

Sondra (Greek) defender of mankind

Sonel (Hindi) form of Sonal: golden girl of the sun
Sonell

Sonesse (American) sings

Song (Chinese) independent

Songsira (American) sings

Sonia (Slavic) effervescent
Soni, Sonnie, Sonny, Sonya

Sonja (Scandinavian) bright woman

Sonnet (American) poetic
Sonnett, Sonni, Sonny

Sonnie (Slavic) wise

Sonoe (Asian) bright

Sonoma (Place name) city in California; wine-loving
Sonomah

Sonora (English) easygoing
Sonorah

Sonova (Spanish) nice

Sonseria (American) giving
Seria, Sonsere, Sonsey

Sonya (Greek) wise
Sonia, Sonje

Soo (Korean) gentle spirit

Soon-Yi (Chinese) delightful; assertive

Soozi (American) form of Suzy: lily; pretty flower
Soos, Sooz, Souz, Souze, Souzi, Soozy

Sophath (American) form of Sophie: wise one

Sophia ○ ❶ (Greek) wise one
Sofeea, Sofi, Sofia, Sofie, Sophea, Sopheea, Sophie, Sophy

Sophia-Loren (Italian) namesake of movie star

Sophie (Greek) form of Sophia: wise one
Sophee, Sophey, Sophi, Sophy

Sophorn (American) form of Sophie: wise one

Sora (Native American) chirping bird
Sorra

Sorangel (Spanish) heavenly
Sorange

Soraya (Persian) royal

Sorayal (Russian) princess

Sorayalle (Russian) princess

Sorcha (Irish) bright
Shorshi, Sorsha, Sorshie

Sorek (Biblical) place name

Sorel (French) reddish-brown

Sorele (French) reddish-brown hair

Sorphal (Asian) speaks well

Sorrel (English) delicate
Sorel, Sorell, Sorie, Sorree, Sorrell, Sorri, Sorrie

Sosamma (Hindi) pretty

Sosannah (Hebrew) form of
Susannah: gentle
Sosana, Sosanah, Sosanna

Soshana (Hebrew) lily
Soshanah

Sosy (Indian) health

Sotee (Greek) saved

Soulah (American) afire

Souza (Persian) fiery

Sowanna (Hindi) peaceful

Soynia (American) form of
Sonya: wise

Sozos (Hindi) clingy
Sosos

Spaulding (English) divided
field
Spalding

Spencer (English)
sophisticate
Spence, Spenser

Spirit (American) lively;
spirited
Spirite, Spyrit

Sprague (American)
respected
Sprage

Sprandee (Invented) spry

Spring (English) springtime;
fresh
Spryng

Sri (Hindi) glorious
Shree, Shri, Sree

Srikantha (Hindi) goddess

Srini (Hindi) feminine

Srinivas (Hindi) goddess

Srividya (Hindi) praised

Stacey (Greek) hopeful and
spiritual
*Stace, Staci, Stacie, Stacy,
Staycee*

Stacha (English) form of
Anastasia: resurrection

Stacia (English) form of
Anastasia: devout
Stace, Stacie, Stasia, Stayshah

Stahsha (Slavic) form of
Stacia; form of Anastasia:
devout

Stana (American) form of
Stacia; form of Anastasia:
devout

Stancie (American) adored

Stanise (American) darling
*Stanee, Staneese, Stani,
Stanice, Staniece*

Star (English) a star
Starr

Starla (American) shining
Starlah, Starlie

Starlene (American) star

Starling (English) glossy bird

Starlite (American)
extraordinary
Starlight, Starr

Starne (American) star

Stasia (Greek/Russian)
ressurection
Stacie, Stasie, Stasya

Stefanie (Greek) form of
Stephanie: regal
*Stafanie, Stefannye, Stefany,
Steff, Steffany, Steffie,
Stephanie*

Stefee (Greek) crowned

Steff (Greek) form of
Stephanie: regal

Steffi (Greek) form of
Stephanie: regal
Steffie, Steffy, Stefi

Stefnee (American) form of
Stephanie: regal
Stef, Steffy

Stelanie (American) crowned

Stella (Latin) bright star
Stele, Stelie

Stephanie ○ (Greek) regal
*Stefanie, Steff, Steffie,
Stephenie, Stephney*

Stephel (American) crowned

Stephene (French/Greek)
dignified
Steph, Stephie, Stephine

Stephine (French) crowned

Stephney (Greek) crowned
Stef, Steph, Stephie, Stephnie

Sterla (American) quality
Sterl, Sterlie, Stirla

Sterry (Dutch) star child
Sterree

Stevie (Greek/American)
jovial
Steve, Stevee, Stevey, Stevi

Stevina (Slavic) crowned

Stina (Scandinavian) believer

Stockard (English) stockyard;
sturdy
Stockerd, Stockyrd

Storelle (Invented) legend
Storee, Storell, Storey, Stori

Storm (English) powerful

Stormy (American) impulsive
Storm, Stormi, Stormie

Story (American) creative
Stori, Storie, Storee, Storey

Stuti (Hindi) goddess

Sua (Spanish) loved

Suazo (Spanish) loved

Subha (Indian) lucky

Sublime (Word as name)

Suchi (Indian) lovely

Sudha (Indian) nectar

Sue (Hebrew) form of Susan:
lily; pretty flower

Suelita (Spanish) comforts

Suez (Place name)

Suganda (Slavic) cedar

Sugar (American) sweet
Shug

Sugy (Spanish) form of the
name Sugar: sweet
Sug, Sugey, Sugie

Suha (Indian) nectar
Sudha

Suhas (Hindi) jovial

Sujata (Indian) wellborn

Sujey (Asian) loved

Sukanya (Hindi) lovely

Sukhee (Asian) wise

Suki (Japanese) beloved
Suke, Sukie, Suky

Sula (Greek) sea-going
Soola, Sue, Suze

Sulafah (Muslim) best

Sulanie (American) sea

Sulay (Arabic) pleased

Sulema (Spanish) pleasant

Sullivan (Last name as first
name) bravehearted
Sulli, Sullie, Sullivin, Sully

Sumati (Indian) strong mind

Sumayah (Indian) good
temperament
Sumana, Sumaaya

Sumi (Asian) distinguished

Summer (English) summery; fresh
Somer, Sommer, Sum, Summie

Summerly (American) vivid summer

Sumona (Hindi) calm

Sun (Korean) obedient girl
Suna, Suni, Sunnie

Sunanda (American) sunny

Sunda (Slavic) form of Sanda: helpful; protective

Sundancer (American) easygoing
Sunndance

Sunday (Latin) day of the week; sunny
Sun, Sundae, Sundaye, Sundee, Sunney, Sunni, Sunnie, Sunny, Sunnye

Sunil (American) sunny

Sunila (Hindi) blue sky

Sunita (Hindi) dharma's child
Suniti

Sunna (American) sunny
Sun, Suna

Sunny (English) bright attitude
Sonny, Sun, Sunni, Sunnye

Sunshine (American) sunny

Supree (Indian) loved
Supriya

Suprema (Hindi) affectionate

Suprina (American) supreme
Suprinna

Suprita (Hindi) pleasant

Surbhi (Indian) sweet smelling

Surekha (Indian) fragrant

Suren (American) delivers

Surene (American) delivers

Suri (Hebrew) princess

Surina (Hindi) wise

Surrender (Word as name) dramatic
Surren

Suruchi (Hindi) pleasant

Surupa (Hindi) beauty

Surya (Indian) sun

Susa (Biblical) place name

Susan (Hebrew) lily; pretty flower
Soozan, Sue, Susahn, Susanne, Susehn, Susie, Suzan

Susaneca (Hebrew) lily

Susannah (Hebrew) gentle
Sue, Susah, Susanna, Susie, Suzannah

Susene (French) pretty girl

Susette (French) form of Susan: lily; pretty flower
Susett

Susha (Hindi) beauty

Sushma (Hindi) gorgeous

Sushmita (Indian) pretty smile

Susiana (Biblical) place name

Susie (American) form of Susan: lily; pretty flower
Susey, Susi, Susy, Suze, Suzi, Suzie, Suzy

Susila (Hindi) sensual

Susita (Hindi) white

Susithah (Biblical) place name

Suszane (Slavic) form on Susan: lily; pretty flower

Sutanu (Hindi) pretty

Sutapa (Hindi) follows God

Sutton (Last name as first name) southern town
Suten, Sutten, Suton

Suvi (Hindi) excels

Suz (American) form of Susan; lily; pretty flower
Suze

Suzan (American) form of Susan: lily; pretty flower
Suzen

Suzanne (English) fragrant
Susanne, Suzan, Suzane, Suzann, Suze

Suzette (French) pretty little one
Sue, Susette, Suze

Suzy (French) form of Susan: lily; pretty flower
Susy, Suze

Svana (Hindi) noisy

Svea (Swedish) patriotic
Svay

Svetlana (Russian) star bright
Sveta, Svete

Swaga (Hindi) gracious

Swan (Scandinavian) swan-like

Swanhildda (Teutonic) swan-like; graceful
Swan, Swanhild, Swann, Swanney, Swanni, Swannie, Swanny

Swarna (Hindi) lustrous

Swaru (Hindi) honest

Sweeney (Irish) young and rambunctious
Sweenee, Sweeny

Sweetpea (American) sweet
Sweet-Pea, Sweetie

Swell (Invented) good
Swelle

Sweta (Hindi) fair

Swetha (Indian) light

Swift (word as name) bold
Swiftie, Swifty

Swoosie (American) unique
Swoose, Swoozie

Syama (Sanskrit) dark

Syantha (American) form on Cynthia: moon goddess

Syb (Greek) form of Sybil: future-gazing
Sybb

Sybil (Greek) future-gazing
Sibel, Sibyl, Syb, Sybill, Sybille, Sybyl

Syble (American) foresees

Syd (French) form of Sydney: enthusiastic
Sydd

Sydel (Hebrew) princess

Sydlyn (American) quiet
Sidlyn, Sydlin, Sydlinne

Sydne (French) enthusiastic

Sydney ✿ (French) enthusiastic
Sidney, Syd, Sydnee, Sydnie

Syene (Biblical) place name

Syfronia (Slavic) serious

Syka (Slavic) studious

Syl (Latin) loves the woods
Sill

Sylvah (Slavic) form of Sylvia: sylvan; girl of the forest

Sylvan (Latin) from the forest
Silvan, Silven, Silvyn, Sylven, Sylvyn

Sylvana (Latin) forest; natural woman
Silvanna, Syl, Sylvie

Sylvenita (Spanish) sylvan

Sylvestra (English) lives in the woods

Sylvia (Latin) sylvan; girl of the forest
Syl, Sylvea

Sylvie (Latin) sylvan; peacefulness
Sil, Silvie, Silvy, Syl, Sylvey, Sylvi, Sylvy

Sylwia (Polish) serene; in the woods
Silwia

Sylwia (Latin) form of Sylvia

Symira (American) enthusiastic
Sym, Symra, Syms, Symyra

Symone (Hebrew) good listener
Sym

Symphony (American) musical
Simphony, Symfonie, Symfony, Symphonee, Symphonie

Syna (Invented) sweet
Sina

Synde (American) form of Sydney: enthusiastic
Cindy

Synora (American) languid
Cinora, Sinora, Synee, Syni, Synor, Synore

Synov (Scandinavian) sun girl

Synpha (American) capable
Sinfa, Sinpha, Synfa

Syntiche (Biblical) shared goal

Syreeta (Hindi) orderly

Syreta (American) assertive
Sireta

Tabbath (Greek) gazelle

Tabea (German) lithe

Tabeen (American) pretty

Tabel (Biblical) happy

Tabia (African) talented girl

Tabina (Arabic) follower of Muhammed

Tabitha (Greek) graceful; gazelle
Tabatha, Tabbatha, Tabbi, Tabytha

Tabla (Native American) wears a tiara; regal

Tacey (American) precious
Tace, Tacita

Tacha (American) form of Tasha: born on Christmas
Tach

Tacho (American) form of Tasha: born on Christmas

Taci (American) strong

Tacie (American) healthy
Tace, Taci, Tacy

Tadewi (Native American) wind

Tadi (Native American) variation of Tadewi: wind

Tadit (Native American) fast

Tadita (Native American) runner
Tadeta

Taesha (American) sterling character
Tahisha, Taisha, Taisha, Tisha

Taffese (Welsh) loved

Taffeta (American) shiny
Tafeta, Taffetah, Taffi, Taffy

Taffy (Welsh) sweet and beloved
Taffee, Taffey, Taffi

Tafin (American) loved

Taft (English) loved
Tafie

Tafta (American) loved

Taghrid (Arabic) singing bird

Tahcawin (Native American) doe

Tahira (Arabic) pure
Tahirah

Tahiyya (Arabic) welcome
Tahiyyah

Tahmeena (Arabic) form of Tamina: psalms

Tahnee (English) little one

Tai (American) fond
Tie, Tye

Taima (Native American) thunder
Taimah, Taiomah

Tain (Native American) new moon

Taina (Spanish) form of Taima: thunder

Taipa (Native American) quail

Tairra (Irish) towers high

Taisha (American) form of Tasha: Christmas-born baby

Taiwo (African) firstborn of twins

Tajanan (American) regal bearing

Tajarah (Hindi) crowned

Tajie (American) highborn

Tajudeen (Spanish) clingy
Taj, Tajjy, Taju

Taka (Japanese) honorable

Takala (Native American) cornstalk
Takalah

Takara (Japanese) beloved gem
Taka, Taki

Takayren (Native American) commotion

Takeko (Japanese) child of the bamboo

Takenya (Native American) falcon in flight

Takeya (African American) knowing
Takeyah

Taki (Japanese) waterfall

Takia (Arabic) spiritual
Taki, Tikia, Tykia

Takiyah (Arabic) devout
Takeya, Takiya

Takona (American) special

Taku (Asian) worshipful

Takuhi (Armenian) queen

Tala (Native American) wolf

Talal (Hebrew) dew

Talasi (Native American) cornflower

Tale (African) green

Taleen (American) golden

Talent (American) self-assured
Talynt

Talesha (African American)
friendly
*Tal, Taleesh, Taleisha, Talisha,
Tallie, Telesha*

Tali (Hebrew) confident

Talia (Greek) golden; dew
from heaven
*Tahlia, Tali, Tallie, Tally, Talya,
Talyah*

Talian (American) golden

Talian (American) golden girl

Talibah (African) intellectual
Tali, Talib, Taliba

Talila (Hebrew) dew

Talisa (African American)
variation of Lisa: dedicated
and spiritual
Telisa

Talise (Native American)
beautiful creek

Talitha (African American)
inventive
*Taleetha, Taleta, Taletha,
Talith, Tally*

Taliyah (American) blooms

Tallis (English) forest

Tallulah (Native American)
leaping water; sparkling girl
*Talie, Talley, Tallula, Talula,
Talulah*

Talluse (American) bold
Talloose, Tallu, Taluce

Tally (Native American)
heroine
Tallee, Talley, Talli, Tally, Taly

Talma (Hebrew) hill

Talou (American) saucy
Talli, Tallou, Tally

Talutah (Native American)
red

Talya (Hebrew) lamb
Talia

Tam (Japanese) decorative
Tama

Tamah (Hebrew) marvel
Tama

Tamajer (American) palms

Tamaka (Japanese) bracelet;
adorned female

Tamaki (Japanese) bracelet

Tamala (American) kind
*Tam, Tama, Tamela, Tammie,
Tammy*

Tamani (Hindi) desirable

Tamanna (Hindu) desire

Tamar (Hebrew) palm; breezy
Tama, Tamarr

Tamara (Hebrew) royal
female
*Tamera, Tammy, Tamora,
Tamra*

Tamas (Hindu) palm tree
Tamasa, Tamasi, Tamasvini

Tamasailau (Hawaiian) gem

Tamasine (English) twin;
feminine of Thomas
*Tamasin, Tamsin, Tamsyn,
Tamzen, Tamzin*

Tamatha (American) palms

Tamaura (American) palms

Tamay (American) form of
Tammy: sweetheart
Tamae,Tamaye

Tamaya (Native American)
grounded

Tambara (American) high-
energy
*Tam, Tamb, Tambra, Tamby,
Tammy*

Tambra (American) palms

Tambre (American) high
energy

Tambusi (African) frank
Tam, Tambussey, Tammy

Tame (American) calm

Tamefa (African American)
form of Tamika: lively
Tamefah, Tamifa

Tameria (Hebrew) palms

Tamesha (African American)
open face
*Tamesh, Tamisha, Tammie,
Tammy*

Tamesis (Spanish) name for
the Thames River
Tam, Tamey

Tami (Japanese) people
Tamie, Tamiko

Tamia (Japanese) little gem
Tameea, Tamya

Tamiah (Hebrew) palms

Tamika (African American)
lively
*Tameca, Tameeka, Tameka,
Tamieka, Tamikah, Tammi,
Tammie, Tammy, Temeka*

Tamiko (Japanese) the
people's child
Tami, Tamico, Tamika

Tamina (Hebrew) palms

Tamirisa (Indian) night; dark
*Risa, Tami, Tamirysa, Tamrisa,
Tamyrisa*

Tammy (American)
sweetheart
*Tam, Tammie, Tammi,
Tammye*

Tamohara (Hindu) the sun

Tamony (Hebrew) form of
Tamara: royal female
*Tamanee, Tamaney, Tamani,
Tamanie, Tamany, Tamonee,
Tamoney, Tamoni, Tamonie*

Tamra (Hebrew) sweet girl
Tammie, Tamora, Tamrah

Tamrika (African) newly
created
Tamreeka

Tamsin (English) benevolent
*Tam, Tami, Tammee, Tammey,
Tammy, Tammye, Tamsa,
Tamsan, Tamsen*

Tamsinn (English) form of
Thomasina: twin

Tamula (American) giving

Tamyrah (African American)
vocalist
Tamirah

Tamyren (Hebrew) form of
Tamyra: vocalist

Tamzin (American) palms

Tana (Slavic) petite princess
Taina, Tan, Tanah, Tanie

Tanaga (American) form of
Tanya: queenly

Tanai (American) thorough

Tanaka (Japanese) swamp
dweller

Tanay (African American)
new
Tanee

Tanaya (Hindu) daughter

Tanda (English) altogether

Tanden (English) altogether

Tandra (English) altogether

Tandria (English) altogether

Tandy (English) team player
Tanda, Tandi, Tandie

Tane (Polynesian) fertile

Tanesha (African) strong
Tanish, Tanisha, Tannesha, Tannie

Tangelia (Greek) angel
Gelia, Tange, Tangey

Tangenika (American) form of former country Tanganyika
Tange, Tangi, Tangy

Tangerla (American) of the fairies

Tangi (American) tangerine
Tangee

Tango (Spanish) dance
Tangoh

Tangyla (Invented) form of Tangela: combo of Tan and Angela
Tange, Tangy

Tani (Slavic) glorious
Tahnie, Tanee, Tanie

Tania (Russian/Slavic) queenly
Tannie, Tanny, Tanya

Tanikella (American) of the fairies

Tanimu (American) of the fairies

Tanina (American) bold
Tan, Tana, Tanena, Taninah, Tanney, Tanni, Tannie, Tanny, Tanye, Tanyna

Tanis (Slavic) form of Tania: queenly
Taniss, Tanys, Tanyss

Tanise (American) unique
Tanes, Tanis

Tanish (Greek) eternal
Tan, Tanesh, Tanny

Tanisha (African American) talkative
Taniesha, Tannie, Tenisha, Tinishah

Tanit (American) goddess

Tanith (Irish) estate
Tanita, Tanitha

Taniyah (Slavic) form of Tanya: queenly

Taniyen (Slavic) form of Tanya: queenly

Tanja (American) queen of fairies

Tanjiela (American) queen of fairies

Tannelle (English) tans leather

Tanra (English) tans leather

Tanrik (Hindi) flowers

Tansy (Latin) pretty
Tan, Tancy, Tansee, Tanzi

Tanuneka (African American) gracious
Nuneka, Tanueka, Tanun

Tanvi (Indian) fragile

Tanvi (Hindu) young woman

Tanya (Russian) queenly bearing
Tahnya, Tan, Tanyie, Tawnyah, Tonya

Tanyav (Slavic) regal
Tanyev

Tanyette (Italian) talkative
Tanye, Tanyee, Tanyett

Tanze (Greek) form of Tansy: pretty
Tans, Tansee, Tanz, Tanzee, Tanzey, Tanzi

Tanzy (Greek) eternal

Tao (Vietnamese) apple

Tapa (Spanish) little snack
Tapas

Tapasya (Hindu) bitter

Tapia (Spanish) small

Tapice (Spanish) covered
*Tapeece, Tapeese, Tapese,
Tapiece, Tapp, Tappy*

Tappuah (Biblical) place name

Tapus (Sanskrit) deliberate

Taquanna (African
American) noisy
*Takki, Takwana, Taquana,
Taque, Taquie*

Taquesha (African
American) joyful
Takie, Takwesha

Taquilla (American) from the
Spanish word tequila; lively
*Takela, Takelah, Taque, Tuquella,
Taqui, Taquile, Taquille*

Tara (Gaelic) towering
Tarah, Tari, Tarra

Tarafena (Biblical) gentle

Tarakini (Hindi) nighttime
with stars

Taral (Hindu) rippling

Taralah (Biblical) place name

Taran (American) earthy
*Taren, Tarran, Tarren, Tarryn,
Taryn*

Tarani (Hindu) light

Taree (Japanese) tree branch

Tarena (Slavic) melodic

Taricheae (Biblical) place
name

Tarika (Hindu) star

Tarina (Slavic) kind

Tarita (American) starry

Tarla (American) flamboyant

Tarlam (Hindu) flowering

Tarlease (American)
flamboyant

Tarleen (American)
flamboyant

Tarmica (American)
flamboyant

Tarnettia (American) from
the lake

Taro (Invented) card name;
farsighted

Tarona (American) form of
Tara: towering

Tarracina (Biblical) place name

Tarub (Arabic) cheerful

Taryn (English) county in
Northern Ireland
*Taran, Taren, Tarran, Tarrin,
Tarron*

Tasha (Russian) form of
Natasha: born on Christmas
*Tacha, Tahshah, Tash, Tashie,
Tasia, Tasie, Tasy, Tasya*

Tashanah (African
American) spunky
Tash, Tashana

Tashanee (African American)
lively
Tashaunie

Tashawndra (African
American) bright smiling
Tasha, Tashaundra, Tashie

Tashel (African American)
studious
*Tasha, Tashelle, Tashelle,
Tochelle*

Tashina (African American)
sparkles
Tasheena, Tasheenah, Tashinah

Tashka (Russian) together
Tashca, Tashcka

Tashua (American) cherishes

Tashza (African American) form of Tasha: born on Christmas
Tashi, Tashy, Tashzah

Tasia (American) Christmas baby

Tasida (Native American) rides a horse

Taska (American) Christmas baby

Tasma (American) twin
Tasmah

Tasmin (Pakistani) twin

Tasmind (American) twin

Tasmine (English) twin
Tasmin

Tasni (Arabic) spring

Tassi (Slavic) bold
Tassee, Tassey, Tassy

Tassie (English) twin

Tatanika (Slavic) fairy queen

Tataren (Slavic) fairy queen

Tate (English) short

Tateeahna (Invented) form of Tatiana: snow queen

Tatenda (Indian) fanciful

Tatiana (Russian) snow queen
Tanya, Tatania, Tatia, Tatianna, Tatiannia, Tatie, Tattianna, Tatyana, Tatyanna

Tatiyama (Asian) joyful

Tatjana (Slavic) vibrant

Tatrika (American) playful

Tatsu (Japanese) dragon

Tatum (English) cheery; high-spirited
Tata, Tate, Tatie, Tayte

Tauni (American) tawny; little

Taunja (American) form of Tonya: queenly

Taunya (American) form of Tonya: queenly

Taura (Latin) bull-like; stubborn

Tauvia (American) form of Octavia: eighth child; born on the eighth day of the month; musical

Tavia (Latin) form of Octavia: eighth child; born on the eighth day of the month; musical
Tava, Taveah, Tavi

Tavina (American) form of Tavia; form of Octavia: eighth child

Tavishi (Hindi) brave

Tavonia (American) form of Tavia; form of Octavia: eighth child

Tawannah (African American) talkative
Tawana, Tawanda, Tawanna, Tawona

Tawanner (American) loquacious
Tawanne, Twanner

Tawanta (African American) smart
Tawan, Tawante

Tawia (African) born after twins

Tawn (English) small girl

Tawnida (American) small

Tawny (American) tan-skinned
Tawn, Tawnee, Tawni, Tawnie

Tawnya (American) form of
Tanya: queenly bearing
Tawnie, Tawnyah, Tonya,
Tonyah

Tawyn (American) reliable;
tan
Tawenne, Tawin, Tawynne

Taya (English) tailor

Tayanita (Native American)
beaver

Tayla (American) doll-like
Taila, Taylah

Taylor ○ ❶ (English) tailor
by trade; style-setter
Tailor, Talor, Tay, Taye, Taylar,
Tayler

Tazmin (American) form of
Jasmine: fragrant; sweet
Tazminn, Tazmyn, Tazmynn

Tazmind (American) form of
Jasmine: fragrant; sweet

Tazu (Japanese) stork

Teagan (Irish) worldly;
creative
Teague, Teegan, Tegan

Teague (Irish) creative
Tee, Teegue, Tegue

Teah (Greek) goddess
Tea

Teale (English) blue-green;
bird
Teal, Teala

Tealisha (American) good
heart
Tee

Teamhair (Irish) hill

Teamikka (African American)
form of Tamika: lively
Teamika

Teana (American) form of
Tina: little and lively
Teanah, Teane

Teasa (Slavic) calm

Techa (Greek) of God

Tecoa (American) precocious
Tekoa

Teddi (Greek) cuddly
Ted, Teddie, Teddy

Tedra (Greek) outgoing
Teddra, Tedrah

Teen (Spanish) form of Tina:
little and lively

Tegin (Welsh) pretty

Tegvyen (Welsh) lovely

Tehara (Native American)
darling
Tihara, Tyhara

Teishya (American) joyful

Tejuana (Place name)
Tijuana, Mexico
T'Juana, Tijuana

Tekira (American) legendary
Tekera, Teki

Tekla (Greek) legend; divine
glory
Tekk, Teklah, Thekla, Tikla,
Tiklah

Tela (Greek) wise
Tella

Teleri (Welsh) variation of
Eleri: smooth

Telery (Welsh) delight

Teletha (American) loving
child

Teleza (African) slippery

Telina (American) storyteller
Teline, Telyna, Telyne, Tilina

Telma (Greek) ambitious

Telmah (American) capable

Telsa (American) form of
Tessa: reaping a harvest
Telly

Tema (Biblical) place name; orderly

Temetris (African American) respected
Teme, Temi, Temitris, Temmy

Temika (American) form of Tamika: lively

Temike (American) form of Tamika: lively

Temira (Hebrew) tall
Temora, Timora

Temperance (Latin) moderation

Tempest (French) tempestuous; stormy
Tempeste, Tempie, Tempyst

Templa (Latin) spiritual; moderate
Temp, Templah

Tenay (American) praised
Tendai

Tenday (African) praiseworthy

Tenesha (African American) clever
Tenesia, Tenicha, Tenisha, Tennie

Tenia (Spanish) tenuous

Tenika (American) cautious

Tennie (American) cautious

Tennille (American) innovative
Tanielle, Tanile, Ten, Teneal, Tenile, Tenneal, Tennelle, Tennie

Tenuvah (Hebrew) fruit and vegetables

Teo (Spanish) form of masculine name Teodoro: God's gift
Teeo, Teoh

Teodomira (Spanish) important

Teodora (Scandinavian) God's gift
Teo, Teodore

Teodula (Spanish) gives

Tequila (Spanish) intoxicating
Tequela, Tequilla, Tiki, Tiquilia

Terah (Latin) earth's child

Tereena (American) earth

Terena (English) feminine version of Terence
Tereena, Terenia, Terina, Terrena, Terrina, Teryna

Teresa (Greek) gardener
Taresa, Terese, Terhesa, Teri, Terre, Tess, Tessie, Treece, Tressa, Tressae

Terese (Greek) nurturing
Tarese, Therese, Treece

Teresille (American) earth

Teresita (Spanish) form of Teresa: gardener

Tereso (Spanish) reaper
Tere, Terese

Teressa (English) reaps what she sows

Teri (Greek) reaper
Terre, Terri, Terrie

Terlah (Arabic) of the earth

Teronica (American) form of Veronica: girl's image; real

Terra (Latin) earthy; name for someone born under an astrological earth sign
Tera, Terrie

Terrea (Spanish) earth

Terrell (Greek) hardy
Ter, Teral, Terell, Terrelle, Terrie, Teryl

Terrena (Latin) smooth-talking
Terina, Terrina, Terry

Ter-Ri (American) form of Terri: reaper

Terrian (American) earth

Terry (Greek) form of Theresa: gardener
Teri, Terre, Terrey, Terri, Tery

Terson (Last name used as first name) child of earth

Tertia (Latin) third
Ters, Tersh, Tersha, Tersia

Teshuah (Hebrew) reprieve
Teshua, Teshura

Tess (Greek) harvesting life
Tesse

Tessa (Greek) reaping a harvest
Tesa, Tessie, Teza

Tessella (Italian) countess
Tesela, Tesella, Tessela

Tessica (American) form of Jessica: rich
Tesica, Tess, Tessa, Tessie, Tessika

Tessie (Greek) form of Theresa: gardener
Tessey, Tessi, Tezi

Tetsu (Japanese) iron

Teuila (Spanish) young

Tevy (Cambodian) angel

Texie (American) form of Texas: U.S. state; cowboy

Tezuma (Spanish) form of the word Montezuma

Thada (Greek) appreciative
Thadda, Thaddeah

Thadyne (Hebrew) worthy of praise
Thadee, Thadine, Thady

Thalassa (Greek) sensitive
Talassa, Thalassah, Thalasse

Thalia (Greek) joyful; fun
Thalya

Thana (Arabic) happy

Thana (Arabic) thanksgiving

Thandiwe (African) affectionate

Thanh (Vietnamese) brilliant

Thao (Vietnamese) respect

Tharamel (Invented) form of the word caramel: dedicated
Thara

The (Vietnamese) pledged

Thea (Greek) goddess
Teah, Teeah, Theah, Theeah, Theo, Tiah

Theadora (Greek) God's gift

Theadra (Greek) goddess

Thebes (Biblical) place name

Theda (American) confident
Thada, Thedah

Theia (Greek) divine one

Thekia (Greek) famous

Thekla (Greek) famous; divine
Tecla, Tekla, Thecla

Thel (American) opinionated

Thelia (Greek) form of Thalia: joyful; fun

Thelina (American) musical

Thelma (Greek) giver
Thel

Thema (African) queen

Themba (African) trusted

Themis (Greek) just

Themla (Greek) just

Theodora (Greek)
sweetheart; God's gift
*Dora, Teddi, Teddie, Teddy,
Tedi, Tedra, Tedrah, Theda,
Theo, Theodorah, Theodrah*

Theola (Greek) excellent
Theo, Theolah, Thie

Theone (Greek) serene
Theona, Theonne

Theoni (Greek) God's child

Theonus (American) calm

Theophania (Greek) God's
features
Theophanie

Theophila (Greek) loved by
God
Theofila

Theora (Greek) God's gift
Theorah, Theorra, Theorrah

Theres (Greek) reaps what
she sows

Theresa (Greek) gardener
Reza, Teresa, Terri, Terrie, Terry

Therese (Greek) bountiful
harvest
Tereece, Terese, Terise, Terry

Theresia (Spanish) harvests

Theressa (Spanish) harvests

Therna (Greek) wild
Thera

Thersa (Hebrew) pleases
Therza, Thirza

Thesina (American) creates

Thessalonica (Biblical) place
name

Thessaly (Biblical) place name

Theta (Greek) letter in Greek
alphabet; substantial
Thayta, Thetah

Thetis (Greek) mother of
Achilles

Theya (American) pleases

Thi (Vietnamese) poem

Thia (Greek) goddess

Thim (Thai) ice cream; sweet

Thirzah (Hebrew) pleasant
Thirza, Thursa, Thurza

Thoa (Asian) hopeful

Thocmetony (Native
American) flower
Tocmetone

Thomasina (Hebrew) twin
*Tom, Toma, Tomasa,
Tomasina, Tomina, Tommie,
Toto*

Thomia (Hebrew) twin

Thonie (American) prepared

Thonne (American) prepared

Thora (Scandinavian) like
thunder
Thorah

Thrixia (American) kindness

Thu (Vietnamese) autumn

Thuy (Vietnamese) gentle

Thyatira (Biblical) place name
Tiamat, Tiam, Tya

Thyra (Scandinavian) loud
Thira

Tia (Greek/Spanish) princess;
aunt
Teah, Tee, Teia, Tiah

Tiama (Mythology) ocean-
loving

Tian (Greek) lovely
*Ti, Tiane, Tiann, Tianne,
Tyan, Tyann, Tyanne, Tye*

Tiana (Greek) highest beauty
Tana, Teeana, Tiane, Tiona

Tiandye (American) princess

Tianth (American) pretty and impetuous
Teanth, Tia, Tian, Tianeth

Tiara (Latin) crowned goddess
Teara, Tearra, Tee, Teearah, Tierah, Tira

Tiare (French) ornamented

Tiaret (French) wears a crown

Tiarna (American) tiara

Tiaura (American) form of Tiara: crowned goddess

Tibby (American) frisky
Tib, Tibb, Tybbee

Tiberia (Latin) majestic
Tibbie, Tibby

Tibisay (American) uniter
Tibi, Tibisae

Tichanda (African American) stylish
Tichaunda, Tishanda

Tiena (Spanish) earthy
Teena

Tierah (Latin) jeweled; ornament
Tia, Tiarra, Tiera

Tiernan (English) lord

Tierney (Irish) wealthy
Teern, Teerney, Teerny, Tiern

Tierra (Latin) tiara

Tifara (Hebrew) festive
Tiferet, Tifhara

Tifaya (Greek) form of Tiffany: lasting love
Tifaya, Tifayane, Tiff, Tiffy

Tiffa (American) holy trinity

Tiffany (Greek) lasting love
Tifanie, Tiff, Tiffanie, Tiffenie, Tiffi, Tiffie, Tiffy, Tiphanie, Tyfannie

Tiffin (American) form of Tiffany: lasting love

Tig (American) tigress

Tigerlilly (American) flower

Tigress (Latin) wild
Tigris, Tye, Tygris

Tigris (Irish) tiger

Tigris (Biblical) place name

Tija (Spanish) form of Tijuana, Mexico

Tijana (American) form of Tijuana, Mexico

Tiki (Polynesian) ancestor; image
Tekee

Tikoletta (American) frivolous

Til (American) form of Matilda: powerful fighter

Tilana (Spanish) truth

Tilda (German) form of Matilda: powerful fighter
Telda, Tildie, Till, Tylda

Tiliera (American) strong

Tilira (American) strong

Tilla (German) industrious
Tila

Tilly (German) cute; strong
Till, Tillee, Tillie

Timerra (American) timid

Timia (American) timid

Timmie (Greek) form of Timothie: honorable
Tim, Timi, Timmy

Timna (Biblical) Anah's sister

Timothea (Greek) honoring God
Timaula, Timi, Timie, Timmi, Timmie

Timothie (Greek) honorable
Tim, Timmie, Timothea, Timothy

Timsuh (Biblical) place name

Tina (Latin/Spanish) little and lively
Teena, Teenie, Tena, Tiny

Tinker (American) animated

Tinkette (American) form of Tinker: animated

Tinna (American) form of Tina: little and lively

Tinsia (American) form of Tina: little and lively

Tiofila (Spanish) friend

Tionne (American) hopeful
Tionn

Tiphanie (Spanish) form of Tiffany: lasting love

Tiphsuh (Biblical) place name

Tiponya (Native American) owl; watchful

Tippah (Hindi) form of Tipo: tiger; ferocious

Tipper (Irish) pourer of water; nurturing
Tip, Tippy, Typper

Tippett (American) giving

Tippie (American) generous
Tippi, Tippy

Tira (Hebrew) camp

Tirathana (Biblical) place name

Tiri (Welsh) sweet

Tirica (American) form of Erica: honorable; leading others

Tirion (Welsh) gentle

Tirrza (Hebrew) sweet; precious
Thirza, Thirzah, Tirza, Tirzah

Tirtha (Hindu) ford

Tirza (Hebrew) kindness
Thirza, Tirza, Tirzah

Tisa (African) ninth child
Tesa, Tesah, Tisah

Tish (Latin) happy
Tysh

Tisha (Latin) joyful
Tesha, Ticia, Tishah, Tishie

Tishbe (Biblical) place name

Tishema (American) joyful

Tishka (American) joyful

Tishra (African American) original
Tishrah

Tishunette (African American) happy girl
Tish, Tisunette

Tita (Greek) giant; large

Titania (Greek) giant

Tivona (Hebrew) lover of nature

Tiwa (Native American) onion

Tobago (Place name) west Indies island; islander
Bago, ToTo

Tobarista (American) believer

Tobi (Hebrew) good
Tobie, Toby

Toblene (American) believer

Toffey (American) spirited
Toff, Toffee, Toffi, Toffie, Toffy

Tohuia (Polynesian) flower

Toinette (Latin) wonderful
Toin, Toinett, Toney, Tony, Toynet

Toireasa (Irish) strong
Treise

Toki (Japanese) chance

Tokiwa (Japanese) steady

Tolice (American) creative

Tolikna (Native American) coyote ears

Tollie (Hebrew) confident
Toll, Tollee, Tolli, Tolly, Tollye

Toloisi (French) ingenious

Tomazja (Polish) twin

Tomea (American) twin

Tomeka (African American) form of Tamika: lively
Tomeke

Tomiko (Japanese) wealthy
Miko, Tamiko, Tomi

Tomitria (African American) form of Tommie: sassy
Toml

Tommie (Hebrew) sassy
Tom, Tomi, Tommy

Tomo (Japanese) intelligence

Tonaya (American) valuable
Tona, Tone

Tonesa (Greek) thriving

Tonet (French) form of Tony: meritorious

Tonetta (American) thriving

Toney (American) form of Tony: meritorious

Toni (Latin) form of Tony: meritorious
Tone, Tonee, Tonie, Tony

Tonia (Latin) a wonder
Toneah, Tonya, Tonyah, Toyiah

Tonia (Latin) daring
Tonni, Tonnie, Tony, Tonya

Tonicia (American) form of Tony: meritorious

Tonisha (African American) lively
Nisha, Tona, Toneisha, Tonesha, Tonie, Tonish

Tonla (American) form of Tonya: queenly

Tonna (American) form of Tony: meritorious

Tooka (Japanese) ten days

Topaz (Latin) gemstone; sparkling
Tophaz

Topher (Greek) feminine form of Christopher: the bearer of Christ

Tophery (Greek) form of Topher; form of Christopher: Christian

Tophie (Greek) form of Sophie: intelligent

Topsy (English) topnotch
Toppie, Toppsy, Topsey, Topsi, Topsie

Tora (Scandinavian) thunder

Toranda (American) wins

Torborg (Scandinavian) thunder
Thorborg, Torbjorg

Tordis (Scandinavian) thor's goddess

Tori (Scottish) rich and winning
Toree, Torri, Torrie, Torry, Tory

Torill (Scandinavian) loud
Toril, Torille

Torrance (Place name) town in California; confident
Torr, Torri

Torsha (American) wins

Torta (American) wins

Torunn (Scandinavian) loved by Thor

Toscha (Slavic) prepared

Tosha (Slavic) priceless
Tosh, Toshia

Toshala (Hindu) satisfied

Toshio (Japanese) year-old child
Toshi, Toshie, Toshiko, Toshikyo

Toski (Native American) bug

Tossia (Slavic) prepared

Toti (English) form of Charlotte: little woman

Totsi (Native American) moccasins

Toula (American) athletic

Tova (Hebrew) good woman
Tovah

Toxie (American) athletic

Toy (American) playful
Toia, Toya, Toye

Tozie (American) friendly

Trace (French) takes the right path
Traice, Trayce

Tracey (Gaelic) aggressive
Trace, Tracee, Traci, Tracie, Tracy

Tracinal (American) form of Tracy: summer

Tracy (English) summer
Trace, Tracee, Tracey, Traci, Tracie, Trasey, Treacy, Treesy

Traina (American) thinker

Trana (American) thoughtful

Trancine (American) form of Francine: beautiful

Tranell (American) confident
Tranel, Tranelle, Traney, Trani

Trang (Vietnamese) smart

Trangera (American) smart

Traniqua (African American) hopeful
Tranaqua, Tranekwa, Tranequa, Trani, Tranikwa, Tranney, Tranniqua, Tranny

Trava (Czech) grass

Traviata (Italian) woman who wanders

Travistene (American) feminine form of Travis: conflicted

Tray (American) form of Trey: third-born; creatively brilliant

Trayceez (American) form of Tracy: summer

Traysha (American) form of Tricia: humorous

Trazanna (African American) talented
Traz, Trazannah, Traze

Treana (American) pure

Treann (American) pure

Treasah (American) pure

Treat (Word as name)

Trecia (American) form of Tricia: humorous

Tree (American) sturdy

Treece (American) form of Terese: nurturing
Treese, Trice

Treena (American) form of Trina: perfect; scintillating
Treen

Treesjie (American) distinctive

Trella (Spanish) star; sparkles
Trela

Tremira (African American) anxious
Tremera, Tremmi

Treneth (American) smiling
Trenith, Trenny

Trenia (American) form of Trina: perfect; scintillating

Trenica (African American) smiling
Trenika, Trinika

Trenise (African American) songbird
Tranese, Tranise, Trannise, Treenie, Treneese, Treni, Trenniece, Trenny

Trenllita (Spanish) form of Trina: perfect; scintillating

Trentine (American) pure

Trenyce (American) smiling
Trienyse, Trinyce

Tres (Greek) form of Theresa: gardener

Tresca (American) form of Theresa: gardener

Treseme (American) form of Theresa: gardener

Tressa (Greek) reaping life's harvest
Tresa, Tresah, Tress, Trisa

Tressel (American) form of Theresa: gardener

Tressem (American) form of Theresa: gardener

Tressie (American) successful
Tress, Tressa, Tressee, Tressey, Tressi, Tressy

Tressy (American) form of Theresa: gardener

Tresure (Invented) giving
Treasure, Tress

Treva (English) homestead by the sea

Trevei (American) wise

Trevina (English) variation of Treva: homestead by the sea

Treyvin (American) form of Trevin: strong

Tricia (Latin) humorous
Treasha, Tresha, Trich, Tricha, Trish, Trisha

Trido (American) threefold

Trilby (English) literary
Trilbie, Trilby

Trill (American) excitable

Trin (American) pure

Trina (Greek) perfect; scintillating
Tina, Treena, Trine, Trinie

Trinda (American) pure

Trinesse (American) pure

Trinh (Vietnamese) virgin

Trinida (Spanish) trinity

Trinidad (Place name) island off of Venezuela; spiritual person
Trini, Trinny

Trinity ✪ (Latin) triad
Trini, Trinita

Trinka (American) ideal

Trinlee (American) genuine
Trinley, Trinli, Trinly

Trionelle (Scottish) pure

Tripti (Hindi) content

Tris (American) form of Patricia: woman of nobility; unbending

Trish (American) form of Patricia: woman of nobility; unbending
Trysh

Trisha (American) form of Patricia: woman of nobility; unbending
Tricia

Trishelle (African American) humorous girl
Trichelle, Trichillem, Trish, Trishel, Trishie

Trishna (Indian) desired

Trissy (American) tall
Triss, Trissi, Trissie

Trista (Latin) pensive; sparkling love
Tresta, Trist, Tristie, Trysta

Tristen (Latin) bold
Tristan, Tristie, Tristin, Trysten

Tristica (Spanish) form of Trista: pensive; sparkling love
Trist, Tristi, Tristika

Trixie (Latin) personable
Trix, Trixi, Trixy

Tru (English) form of Truly: honest
True

Truc (Vietnamese) desire

Trudin (American) form of Trudy: hopeful

Trudis (German) optimist

Trudy (German) hopeful
Trude, Trudi, Trudie

True (American) truthful
Truee, Truie, Truth

Truette (American) truthful
Tru, True, Truett

Truffle (French) delicacy
Truff, Truffy

Trulea (American) honest

Trulencia (Spanish) honest
Lencia, Tru, Trulence, Trulens, Trulense

Truly (American) honest
true, Trulee, Truley

Trusteen (American) trusting
Trustean, Trustee, Trustine, Trusty, Trusyne

Truth (American) honest
Truthe

Try (American) earnest
Tri, Trie

Tryna (Greek) form of Trina: perfect; scintillating
Trine, Tryne, Trynna

Tsifira (Hebrew) crown

Tsomah (Native American) rose

Tsonka (American) capricious
Sonky, Tesonka, Tisonka, Tsonk

Tsuhgi (Japanese) second daughter

Tsula (Native American) fox

Tteirrah (American) form of Tara: towering

Tua (Polynesian) outdoors

Tualau (Polynesian) outdoors

Tucker (English) tailor
Tukker

Tuenchit (Thai) mysterious

Tuesday (English) weekday

Tuhina (Hindu) snow

Tuki (Japanese) moon

Tula (Native American) moon

Tulasi (Indian) basil sacred

Tulia (Spanish) glorious
Tuli, Tuliana, Tulie, Tuliea, Tuly

Tuliki (Mythology) of the wind

Tully (Irish) powerful;
dark spirit
Tull, Tulle, Tulli, Tullie

Tulse (Hindi) growing

Tulsi (Hindu) basil

Tunishua (American) place
name Tunisia

Tunisia (Place name)

Turin (American) creative
Turan, Turen, Turrin, Turun

Turney (Latin) wood worker
Turnee, Turni, Turnie, Turny

Turquoise (French) blue-
green
Turkoise, Turquie, Turrkoise

Tursha (Slavic) warm
Tersha

Turush (Biblical) place name

Turya (Hindi) spiritual

Tusa (Native American) prarie
dog

Tusti (Indian) peace

Tuwa (Native American) earth

Tuyen (Vietnamese) angel
Tuyet

Twaina (English) divided
Twayna

Twanda (African) dual

Tweetie (American) vivacious
Tweetee, Tweetey, Tweeti

Twiggy (English) slim
Twiggie, Twiggee, Twiggey

Twyla (English) creative
Twila, Twilia

Twynceola (African
American) bold
Twin, Twyn, Twynce

Tyana (African American)
new

Tyberia (Place name)

Tyce (American) Ty's child

Tye (American) talented

Tyeoka (African American)
rhythmic
Tioka, Tyeo, Tyeoke

Tyesha (African American)
duplicitous
*Tesha, Tisha, Tyeisha, Tyiesha,
Tyisha*

Tyisha (African American)
sweet
Isha, Tisha, Ty, Tyeisha, Tyish

Tyla (American) form of Tyler:
stylish; tailor

Tyler (American) stylish;
tailor
Tielyr, Tye

Tymitha (African American)
kind
*Timitha, Tymi, Tymie, Tymith,
Tymy, Tymytha*

Tyndall (Irish) dark
*Tyndal, Tyndel, Tyndell, Tyndyl,
Tyndyll*

Tyne (American/English)
dramatic; sylvan
Tie, Tine, Tye

Tynisha (African American)
fertile
Tinisha, Tynesha, Tynie

Tyonia (American) of the
river

Tyra (Scandinavian) assertive
woman
Tye, Tyrah, Tyre, Tyrie

Tyrea (African American)
form of Thora: like thunder
Tyree, Tyria

Tyredda (American) form of
Tyra: assertive woman

Tyrina (American) ball of fire
Tierinna, Tye, Tyreena, Tyrinah

Tyrra (Scandinavian)
aggressive

Tyson (French) son of Ty
Ty, Tysen

Tyzna (American) ingenious;
assertive
Tyze, Tyzie

Tzadika (Hebrew) loyal
Zadika

Tzafra (Hebrew) morning
Tzefira, Zafra, Zefira

Tzahala (Hebrew) happy
Zahala

Tzeira (Hebrew) young

Tzemicha (Hebrew) in bloom
Zemicha

Tzeviya (Hebrew) gazelle
*Civia, Tzevia, Tzivia, Tzivya,
Zibiah, Zivia*

Tzigane (Hungarian) gypsy
Tsigana, Tsigane

Tzila (Hebrew) darkness
Tzili, Zila, Zili

Tzina (Hebrew) shelter
Zina

Tzipiya (Hebrew) hope
Tzipia, Zipia

Tziyona (Hebrew) hill
Zeona, Ziona

Tzofi (Hebrew) scout
*Tzofia, Tzofit, Tzofiya, Zofi,
Zofia, Zofit*

Tzuriya (Hebrew) God is
powerful
Tzuria, Zuria

Uberta (Italian) bright

Uchechi (African) God's will

Udavine (American) thriving
Uda

Udele (English) prospering
woman
*Uda, Udela, Udell, Udella,
Udelle*

Uela (Unknown) dedicated to
God
Uella

Ufrosinne (Mythology) jovial
Euphrosyne

Uganda (Place name) African
nation

Ujhala (Hindi) shines

Ula (Celtic) jewel-like beauty
Eula, Ulah, Ule, Ulla, Ylla

Ulanda (American) confident
Uland, Ulandah, Ulande

Ulani (Hawaiian/Polynesian)
happy
Ulanee

Ulatha (Biblical) place name;
happy

Ulda (Unknown origin)
prophetess

Ule (Unknown origin)
burdens

Ulielmi (Unknown origin)
intelligent

Ulima (Unknown origin)
smart

Ulla (German) powerful and
rich

Ulphi (Unknown origin)
lovely
Ulphia, Ulphiah

Ulrika (Teutonic) leader
*Rica, Ulree, Ulric, Ulrica,
Ulrie, Ulry, Urik*

Ultima (Latin) aloof

Ulupi (Hindi) pretty

Ulva (German) wolf; courage

Ulyssia (Invented) form of
Ulysses: forceful
Lyss, Lyssia, Uls, Ulsy, Ulsyia

Uma (Hebrew) nation;
worldview
Umah

Umberlina (Unknown
origin) feminine form of
Umberto

Umeko (Unknown origin)
blossom

Umma (Hindi) mother
Uma, Umah

Umnia (Arabic) desirable
Umniah, Umniya, Umniyah

Una (Latin) unique
Ona, Oona, Unah

Unda (Scandinavian) water
child

Undine (Latin) from the
ocean
Ondine, Undene, Undyne

Undra (American) one;
longsuffering

Unet (French) the one

Unette (American) the one

Unice (English) sensible
Eunice, Uniss

Unika (Slavic) different

Unique (Latin) singular
Uneek

Unity (English) unity of spirit
Unitee

Unn (Scandinavian) loving
Un

Ural (Place name) ural
Mountains
Ura, Uralle, Urine, Uris

Urania (Greek) universal
beauty
*Ranie, Uraine, Urana,
Uraneah, Uranie*

Urbai (Unknown origin)
gentle

Urbana (Latin) born in the
city
Urbani, Urbanna, Urbannai

Urbi (Egyptian) princess

Urena (Slavic) lights the way

Urgita (Hindi) energetic

Uria (Hebrew) God is my
flame
Ria, Uri, Uriah, Urial, Urissa

Uridia (Slavic) light

Uriela (Hebrew) God's light
Uriella, Uriyella

Urit (Hebrew) candle

Urith (Hebrew) bright
Urit

Urmia (Biblical) place name

Ursa (Greek/Latin) star;
bearlike
Urs, Ursah, Ursie

Ursula (Latin) little female
bear
Ursa, Urse, Ursela, Ursila

Urta (Latin) spiny plant

Usha (Indian) dawn;
awakening

Usher (Word as name)
helpful
Ush, Ushar, Ushur

Usiana (Biblical) place name

Uta (Teutonic) battle heroine

Utas (Unknown origin) glorious

Ute (German) rich and powerful

Utica (Native American)
Uticas, Uttica

Utopia (American) idealistic
Uta, Utopiah

Uttasta (Unknown origin) from the homeland

Uzbek (Place name) for Uzbekistan
Usbek

Uzetta (American) serious
Uzette

Uzia (Hebrew) God is my strength
Uzial, Uzzia, Uzzial

Uzma (Spanish) capable
Usma, Uz, Uzmah

Uzoma (African) the right way

Vacla (Origin unknown) vain

Vaclava (Origin unknown) conceited

Vada (German) form of Valda: high spirits
Vaida, Vay

Vadnee (Origin unknown) gives

Vairie (Spanish) versatile child

Val (Latin) form of Valerie: robust

Vala (German) chosen one

Valaida (German) chosen

Valaine (French) chooses

Valarie (Latin) strong
Val, Valaria, Valerie

Valda (German) high spirits
Val, Valdah, Valida, Velda

Vale (English) valley; natural
Vail, Vaylie

Valecia (Spanish) form of Valencia: city in Spain; strong-willed

Valeda (Latin) strong woman
Val, Valayda, Valedah

Valencia (Place name) city in Spain; strong-willed
Val, Valecia, Valence, Valenica, Valensha, Valentia, Valenzia, Valincia

Valene (Latin) strong girl
Valaine, Valean, Valeda, Valeen, Valen, Valena, Valeney, Vallen, Valina, Valine, Vallan, Vallen

Valensia (Spanish) strong

Valenteen (American) strong

Valentina (Latin) romantic
Val, Vala, Valantina, Vale Valentin, Valentine, Valiaka, Valtina, Valyn, Valynn

Valeny (American) hard
Val, Valenie

Valera (American) form of Valerie: robust

Valeria (Spanish) having valor
Valeri, Valerie, Valery

Valerie (Latin) robust
*Vairy, Val, Valarae, Valaree,
Valarey, Valari, Valarie, Vale,
Valeree, Valeri, Valeriane,
Valery, Vallarie, Valleree,
Valleri, Vallerie, Vallery, Valli,
Vallie, Vallirie, Valora, Valry,
Veleria, Velerie*

Valerta (Invented) form of
Valerie: robust
Valer, Valert

Valesca (Slavic) rules

Valeska (Polish) joyous leader
*Valese, Valeshia, Valeske,
Valezka, Valisha*

Valetta (Italian) feminine
Valettah, Valita, Valitta

Valida (Spanish) right

Valince (American) valiant

Valinda (American) valiant

Valindae (American) valiant

Valkie (Scandinavian)
fantastic
*Val, Valkee, Valki, Valkry,
Valky*

Valley (Word as name)

Vallie (Latin) natural
Val, Valli, Vally

Vallie-Mae (Latin) form of
Valentina and Mae: romantic
Valliemae, Vallimae, Vallimay

Valluri (Slavic) form of
Valerie: robust

Valma (Scandinavian) loyal

Valmay (American) spring

Valonia (Scandinavian) loyal
Vallon, Valona

Valora (Latin) intimidating
*Val, Valorah, Valori, Valoria,
Valorie, Valory, Valorya*

Valore (Latin) courageous
Val, Valour

Valoria (Spanish) brave
Vallee, Valora, Valore

Valrie (American) form of
Valerie: robust

Value (Word as name) valued
Valu, Valyou

Valyn (American) perky
Valind, Valinn, Valynn

Vamia (Hispanic) energetic
Vamee, Vamie

Vanay (American) honor

Vanda (German) smiling
beauty
*Vandah, Vandana, Vandelia,
Vandetta, Vandi, Vannda*

Vandan (American) honors

Vandana (Hindi) honor
Vandani

Vandeen (Sanskrit) prayerful

Vandyke (Dutch) lives by the
water

Vaneecai (Slavic) form of
Vanessa: flighty

Vanessa ☉ (Greek) flighty
*Nessa, Van, Vanassa, Vanesa,
Vanesah, Vanesha, Vaneshia,
Vanesia, Vanessah, Vanesse,
Vanessia, Vanessica, Veneza,
Vaniece, Vaniessa, Vanisa,
Vanissa, Vanita, Vanna,
Vannessa, Vanneza, Vanni,
Vannie, Vanny, Varnessa,
Venesa, Venessa*

Vani (Russian) form of Vania:
gifted

Vania (Hebrew) gifted
Vaneah, Vanya

Vanille (American) simplistic
*Vana, Vani, Vanila, Vanile,
Vanna*

Vanity (English) vain girl
Vanita, Vaniti

Vanna (Greek) golden girl
Van, Vana, Vanae, Vannah,
Vannalee, Vannaleigh

Vanniea (American)
capricious

Vanora (Welsh) wave;
mercurial
Vannora

Vantha (Greek) yellow hair

Vanthe (Greek) form of
Xanthe: beautiful blonde

Vantje (Scandinavian) blonde

Vanya (American) form of
Vanna: golden girl
Vani, Vanja, Vanni, Vanyuh

Vara (Greek) strange
Varah, Vare

Varaina (Invented) form of
Lorraine: sad-eyed

Varda (Hebrew) rosy
Vadit, Vardah, Vardia, Vardice,
Vardina, Vardis, Vardit

Varetta (American)
methodical

Varina (Czech) form of
Barbara: traveler from a
foreign land

Varna (Origin unknown) no
trace of vanity

Vasa (Slavic) pretty

Vashi (Slavic) pretty

Vashti (Persian) beauty
Vashtee, Vashtie

Vasta (Persian) pretty
Vastah

Vasteen (American) capable
Vas, Vastene, Vastine, Vasty

Vateyo (American) pious

Vatima (Slavic) form of
Fatima: wise woman

Vaughan (Last name as first
name) smooth talker
Vaughn, Vawn, Vawne

Veanetta (American)
knowing

Veanu (American) knowing

Veata (Cambodian) smart;
organized
Veatah

Veaunarda (Slavic) vineyard

Veda (Sanskrit) wise woman
Vedad, Vedah, Vedis, Veeda,
Veida, Vida, Vita

Veddy (Slavic) jubilant

Vedea (Slavic) spirited child

Vedette (French) watchful
Veda, Vedett, Vedetta

Vedi (Sanskrit) wisdom

Vedis (Slavic) lively

Vedrana (Slavic) pleasant

Veena (Indian) musical
instrument

Veera (Spanish) form of Vera:
faithful friend

Vega (Scandinavian) star
Vay, Vayga, Vegah, Veguh

Velacy (Origin unknown)
delicate

Velda (German) famous
leader
Veleda, Valeda

Veleda (German) intelligent
Vel, Veladah, Velayda

Veletta (American) secretive

Velia (American) secretive

Velika (Slavic) wonder

Velina (American) secretive

Velinda (American) form of
Melinda: honey; sweetheart
*Vel, Velin, Velind, Vell, Velly,
Velynda*

Vell (American) form of
Velma: hardworking
Vel, Velly, Vels

Vellamo (Mythology)
attractive

Velma (German)
hardworking
*Valma, Vel, Vellma, Velmah,
Vilma, Vilna*

Velonne (Spanish) capable

Velore (Origin unknown)
poised

Veltria (American) secretive

Velvet (French) luxurious
Vel, Vell, Velvete, Velvett

Vendy (American) respects

Venecia (Italian) girl from
Venice; sparkles
*Vanecia, Vanetia, Veneise,
Venesa, Venesha, Venesher,
Venesse, Venessia, Venetia,
Venette, Venezia, Venice,
Venicia, Veniece, Veniesa,
Venise, Venisha, Venishia,
Venita, Venitia, Venize,
Vennesa, Vennice, Vennisa,
Vennise, Vonitia, Vonizia*

Veneradah (Spanish)
honored; venerable
Ven, Venera, Venerada

Veneranda (Spanish)
venerated; respected

Venetia (Latin) girl from
Venice

Veney (American) respects

Venice (Place name) city in
Italy; coming of age
*Vanice, Vaniece, Veneece,
Veneese*

Venitia (Italian) forgiving
*Esha, Venesha, Venn, Venney,
Venni, Vennie, Venny*

Venka (Indian) hunter

Venkata (Indian) hunter

Venke (Polish) form of
Venice: city in Italy; coming
of age

Vennita (Italian) form of
Venice: city in Italy; coming
of age
*Nita, Vanecia, Ven, Venesha,
Venetia, Venita, Vennie,
Vinetia*

Ventura (Spanish) fortunate

Venus (Latin) loving; goddess
of love
*Venis, Venise, Vennie, Venusa,
Vinny*

Veola (American) form of
Viola: violet; lovely lady
Violet

Veoline (American) violet

Veonia (American) form of
Venus: loving; goddess of
love

Veonialle (American) form of
Venus:loving; goddess of love

Vera (Russian) faithful friend
*Vara, Veera, Veira, Veradis,
Verah, Vere, Verie, Vira*

Verbena (Latin) natural
beauty

Verchema (American) honest

Verda (Latin) breath of spring
*Ver, Vera, Verdah, Verde, Verdi,
Verdie, Viridiana, Viridis*

Verdad (Spanish) verdant;
honest
*Verda, Verdade, Verdie,
Verdine, Verdite*

Verdelina (American) verdant

Verdia (American) verdant

Verdie (Latin) fresh as springtime
Verd, Verda, Verdee, Verdi, Verdy

Verena (English) honest
Veren, Verenah, Verene, Verenis, Vereniz, Verina, Verina, Verine, Virena, Virna

Verenase (Swiss) flourishing; truthful
Ver, Verenese, Verennase, Vy, Vyrenase, Vyrennace

Verity (French) truthful
Verety, Verita, Veritee, Veriti, Veritie

Verla (Latin) truthful

Verlene (Latin) vivacious
Verleen, Verlena, Verlie, Verlin, Verlina, Verlinda, Verline, Verlyn, Verlynne

Verlita (Spanish) growing

Vermekia (African American) natural
Meki, Mekia, Verme, Vermekea, Vermy, Vermye

Verna (Latin) springlike
Vernah, Verne, Vernese, Vernesha, Verneshia, Vernessa, Vernetia, Vernetta, Vernette, Vernia, Vernice, Vernis, Vernisha, Vernishela, Vernita, Verusya, Viera, Virida, Virna, Virnell

Verneake (American) spring

Verneta (Latin) verdant
Vernita, Verna, Virena, Virna

Vernice (American) natural
Verna, Vernica, Vernicca, Vernie, Verniece, Vernique

Vernicia (Spanish) form of Vernice: natural
Vern, Verni, Vernisia

Vernita (Latin) of the spring

Verona (Place name) city in Italy; flourishes; honest

Veronica (Latin) girl's image; real
Nica, Ronica, Varonica, Veron, Verhonica, Verinica, Verohnica, Veron, Verone, Veronic, Veronice, Veronika, Veronne, Veronnica, Vironica, Vonni, Von, Vonni, Vonnie, Vonny, Vron, Vronica

Veronican (American) form of Veronica: girl's image; real

Veronique (French) form of Veronica: girl's image; real
Veroneek, Veroneese, Veroniece

Veroniquea (French) form of Veronica: girl's image; real
Vesna, Vezna

Versperah (Latin) evening star
Vesp, Vespa, Vespera

Vertrelle (African American) organized
Vertey, Verti, Vertrel, Vetrell

Vesela (Origin unknown) open
Vess

Vesnah (Slavic) spring goddess

Vespera (Latin) evening star

Vesta (Latin) home-loving; goddess of the home
Vess, Vessie, Vessy, Vest, Vestah, Vesteria

Veste (Latin) keeps home fires burning
Esta, Vesta

Vetaria (Slavic) regal woman

Vevay (Latin) form of Vivian: bubbling with life
Vevah, Vi, Viv, Vivay, Vivi, Vivie

Vevila (Irish) vivacious

Vevina (Latin) sweetheart

Vi (Latin) form of Viola: violet; lovely lady
Vy, Vye

Viana (Italian) vital

Vianca (American) form of Bianca: white

Vianey (Spanish) form of Vivian: bubbling with life
Via, Viana, Viane, Viani, Vianne, Vianney, Viany

Vianne (French) striking
Vi, Viane, Viann

Viara (American) vibrant

Vibeke (Hindi) vibrant

Vickay (American) form of Vicky: winner

Vicky (Latin) form of Victoria: winner
Vic, Viccy, Vick, Vickee, Vickey, Vicki, Vickie, Vikkey, Vikki, Viky

Victoria ○ (Latin) winner
Vic, Vicki, Vicky, Victoriah, Victoriana, Victorie, Victorina, Victorine, Victory, Vikki, Viktoria, Vyctoria

Victorine (French) winner

Victory (Latin) a winning woman
Vic, Viktorie

Vida (Hebrew) form of Davida: beloved one
Veeda

Vidella (Spanish) life
Veda, Vida, Videline, Vydell

Vidette (Hebrew) loved
Viddey, Viddi, Viddie, Vidett, Videy

Vidonia (Portuguese) vine; winding

Vidrine (Last name as first name) life

Vie (American) competitor

Vienna (Place name) a city in Austria
Veena, Vena, Venna, Viena, Viennah, Vienne, Vienette, Vina

Viennese (Place name) form of Vienna: a city in Austria
Vee, Viena, Vienne

Viera (Spanish) smart; alive

Vieyra (Spanish) lively

Vigdis (Scandinavian) war goddess

Vigilia (Latin) vigilant

Vignette (American) special scene

Villoria (Spanish) valor

Vijaya (Indian) wins

Vilhelmina (Scandinavian) form of Wilhelmina: able protector
Velma, Vilhelmine, Vilma

Villa (American) of the village

Villette (French) little village girl
Vietta

Villian (American) form of Lillian: pretty as a lilly

Vilma (Spanish) form of Velma: hardworking
Vi, Vil

Vilmean (American) form of Velma: hardworking

Vimala (Hindi) attractive

Vina (Hindi) musical instrument
Veena, Vena, Vin, Vinah, Vinesha, Vinessa, Vinia, Viniece, Vinique, Vinisha, Vinita, Vinna, Vinni, Vinnie, Vinny, Vinora, Vyna

Vinah (American) up-and-coming
Vi, Vyna

Vincentia (Latin) winner
Vicenta, Vin, Vincenta, Vincentena, Vincentina, Vincentine, Vincenza, Vincy, Vinnie

Vinci (Spanish) wins

Vincia (Spanish) forthright; winning
Vincenta, Vincey, Vinci

Vinee (Spanish) welcomed

Vineeta (Indian) modest

Vinefrida (Scandinavian) bold

Vinelle (English) wine

Vineta (Indian) modest
Vinata

Vinetae (English) wine

Vinia (Spanish) vineyard woman

Vinishia (English) wine

Vinita (Hindi) she comes home

Vinital (Indian) asks

Vinne (American) from the vineyard

Vinuela (Spanish) longsuffering

Viola (Latin) violet; lovely lady
Vi, Violah, Violaine, Violanta, Viole, Violeine

Violanth (Latin) from the purple flower violet
Vi, Viol, Viola, Violanta, Violante

Violet (English/French) purple flower
Vi, Viole, Violette, Vylolet, Vyoletta, Vyolette

Violeta (Spanish) form of Violet: purple flower

Violia (Italian) form of Violet: purple flower

Violin (American) instrument

Violyne (Latin) form of Violet: purple flower
Vi, Vio, Viola, Violene, Violine

Viorica (Spanish) views

Virendra (Spanish) alive

Virethal (American) vibrant

Virgilia (Latin) bears all; stoic
Virgillia

Virginia (Latin) pure female
Giniah, Verginia, Verginya, Virge, Virgen, Virgenia, Virgenya, Virgie, Virgine, Virginio, Virginnia, Virginya, Virgy, Virjeana

Viridas (Latin) green; growing
Viridis

Viridis (Latin) green and verdant
Virdis, Virida, Viridia, Viridiana

Virjean (American) virginal

Virtue (Latin) strong; pure

Virzie (American) virginal

Visala (Indian) heavenly

Visidora (Spanish) clear view; storng

Vision (Word as name) visionary

Visitacion (Spanish) a visit

Vita (Latin) animated; lively; life
Veda, Veeta, Veta, Vete, Vitaliana, Vitalina, Vitel, Vitella, Vitia, Vitka, Vitke

Viv (Latin) form of Vivian: bubbling with life

Viva (Latin) alive; lively
Veeva, Vivan, Vivva

Vivadell (Combo of Viva and Dell) lively

Vivecca (Scandinavian) lively; energetic
Viv, Viveca, Vivecka, Viveka, Vivica, Vivie, Vyveca

Vivi (Hindi) vital
Viv

Vivian (Latin) bubbling with life
Viv, Viva, Vive, Vivee, Vivi, Vivia, Viviana, Viviane, Vivie, Vivien, Vivienne, Vivina, Vivion, Vivyan, Vyvyan

Vivianeth (American) form of Vivian: bubbling with life

Vivianetta (American) form of Vivian: bubbling with life

Vivianna (American) inventive
Viviannah, Vivianne

Vivilyn (American) vital
Viv, Vivi

Vivka (Slavic) form of Vivian: bubbling with life

Vix (American) form of Vixen: flirt
Vixa, Vixie, Vyx

Vixen (American) flirt
Vix, Vixee, Vixie

Vlada (Slavic) admired

Vladmirea (Slavic) admired

Vlasta (Slavic) likeable

Voila (French) attention; seen
Vwala

Volante (Italian) veiled

Voletta (French) mysterious
Volette, Volettie

Volette (Greek) hidden; veiled

Volina (American) form of Violin: instrument

Vona (French) pretty woman

Vona (French) pretty woman

Vonceil (Spanish) form of Yvonne: athletic

Voncille (American) form of Yvonne: athletic; form of Vonna: graceful

Vonda (Czech) loving; talented
Vondah, Vondi

Vonda (Czech) loving; talented
Vondah, Vondi

Vondrah (Czech) loving

Vondrah (Czech) loving
Vond, Vonda, Vondie, Vondra, Vondrea

Vonese (American) form of Vanessa: flighty
Vonesa, Vonise, Vonne, Vonnesa, Vonny

Voni (Slavic) affectionate
Vonee, Vonie

Vonna (French) graceful
Vona, Vonah, Vonne, Vonni,
Vonnie, Vonny

Vonnala (American) sweet
Von, Vonala, Vonnalah, Vonnie

Vonzetta (American) form of
Yvonne: athletic

Voula (Greek) sly

Voyage (Word as name) trip;
wanderer
Voy

Vrant (American) truth

Vrenean (American) truth

Vyera (Spanish) form of
Viera: alive

Wade (American) campy

Wafa (Arabic) loyal

Wakana (Japanese) plant;
thriving

Wakanda (Native American)
magical
Wakenda

Wakebia (African) strong

Wakeen (American) spunky
Wakeene, Wakey, Wakine

Wakeishah (African
American) happy
Wake, Wakeisha, Wakesha

Walburga (German)
protective
Walberga, Wallburga,
Walpurgis

Walda (German) powerful
woman
Waldah, Waldena, Waldette,
Waldina, Wallda, Wally,
Welda, Wellda

Waldeen (American) strong

Waleria (Polish) sweet

Waleska (Last name as first
name) effervescent
Wal, Walesk, Wally

Walker (English) active;
mover
Wallker

Walkiria (Mythology)
fantastic

Wallis (English) open-minded
Walis, Wallace, Walless, Wallie,
Walliss, Wally, Wallys

Walsie (American) form of
Waltz: graceful

Waltz (American) graceful

Wana (American) wandering

Wanakee (Native American)
innovative

Wanda (Polish) wild;
wandering
Vanda, Wahnda, Wandah,
Wandie, Wandis, Wandy,
Wannda, Wenda, Wendaline,
Wendall, Wendeline, Wendy,
Wohnda, Wonda, Wonnda

Wandelka (Slavic) praised

Wanetta (English) fair
Waneta, Wanette, Wanita

Wanicka (American) form of
Juanita: believer in a gracious
God; forgiving

Wanita (American) form of
Juanita: believer in a gracious
God; forgiving

Warda (German) guards her own
Wardia, Wardine

Warma (American) warmth-filled
Warm

Warna (German) defends her own

Warner (German) outgoing; fighter
Warna, Warnar, Warnir

Wasana (Native American) good health

Washina (Native American) good health

Waun (Native American) vocal

Wauneta (American) form of Juanita: believer in a gracious God; forgiving

Waverly (English) wavers in the meadow of swaying aspens
Waverley

Wayla (African) young child

Waynette (English) makes wagons; crafts wood
Waynel, Waynelle, Waynlyn

Waywan (Native American) little girl

Weeko (Native American) pretty

Wehilani (Hawaiian) heaven

Weinsia (American) of the heavens

Wenda (German) adventurer
Wend, Wendah, Wendy

Wendell (English) has wanderlust
Wendaline, Wendall, Wendelle

Wendy (English) friendly; childlike
Wenda, Wendaline, Wende, Wendee, Wendeline, Wendey, Wendi, Wendie, Wendye

Weneta (American) of the heavens

Wenetta (American) of the heavens

Weslee (English) girl from meadows of the west
Weslea, Weslene, Wesley, Weslia, Weslie, Weslyn

Weslia (English) meadow in the west
Wesleya, Weslie

Weslie (English) woman in the meadow
Wes, Weslee, Wesli

Wheeler (English) inventive
Wheelah, Wheelar

Whitley (English) outdoorsy
Whitelea, Whitlea, Whitlee, Whitly, Whittley, Witlee

Whitman (English) white-haired
Whit, Wittman

Whitney (English) white; fresh
Whit, Whiteney, Whitne, Whitnea, Whitnee, Whitneigh, Whitni, Whitnie, Whitny, Whittaney, Whittany, Whittney, Whytnie

Whitson (Last name as first name) white
Whits, Whitty, Witte, Witty

Whittier (Literature) for the poet John Greenleaf Whittier; distinguished
Whitt

Whoopi (English) excitable
Whoopee, Whoopie, Whoopy

Whynesha (African American) kindhearted
Whynesa, Wynes, Wynesa, Wynesha

Wibeke (Scandinavian) vibrant
Wiebke, Wiweca

Wiktoria (Polish) victor
Wikta

Wilda (English) wild-haired girl
Willda, Willie, Wylda, Wyle

Wildress (American) form of the wilderness

Wile (American) coy; wily
Wiles, Wyle

Wilemma (English) determined

Wilene (English) determined

Wilfreda (English) goal-oriented
Wilfridda, Wilfrieda

Wilfrid (Spanish) willful

Wilhelmina (German) feminine form of William: staunch protector
Willa, Willhelmena, Willie, Wilma

Willa (English) desirable
Will, Willah

Willette (American) open
Wilet, Wilett, Will, Willett

Willima (Spanish) protective

Willine (American) form of will: willowy
Will, Willene, Willy, Willyne

Willis (American) sparkling
Wilice, Will, Willice

Willistine (French) form of Willis: sparkling

Willough (American) form of Willow: free spirit; willow tree

Willow (American) free spirit; willow tree
Willo

Willsie (American) form of Willow: free spirit; willow tree

Wilma (German) sturdy
Willma, Wilmah, Wilmina, Wylm, Wylma

Wilmot (English) form of William: staunch protector

Wilona (English) desirable
Wilo, Wiloh, Wilonah, Wylona

Wilona (English) desired child
Willonoa, Willone, Wilone

Win (German) flirty
Winnie, Wyn, Wynne

Winata (American) form of Juanita: believer in a gracious God; forgiving

Wind (American) breezy
Winde, Windee, Windey, Windi, Windy, Wynd

Winda (African) hunts for prey

Windy (English) likes the wind
Windee, Windey, Windi, Windie, Wyndee, Wyndy

Winella (American) form of Juanita: believer in a gracious God; forgiving

Winema (Native American) leader

Winesa (American) winning

Winetta (American) peaceful; country girl
Winette, Winietta, Wyna, Wynette

Winifred (German) peaceful
woman
*Win, Wina, Winafred, Windy,
Winefred, Winefride, Winefried,
Winfreda, Winfrieda, Winifryd,
Winne, Winnie, Winniefred,
Winnifreed, Wynafred,
Wynifred, Wynn, Wynne,
Wynnifred*

Winkie (American) vital
Winkee, Winky

Winna (African) friendly
Winnah

Winner (American)
outstanding

Winnie (English) winning
Wini, Winny, Wynnie

Winnielle (African) victorious
female
Winielle, Winnicle, Wynnielle

Winnien (American) saintly

Winola (German) vivacious

Winona (Native American)
firstborn girl
*Wenona, Wenonah, Winnie,
Winnona, Winoena, Winonah,
Wye, Wynnona, Wynona,
Wynonah, Wynonna*

Winonia (American) oldest
girl

Winsome (English) nice;
beauty
Wynsome

Winter (English) child born
in winter
Wynter

Wisdom (English) discerning

Wistar (German) respected
Wistarr, Wister

Wisteria (Botanical) vine;
entangles
Wistaria

Witera (American) dramatic

Wonder (American) filled
with wonder
*Wander, Wonda, Wondee,
Wondy, Wunder*

Wonila (African American)
swaying
Waunila, Wonilla, Wonny

Wood (American) smooth
talker
*Woode, Woodee, Woodie,
Woody, Woodye*

Woodett (English) of the
woods

Woodine (English) of the
woods

Worship (Word as name)
religious

Wova (American) brassy
Whova, Wovah

Wowena (American) form of
Rowena: blissful; beloved
friend

Wren (English) flighty girl;
bird
Renn, Wrin, Wryn, Wrynne

Wrenny (American) wren

Wurei (American) combative

Wyanda (American) form of
Wanda: wild; wandering
Wyan

Wyanet (Native American)
lovely
Wyanetta, Wyonet, Wyonetta

Wyetta (French) feisty
Wyette

Wyld (American) spirited

Wyldanen (American) spirited

Wyleen (American) spirit

Wylie (American) wily
Wylee, Wyley, Wyli

Wymette (American) vocalist
*Wimet, Wimette, Wymet,
Wynette*

Wyna (American) oldest

Wynell (American) oldest

Wynelle (American) oldest

Wynndi (American) friend
Wendy

Wynne (Welsh) fair-haired
*Win, Winne, Winnie, Winny,
Winwin, Wyn, Wynee, Wynn,
Wynnie*

Wynnika (American) friend

Wynstelle (Latin) chaste; star
*Winstella, Winstelle,
Wynnestella, Wynnestelle*

Wyntress (American) friend

Wyomie (Native American)
horse-rider on the plains
*Why, Wyome, Wyomee,
Wyomeh, Wyomia*

Wyoming (Native American)
u.S. state; cowgirl
Wy, Wye, Wyoh, Wyomia

Wyrene (American) helps

Wysandra (Greek) fair;
protects

Wyss (Welsh) spontaneous;
fair
Whyse

Xandra (Greek) protective
Xandrae, Zan, Zandie, Zandra

Xanthe (Greek) beautiful
blonde; yellow
*X, Xanth, X-Anth, Xantha,
Xanthie, Xes, Zane, Zanthie*

Xanthippe (Greek) form of
Xanthe: beautiful blonde;
yellow

Xara (Hebrew) form of Sara:
God's princess

Xavia (Origin unknown)
feminine form of Xavier:
familiar

Xaviera (French) smart
*Zavey, Zavie, Zaviera,
Zavierah, Zavy*

Xena (Greek) girl from afar
Xenia, Zen, Zena, Zennie

Xeniah (Greek) gracious
entertainer
Xen, Xenia, Zenia, Zeniah

Xianona (American) fragrant

Ximena (Greek) greets

Ximenia (Spanish) form of
Serena: calm

Xiomara (Spanish) congenial

Xloie (American) form of
Chloe: flowering

Xylene (Greek) outdoorsy
*Leen, Lene, Xyleen, Xyline,
Zylee, Zyleen, Zylie*

Xylia (Greek) woods-loving
Zylea, Zylia

Xylophila (Greek) lover of
nature

Y

Yacoa (American) form of Coco: coconut

Yadavendra (Indian) friendly

Yadira (Hindi) dearest

Yael (Hebrew) strength of God
Yaele, Yayl, Yayle

Yaffa (Hebrew) beautiful girl
Yafa, Yafah, Yaffah, Yapha

Yagna (Slavic) giving

Yahaira (Hebrew) precious
Yajaira

Yahnnie (Greek) giving
Yahn, Yanni, Yannie, Yannis

Yahsah (American) dear one

Yajaira (Spanish) dear one

Yaki (Japanese) tenacious
Yakee

Yakira (Hebrew) adored baby

Yalcin (American) violet

Yale (English) fertile moor
Yaile, Yayle

Yalonda (American) form of Yolanda: pretty as a violet flower

Yamayo (Asian) lovely

Yamileth (American) form of Yamila: beautiful

Yamileth (Spanish) girl of grace
Yami

Yamilla (Arabic) form of Jamila: beautiful female; form of Camilla: wonderful
Yamila, Yamyla, Yamylla

Yamille (Arabic) beautiful
Yamill, Yamyl, Yamyle, Yamylle

Yamin (Hebrew) near to God

Yamini (Indian) nighttime

Yamya (Hindi) nighttime

Yan (Slavic) forgiving

Yana (Slavic) lovely
Yanah, Yanna, Yanni, Yannie, Yanny

Yancy (Native American) yankee; sassy
Yancee, Yancey, Yanci, Yancie

Yanessa (American) form of Vanessa: flighty
Yanesa, Yanisa, Yanissa, Yanysa, Yanyssa

Yanet (Spanish) form of Janet: small; forgiving

Yaney (American) form of Janey: believer in a gracious God

Yanine (American) form of Janine: kind

Yanni (Australian) peaceful

Yaquelin (Spanish) form of Jacqueline: supplanter; substitute
Yackie, Yacque, Yacquelyn, Yaki, Yakie, Yaque, Yaquelinn, Yaquelinne

Yara (Spanish) expansive; princess
Yarah, Yare, Yarey

Yarai (African) modest
Nyarai

Yardena (Hebrew) flows naturally

Yardley (English) open-minded
Yardlee, Yardleigh, Yardli, Yardlie, Yardly

Yareli (American) grateful

Yarine (Russian) peaceful
Yari, Yarina

Yarita (Spanish) flashy

Yarkona (Hebrew) growing

Yas (Hindi) scented

Yasha (Indian) maternal

Yashita (Indian) famous

Yashona (Hindi) rich
*Yaseana, Yashauna, Yashawna,
Yeseana, Yeshauna, Yeshawna,
Yeshona*

Yasmina (Hindi) form of
Jasmine: fragrant; sweet
Yasmeena, Yasmyna

Yasmine (Arabic) pretty
*Yasmeen, Yasmen, Yasmin,
Yasminn, Yasmyn, Yasmynn*

Yati (Indian) careful

Yaura (American) desirous
Yara, Yaur, YaYa

YaVonne (Indian) beautiful
girl

Yazith (Biblical) place name

Yazmin (Persian) pretty
flower
*Yazmen, Yazminn, Yazmyn,
Yazmynn*

Yeardley (English) home
enclosed in meadow
*Yeardlee, Yeardleigh, Yeardli,
Yeardlie, Yeardly*

Yebenette (American) little
Yebe, Yebey, Yebi

Yechiel (Spanish) helps

Yelba (Spanish) form of
Melba: talented; light-hearted

Yelena (Russian) friendly

Yelisabeta (Russian) form of
Elizabeth: God's promise
Yelizabet

Yemaya (African) smart;
quirky
Yemye

Yenisey (French) spellbound

Yepa (Native American)
traditional

Yeriel (Hebrew) God's child

Yesica (Hebrew) form of
Jessica: rich

Yeskia (Spanish) yesida
Yesika

Yesmin (Spanish) Jasmine
flower

Yessenia (Spanish) devout
Jesenia, Yesenia

Yessi (Hebrew) God-loving

Yesun (Turkish) jade
Yesim, Jesin

Yetta (English) head of home

Yeva (Russian) lively; loving
Yevka

Yevettea (Slavic) form of
Yvette: lively archer

Yevgeniya (Slavic) highborn

Yildiz (Spanish) star

Yilma (Spanish) form of
Wilma: sturdy

Yilmalla (Spanish) form of
Wilma: sturdy

Yina (Spanish) winning
Yena

Yinyin (Asian) silver hair

Yitta (Hebrew) lightness

Ynez (Spanish) form of Inez:
lovely

Yoanna (Hebrew) feminine form of John: God is gracious
Yoana, Yoanah, Yoannah

Yochana (Indian) thoughtful

Yodelle (American) old-fashioned
Yode, Yodell, Yodelly, Yodette, Yodey

Yoella (Hebrew) loves Jehovah
Yoela, Yoelah, Yoellah

Yogee (American) bright

Yogeta (American) bright

Yogini (Indian) centered

Yogita (Indian) smart

Yohanna (Greek) violet; textured
Yohuna, Yohanah, Yohannah

Yoka (Native American) bird song

Yokasta (Greek) form of Jocasta: light

Yoko (Japanese) good; striving
Yokoh

Yola (Spanish) form of Yolanda: pretty as a violet flower
Yolanda, Yoli

Yolada (Spanish) form of Yolanda: pretty as a violet

Yolanda (Greek) pretty as a violet flower
Yola, Yolana, Yolandah, Yolie, Yoyly

Yolia (Spanish) form of Julia: forever young

Yolie (Greek) violet; flower
Yolee, Yoley, Yoli, Yoly

Yomi (Spanish) sun child

Yon (Korean) lotus; lovely
Yonn

Yona (Hebrew) dove; calm
Yonah, Yonna, Yonnah

Yonaide (American)
Yonade, Yonaid

Yonina (Hebrew) dove; calm
Yonyna

Yonit (Hebrew) passive
Yonitt, Yonyt, Yonytt

Yorba (Place name)

Yordaine (French) form of Jordan: excellent descendant
Yordane, Yordayne

Yordan (Hebrew) form of Jordan: excellent descendant
Yorden, Yordyn

Yordana (Hebrew) humble
Yordanah, Yordanna, Yordannah

Yoreni (Place name)

Yori (Japanese) dependable
Yoree, Yorey, Yorie, Yory

York (English) forthright
Yorkie, Yorkke

Yoselin (Spanish) form of Joselin: happy girl

Yosepha (Hebrew) form of Josephine: blessed

Yoshe (Japanese) form of Yoshi: good girl
Yoshee, Yoshey, Yoshi, Yoshie, Yoshy

Youhanna (Slavic) form of Johanna: believer in a gracious God

Young (Korean) forever

Yousha (Indian) girl

Yousheika (Slavic) joyful

Youvet (French) form of Yvette: lively archer

Youvone (American) form of
Yvonne: athletic

Yovana (Slavic) joy

Yovelle (Hebrew) joy

Yovona (African American)
form of Yvonne: athletic
*Yovaana, Yovanna, Yovhana,
Yovhanna, Yoviana, Yovianna*

Ysabel (Spanish) form of
Isabel: clever
*Ysabell, Ysabelle, Ysebel, Ysebell,
Ysebelle, Ysybel, Ysybell, Ysybelle*

Ysabella (Spanish) smart and
witty
*Ysabela, Ysebela, Ysebella,
Ysybela, Ysybella*

Ysanne (English) graceful
*Esan, Esanne, Essan, Ysan,
Ysann*

Yseult (Irish) prettiness
Yseulte

Yu (Asian) jade; a gem

Yue (Asian) happy

Yuette (American) capable
Yue, Yuete, Yuetta

Yuki (Japanese) snow child

Yukolina (Slavic) form of
Julia: forever young

Yulan (Spanish) splendid

Yuldene (Slavic) form of
Juliana: youthful; Jove's child

Yule (Spanish) competitive

Yulondita (Spanish) form of
Juliana: youthful; Jove's child

Yuna (African) gorgeous
Yunah

Yuri (Chinese) lily

Yuridia (American) lily

Yuta (American) dramatic
Uta

Yutaca (Spanish) dramatic

Yuti (Indian) united as one

Yuvati (Indian) girl

Yuventia (Spanish) archer

Yuvette (English) petite
archer

Yuvrani (Indian) princess

Yves (French) clever

Yvette (French) lively archer
Yavet, Yevette, Yvete, Yvett

Yvonnda (American) form of
Yvonne: athetic

Yvonne (French) athletic
*Vonne, Vonnie, Yavonne,
Yvone, Yvonna*

Yvonnig (Invented) athlete

Yzabel (Hebrew) form of
Isabel: God-loving
*Yzabell, Yzabelle, Yzebel,
Yzebell, Yzebelle, Yzybel,
Yzybell, Yzybelle*

Zabrina (American) form of
Sabrina: passionate
Zabreena, Zabryna

Zac (American) God
remembers her

Zachah (Hebrew) lord
remembered; bravehearted
Zach, Zacha, Zachie, Zachrie

Zachree (Hebrew) loves God

Zada (Arabic) fortunate
Zaida, Zayda

Zadie (American) form of
Sadie: charmer; princess

Zafira (Arabic) successful
Zafirah

Zahara (African) flower
Zahari, Zaharit

Zahavah (Hebrew) golden
girl
Zahava, Zeheva, Zev

Zahidee (Arabic) white

Zahira (African) flower
*Zahara, Zahirah, Zahrah,
Zara, Zuhra*

Zahra (African) blossoming
Zara, Zarah

Zaibunissa (Spanish)
peaceful

Zaida (Spanish) peacemaker
Zada, Zai

Zaina (Muslim) beautiful girl

Zaina (Arabic) lovely

Zainab (Arabic) brave

Zaira (Arabic) flower
Zara, Zarah, Zaria, Zayeera

Zaire (Place name) country in
Africa
Zai, Zay, Zayaire

Zakah (African) smart
Zaka, Zakia, Zakiah

Zakiya (Arabic) chaste
Zakiyah

Zakiyyah (Hebrew) pure

Zakria (Hebrew) pure

Zaky (Hebrew) pure

Zakya (Hebrew) chaste

Zale (Greek) strong force of
the sea
Zaile, Zayle

Zalika (African) born to
royalty

Zaltana (Native American)
high mountain

Zaltene (American) highborn

Zambee (Place name) form
of Zambia
*Zambi, Zambie, Zamby,
Zamby*

Zamilla (Greek) strong force
of the sea
Zamila, Zamyla, Zamylla

Zamir (Hebrew) intelligent
leader
Zameer, Zamyr

Zan (Greek/Chinese)
supportive; praiseworthy
Zander, Zann

Zana (Greek) defender;
energetic
Zanah

Zanabria (Greek) defends

Zandile (American) pure

Zandra (Greek) shy; helpful
Zan, Zondra

Zane (Scandinavian) bold girl
Zain

Zaneta (Spanish) God is good

Zanita (American) gifted
*Zaneta, Zanetta, Zanette,
Zanitt, Zeneta*

Zanna (Hebrew) lily
Zana, Zanah, Zannah

Zanoah (Biblical) place name

Zanth (Greek) leader
*Zanthe, Zanthi, Zanthie,
Zanthy*

Zara (Hebrew) dawn; glorious
Zahra, Zarah, Zaree

Zaray (Arabic) going strong

Zareen (Hebrew) form of
Sareen: strong

Zarena (Hebrew) dawn
Zareena, Zarina, Zaryna

Zarephath (Biblical) place name

Zaria (Hebrew) form of Zara: dawn; glorious

Zarieh (Hebrew) form of Zara: dawn; glorious

Zarifa (Arabic) successful

Zarina (Hebrew) form of Sarika: thrush; sings

Zarita (Hebrew) form of Sarah: God's princess

Zarmina (Origin unknown) bright
Zar, Zarmynna

Zarney (American) progressive

Zarni (American) direct

Zarreta (American) form of Zara: dawn; glorious

Zarria (Arabic) splendid

Zavina (Spanish) flower

Zawadi (African) gift

Zayba (Muslim) lovely

Zayit (Hebrew) olive

Zaylee (English) heavenly
Zay, Zayle, Zayley, Zayli, Zaylie

Zayna (Arabic) pretty girl

Zayna (Arabic) wonderful
Zayne

Zaynab (Iranian) child of Ali
Zainab

Zaza (Hebrew) golden

Zazalesha (African American) zany
Lesha, Zaza, Zazalese, Zazalesh

Zazula (Polish) outstanding

Zdenka (Czech) one from Sidon; winding sheet
Zdena, Zdenicka, Zdenina, Zdeninka, Zdenuska

Zdeslava (Czech) present glory
Zdevsa, Zdisa, Zdiska, Zdislava

Zea (Latin) grain
Zia

Zeandrea (American) form of Deandra: divine
Zeandraea, Zeandraya, Zeandria, Zeandrya

Zeb (Hebrew) Jehovah's gift

Zebrine (American) form of Sabrina: passionate

Zecua (American) loyal

Zeezee (American) sunny

Zef (Polish) moves with the wind
Zeff

Zeffa (Origin unknown) breezy

Zefiryn (Polish) a form of Zephyr: windlike

Zehara (Hebrew) light

Zehava (Hebrew) gold
Zahava, Zehovit, Zehuva, Zehuvit

Zehira (Hebrew) careful

Zel (Persian) cymbal

Zela (Greek) blessed; smiling

Zelana (American) sunny

Zelda (German) practical
Zell, Zellie

Zeldia (Spanish) form of Zelda: practical

Zelenka (Czech) fresh

Zelfa (African American) in control

Zelia (Spanish) sunshine
Zeleah

Zella (German) resistant

Zelma (German) divine

Zelpha (American) confident

Zemira (Hebrew) song

Zemorah (Hebrew) tree branch
Zemora

Zena (Greek) holy

Zenae (Greek) helpful
Zen, Zenah, Zennie

Zenaida (Greek) daughter of Zeus

Zenana (Hebrew) woman
Zena, Zenia

Zenda (Hebrew) holy

Zeni (Slavic) gracious

Zenia (Greek) open
Zeniah, Zenney, Zenni, Zennie, Zenny, Zenya

Zenobia (Greek) strength of Zeus

Zenobietta (Spanish) form of Zenobia: strength of Zeus

Zenorina (Spanish) holy

Zenov (Slavic) gracious

Zenzi (German) crescent

Zephirin (English) form of Zephyr: the west wind; wandering girl

Zephirinia (English) form of Zephyr: the west wind; wandering girl

Zephyr (Greek) the west wind; wandering girl
Zefir, Zeph, Zephie, Zephir, Zephira, Zephyra

Zeppelina (English) beautiful storm

Zera (Hebrew) seeds

Zerafina (Greek) the west wind; zephyr
Zerafeena, Zerafyna

Zeraldina (Polish) spear ruler

Zerdali (Turkish) wild apricot

Zeredah (Biblical) place name

Zerel (Hindi) brave

Zerena (Turkish) golden woman
Zereena, Zerina, Zeryna

Zerlinda (Hebrew) dawn
Zerlina

Zerly (Hebrew) morning

Zerren (English) flower

Zesiro (African) first of twins

Zesta (American) zestful
Zestah, Zestie, Zesty

Zeta (Greek) born last
Zetah, Zetta

Zett (Hebrew) olive; flourishing
Zeta, Zetta

Zetulio (Spanish) from the rose

Zevida (Hebrew) current
Zevuda

Zezziska (Slavic) form of Jessica: rich

Zhane (African American) feminine of Shane

Zhanna (Slavic) form of Janet: small; forgiving

Zhen (Chinese) pure

Zhenia (Latin) bright
Zennia, Zhen, Zhenie

Zhi (Chinese) of high character; ethical

Zho (Chinese) character

Zhong (Chinese) honorable

Zhuo (Chinese) smart; wonderful
Zuo

Zi (Chinese) flourishing; giving

Zia (Latin) textured
Zea, Ziah

Zibah (Biblical) delights

Zibute (Lithuanian) shines

Zigana (Hungarian) gypsy

Zihna (Native American) spinning

Zila (Hebrew) shadowy
Zilah, Zilla, Zillah, Zylla

Zildjian (Slavic) God judges her

Zilias (Hebrew) shadow
Zillia, Zillya, Zilya

Zillah (Biblical) in the shade

Zilpah (Hebrew) dignity
Zillpha, Zilpha, Zulpah, Zylpha

Zilu (Biblical) place name

Zilvinas (Spanish) hidden

Zimbab (Place name) form of Zimbabwe
Zimbob

Zimriah (Hebrew) songs
Zimria, Zimriya

Zina (Greek) hospitable woman
Zena, Zinah, Zine, Zinnie

Zindi (Spanish) form of Cindy: moon goddess

Ziniah (Muslim) prepared

Zinnia (Botanical) flower
Zenia, Zinia, Zinny, Zinnya, Zinya

Zinzi (American) flower

Zinzida (African) gracious

Ziona (Hebrew) symbol of good
Zionah, Zyona, Zyonah

Zipory (Hebrew) bird

Zipporah (Hebrew) bird in flight
Ziporah, Zippi, Zippie, Zippora, Zippy

Ziracuny (Native American) water

Zirah (Hebrew) coliseum
Zira

Zisla (Slavic) rose

Zita (Spanish) rose girl

Zita (Greek) seeker
Zeeta, Zitah

Ziv (Hebrew) radiant

Ziva (Hebrew) brilliant
Zeeva, Ziv

Ziz (Hungarian) dedicated
Zizz, Zyz, Zyzz

Zlata (Czech) golden

Zoa (Greek) life; vibrant

Zocha (Polish) wisdom

Zoe ⊙ (Greek) lively; vibrant
Zoee, Zoey, Zoie, Zooey

Zoelle (Spanish) form of Noelle: Christmas baby

Zofia (Polish) skilled

Zofie (Czech) wise

Zoheret (Hebrew) shining

Zohreh (Hebrew) shines

Zoila (Italian) earthy

Zola (French) earthy
Zolah

Zolema (American) confessor
Zolem

Zona (Latin) funny; brash
Zonah, Zonia, Zonna

Zonia (English) flower

Zonice (American) form of Zona: funny; brash

Zonta (Native American) honest

Zooey (Greek) life

Zoom (American) energetic
Zoomi, Zoomy, Zoom-Zoom

Zora (Slavic) beauty of dawn
Zara, Zorah, Zorrah, Zorre, Zorrie

Zoralle (Slavic) ethereal
Zoral, Zoralye, Zorre, Zorrie

Zore (Slavic) dawn of day

Zorina (Slavic) golden
Zorana

Zorka (Slavic) dawn
Zorke, Zorky

Zorna (Slavic) golden

Zorrie (American) gold

Zosa (Greek) lively
Zosah

Zosima (Greek) vibrant

Zowie (Irish) vibrant
Zowee, Zowey, Zowi, Zowy

ZsaZsa (Hungarian) wild-spirited
Zsa, Zsaey

Zuba (English) musical

Zubaida (Arabic) laborer
Zubaidah, Zubeda

Zubeen (American) excellent

Zubida (Spanish) singer

Zubinelle (Spanish) vocal

Zudora (Sanskrit) laborer

Zulah (African) country-loving
Zoola, Zoolah, Zula

Zulaila (African) smart

Zyan (Native American) everlasting

Zydeco (French) musical

Bibliography

20,000+ Names Page. "20,000+ Names from Around the World." 1 Nov. 2002. http://www.20000-names.com.

Baby Center Baby Name Finder Page. 1 Dec. 2002. http://www.babycenter.com/babyname.

Baby Chatter Page. 1 Dec. 2002. http://www.babychatter.com.

Baby Names/Birth Announcements Page. 1 Oct. 2002. http://www.princessprints.com.

Baby Names Page. 1 Oct. 2002. http://www.babyshere.com.

Baby Names Page. 1 Nov. 2002. http://www.babynames.com.

Baby Names Page. 1 Dec. 2002. http://www.yourbabysname.com.

Baby Names World Page. 15 Jan. 2003. http://www.babynameworld.com.

Baby Zone Page. "Around-the-World Names." 15
    Jan. 2003. http://www.babyzone.com/babynames.

Behind the Name Page 1. Sep. 2006.
http://www.behindthename.com.

"Biographical Names." *The Merriam-Webster
    Dictionary.* Springfield, Mass: Merriam Webster,
    Inc., 1998.

Capeci, Jerry. This Week in Gangland, The Online
    Column Page. "Gambino Capos Held in 1989
    Mob Hit." 1 Aug. 2002.
    http://www.ganglandnews.com/column289.htm.

Celebrity Names Page. 1 Nov. 2002.
    http://www.celebnames.8m.com.

Collin, P.H., ed. "The American States." *Webster's
    Concise Desk Dictionary.* New York: Barnes &
    Noble Books, 2001.

Collin, P.H., ed. "The Animal Kingdom." *Webster's
    Concise Desk Dictionary.* New York: Barnes &
    Noble Books, 2001.

Collin, P.H., ed. "Biographical Names." *Webster's
    Concise Desk Dictionary.* New York: Barnes &
    Noble Books, 2001.

Collin, P.H., ed. "Books of the Bible." *Webster's Concise Desk Dictionary*. New York: Barnes & Noble Books, 2001.

Collin, P.H., ed. "The Plant Kingdom." *Webster's Concise Desk Dictionary*. New York: Barnes & Noble Books, 2001.

Collin, P.H., ed. "Presidents of the United States." *Webster's Concise Desk Dictionary*. New York: Barnes & Noble Books, 2001.

Collin, P.H., ed. "Prime Ministers of the U.K." *Webster's Concise Desk Dictionary*. New York: Barnes & Noble Books, 2001.

"Common English Given Names." *The Merriam-Webster Dictionary*. Springfield, Mass: Merriam Webster, Inc., 1998.

Death Penalty Info Page. "Current Female Death Row Inmates." 1 Feb. 2003. http://www.deathpenaltyinfo.org/womencases.html

Dunkling, Leslie. *The Guinness Book of Names*. Enfield, UK: Guinness Publishing, 1993.

eBusinessRevolution Page. 1 Nov. 2002. http://www.ebusinessrevolution.com/babynames/a.html.

ePregnancy Page. 1 Dec. 2002.
http://www.Epregnancy.com/directory/Baby_Names.

Fortune Online. "America's 40 Richest Under 40."
16 Sept. 2002. http://www.fortune.com.

Fortune Online. "Most Powerful Women in
Business." 14 Oct. 2002. http://www.fortune.com.

Gove, Philip Babcock, ed. "Fifty Important Stars."
*Webster's Third New International Dictionary of the
English Language Unabridged.* Springfield, Mass:
Merriam-Webster, Inc., 1981.

Gove, Philip Babcock, ed. "Months of the Principal
Calendars." *Webster's Third New International
Dictionary of the English Language Unabridged.*
Springfield, Mass: Merriam-Webster Inc., 1981.

Gove, Philip Babcock, ed. "Signs of the Zodiac."
*Webster's Third New International Dictionary of the
English Language Unabridged.* Springfield, Mass:
Merriam-Webster Inc., 1981.

Hanks, Patrick, and Flavia Hodges. *A Dictionary of
First Names.* Oxford: Oxford University Press, 1992.

Hanley, Kate, and the Parents of Parent Soup. *The
Parent Soup Baby Name Finder: Real Advice from*

Real Parents Who Have Named Their Babies and Lived to Tell about It—with More Than 15,000 Names. Lincolnwood, Illinois: Contemporary Books, 1998.

Harrison, G.B. ed. *Major British Writers.* New York: Harcourt, Brace & World, Inc., 1959.

HypoBirthing Page. "Baby Names." 1 Oct. 2002. http://www.hypobirthing.com.

Indian Baby Names Page. 1 Nov. 2002. http://www.indiaexpress.com/specials/babynames.

Internet Movie Database online. "Movie-Star Names." 1 Nov. 2002. http://www.imdb.com.

Irish Names Page. 15 Jan. 2003. http://www.hylit.com/info.

Jewish Baby Names Page. 15 Jan. 2003. http://www.jewishbabynames.net.

Kaplan, Justin, and Anne Bernays. *The Language of Names: What We Call Ourselves and Why It Matters.* New York: Simon & Schuster, 1997.

Lansky, Bruce. *The Mother of All Baby Name Books: Over 94,000 Baby Names Complete with Origins and Meanings*. New York: Meadowlark Press (Simon and Schuster), 2003.

Norman, Teresa. *A World of Baby Names: A Rich and Diverse Collection of Names from Around the World*. New York: Perigee (Penguin Putnam), 1996.

Origins/Meanings of Baby Names from Around the World Page. 1 Nov. 2002. http://www.BabyNamesOrigins.com.

Oxygen Page. "Baby Names." 1 Nov. 2002. http://www.oxygen.com/babynamer.

Parenthood Page. 1 Nov. 2002. http://www.parenthood.com/parent_cfmfiles/babynames.cfm.

Popular Baby Names Page. 1 Nov. 2002. http://www.popularbabynames.com.

Racketeering and Fraud Investigations Page. 4 Feb. 2003. http://www.oig.dol.gov/public/media/oi/mainz01.htm.

Rick Porelli's AmericanMafia.com Page. 21 June 2002. http://www.americanmafia.com/news/6-21-02_Feds_Bust.html.

Rosenkrantz, Linda, and Pamela Redmond Satran. *Baby Names Now*. New York: St. Martin's Press, 2002.

Rosenkrantz, Linda, and Pamela Redmond Satran. *Beyond Charles and Diana: An Anglophile's Guide to Baby Naming.* New York: St. Martin's Press, 1992.

Rosenkrantz, Linda, and Pamela Redmond Satran. *Beyond Jennifer and Jason.* New York: St. Martin's Press, 1994.

Ryan, Joal. *Puffy, Xena, Quentin, Uma: And 10,000 Other Names for Your New Millenium Baby.* New York: Plume (Penguin Putnam), 1999.

Schwegel, Janet. *The Baby Name Countdown.* New York: Marlowe & Company (Avalon), 2001.

Shaw, Jessica. *The Everything Baby Names Book.* Massachusetts: Adams Media Corporation, 1996.

Social Security Administration Online. "Most Popular Names of the 1950s." 1 Nov. 2002. http://www.ssa.gov/OACT/babynames.

Social Security Administration Online. "Most Popular Names of the 1960s." 1 Nov. 2002. http://www.ssa.gov/OACT/babynames.

Social Security Administration Online. "Most Popular Names of the 1970s." 1 Nov. 2002. http://www.ssa.gov/OACT/babynames.

Social Security Administration Online. "Most Popular Names of the 1980s." 1 Nov. 2002. http://www.ssa.gov/OACT/babynames.

Social Security Administration Online. "Most Popular Names of the 1990s." 1 Nov. 2002. http://www.ssa.gov/OACT/babynames.

Social Security Administration Online. "Most Popular Names of 2001." 1 Nov. 2002. http://www.ssa.gov/OACT/babynames.

Television show credits. 1 Oct. 2002–25 Feb. 2003.

Texas Department of Criminal Justice Page. "Offenders on Death Row." 1 Feb. 2003. http://www.tdcj.state.tx.us/stat/offendersondrow.htm.

Trantino, Charlee. *Beautiful Baby Names from Your Favorite Soap Operas*. New York: Pinnacle Books, 1996.

United Kingdom Baby Name Page. 15 Jan. 2003. http://www.baby-names.co.uk.

Wallace, Carol McD. *The Greatest Baby Name Book Ever*. New York: Avon, 1998.

About the Author

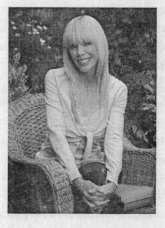

Author of the wildly popular book *40,001 Best Baby Names*, magazine editor (five times running), and creative-agency writer, Diane Stafford has twenty-five years of experience in writing and editing—but nothing has rivaled the indecent amount of fun involved in turning out a new book, called *50,001 Best Baby Names*, with 10,000 more names for readers.

Adding names from numerous sources, including radio talk-show listeners who called in when Stafford did first-edition interviews, this high-energy author gamely enlarged the scope of a book already filled with great names, fun anecdotes, and baby-naming tips.

"Today people are more creative than ever when it comes to naming their babies," notes Stafford.

"Though it may be hard to believe, the fact is, every name in this book belongs to someone out there—even ones as off-the-wall as Blanket, Zero, and Conk. Although the traditional favorites like Emma and Joshua still reign supreme, lots of people enjoy making up names for their kids, thus adding to the huge universe of options. While name inventing is controversial—people even talk about it at cocktail parties—my feeling is that you have every right to relish choosing a name for your baby. Sure, take it seriously, but not too seriously."

Stafford adds, "Having a baby is absolutely the most wonderful thing that can happen to a person, and I hope this book reflects my enormous respect for parents and my celebration of the special privilege of parenting."

Living in sunny Newport Beach, California, Stafford—a transplant from Houston, Texas—writes books and works for a creative agency. Her published books include: *Migraines for Dummies, Potty Training for Dummies, The Encyclopedia of STDs, No More Panic Attacks, 1000 Best Job Hunting Secrets*, and her latest, *The Big Book of 60,000 Baby Names*. Four of these books were coauthored with Stafford's daughter, Jennifer Shoquist, MD; her job hunting book coauthor was Moritza Day.

Notes

Mom's Picks

_____

_____

_____

_____

_____

_____

_____

_____

_____

_____

_____

_____

Dad's Picks

_____

_____

_____

_____

_____

_____

_____

_____

_____

_____

_____

_____

Our Picks

_____

_____

_____

_____

_____

_____

_____

_____

_____

_____

_____

_____

Our Picks

_____

_____

_____

_____

_____

_____

_____

_____

_____

_____

_____

_____

_____

Our Picks

_____

_____

_____

_____

_____

_____

_____

_____

_____

_____

_____

_____